Legumes for Soil Health and Sustainable Management

Mastering ICU Care

Shakti Bedanta Mishra • Samir Samal
Sagarika Panda

Mastering ICU Care

Algorithms and Clinical Decision-Making for Residents

Springer

Shakti Bedanta Mishra
Department of Critical Care Medicine
Institute of Medical Sciences
and SUM Hospital
Bhubaneswar, Odisha, India

Samir Samal
Department of Critical Care Medicine
Institute of Medical Sciences
and SUM Hospital
Bhubaneswar, Odisha, India

Sagarika Panda
Department of Critical Care Medicine
Institute of Medical Sciences
and SUM Hospital
Bhubaneswar, Odisha, India

ISBN 978-981-95-0178-6 ISBN 978-981-95-0179-3 (eBook)
https://doi.org/10.1007/978-981-95-0179-3

This Springer imprint is published by the registered company Springer Nature Singapore Pte Ltd.
The registered company address is: 152 Beach Road, #21-01/04 Gateway East, Singapore 189721, Singapore

Contents

About the Authors

Shakti Bedanta Mishra is an Indian anesthesiologist and critical care specialist. He is also a certified palliative care provider. His areas of interest include Acute Trauma Life Support (ATLS) and Acute Advanced Cardiac Life Support (ACLS), renal replacement therapy, and Acute Respiratory Distress Syndrome (ARDS). He has published many papers on topics such as renal replacement therapy, ARDS, and infection control in ICU settings in peer-reviewed national and international journals, and several chapters in various books. His published titles include work on ventilator-associated complications, ultrasound-guided approaches for internal jugular vein cannulations, and management of acute kidney injury with septic shock.

Samir Samal is a critical care medicine and emergency medicine specialist. He has published many papers in peer-reviewed national and international journals. His research includes work on balanced crystalloids in acutely ill patients, antimicrobial utilization, cost of therapy in medicine intensive care units, and targeted temperature management in unconscious survivors of postcardiac arrest. He is an active member of educational programs for healthcare professionals and aims to improve patient care and reduce rates of healthcare-associated infections.

Sagarika Panda is an Associate Professor at IMS and SUM Hospital, Bhubaneswar, India, with expertise in critical care medicine. She earned her DM in critical care medicine and has a strong background in clinical practice, medical education, and research. Committed to patient care and academic excellence, she has authored multiple peer-reviewed publications and presented her research at national and international conferences. Recognized for her contributions to healthcare and research, she continues to foster innovation and excellence in her field, striving to enhance critical care practices and medical education through her work.

Part I
Neurology

Chapter 1
Altered Sensorium in the ICU

1.1 Introduction

Altered sensorium is a broad term encompassing various levels of impaired consciousness, ranging from confusion to complete unresponsiveness. This condition can be caused by numerous underlying pathologies, including metabolic disorders, infections, neurological injuries, and psychological factors. Prompt identification and management are crucial in the intensive care unit (ICU) to prevent morbidity and mortality. This write-up elaborates on the step-by-step approach depicted in the flowchart for managing patients with altered sensorium in the ICU (Ref. Algorithm 1.1).

1.2 Immediate Assessment and Stabilization (Fig. 1.1)

1.2.1 Ensure Oxygenation, Airway, and Ventilation

The first step is to ensure that the patient's airway is open and that they are adequately ventilated. Use suction if necessary, administer oxygen to maintain $SpO2 > 94\%$, or intubate if the Glasgow Coma Scale (GCS) is less than 8 or if there are signs of airway obstruction such as pooling of secretions. Maintaining proper oxygenation prevents hypoxic brain injury, which can exacerbate altered sensorium [1].

S. B. Mishra et al., *Mastering ICU Care*,
https://doi.org/10.1007/978-981-95-0179-3_1

Call-Out Box

Critical Action: If a patient presents with altered sensorium and a GCS ≤ 8, immediate preparation for intubation is necessary to secure the airway and prevent hypoxia.

Mnemonic: "AEIOU TIPS"
The common causes of altered mental status:

- **A: Alcohol**
- **E: Epilepsy**
- **I: Insulin**
- **O: Overdose/Oxygen deficiency**
- **U: Uremia**
- **T: Trauma/Temperature**
- **I: Infection**
- **P: Psychogenic/Poisoning**
- **S: Stroke/Shock**

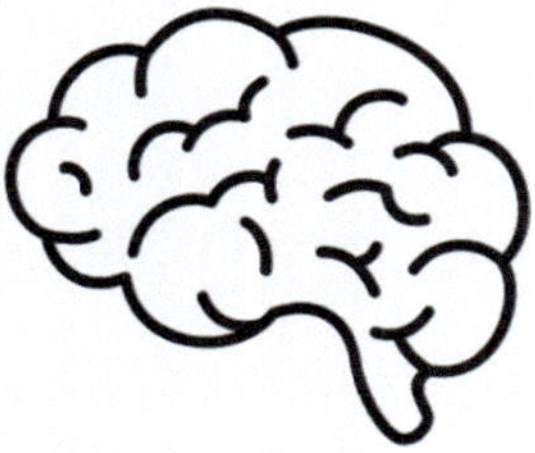

Mnemonic: "DON'T": Key Steps in Initial Management

- **D: Dextrose (check and correct glucose)**
- **O: Oxygen (ensure adequate oxygenation)**
- **N: Naloxone (consider in opioid overdose)**
- **'T': Thiamine (administer before glucose in suspected deficiency like alcoholic)**

Fig. 1.1 Call-out box

1.2.2 Maintain Circulation

It is vital to ensure hemodynamic stability with a systolic blood pressure (SBP) > 100 mmHg or a mean arterial pressure (MAP) > 65 mmHg. This can be achieved using intravenous fluids and vasopressors if needed. Adequate perfusion is essential to prevent further neurological deterioration.

1.2.3 Measure Glucose

Hypoglycemia can cause altered sensorium, so blood glucose levels should be checked immediately and maintained above 70 mg/dL. Administer intravenous glucose if necessary to correct hypoglycemia quickly [2].

1.2.4 Look for Seizures

If seizures are present, follow a specific seizure management algorithm. Seizures can significantly impact neurological status and require immediate intervention with antiepileptic medications.

1.3 Rapid Examination

1.3.1 Conduct a Thorough Physical Examination

A comprehensive physical examination should be conducted to identify possible causes (Fig. 1.1):

Trauma: Check for external injuries, bruises, or signs of head trauma.
Infection: Look for fever, neck stiffness (signs of meningitis), skin rashes, or other signs of systemic infection.
Other Visible Clues: Needle marks, breath odor (indicative of alcohol), or jaundice can provide critical insights into the underlying cause.
Neurological Status: Refer to Table 1.1 for a detailed assessment of the comatose patient, including pupillary reactions, spontaneous eye movements, and deep tendon reflexes [3].

Apply Specific Antidotes As outlined in Table 1.2, antidotes should be administered if specific toxicological causes are suspected, such as thiamine for suspected thiamine deficiency, naloxone for opioid overdose, and flumazenil for benzodiazepine overdose [4–7].

Table 1.1 A score sheet for examination of the comatose patient

History: (from relatives or friends)

Onset of coma

Recent complaints

Previous medical illness

Previous psychiatric history

Access to drugs

Occupation

Exposure to pathogens

General physical examination:

Vital signs

Evidence of trauma

Evidence of acute or chronic systemic illness.

Evidence of drug ingestion

Nuchal rigidity

Neurologic profile:

Respiratory pattern:

Regular

Periodic

Ataxic

Pupillary reactions:

Present

Asymmetric (describe)

Absent

Spontaneous eye movements:

Orienting

Roving conjugate

Roving dysconjugate

Abnormal movements (describe)

None

Oculocephalic responses:

Normal awake (nystagmus)

Full comatose

Abnormal (describe)

Minimal

None

Oculovestibular responses:

Normal awake

Tonic conjugate

Abnormal

Minimal

None

Corneal responses:

Present

Absent

Deep tendon reflexes:

Normal

Increased

Absent

Skeletal muscle tone:

Normal

Paratonic

Flexor

Extensor

Flaccid

Table 1.2 Antidotes

Thiamine and glucose	Administer 100 mg IV thiamine, followed by glucose if blood glucose is less than 70 mg/dL. Provide 100 ml aliquots of a 25% glucose solution until blood glucose exceeds 70 mg/dL
Naloxone	If opioid overdose is suspected, administer 0.4–2.0 mg IV every 3 minutes as needed, or use a continuous IV infusion
Flumazenil	If benzodiazepine overdose is suspected, administer 0.2 mg/min IV, with a maximum total dose of 1 mg
Hyperventilation	Apply hyperventilation if there is clinical evidence of increased intracranial pressure (ICP) or herniation
Gastric lavage with activated charcoal	Perform gastric lavage with activated charcoal after intubation if drug intoxication is suspected

Table 1.3 Emergency laboratory evaluation of metabolic coma

Immediate tests:	
1	Kidney function test
2	Complete blood count (CBC)
3	Coagulation test
4	Arterial blood gas (ABG)
5	Electrocardiogram (ECG)
If required:	
1	Liver function test
2	Thyroid and adrenal function tests
3	Blood culture
4	Lumbar puncture

1.4 Obtain Immediate Diagnostic Imaging

1.4.1 Non-contrast CT Brain

A non-contrast CT scan of the brain should be performed to rule out structural causes such as hemorrhage, stroke, or mass effect.

1.4.2 Laboratory Tests

Refer to Table 1.3 for a comprehensive list of laboratory tests, including kidney function tests, electrolytes, complete blood count (CBC), coagulation tests, arterial blood gas (ABG), and electrocardiogram (ECG). These tests help identify metabolic or systemic causes of altered sensorium [8].

1.5 Measure Optic Nerve Sheath Diameter

This measurement can help assess intracranial pressure, which is critical in evaluating patients with suspected increased intracranial pressure or herniation [9].

1.6 Diagnostic Categories

1.6.1 Infection

Signs of infection include fever, neck stiffness, skin rashes, elevated white blood cell count, and positive blood cultures or lumbar puncture findings. Management involves antimicrobial therapy tailored to the suspected pathogen.

1.6.2 Metabolic

Metabolic causes are indicated by abnormal lab values, evidence of organ failure, and history of diseases such as diabetes, liver, or renal disease. Treatment focuses on correcting metabolic imbalances and supporting organ function.

1.6.3 Cerebral Injury

Sudden onset of focal neurological deficits, asymmetrical findings, and abnormal imaging results suggest a cerebral injury. Management includes addressing the underlying cause, such as stroke or trauma, and supporting neurological recovery.

1.6.4 Psychogenic

History of psychiatric disorders or recent psychological stressors, along with the absence of other abnormalities, points to a psychogenic cause. Management involves psychiatric evaluation and appropriate mental health interventions.

1.7 Conclusion

The management of altered sensorium in the ICU requires a systematic approach to identify and treat the underlying cause. Immediate stabilization, thorough examination, and prompt diagnostic testing are essential steps. Understanding the rationale behind each decision point ensures comprehensive care and improves patient outcomes.

1.7.1 Glasgow Coma Scale (GCS)

The Glasgow Coma Scale (GCS) is a widely used scoring system for assessing the level of consciousness in patients with altered sensorium, particularly those with head injuries or neurological conditions. The GCS provides a reliable and objective way of recording the conscious state of a person and helps guide initial management decisions [10, 11].

The GCS assesses three aspects of a patient's responsiveness:

1. **Eye Opening (E)**
   - **Spontaneous (4 points)**: Eyes open spontaneously without any external stimulus.
   - **To Speech (3 points)**: Eyes open in response to verbal commands or speech.
   - **To Pain (2 points)**: Eyes open in response to a painful stimulus.
   - **None (1 point)**: No eye opening, even with painful stimuli.
2. **Verbal Response (V)**
   - **Oriented (5 points)**: Patient is oriented to time, place, and person and can converse coherently.
   - **Confused (4 points)**: Patient is able to speak but is confused and disoriented.
   - **Inappropriate Words (3 points)**: Patient uses inappropriate words or phrases that are unrelated to the conversation.
   - **Incomprehensible Sounds (2 points)**: Patient makes incomprehensible sounds or groans.
   - **None (1 point)**: No verbal response, even to painful stimuli.

3. **Motor Response (M)**
    - **Obeys Commands (6 points)**: Patient follows simple commands.
    - **Localizes Pain (5 points)**: Patient localizes and attempts to remove the source of pain.
    - **Withdraws from Pain (4 points)**: Patient withdraws or pulls away from the source of pain.
    - **Flexion to Pain (Decorticate Posturing) (3 points)**: Abnormal flexion in response to pain (bending of the arms at the elbow, bringing the arms to the chest).
    - **Extension to Pain (Decerebrate Posturing) (2 points)**: Abnormal extension in response to pain (straightening of the arms and legs, downward pointing of the toes).
    - **None (1 point)**: No motor response, even to painful stimuli.

The total GCS score is the sum of the scores for eye opening, verbal response, and motor response. The maximum score is 15, indicating a fully alert and oriented person, and the minimum score is 3, indicating deep unconsciousness or coma.

1.7.2 Interpretation of GCS Scores

- **13–15**: Mild brain injury
- **9–12**: Moderate brain injury
- **3–8**: Severe brain injury (coma).

Algorithm 1.1: Altered sensorium in the ICU

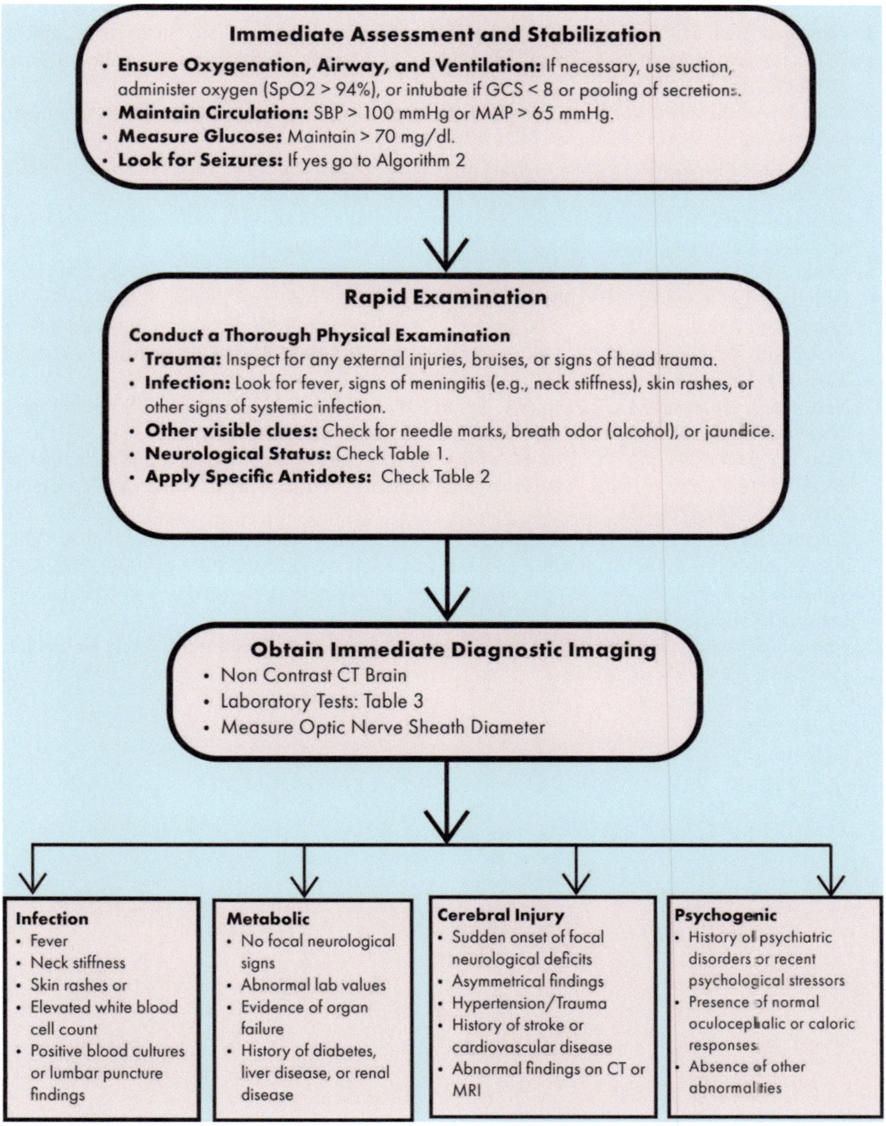

Bibliography

1. Galvagno SM Jr, Nahmias JT, Young DA. Advanced trauma life support(®) update 2019: management and applications for adults and special populations. Anesthesiol Clin. 2019;37(1):13–32.
2. Nakhleh A, Shehadeh N. Hypoglycemia in diabetes: an update on pathophysiology, treatment, and prevention. World J Diabetes. 2021;12(12):2036–49.
3. Simon RP, Aminoff MJ, Greenberg DA. Clinical neurology, 10e. New York, NY: McGraw-Hill Education; 2017.
4. Sechi G, Serra A. Wernicke's encephalopathy: new clinical settings and recent advances in diagnosis and management. Lancet Neurol. 2007;6(5):442–55.
5. Boyer EW. Management of opioid analgesic overdose. N Engl J Med. 2012;367(2):146–55.
6. Penninga EI, Graudal N, Ladekarl MB, Jürgens G. Adverse Events Associated with Flumazenil Treatment for the Management of Suspected Benzodiazepine Intoxication--A Systematic Review with Meta-Analyses of Randomised Trials. Basic Clin Pharmacol Toxicol 2016;118(1):37–44.
7. Nelson LS, Howland MA, Lewin NA, Smith SW, Goldfrank LR, Hoffman RS. Goldfrank's Toxicologic emergencies, 11e. New York, NY: McGraw-Hill Education; 2019.
8. Xiao HY, Wang YX, Xu TD, Zhu HD, Guo SB, Wang Z, et al. Evaluation and treatment of altered mental status patients in the emergency department: life in the fast lane. World J Emerg Med. 2012;3(4):270–7.
9. Soldatos T, Karakitsos D, Chatzimichail K, Papathanasiou M, Gouliamos A, Karabinis A. Optic nerve sonography in the diagnostic evaluation of adult brain injury. Crit Care. 2008;12(3):R67.
10. Teasdale G, Jennett B. Assessment of coma and impaired consciousness. A practical scale. Lancet. 1974;2(7872):81–4.
11. Teasdale G, Jennett B. Assessment and prognosis of coma after head injury. Acta Neurochir. 1976;34(1–4):45–55.

Chapter 2
Management of Seizures in the ICU

2.1 Introduction

Seizures are common neurological emergencies in the intensive care unit (ICU), requiring immediate recognition and intervention to prevent significant morbidity and mortality. Status epilepticus (SE) is a particularly severe condition defined by the International League Against Epilepsy (ILAE) as a seizure lasting longer than five minutes (t_1), beyond which normal seizure termination mechanisms are unlikely, necessitating prompt treatment. Prolonged seizures beyond 30 minutes (t_2) can lead to long-term neurological consequences, including neuronal injury and death [1, 2].

SE is further classified into convulsive and nonconvulsive types, each requiring specific diagnostic and management strategies. Early and effective intervention is crucial, especially within the first five minutes of seizure onset to improve outcomes and reduce the risk of progression to refractory or super-refractory SE.

This chapter provides an evidence-based, systematic approach to the management of seizures in the ICU, emphasizing rapid stabilization, timely pharmacologic interventions, diagnostic evaluations, and consideration of underlying causes, including special populations and emerging therapies (Ref. Algorithm 2.1).

2.2 Definition and Classification of Status Epilepticus

- **Status Epilepticus (SE):** Seizure activity lasting longer than five minutes or recurrent seizures without recovery of consciousness between episodes.
- **Refractory Status Epilepticus (RSE):** SE that persists despite administration of adequate doses of at least two appropriate antiseizure medications, typically a benzodiazepine and a second-line agent.

S. B. Mishra et al., *Mastering ICU Care*,
https://doi.org/10.1007/978-981-95-0179-3_2

- **Super-Refractory Status Epilepticus (SRSE):** SE that continues or recurs 24 hours or more after the onset of anesthesia, including cases where SE recurs upon the reduction or withdrawal of anesthesia [3].

2.3 Initial Assessment and Stabilization (0–5 Min)

The first priority is rapid stabilization to ensure airway patency, adequate breathing, and circulation while initiating a focused neurologic assessment. Early treatment initiation within the first five minutes (t_1) is critical to prevent progression to prolonged SE [2].

1. **Airway, Breathing, Circulation (ABCs)**
   - Airway: Ensure airway patency. If the patient is unconscious or has impaired protective reflexes, consider endotracheal intubation to prevent aspiration. Position the patient in the lateral decubitus position if possible.
   - Breathing: Administer supplemental oxygen to maintain saturation above 94%. Monitor respiratory rate and effort continuously. Be prepared to provide ventilatory support in cases of hypoventilation or apnea.
   - Circulation: Establish intravenous (IV) access promptly for medication administration. Monitor blood pressure and heart rate continuously. Treat hypotension with isotonic fluids and vasopressors if necessary.
2. **Neurologic Assessment**
   Conduct a rapid neurologic examination:
   - Level of Consciousness: Assess using the Glasgow Coma Scale (GCS).
   - Pupillary Response: Evaluate for size, symmetry, and reactivity.
   - Motor Function: Check for focal neurological deficits or lateralizing signs.
   - Seizure Documentation: Note onset time, duration, type (convulsive vs. nonconvulsive), and characteristics to guide management and assess treatment response.
3. **Laboratory and Diagnostic Workup**
   - Blood Glucose: Check immediately; correct hypoglycemia with 50% dextrose IV if present.
   - Electrolytes: Obtain serum levels of sodium, calcium, and magnesium.
   - Renal and Liver Function Tests: Assess for metabolic derangements.
   - Complete Blood Count (CBC): Evaluate for infection or anemia.
   - Toxicology Screen: Consider in suspected overdose or poisoning.
   - Antiepileptic Drug Levels: If the patient is on maintenance therapy, check serum levels.
   - Continuous Monitoring: Initiate cardiac monitoring and obtain an electrocardiogram (ECG) to detect arrhythmias or conduction abnormalities [4].

4. **Diagnostic Evaluation**
    - Electroencephalography (EEG): Early EEG is essential, especially to detect nonconvulsive SE, which may not have overt clinical signs but can cause significant morbidity.
    - Neuroimaging: Obtain emergent brain imaging (CT or MRI) to identify structural causes such as hemorrhage, infarction, tumor, or cerebral edema.
5. **Consideration of Special Populations**
    - Older Adults: Higher risk of SE due to comorbidities like stroke or neurodegenerative diseases. Adjust medication doses to avoid adverse effects and consider drug interactions.
    - Pregnant Women: Be cautious with teratogenic medications like valproic acid. Balance maternal and fetal risks when selecting antiseizure medications. (Table 2.1).

Table 2.1 Pharmacological management of seizures: dosing, routes, and considerations for clinical practice

Drug	Dose	Route	Maximum dose	Considerations/ contraindications
Benzodiazepines				
Lorazepam	0.1 mg/kg	IV	Up to 4 mg/dose, may repeat once after 5–10 min	Preferred for initial control, monitor for respiratory depression
Diazepam	0.15–0.2 mg/kg	IV	Up to 10 mg/ dose, may repeat once	Quick onset but shorter duration, monitor for hypotension
Midazolam	0.2 mg/kg	IM, buccal intranasal	Up to 10 mg, single dose	Suitable for non-IV routes, watch for respiratory effects
Clonazepam	0.01–0.02 mg/ kg	IV	Up to 1 mg	For adjunctive use, caution in respiratory and liver diseases
Second-line anticonvulsants				
Phenytoin	20 mg/kg	IV	Max. Rate 50 mg/min	Avoid in cardiac arrhythmias, monitor for hypotension
Fosphenytoin	20 mg PE/kg	IV	Max. Rate 150 mg PE/min	Converted to phenytoin, safer for veins, same considerations
Valproic acid	40 mg/kg	IV	Up to 3000 mg	Caution in liver disease, can cause hyperammonemia
Levetiracetam	60 mg/kg	IV	Up to 4500 mg	Few drug interactions, adjust dose in renal impairment

(continued)

Table 2.1 (continued)

Drug	Dose	Route	Maximum dose	Considerations/ contraindications
Phenobarbital	15–20 mg/kg	IV	Up to 1000 mg	Long-acting, monitor for sedation and respiratory depression
Third-line anticonvulsants and sedatives				
Propofol	1–2 mg/kg loading	IV	Maintenance 2–10 mg/kg/hr	Risk of propofol infusion syndrome (PRIS), monitor hemodynamics
Ketamine	1–2 mg/kg loading	IV	Maintenance 1–2 mg/kg/hr	Useful for refractory cases, monitor for psychomimetic effects
Thiopental	3–5 mg/kg loading	IV	Maintenance 0.5–3 mg/kg/hr	Barbiturate, monitor for hypotension and prolonged sedation
Alternative antiepileptic drugs (AEDs)				
Lacosamide	200–400 mg loading	IV	Up to 600 mg	Avoid in severe cardiac conditions (e.g., AV block)
Topiramate	200 mg loading	Oral, NG tube	Up to 600 mg/kg	Slow titration needed, monitor for metabolic acidosis
Supportive and adjunctive therapies				
Magnesium sulfate	2–4 g loading	IV	Maintenance 1–2 g/hr	For seizures due to eclampsia, monitor for respiratory depression
Thiamine	100 mg	IV	–	For alcohol-related SE, give before glucose to prevent Wernicke's encephalopathy.
Dextrose	500 ml of 50% solution	IV	–	To correct hypoglycemia, monitor blood glucose levels

2.4 Initial Medication Administration (5–20 Min)

If seizure activity persists beyond five minutes, initiate pharmacologic treatment promptly with first-line agents. Early administration of benzodiazepines significantly improves outcomes [5].

1. **Benzodiazepines (First-Line Therapy)**
   - Intravenous Lorazepam: 0.1 mg/kg IV (maximum 4 mg per dose). Preferred for its longer duration of action. May repeat once after 5–10 min if seizures persist.
   - Intravenous Diazepam: 0.15–0.2 mg/kg IV (maximum 10 mg per dose). Rapid onset but shorter duration; may require repeated dosing.
   - Intramuscular Midazolam: 10 mg IM for adults if IV access is unavailable. Alternative routes include intranasal or buccal administration.

   - Reassessment: Monitor for seizure cessation and adverse effects. If seizures have stopped, proceed to maintenance therapy. If seizures continue, advance to second-line agents.

2.5 Second-Line Anticonvulsants (20–60 Min)

Administer second-line antiepileptic drugs if seizures are refractory to benzodiazepines. Choice of agent depends on availability, patient-specific factors, and contraindications.

1. Intravenous Levetiracetam
   - Levetiracetam: 60 mg/kg IV (maximum 4500 mg) over 15 min. Increasingly favored due to rapid administration, minimal drug interactions, and few side effects.
2. Intravenous Valproic Acid
   - Valproic Acid: 40 mg/kg IV (up to 3000 mg) over 10–15 min. Effective with minimal hemodynamic effects. Contraindicated in pregnant women and women of childbearing potential not using effective contraception due to teratogenicity.
3. Intravenous Phenytoin or Fosphenytoin
   - Fosphenytoin: 20 mg phenytoin equivalents (PE)/kg IV (maximum rate 150 mg PE/min). Preferred over phenytoin for safer infusion profile.
   - Phenytoin: 20 mg/kg IV (maximum rate 50 mg/min). Requires cardiac monitoring due to risk of hypotension and arrhythmias.
4. Intravenous Phenobarbital
   - Phenobarbital: 15–20 mg/kg IV (rate of 50–100 mg/min). Effective but may cause significant sedation and respiratory depression.

Check Table 2.2 for details on doses and other considerations.

Table 2.2 Seizure management in pregnancy: therapeutic approaches and special considerations

Aspect	Considerations for pregnant women
Medication selection	Prefer drugs with low teratogenic risk (e.g., Levetiracetam, lamotrigine) Avoid valproic acid and phenytoin if possible due to teratogenic risks. Use magnesium sulfate specifically for eclampsia-related seizures
Dosage adjustments	Adjust for altered pharmacokinetics (increased clearance, volume of distribution) Regularly monitor and adjust drug levels to maintain efficacy and safety
Monitoring	Continuous fetal monitoring to assess Well-being Monitor maternal drug levels more frequently to avoid fetal exposure to high doses
Supportive care	Position in left lateral decubitus to improve uteroplacental blood flow Avoid supine position to prevent compression of the inferior vena cava
Underlying causes	Manage pregnancy-specific conditions like eclampsia with magnesium sulfate Consider and treat pregnancy-related complications promptly
Delivery planning	Seizures alone are not an automatic indication for cesarean section Coordinate with obstetric care to plan for high-risk delivery if needed
Postpartum care	Adjust anticonvulsant therapy as pharmacokinetics change post-delivery Assess the safety of breastfeeding with current medications
Counseling and education	Provide detailed counseling on seizure management during pregnancy and postpartum Discuss the safety of anticonvulsants during breastfeeding

Reassessment: Monitor for seizure control and adverse effects. If seizures persist after adequate dosing of two appropriate medications (benzodiazepine and a second-line agent), the patient is considered to have refractory status epilepticus (RSE).

2.6 Third-Line Anticonvulsants and Sedatives (Beyond 60 Min)

In RSE, more aggressive treatment is required, including the use of anesthetic agents and advanced monitoring [5].

1. Refractory Status Epilepticus (RSE).
   - Definition: Seizures persisting after administration of a benzodiazepine and a second-line antiepileptic drug.
   - Management: Initiate continuous infusion of anesthetic agents and continuous EEG monitoring.
2. Anesthetic Agents

   Intravenous Midazolam
   - Dosage: Loading dose of 0.2 mg/kg IV, followed by maintenance infusion of 0.05–2 mg/kg/hr. Titrate to burst suppression or seizure cessation on EEG.

- Intravenous Propofol
- Dosage: Loading dose of 1–2 mg/kg IV, maintenance infusion of 2–10 mg/kg/hr. Monitor for hypotension and propofol infusion syndrome, especially with prolonged use.
- Intravenous Ketamine
- Dosage: Loading dose of 1–3 mg/kg IV, maintenance infusion of 1–5 mg/kg/hr. NMDA receptor antagonist beneficial in refractory cases, particularly when GABAergic agents fail [6, 7].
- Intravenous Thiopental/Pentobarbital
- Dosage: Loading dose of 3–5 mg/kg IV, maintenance infusion of 0.5–3 mg/kg/hr. Requires intensive hemodynamic and respiratory support due to profound sedation and hypotension.

3. **Super-Refractory Status Epilepticus (SRSE)** [6]

- Definition: SE that continues or recurs 24 hours or more after the onset of anesthetic therapy.
- Management: Consider additional therapies such as:
- Hypothermia: Therapeutic hypothermia may reduce metabolic demand and neuronal injury [8].
- Ketogenic Diet: High-fat, low-carbohydrate diet shown to reduce seizure frequency in some cases [9].
- Immunotherapy: In cases of suspected autoimmune encephalitis, consider steroids, intravenous immunoglobulin (IVIG), or plasmapheresis [10].

4. **Complications and Prognosis**

- Neuroinflammatory Conditions: Autoimmune encephalitis is a recognized cause of RSE and SRSE. Early identification and immunotherapy are crucial.
- Mortality: SRSE is associated with high mortality rates; early aggressive management may improve outcomes.

EEG Monitoring and Diagnostic Considerations

1. Continuous EEG Monitoring

- Purpose: Detect ongoing seizure activity, especially nonconvulsive seizures masked by sedation.
- Guidance: Adjust therapy based on EEG findings, aiming for seizure cessation or burst suppression patterns.

2. Neuroimaging

- CT/MRI: Essential to identify structural lesions, hemorrhages, infarctions, tumors, or cerebral edema contributing to seizures.

3. Additional Diagnostic Tests

- Lumbar Puncture: Perform if infection or autoimmune etiology is suspected.
- Autoimmune Panels: Consider testing for neuronal antibodies in cases of unexplained RSE or SRSE.

2.7 Maintenance Antiepileptics

After seizure control, transition to maintenance antiepileptic therapy to prevent recurrence. The choice depends on the underlying etiology, patient factors, and potential side effects [11].

Considerations
- Reversible Causes: If SE is due to reversible metabolic derangements, short-term therapy may suffice.
- Structural or Chronic Epilepsy: Patients with underlying brain abnormalities or chronic epilepsy may require long-term therapy.
- Drug Interactions: Consider potential interactions with other medications, especially in older adults with polypharmacy.

Common Maintenance AEDs
- Levetiracetam: Favorable side effect profile and minimal interactions. Dose adjustment may be needed in renal impairment.
- Phenytoin/Fosphenytoin: Requires monitoring of serum levels and attention to drug interactions.
- Valproic Acid: Broad-spectrum efficacy; avoid in women of childbearing potential unless no alternatives.
- Phenobarbital: Effective but associated with sedation and cognitive impairment.

Long-Term Management and Prognosis
1. Recurrence Risks
   - Structural Abnormalities: Higher risk of seizure recurrence in patients with stroke, tumors, or traumatic brain injuries [12].
   - Chronic Epilepsy: May require adjustment of maintenance therapy and close follow-up.
2. Special Populations
   - Older Adults: Monitor for cognitive side effects and adjust dosages accordingly.
   - Women of Childbearing Potential: Avoid teratogenic medications; provide counseling on contraception.
3. Rehabilitation and Support
   - Multidisciplinary Approach: Involve neurology, rehabilitation services, and social support for optimal recovery.
   - Education: Educate patients and families about seizure precautions, medication adherence, and follow-up care [13].

2.8 Conclusion

The management of seizures in the ICU is a time-sensitive, systematic process focusing on rapid stabilization, seizure termination, and prevention of complications. Early intervention within the first five minutes is critical to prevent progression to refractory stages. The use of benzodiazepines as first-line agents, followed by appropriate second-line antiepileptics, is supported by current evidence. In refractory cases, anesthetic agents and advanced therapies may be necessary.

Identifying and addressing underlying etiologies, including metabolic disturbances, structural lesions, infections, and autoimmune conditions, are essential components of care. Continuous EEG monitoring aids in guiding therapy, especially in nonconvulsive and refractory cases. Transitioning to appropriate maintenance therapy and considering patient-specific factors, such as age and comorbidities, are crucial for long-term management and improving patient outcomes.

Early and decisive intervention, coupled with comprehensive care, is paramount in preventing the severe consequences associated with prolonged seizure activity.

Algorithm 2.1: Management of seizures in the ICU

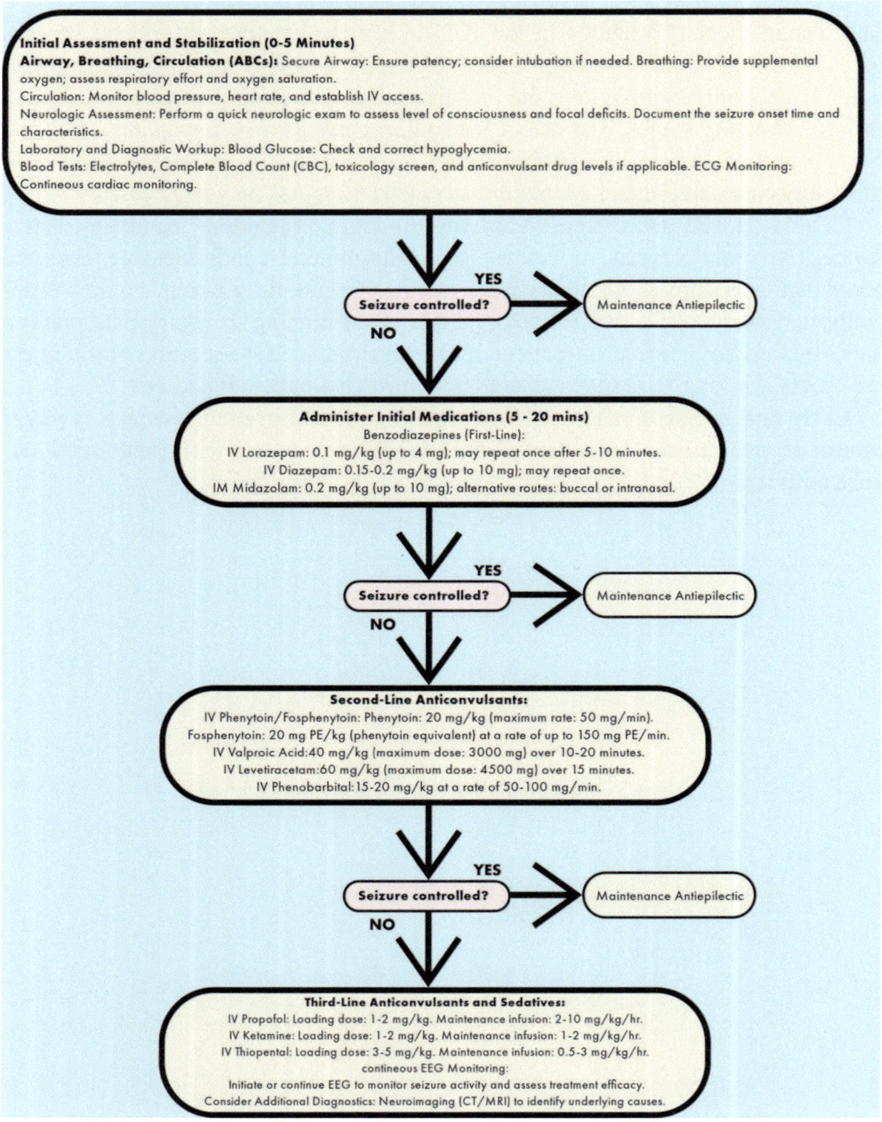

Bibliography

1. Glauser T, Ben-Menachem E, Bourgeois B, Cnaan A, Chadwick D, Guerreiro C, et al. ILAE treatment guidelines: evidence-based analysis of antiepileptic drug efficacy and effectiveness as initial monotherapy for epileptic seizures and syndromes. Epilepsia. 2006;47(7):1094–120.
2. Brophy GM, Bell R, Claassen J, Alldredge B, Bleck TP, Glauser T, et al. Guidelines for the evaluation and management of status epilepticus. Neurocrit Care. 2012;17(1):3–23.
3. Shorvon S, Ferlisi M. The treatment of super-refractory status epilepticus: a critical review of available therapies and a clinical treatment protocol. Brain. 2011;134(10):2802–18.
4. Almohaish S, Tesoro EP, Brophy GM. Status epilepticus: an update on pharmacological management. Semin Neurol. 2024;44(03):324–32.
5. Neligan A, Rajakulendran S, Walker MC. Advances in the Management of Generalized Convulsive Status Epilepticus: what have we learned? Brain. 2021;144(5):1336–41.
6. Rai S, Drislane FW. Treatment of refractory and super-refractory status epilepticus. Neurotherapeutics. 2018;15(3):697–712.
7. Gaspard N, Foreman B, Judd L, Brenton JN, Nathan BBR, McCoy B, et al. Intravenous ketamine for the treatment of refractory status epilepticus: a retrospective multicenter study. Epilepsia. 2013;54(8):1498–503.
8. Shorvon S, Ferlisi M. The treatment of super-refractory status epilepticus: a critical review of available therapies and a clinical treatment protocol. Brain. 2011;134(Pt 10):2802–18.
9. Neal EG, Chaffe H, Schwartz RH, Lawson MS, Edwards N, Fitzsimmons G, et al. The ketogenic diet for the treatment of childhood epilepsy: a randomised controlled trial. Lancet Neurol. 2008;7(6):500–6.
10. Dalmau J, Rosenfeld MR. Autoimmune encephalitis update. Neuro-Oncology. 2014;16(6):771–8.
11. Lamsal R, Bista NR. Management of Status Epilepticus. J Neuroanaesthesiol Crit Care. 2019;06(03):267–74.
12. Sutter R, Kaplan PW, Marsch S, Hammel EM, Rüegg S, Ziai WC. Early predictors of refractory status epilepticus: an international two-center study. Eur J Neurol. 2015;22(1):79–85.
13. Legriel S, Azoulay E, Resche-Rigon M, Lemiale V, Mourvillier B, Kouatchet A, et al. Functional outcome after convulsive status epilepticus. Crit Care Med. 2010;38(12):2295–303.

Chapter 3
Management of Patients with Focal Neurological Deficits in the ICU

3.1 Introduction

Patients in the intensive care unit (ICU) who present with focal neurological deficits require immediate and precise assessment to prevent further deterioration and to optimize outcomes. These deficits may stem from various underlying conditions, including hemorrhagic and ischemic strokes, subarachnoid hemorrhage, hydrocephalus, brain tumors, or abscesses. This chapter provides a step-by-step algorithm for managing such patients, emphasizing critical clinical evaluations, diagnostic procedures, and initial treatment strategies (Ref. Algorithm 3.1).

3.2 Conduct a Comprehensive Neurological Assessment

A. **National Institutes of Health Stroke Scale (NIHSS) (Table 3.1)**

- Purpose: The NIHSS is a systematic tool used to measure the severity of a stroke by assessing specific neurological functions [1, 2].
- Components:

1. Level of Consciousness: Alertness and ability to respond to questions and commands.
2. Best Gaze: Horizontal eye movements.
3. Visual Fields: Presence of visual field cuts.
4. Facial Palsy: Facial muscle movement.

S. B. Mishra et al., *Mastering ICU Care*,
https://doi.org/10.1007/978-981-95-0179-3_3

Table 3.1 National Institutes of Health Stroke Scale (NIHSS) components

1. Level of consciousness: alertness and ability to respond to questions and commands	
(A)	
Scale definition	
Alert; keenly responsive	0
Not alert; but arousable by minor stimulation to obey, answer, or respond	1
Not alert; requires repeated stimulation to attend, or is obtunded and requires strong or painful stimulation to make movements (not stereotyped)	2
Responds only with reflex motor or autonomic effects, or totally unresponsive, flaccid, and areflexic	3
Score	
(B)	
Scale definition	
Answers both questions correctly	0
Answers one question correctly	1
Answers neither question correctly	2
Score	
(C)	
Scale definition	
Performs both tasks correctly	0
Performs one task correctly	1
Performs neither task correctly	2
Score	
2. Best gaze: horizontal eye movements	
Scale definition	
Normal	0
Partial gaze palsy; gaze is abnormal in one or both eyes, but forced deviation or total gaze paresis is not present	1
Forced deviation, or total gaze paresis is not overcome by the oculocephalic maneuver	2
Score	
3. Visual fields: presence of visual field cuts	
Scale definition	
No visual loss	0
Partial hemianopia	1
Complete hemianopia	2
Bilateral hemianopia (blind including cortical blindness)	3
Score	
4. Facial palsy: facial muscle movement	
Scale definition	
Normal symmetrical movements	0
Minor paralysis (flattened nasolabial fold, asymmetry on smiling)	1
Partial paralysis (total or near-total paralysis of lower face)	2
Complete paralysis of one or both sides (absence of facial movement in the upper and lower face)	3

(continued)

Table 3.1 (continued)

Score			
Motor function:			
A) Arm: ability to hold arms up			
Scale definition			
No drift; limb holds 90 (or 45) degrees for full 10 seconds			0
Drift; limb holds 90 (or 45) degrees, but drifts down before full 10 seconds; does not hit bed or other support			1
Some effort against gravity; limb cannot get to or maintain (if cued) 90 (or 45) degrees, drifts down to bed, but has some effort against gravity			2
No effort against gravity; limb falls			3
No movement			4
Amputation or joint fusion, explain			UN
Score	5a: left arm	5b: Right arm	
B) Leg: ability to lift legs			
Scale definition			
No drift; leg holds 30-degree position for full 5 seconds			0
Drift; leg falls by the end of the 5-second period but does not hit the bed			1
Some effort against gravity; leg falls to bed by 5 seconds but has some effort against gravity			2
No effort against gravity; leg falls to bed immediately			3
No movement			4
Amputation or joint fusion, explain			UN
Score	5a: left leg	5b: Right leg	
6. Limb Ataxia: Coordination tests (finger-to-nose, heel-to-shin)			
Scale definition			
Absent			0
Present in one limb			1
Present in two limbs			2
Amputation or joint fusion, explain			3
Score			
7. Sensory: Response to pinprick in face, arms, and legs			
Scale definition			
Normal; no sensory loss			0
Mild-to-moderate sensory loss; patient feels pinprick is less sharp or is dull on the affected side; or there is a loss of superficial pain with pinprick, but patient is aware of being touched			1
Severe or total sensory loss; patient is not aware of being touched in the face, arm, and leg			2
Score			
8. Language: ability to name objects, describe pictures, and read			
Scale definition			

(continued)

Table 3.1 (continued)

No aphasia; normal	0
Mild-to-moderate aphasia; some obvious loss of fluency or facility of comprehension, without significant limitation on ideas expressed or form of expression. Reduction of speech and/or comprehension, however, makes conversation about provided materials difficult or impossible. For example, in conversation about provided materials, examiner can identify picture or naming card content from patient's response	1
Severe aphasia; all communication is through fragmentary expression; great need for inference, questioning, and guessing by the listener. Range of information that can be exchanged is limited; listener carries burden of communication. Examiner cannot identify materials provided from patient response	2
Mute, global aphasia; no usable speech or auditory comprehension	3
Score	
9. Speech: clarity of speech and articulation	
Scale definition	
Normal	0
Mild-to-moderate dysarthria; patient slurs at least some words and, at worst, can be understood with some difficulty	1
Severe dysarthria; patient's speech is so slurred as to be unintelligible in the absence of or out of proportion to any dysphasia, or is mute/anarthric	2
Intubated or other physical barrier, explain	3
Score	
10 Extinction and inattention (neglect): awareness of surroundings and stimuli	
Scale definition	
No abnormality	0
Visual, tactile, auditory, spatial, or personal inattention, or extinction to bilateral simultaneous stimulation in one of the sensory modalities	1
Profound hemi-inattention or extinction to more than one modality; does not recognize own hand or orients to only one side of space	2
Score	

5. Motor Function:
    - Arm: Ability to hold arms up.
    - Leg: Ability to lift legs.
6. Limb Ataxia: Coordination tests (finger-to-nose, heel-to-shin).
7. Sensory: Response to pinprick in face, arms, and legs.
8. Language: Ability to name objects, describe pictures, and read.
9. Speech: Clarity of speech and articulation.

10. Extinction and Inattention (Neglect): Awareness of surroundings and stimuli.

- Scoring:
- Total score ranges from 0 to 42.
- Interpretation:
  - 0: No stroke symptoms.
  - 1–4: Minor stroke.
  - 5–15: Moderate stroke.
  - 16–20: Moderate to severe stroke.
  - 21–42: Severe stroke.
- Clinical Use:
  - Establish baseline neurological status.
  - Guide treatment decisions (e.g., eligibility for thrombolytic therapy).
  - Monitor changes over time.

B. **Glasgow Coma Scale (GCS)** (Table 3.2)

- Purpose: Assesses the level of consciousness based on eye, verbal, and motor responses [3, 4].

Table 3.2 Glasgow Coma Scale (GCS)

Scale definition	Score
Eye opening (E)	1–4
Spontaneous	4
To speech (to sound)	3
To noxious stimulation (to pain)	2
No response (none)	1
Verbal response (V)	1–5
Alert and oriented (oriented)—5	5
Confused/disoriented (confused)	4
Inappropriate words (words)	3
Incomprehensible sounds (sounds)	2
No response (none) or in intubated patients	1
Motor response (M)	1–6
Obeys commands—6	6
Localizes to noxious stimuli (localizing)	5
Withdraws from pain	4
Decorticate posture (abnormal flexion)	3
Decerebrate posture (abnormal extension)	2
No response (none)	1

- Scoring:
- Eye Opening (E): 1–4 points.
- Verbal Response (V): 1–5 points.
- Motor Response (M): 1–6 points.
- Total Score: 3 (deep unconsciousness) to 15 (fully alert).
- Interpretation:
- Helps identify patients at risk of deterioration.
- Useful for monitoring trends in consciousness level.

C. **Evaluate for Signs of Brain Herniation**

Recognizing signs of brain herniation is critical for prompt intervention:

- Uncal Herniation:
  - Clinical Signs:
  - Ipsilateral pupil dilation and non-reactivity (due to oculomotor nerve compression).
  - Ptosis and impaired eye movement.
  - Contralateral hemiparesis.
  - Decreased level of consciousness.
- Central (Transtentorial) Herniation:
  - Clinical Signs:
  - Bilateral fixed and dilated pupils.
  - Loss of brainstem reflexes (e.g., corneal, gag reflexes).
  - Decerebrate posturing.
  - Abnormal respiratory patterns.
  - Rapid progression to coma.
- Management:
  - Immediate measures to reduce intracranial pressure (ICP).
  - Potential surgical intervention (e.g., decompressive craniectomy).

3.3 Perform Urgent Neuroimaging

A. **Computed Tomography (CT) Scan or Magnetic Resonance Imaging (MRI)**

- CT Scan:
  - First-line imaging modality.
  - Quick and effective in detecting intracranial hemorrhage, hydrocephalus, and mass effect.

- MRI:
  - Provides detailed images of brain parenchyma.
  - More sensitive for detecting early ischemic changes, brainstem lesions, and demyelinating diseases.

B. **Vascular Imaging**

- CT Angiography (CTA) or Magnetic Resonance Angiography (MRA):
  - Indicated if vascular abnormalities are suspected (e.g., aneurysms, arterial occlusions).
  - Essential for planning surgical or endovascular interventions.

3.4 Identify the Underlying Condition and Initiate Appropriate Management

A. **Intracerebral Hemorrhage (ICH)**

- Management Protocol:
- Blood Pressure Control: Maintain systolic BP < 140 mmHg unless contraindicated.
- Reversal of Anticoagulation: Administer appropriate reversal agents if the patient is on anticoagulant and has deranged coagulation parameters.
- Surgical Consideration: Hematoma evacuation may be necessary for large hemorrhages or those causing significant mass effect (for details, refer to Chap. 7).

B. **Ischemic Stroke**

- Management Protocol:
- Thrombolytic Therapy: Consider intravenous alteplase if within 4.5 h of symptom onset and no contraindications.
- Mechanical Thrombectomy: Indicated for large vessel occlusions within 24 h in selected patients.
- Secondary Prevention: Antiplatelet agents, statins, and management of risk factors (for details, refer to Chap. 8).

C. **Aneurysmal Subarachnoid Hemorrhage (SAH)**

- Management Protocol:
- Securing the Aneurysm: Endovascular coiling or surgical clipping.

- Preventing Vasospasm: Administer nimodipine and monitor with transcranial Doppler.
- ICP Management: Monitor and control intracranial pressure (for details, refer to Chap. 9).

D. **Hydrocephalus**

- Management Protocol:
  - External Ventricular Drainage (EVD): Immediate relief of increased ICP.
  - Long-Term Solutions: Ventriculoperitoneal shunt placement if necessary (for details, refer to Chap. 10).

E. **Brain Tumors or Abscesses**

- Management Protocol:
- Brain Tumors:
  - Surgical Resection: Removal of tumor mass when feasible.
  - Adjunct Therapies: Radiation and chemotherapy as indicated.
- Brain Abscesses:
  - Antimicrobial Therapy: Broad-spectrum antibiotics tailored to culture results.
  - Surgical Drainage: Aspiration or excision if abscess is large or causing mass effect (for details, refer to Chap. 11).

3.5 Conclusion

Managing patients with focal neurological deficits in the ICU requires a prompt, systematic approach to assessment and intervention. Early recognition of signs and symptoms, coupled with rapid diagnostic imaging and identification of the underlying cause, is essential for initiating appropriate treatment. By following this algorithm, healthcare providers can improve patient outcomes through timely and targeted therapies.

Algorithm 3.1: Management of patients with localizing neurological lesions in the ICU

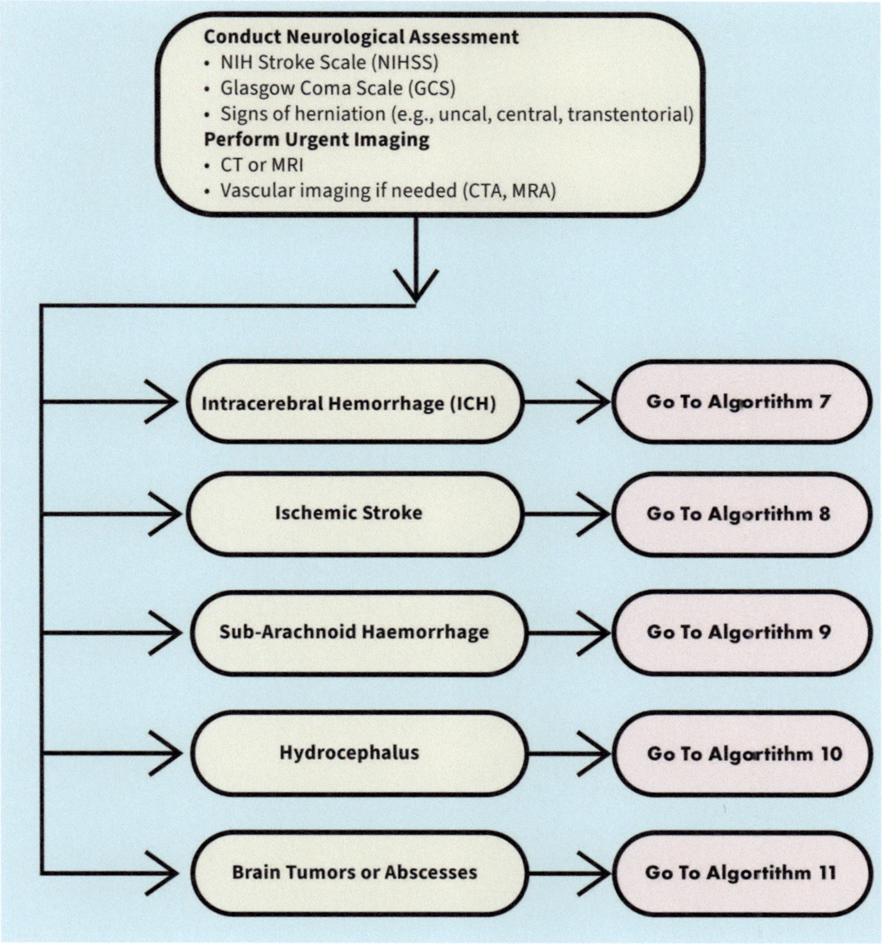

Bibliography

1. Brott T, Adams HP Jr, Olinger CP, Marler JR, Barsan WG, Biller J, et al. Measurements of acute cerebral infarction: a clinical examination scale. Stroke. 1989;20(7):864–70.
2. Goldstein LB, Bertels C, Davis JN. Interrater reliability of the NIH stroke scale. Arch Neurol. 1989;46(6):660–2.
3. Teasdale G, Jennett B. Assessment of coma and impaired consciousness. Pract Scale Lancet. 1974;2(7872):81–4.
4. Teasdale G, Jennett B. Assessment and prognosis of coma after head injury. Acta Neurochir. 1976;34(1–4):45–55.

Chapter 4
Management of Suspected Brain Infection in the ICU

4.1 Introduction

Suspected brain infections, such as encephalitis and meningitis, are critical conditions that require prompt and precise management in the intensive care unit (ICU). These infections can cause severe neurological damage or death if not treated in a timely and appropriate manner. This chapter outlines the management of suspected brain infections, including bacterial, viral, autoimmune, and atypical causes, and is designed to accompany a flowchart for guiding ICU clinicians (Ref. Algorithm 4.1).

4.2 Initial Assessment

Review Patient History and Perform Neurological Examination

- Patient History: Gather detailed information about recent travel, immunocompromised status, exposure to infectious agents, and prior infections or medications.
- Neurological Examination: Assess for signs of meningeal irritation (e.g., neck stiffness, photophobia, positive Kernig's sign, and Brudzinski's sign), focal neurological deficits (e.g., weakness, speech difficulties), and altered mental status (confusion, lethargy).

Lumbar Puncture (LP)

- Indications and Procedure: Perform LP unless contraindicated (e.g., signs of raised intracranial pressure such as focal deficits or papilledema). LP is crucial for diagnosing central nervous system (CNS) infections, analyzing cerebrospinal fluid (CSF) parameters (e.g., cell count, glucose, protein), and detecting specific pathogens via PCR.

S. B. Mishra et al., *Mastering ICU Care*,
https://doi.org/10.1007/978-981-95-0179-3_4

- Neuroimaging Before LP: Perform a CT or MRI before LP if there are indications such as focal neurological signs, papilledema, altered consciousness, new onset seizure, or suspicion of increased intracranial pressure. This helps residents avoid unnecessary imaging delays in patients without contraindications.

4.3 Blood Culture

4.3.1 Empirical Antimicrobial Therapy

Critical Time Windows for Therapy

- Antiviral Treatment: Initiate intravenous acyclovir (10 mg/kg every 8 h) immediately if HSV encephalitis is suspected, as delays can lead to poor outcomes.
- Antibacterial Treatment: Start with ceftriaxone (2 g IV every 12 hours) and vancomycin (15–20 mg/kg IV every 8–12 hours). For patients at risk for *Listeria monocytogenes* (e.g., elderly, immunocompromised), add ampicillin (2 g IV every 4 h).
- Other Antibiotics: Consider doxycycline (100 mg IV every 12 hours) for specific bacterial infections (e.g., rickettsial infections) [1].

Antibiotic Stewardship

- Once culture and PCR results are available, de-escalate antibiotics to targeted therapy based on pathogen sensitivity to prevent unnecessary broad-spectrum use and combat antimicrobial resistance.

Adjunct Therapy

- Corticosteroids: Administer intravenous dexamethasone (0.15 mg/kg q6h 2–4 days) in cases of suspected bacterial meningitis, especially in pneumococcal meningitis, to reduce mortality and prevent neurological complications. The first dose of steroid should be administered 10–20 min before the first dose of antimicrobial therapy.
- Intracranial Pressure Management: Monitor for signs of increased intracranial pressure and manage using hypertonic saline or mannitol. This is especially critical in patients with bacterial or tuberculous meningitis, and HSV encephalitis.

Role of Prophylaxis for Close Contacts

- Chemoprophylaxis: In cases of bacterial meningitis, particularly meningococcal meningitis, consider chemoprophylaxis for close contacts and healthcare workers. Rifampicin or ciprofloxacin may be used, as per local guidelines, for infection control.

4.4 Lumbar Puncture Report and Further Imaging

CSF Analysis

- White Cell Count: Pleocytosis indicates infection, while normal white cell counts often rule out bacterial or viral meningitis.
- Glucose and Protein Levels: Low CSF glucose is indicative of bacterial or tuberculous meningitis, while elevated protein levels suggest CNS inflammation (Table 4.1).

Pathogen Detection

- Use PCR for rapid identification of viral pathogens and culture for bacterial detection. Perform acid-fast staining and culture if *Mycobacterium tuberculosis* is suspected.

Imaging

- MRI: Perform MRI in cases of suspected encephalitis or to exclude alternative diagnoses. MRI is particularly useful in diagnosing HSV encephalitis and autoimmune encephalitis.

Autoimmune Encephalitis Workup

- Panel and Treatment: If autoimmune encephalitis is suspected, send an autoimmune encephalitis panel. Start high-dose methylprednisolone (1 g IV daily for 3–5 days), followed by oral steroids.
- Further Investigations: Involve a neurologist for specific autoantibody testing and management strategies.

Criteria for Discontinuing Empirical Therapy

- Discontinuation of Therapy: Once CSF PCR results are negative and there is clinical improvement, discontinue antiviral or antibacterial therapy to avoid prolonged and unnecessary treatment.

Table 4.1 Cerebrospinal fluid analysis

Condition	Opening pressure	Appearance	CSF white cell count (WBC)	Predominant cell type	CSF protein level	CSF glucose level	CSF/blood glucose ratio
Normal	12–20 cm CSF	Clear	< 5 cells/μL	None	< 0.4 g/L	2.6–4.5 mmol/L	> 0.66
Bacterial meningitis	Raised	Purulent, turbid, cloudy	> 100 cells/μL	Neutrophils	Raised	Very low	< 0.36
Viral meningitis	Normal/mildly raised	Clear	5–1000 cells/μL	Lymphocytes	Mildly raised	Normal/slightly low	Normal/slightly low
Tuberculous meningitis	Raised	Clear or cloudy	5–100 cells/μL	Lymphocytes	Markedly raised	Very low	< 0.36
Fungal meningitis	Raised	Clear or cloudy	5–100 cells/μL	Lymphocytes	Raised	Low	Low
HSV encephalitis	Raised	Clear	10–500 cells/μL	Lymphocytes	Mildly raised	Normal/slightly low	Normal/slightly low
Autoimmune encephalitis	Normal/mildly raised	Clear	5–100 cells/μL	Lymphocytes	Normal/slightly raised	Normal	Normal
Cryptococcal meningitis	Raised	Clear or cloudy	20–200 cells/μL	Lymphocytes	Raised	Low	Low

4.5 Specific Treatment Based on LP Findings

Bacterial Meningitis

- Empirical Antibiotics: Begin with ceftriaxone and vancomycin [2]. Adjust therapy based on identified pathogens:
- *Streptococcus pneumoniae*: Continue ceftriaxone or switch to penicillin G (24 million units/day).
- *Neisseria meningitidis*: Penicillin G or ceftriaxone.
- *Listeria monocytogenes*: Ampicillin plus gentamicin.
- Supportive Care: Manage symptoms, including seizures and increased intracranial pressure.

Viral Meningitis

- Supportive Care: Ensure hydration, manage pain, and control fever [3].
- Antiviral Therapy: Initiate acyclovir for suspected or confirmed HSV infections.
- Monitoring: Regular follow-up for recovery.

Tuberculous Meningitis

- Antitubercular Therapy: Begin the RIPE regimen (isoniazid, rifampicin, pyrazinamide, ethambutol). Adjust based on drug susceptibility [4].
- Adjunctive Therapy: Use corticosteroids like dexamethasone to reduce inflammation. Initial adjuvant corticosteroid therapy with dexamethasone or prednisolone tapered over 6–8 weeks.
- Duration: Treatment lasts 9–12 months, depending on disease severity.

Fungal Meningitis

- Cryptococcal Meningitis: Start with Amphotericin B (0.7–1.0 mg/kg IV daily) plus flucytosine, followed by fluconazole maintenance.
- Other Fungal Infections: Treat according to pathogen and susceptibility using antifungals such as voriconazole or itraconazole.

Autoimmune Encephalitis

- Immunotherapy: Administer high-dose corticosteroids and consider IVIG or plasmapheresis for severe cases [5, 6].
- Long-Term Management: Consider rituximab or cyclophosphamide for refractory or chronic cases.

Detailed Management of Specific Subpopulations

- Immunocompromised Patients: Pay special attention to immunocompromised patients (e.g., HIV/AIDS, transplant recipients) who are at higher risk for atypical infections like fungal, tuberculous, or viral meningitis. Adjust treatment based on the specific risks and pathogen involved.

Rehabilitation and Long-Term Follow-Up

- Rehabilitation: Emphasize the importance of rehabilitation and neurocognitive follow-up for patients recovering from severe encephalitis or meningitis, as many may experience long-term neurological or psychological deficits.
- Long-Term Care: Ensure follow-up with neurologists and rehabilitation specialists to monitor recovery, cognitive function, and potential disability.

4.6 Conclusion

Managing suspected brain infections in the ICU requires a structured approach involving prompt empirical therapy, diagnostic testing, and treatment adjustments based on specific pathogens. Lumbar puncture and timely imaging are essential to guide management. Attention to special populations, such as immunocompromised patients, and conditions like autoimmune encephalitis and tuberculosis, is critical to optimizing outcomes. Long-term rehabilitation and follow-up are vital for addressing residual neurological deficits.

Algorithm 4.1: Management of suspected brain infection in the ICU

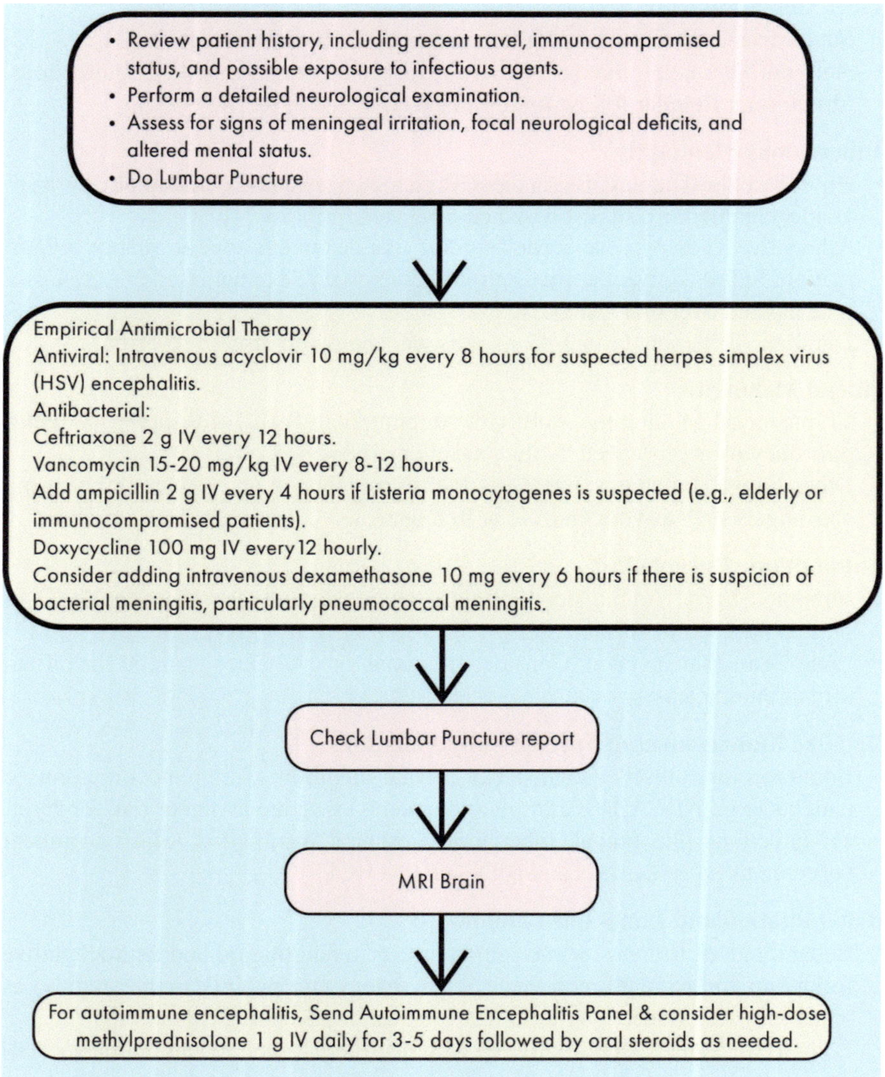

Bibliography

1. Tunkel AR, Hasbun R, Bhimraj A, Byers K, Kaplan SL, Scheld WM, et al. Infectious diseases society of America's clinical practice guidelines for healthcare-associated Ventriculitis and meningitis*. Clin Infect Dis. 2017;64(6):e34–65.
2. van de Beek D, Cabellos C, Dzupova O, Esposito S, Klein M, Kloek AT, et al. ESCMID guideline: diagnosis and treatment of acute bacterial meningitis. Clin Microbiol Infect. 2016;22:S37–62.
3. Costa BK, Sato DK. Viral encephalitis: a practical review on diagnostic approach and treatment. J Pediatr. 2020;96:12–9.
4. Lewinsohn DM, Leonard MK, LoBue PA, Cohn DL, Daley CL, Desmond E, et al. Official American thoracic society/infectious diseases society of America/centers for disease control and prevention clinical practice guidelines: diagnosis of tuberculosis in adults and children. Clin Infect Dis. 2017;64(2):e1–e33.
5. Ellul MA, Wood G, Tooren HVD, Easton A, Babu A, Michael BD. Update on the diagnosis and management of autoimmune encephalitis. Clin Med. 2020;20(4):389–92.
6. Abboud H, Probasco JC, Irani S, Ances B, Benavides DR, Bradshaw M, et al. Autoimmune encephalitis: proposed best practice recommendations for diagnosis and acute management. J Neurol Neurosurg Psychiatry. 2021;92(7):757–68.

Chapter 5
Approach to Psychogenic Coma in the ICU

5.1 Introduction

Psychogenic coma is a condition where a patient appears to be in a comatose state without an identifiable organic cause. This presentation is often linked to psychiatric disorders and can pose significant diagnostic and therapeutic challenges. Effective management requires a structured approach to ensure patient safety, accurate diagnosis, and appropriate treatment. The following write-up details the step-by-step management strategy as outlined in the flowchart, providing comprehensive explanations for each step and decision point [1, 2]. (Ref. Algorithm 5.1).

5.1.1 Establish a Safe Environment

Rationale: The primary step in managing any patient in a comatose state is to ensure their environment is safe. This includes removing any potential hazards that could cause harm to the patient or healthcare providers.

Considerations: Ensure that the patient is in a calm, secure setting, possibly with restraints if they pose a danger to themselves or others.

5.1.2 Monitor Vital Signs and Neurological Reassessment

Rationale: Continuous monitoring of vital signs (heart rate, blood pressure, respiratory rate, and oxygen saturation) is crucial to detect any changes in the patient's physiological status. Regular neurological reassessment helps in tracking any changes in the patient's neurological function.

S. B. Mishra et al., *Mastering ICU Care*,
https://doi.org/10.1007/978-981-95-0179-3_5

Considerations: Utilize tools like the Glasgow Coma Scale (GCS) to systematically assess the patient's level of consciousness. Frequent checks are essential to identify any deterioration that may indicate an organic cause.

5.1.3 Psychiatric Evaluation

Rationale: A thorough psychiatric evaluation is necessary to identify any underlying psychiatric conditions that may contribute to the psychogenic coma. Neurological reassessment continues to ensure no new neurological findings are missed.

Considerations: Engage a psychiatrist early in the evaluation process. Utilize structured interviews and standardized tools to assess the patient's mental state.

5.1.4 Amytal Interview

The Amytal interview, also known as a "sodium Amytal interview" or "truth serum interview," is a diagnostic and therapeutic procedure used primarily in psychiatry and neurology. Sodium Amytal, a barbiturate, is administered intravenously to induce a state of reduced inhibition, relaxation, and mild sedation. This altered state can facilitate communication and uncover psychological conditions that may not be apparent in a fully conscious state [3, 4]. Here is a detailed description of the Amytal interview process:

5.1.5 Purpose and Indications

The Amytal interview is employed to:

- Differentiate between organic and psychogenic disorders.
- Elicit hidden or repressed information.
- Aid in the diagnosis of conditions such as conversion disorder, catatonia, and psychogenic seizures.
- Provide therapeutic insight into unconscious conflicts and psychological issues.

5.1.6 Procedure

1. **Preparation**
    - **Patient Consent**: Obtain informed consent from the patient, explaining the purpose, potential benefits, and risks of the procedure.

- **Environment**: Conduct the interview in a quiet, controlled setting, typically with a psychiatrist or neurologist present. Monitoring equipment should be available to track vital signs.

2. **Administration**

- **Intravenous Injection**: Sodium Amytal is administered intravenously, typically at a dose of 250–500 mg, titrated to effect. The onset of action is usually within a few minutes.
- **Monitoring**: Continuous monitoring of the patient's vital signs, including heart rate, blood pressure, and oxygen saturation, is essential throughout the procedure.

3. **Interview Process**

- **Induction Phase**: As the drug takes effect, the patient enters a state of reduced inhibition and relaxation. The clinician observes for signs of relaxation and responsiveness.
- **Questioning**: The clinician asks open-ended and specific questions to explore the patient's mental state, emotional conflicts, and responses to stimuli. The questions should be gentle and nonconfrontational to encourage the patient to speak freely.
- **Observation**: The clinician carefully notes the patient's responses, emotional reactions, and any emergence of repressed or hidden information.

4. **Post-Interview**

- **Recovery**: After the interview, the patient is monitored until the effects of the drug wear off. This typically takes about 30–60 minutes.
- **Debriefing**: The clinician discusses the findings with the patient once they are fully alert, providing insight and therapeutic guidance based on the information obtained.

5.1.7 Benefits

- **Diagnostic Clarity**: Helps distinguish between psychogenic and organic causes of symptoms.
- **Therapeutic Insight**: Uncovers repressed conflicts and emotions, aiding in therapeutic planning.
- **Enhanced Communication**: Facilitates communication in patients who may be nonresponsive or uncooperative in a fully conscious state.

5.1.8 Risks and Considerations

- **Side Effects**: Possible side effects include drowsiness, dizziness, nausea, and respiratory depression.
- **Contraindications**: Not recommended for patients with a history of severe respiratory conditions, barbiturate allergy, or certain psychiatric disorders.
- **Ethical Concerns**: The use of Amytal interviews should be ethically justified, with a clear clinical indication and patient consent.

5.2 Types of Psychogenic Coma

5.2.1 Conversion Reaction

Psychotherapy: Engaging the patient in psychotherapy helps address the underlying psychological issues.

Cognitive-Behavioral Therapy (CBT): CBT is effective in modifying dysfunctional thoughts and behaviors.

Stress Management: Techniques for managing stress are crucial in preventing recurrence.

Catatonia.

Benzodiazepines: Medications like lorazepam are commonly used to treat catatonia.

Electroconvulsive Therapy (ECT): ECT is effective for patients not responding to benzodiazepines, particularly in severe cases.

5.2.2 Psychogenic Seizures

Education: Informing the patient and their family about the nature of psychogenic seizures is vital.

Psychotherapy: Therapy helps address the psychological triggers.

Avoiding Antiepileptic Drugs: Since these seizures are not epileptic in origin, antiepileptic drugs are generally not indicated.

5.2.3 Cerebellar Cognitive Affective Syndrome

Neuropsychological Rehabilitation: Tailored rehabilitation programs help improve cognitive and affective functions.
Supportive Therapy: Providing emotional and psychological support is crucial for recovery.

5.2.4 Reevaluate for Potential Organic Causes

If all evaluations and interventions indicate no psychogenic cause, reevaluation for potential organic causes is conducted using:

EEG: Electroencephalogram helps in identifying any underlying epileptic activity.
MRI: Magnetic resonance imaging can detect structural brain abnormalities that might contribute to the coma.

- By following this structured approach, clinicians can systematically identify and address the underlying causes of psychogenic coma, ensuring comprehensive and effective patient care.

5.3 Conclusion

Managing psychogenic coma requires a multidisciplinary approach involving careful assessment, monitoring, and intervention. Establishing a safe environment, continuous monitoring, thorough psychiatric and neurological evaluations, and the use of an Amytal interview are crucial steps. Treatment varies based on the specific diagnosis, with psychotherapy, pharmacotherapy, and supportive therapies playing key roles. Reevaluation is necessary if initial tests suggest no psychogenic cause.

Algorithm 5.1: Approach to psychogenic coma in the ICU

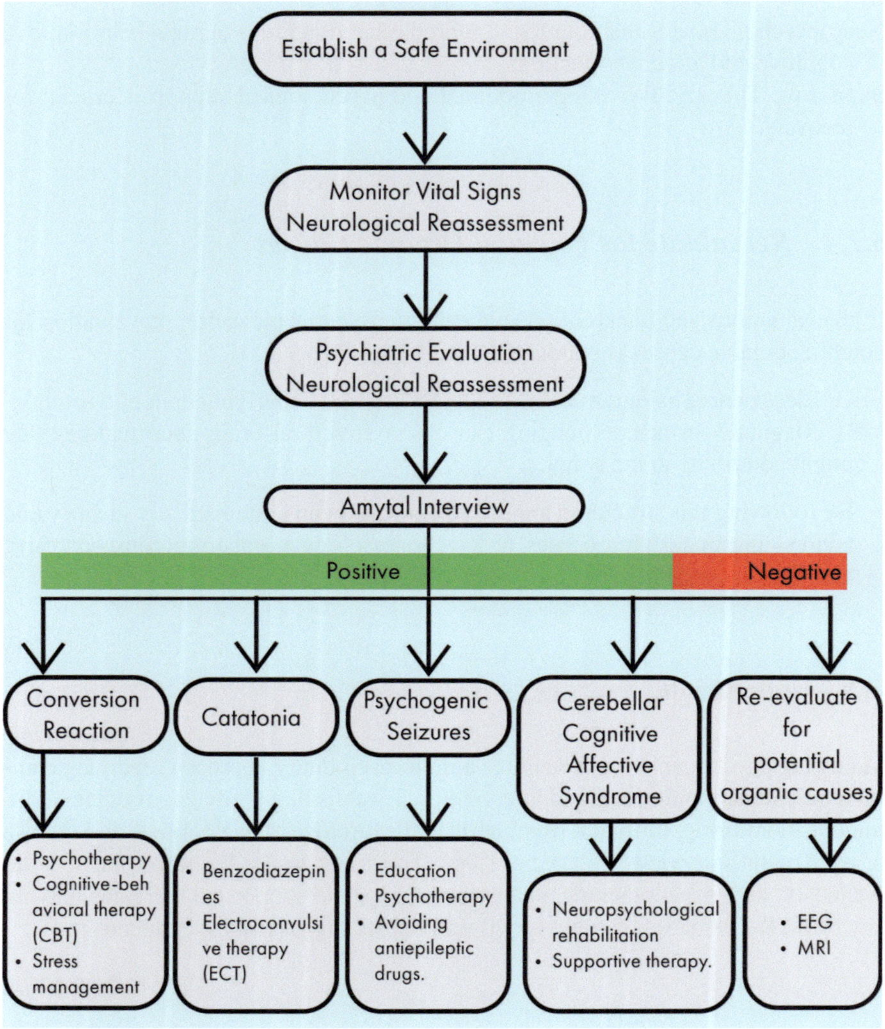

Bibliography

1. Ryznar E, Wilcox D. Functional coma: two case reports and a review of the literature. Psychosomatics. 2019;60(4):343–51.
2. Kim SH, Kim KM, Lim YH, Yoo BH, Cho J, Jun IJ. Psychogenic coma after general anesthesia with remimazolam and remifentanil -a case report. Korean J Anesthesiol. 2022;75(5):449–52.
3. Naples M, Hackett TP. The amytal interview: history and current uses. Psychosomatics. 1978;19(2):98–105.
4. Perry JC, Jacobs D. Overview: clinical applications of the amytal interview in psychiatric emergency settings. Am J Psychiatry. 1982;139(5):552–9.

Chapter 6
Management of Metabolic Encephalopathy in the ICU

6.1 Introduction

Metabolic encephalopathy is a diffuse brain dysfunction caused by systemic illness, characterized by an altered mental state ranging from confusion to coma. Proper management in the ICU is crucial for patient recovery and involves a structured approach to diagnosis, treatment, and continuous monitoring. Early identification of delirium and addressing toxic-metabolic causes are essential to prevent long-term complications [1]. (Ref. Algorithm 6.1).

1. **Initial Evaluation in the ICU**
   Confirm Diagnosis:
   - Action: Review the patient's history, clinical presentation, and initial lab results and imaging from the emergency department.
   - Rationale: It is crucial to rule out structural causes of encephalopathy, such as stroke or hemorrhage, through imaging if not already done. Early identification of the underlying cause helps tailor the treatment approach [2].

   Assess Severity and Monitor Continuously:
   - Action: Use the Glasgow Coma Scale (GCS) to assess the level of consciousness. Monitor vital signs (BP (blood pressure), HR (heart rate), RR (respiratory rate), temperature) and neurological status (level of consciousness, motor responses, pupil reactions). Utilize tools such as the Confusion Assessment Method for the ICU (CAM-ICU) to assess for delirium.
   - Rationale: Continuous assessment allows for timely interventions in response to changes in the patient's condition, with early detection of delirium aiding in preventing progression to more severe encephalopathy.
2. **Laboratory Tests (refer to** Table 6.1)

S. B. Mishra et al., *Mastering ICU Care*,
https://doi.org/10.1007/978-981-95-0179-3_6

Table 6.1 Laboratory tests for metabolic encephalopathy in the ICU

Test	Purpose	Interpretation
Complete blood count (CBC)	Assess overall health, detect a variety of disorders such as infections, anemia, and leukemia	Look for signs of infection, anemia, or other hematologic abnormalities
Electrolyte panel	Measure levels of key electrolytes (sodium, potassium, chloride, calcium, magnesium, bicarbonate)	Detect electrolyte imbalances that can affect neurological function
Blood glucose	Measure blood sugar levels	Identify hypoglycemia or hyperglycemia
Arterial blood gas (ABG)	Evaluate oxygenation, ventilation, and acid-base status	Assess for respiratory or metabolic acidosis/alkalosis, hypoxia
Liver function tests (LFTs)	Evaluate liver function and detect liver damage	Identify hepatic encephalopathy or liver failure
Renal function tests	Assess kidney function	Detect renal failure, uremia
Ammonia levels	Measure ammonia concentration in the blood	Identify hepatic encephalopathy
Toxicology screen	Detect the presence of drugs and toxins	Identify potential toxin exposures
Thyroid function test	Measure levels of thyroid hormones (TSH, T3, T4)	Detect thyroid dysfunction (hypothyroidism or hyperthyroidism)
Lactate levels	Measure lactate concentration	Detect lactic acidosis
Blood cultures	Detect presence of bacterial infection in the blood	Identify systemic infections
Coagulation profile	Assess blood clotting ability (PT, aPTT, INR)	Identify coagulopathies, assess risk of bleeding
Vitamin B12 and folate	Measure levels of these vitamins	Identify deficiencies that can lead to neurological symptoms
Cortisol levels	Measure cortisol concentration	Detect adrenal insufficiency

3. **Identify and Treat Underlying Causes [3–8]**

   Hypoxia:

   - Action: Ensure adequate oxygenation and ventilation. Correct underlying pulmonary issues such as pneumonia or pulmonary edema.

   Ischemia:

   - Action: Optimize cardiac output and treat underlying cardiac conditions like arrhythmias or myocardial infarction.

   Hypoglycemia:

   - Action: Administer IV (intravenous) glucose.

   Electrolyte Imbalance:

   - Action: Correct sodium, potassium, calcium, and magnesium imbalances.

Renal Failure:

- Action: Manage uremia with dialysis if indicated.

Hepatic Encephalopathy:

- Action: Use lactulose to reduce ammonia levels. Consider rifaximin or neomycin to reduce gut ammonia production.

Acid-Base Disorders:

- Action: Correct metabolic and respiratory acidosis or alkalosis

Endocrine Disorders:

- Action: Treat thyroid, adrenal, or pancreatic dysfunction accordingly.

Toxin Exposure:

- Action: Administer appropriate antidotes (e.g., naloxone for opioid overdose, flumazenil for benzodiazepine overdose). Consider hemodialysis for severe toxic ingestions.

4. **Imaging**
   - Action: Repeat CT/MRI if neurological status deteriorates or does not improve as expected. Imaging may be necessary to evaluate for brain edema, increased intracranial pressure, or venous sinus thrombosis.
   - Rationale: Imaging helps in identifying any structural abnormalities or complications that may have developed during the course of treatment.
5. **Electroencephalogram (EEG)**

   EEG is a valuable tool in metabolic encephalopathy for detecting diffuse slowing, triphasic waves, or nonconvulsive seizures, which can aid in diagnosing the severity and differentiating from other causes of altered mental status [9, 10].
6. **Multidisciplinary Approach**
   - Action: Involve neurology, nephrology, hepatology, endocrinology, and toxicology as needed.
   - Rationale: A multidisciplinary team ensures comprehensive care addressing all possible aspects of the patient's condition.
7. **Preventive Strategies**
   - Action: Focus on preventing further episodes of encephalopathy through careful medication management, avoiding polypharmacy, regular monitoring, and optimizing sedation practices.
   - Rationale: Preventive measures reduce the risk of delirium and other complications, improving overall patient outcomes.

8. **Nutritional and Electrolyte Reassessment**
   - Action: Provide adequate nutritional support, especially for patients with hepatic or renal encephalopathy. Closely monitor and correct electrolyte imbalances, particularly in patients undergoing diuresis or renal replacement therapy.
   - Rationale: Optimizing nutrition and electrolyte levels supports metabolic recovery and prevents further deterioration of brain function.

6.2 Conclusion

The management of metabolic encephalopathy in the ICU requires a systematic approach to diagnosis, continuous monitoring, and addressing underlying causes. Timely interventions, including correction of metabolic and toxic imbalances, and a multidisciplinary approach, are essential for improving patient outcomes. Continuous reassessment, early identification of delirium, and preventive strategies play a crucial role in preventing recurrence and promoting recovery.

Algorithm 6.1: Management of metabolic encephalopathy in the ICU

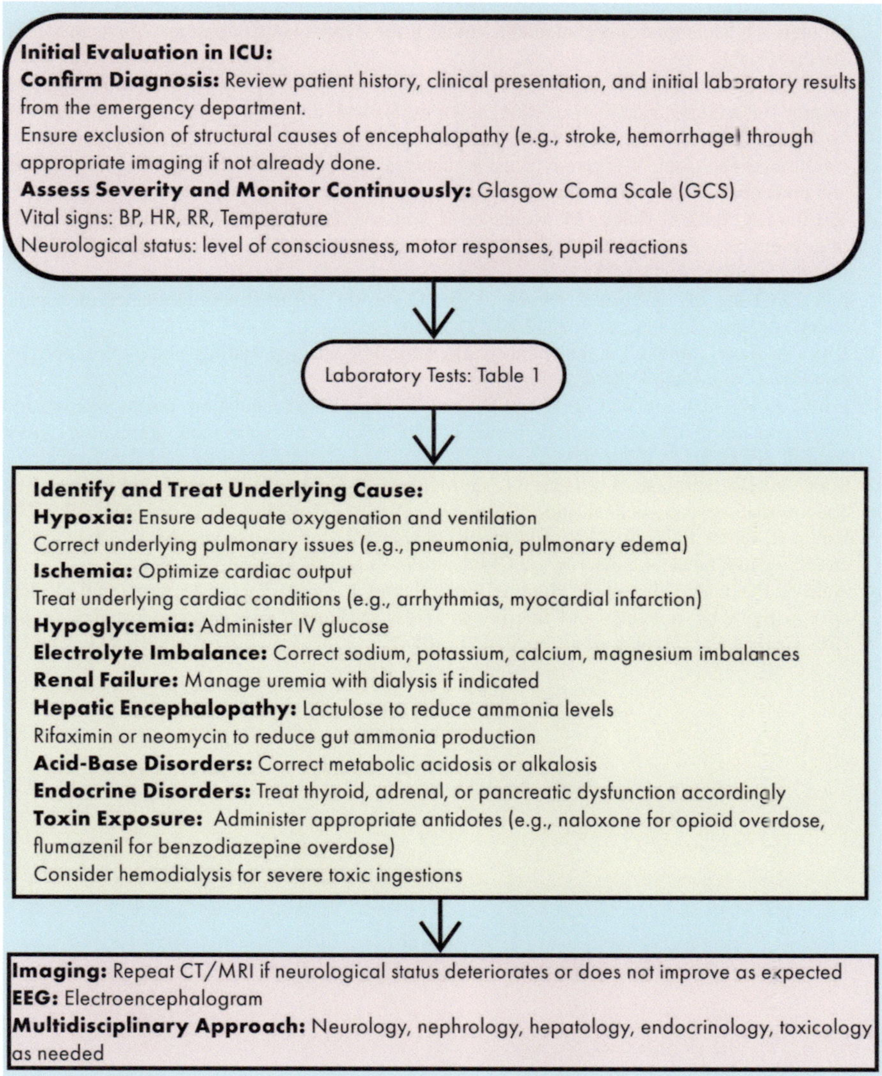

Bibliography

1. Frontera JA. Metabolic encephalopathies in the critical care unit. Continuum (Minneap Minn). 2012;18(3):611–39.
2. Le Guennec L, Marois C, Demeret S, Wijdicks EFM, Weiss N. Toxic-metabolic encephalopathy in adults: critical discussion and pragmatical diagnostic approach. Rev Neurol. 2022;178(1):93–104.
3. Nakhleh A, Shehadeh N. Hypoglycemia in diabetes: an update on pathophysiology, treatment, and prevention. World J Diabetes. 2021;12(12):2036–49.
4. Yassine EA, Sarah S, Najoua M, Mohamed H, Youssouf B, Ahmed B. Psychiatric presentation of a severe vitamin B12 deficiency associated with Biermer's disease: a case report. Int J Med Pharm Case Rep. 2024;17(3):1–4.
5. Poh Z, Chang PE. A current review of the diagnostic and treatment strategies of hepatic encephalopathy. Int J Hepatol. 2012;2012:1–10.
6. Kim DM, Lee I, Song CJ. Uremic encephalopathy: MR imaging findings and clinical correlation. Am J Neuroradiol. 2016;37(9):1604–9.
7. Liu Y, Yu Y, Liu J, Liu W, Cao Y, Yan R, et al. Neuroimmune regulation in sepsis-associated encephalopathy: the interaction between the brain and peripheral immunity. Front Neurol. 2022;13
8. Sonneville R, Benghanem S, Jeantin L, de Montmollin E, Doman M, Gaudemer A, et al. The Spectrum of sepsis-associated encephalopathy: a clinical perspective. Crit Care. 2023;27:27(1).
9. Faigle R, Sutter R, Kaplan PW. Electroencephalography of encephalopathy in patients with endocrine and metabolic disorders. J Clin Neurophysiol. 2013;30(5):505–16.
10. Abid S, Papin G, Vellieux G, Montmollin É, Patrier J, Jaquet P, et al. A simplified electroencephalography montage and interpretation for evaluation of comatose patients in the ICU. Critical Care Explorations. 2022;4(11):e0781.

Chapter 7
Management of Intracerebral Hemorrhage (ICH) in the ICU

Abbreviations

CT	Computed tomography
PCO_2	Partial pressure of carbon dioxide
ICP	Intracranial pressure
CPP	Cerebral perfusion pressure
SBP	Systolic blood pressure
FFP	Fresh frozen plasma
PCC	Prothrombin complex concentrate

7.1 Introduction

Intracerebral hemorrhage (ICH) is a severe and life-threatening condition caused by the rupture of blood vessels within the brain. The management of ICH in the ICU is a critical process involving stabilization, control of intracranial pressure (ICP), management of coagulation, prevention of complications, and rehabilitation. Recent guidelines underscore the importance of a systematic, evidence-based approach in managing patients with ICH, which this guide aims to elaborate for ICU residents, offering practical insights into the management and decision-making process. The chapter follows the flowchart-based management with emphasis on recent updates to optimize patient care and outcomes [1, 2] [Ref. Algorithm 7.1].

7.2 Initial Assessment and Classification

History & CT Suggestive of Trauma?

- Yes: Traumatic ICH
- No: Spontaneous ICH

S. B. Mishra et al., *Mastering ICU Care*,
https://doi.org/10.1007/978-981-95-0179-3_7

7.3 Traumatic ICH

Initial Management

- Follow advanced trauma life support (ATLS) principles.
- Actions: Secure airway, stabilize blood pressure, immobilize the spine, and correct any coagulopathy.
- Perform a rapid neurological exam.
- Actions: Assess Glasgow Coma Scale (GCS) score and pupil response.

Medical Management

ICP Management

- Elevate head of bed to 30 degrees and keep the head straight.
- Osmotic therapy.
- Mannitol (0.25–1 g/kg IV bolus) or hypertonic saline.
- Optimize sedation and analgesia to prevent ICP spikes.
- Maintain euvolemia for adequate cerebral perfusion.
- Target PCO_2: 30–35 mmHg. Avoid hypercapnia, which can increase ICP.
- Target ICP < 20 mmHg, target CPP 60–70 mmHg.
- Target SBP between 100 and 110 mmHg.

Update: It is recommended to maintain smooth, sustained blood pressure control, which has shown to reduce the risk of hematoma expansion.

Coagulation Management

- Administer tranexamic acid (TXA) within 3 hours of injury.
- Reverse anticoagulation.
- Correct platelet count.

Update: For anticoagulation reversal, specific agents such as idarucizumab for dabigatran/RRT (renal replacement therapy), andexanet alfa for factor Xa inhibitors, and prothrombin complex concentrate (PCC) for vitamin K antagonists should be used based on the anticoagulant involved. Activated charcoal should be used if there is history of intake of direct oral anticoagulant in last few hours. PCC may be used if specific antidotes are not available.

Seizure Prophylaxis

- Levetiracetam or phenytoin for early seizure prophylaxis.

Update: Prophylactic use of antiseizure medications without documented evidence of seizures is generally not recommended as it may not improve outcomes.

Surgical Intervention

- Indications: Large hematomas, neurological deterioration, signs of herniation.
- Procedures: Decompressive craniectomy, hematoma evacuation.
- Use of external ventricular drainage (EVD) if hydrocephalus is present.

Update: Minimally invasive surgery for hematoma evacuation may reduce mortality, though improvement in functional outcomes remains neutral. Larger cerebellar hemorrhages (>15 mL) and signs of neurological deterioration require immediate surgical intervention.

7.4 Spontaneous ICH

Initial Management

- Ensure airway control, stabilize blood pressure, and correct impaired coagulation.
- Perform a rapid neurological exam to identify immediate needs and guide further management.

Update: Recognize the importance of early neuroimaging markers to predict hematoma expansion, as this is associated with worse outcomes.

7.5 Medical Management

ICP Management

- Same protocol as in traumatic ICH.

Blood Pressure Control

- Initiate treatment in 2 hours of ICH and achieve target in 1 hour. Target SBP: 130–150 mmHg.
- Rationale: Balances reducing bleeding risk while maintaining cerebral perfusion.

Update: Implementing acute blood pressure lowering with minimal variability appears to improve outcomes and limit hematoma expansion.

Coagulation Management

- Same as in traumatic ICH.
- Platelet may be transfused in ICH due to antiplatelets only if patient undergoes surgical intervention.

Surgical Intervention

- Indications: Patients with GCS of 5–12 and supratentorial ICH of >20 to 30 ml volume.
- Procedures: Minimally invasive surgery for hematoma evacuation.
- Use of external ventricular drainage (EVD) for spontaneous ICH with large IVH and impaired level of consciousness.
- Indications: Posterior fossa ICH with neurological deterioration, brain-stem compression, hydrocephalus or bleed volume $\geq$ 15 ml.
- Procedures: Complete surgical removal of hematoma with or without EVD.

7.6 Ongoing Management and Monitoring in ICH

Regular Assessments

- Neurological: Glasgow Coma Scale (GCS), NIHSS.
- Vital signs, ICP monitoring.
- Rationale: Detects early signs of deterioration.

Prevent Complications

- Infections, DVT, pressure sores.
  LMWH prophylaxis to be started at 24–48 hours from ICH onset after documenting stability on CT.
- Rationale: Reduces morbidity and improves outcomes.

Update: Avoid prophylactic corticosteroids for treatment of elevated ICP and platelet transfusions outside of emergency surgical or severe thrombocytopenia settings as they may worsen outcomes.

Glycemic control (60–180 mg/dL) and avoid hyperthermia.

7.7 Rehabilitation and Secondary Prevention

Early Mobilization and Rehabilitation

- Early mobilization, physical therapy, cognitive/speech therapy.
- Rationale: enhances recovery and minimizes long-term disability.

Update: Early mobilization within 24 hours of ICH has been shown to worsen short-term outcomes; start 24 to 48 hours post-stabilization for moderate ICH.

Patient/Family Education

- Education on stroke prevention, lifestyle modifications, and adherence to rehabilitation programs.

7.8 Conclusion

Managing intracerebral hemorrhage in the ICU requires a structured and evidence-based approach. Recent advancements in blood pressure management, anticoagulation reversal, surgical interventions, and rehabilitation should be incorporated into standard care to optimize outcomes. Adhering to these updated guidelines ensures comprehensive management, reduces morbidity, and enhances recovery in ICH patients.

Algorithm 7.1: Management of intracerebral hemorrhage (ICH) in the ICU

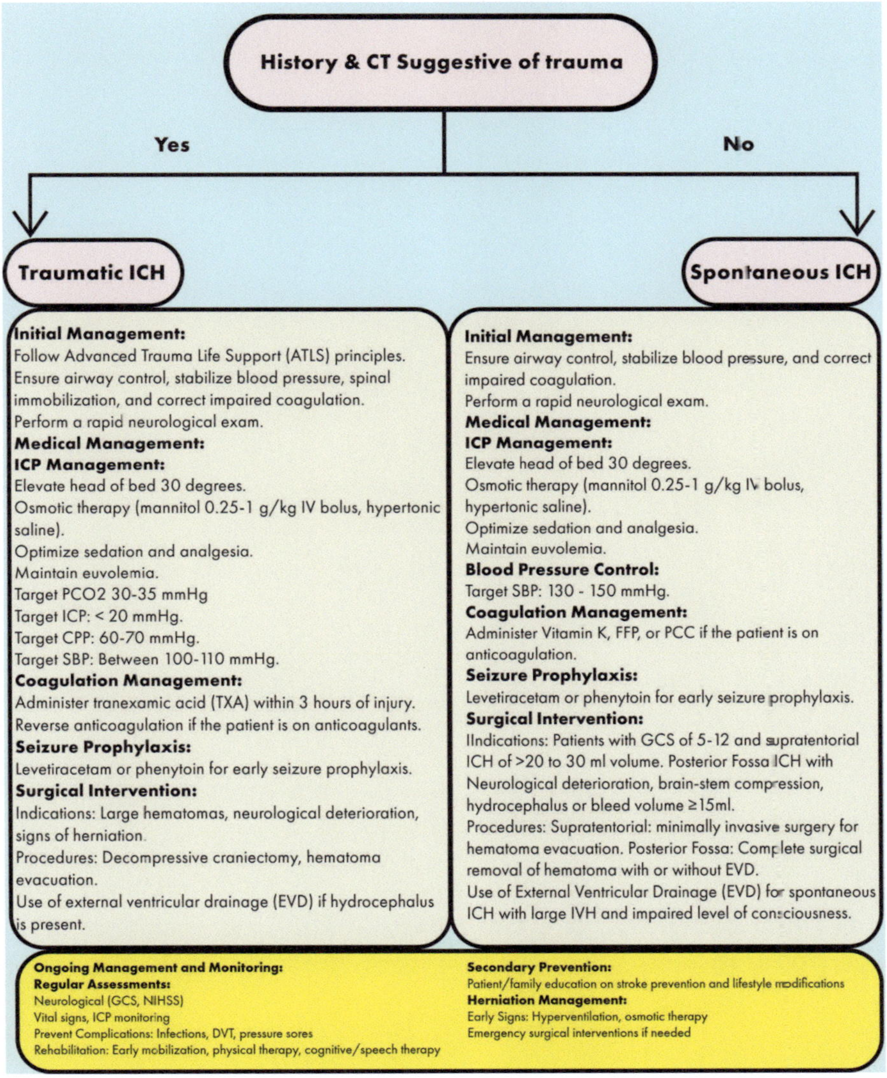

Bibliography

1. Hemphill JC, Greenberg SM, Anderson CS, Becker K, Bendok BR, Cushman M, et al. Guidelines for the management of spontaneous intracerebral hemorrhage. Stroke. 2015;46(7):2032–60.
2. Greenberg SM, Ziai WC, Cordonnier C, Dowlatshahi D, Francis B, Goldstein JN, et al. Guideline for the management of patients with spontaneous intracerebral hemorrhage: a guideline from the American Heart Association/American Stroke Association. Stroke. 2022;53(7):e282–361.

Chapter 8
Management of Ischemic Stroke in the ICU

8.1 Introduction

Ischemic stroke is a medical emergency characterized by the sudden loss of blood circulation to an area of the brain, resulting in neurological dysfunction. It remains the leading cause of disability and a major contributor to mortality worldwide. Effective management of ischemic stroke in the intensive care unit (ICU) requires prompt intervention to restore blood flow, minimize brain damage, and optimize recovery [1, 2] (Ref. Algorithm 8.1).

1. **Assess Time to Symptoms**

The management of ischemic stroke is highly dependent on the time elapsed since symptom onset, as well as patient-specific factors [3, 4].

Time to Symptoms <4.5 H

- Intravenous Thrombolysis:

  (a) Administer intravenous (IV) alteplase (tPA) or, as an alternative, tenecteplase in specific cases such as wake-up strokes, where patients were last known to be well more than 4.5 h earlier (MRI to identify diffusion-positive FLAIR negative lesions).
  (b) Avoid alteplase if patient received LMWH within 24 h.
  (c) Dose: 0.9 mg/kg; maximum dose 90 mg over 60 min. Initial 10% dose-bolus over 1 min.

  Indications: Acute ischemic stroke within 4.5 h of symptom onset.

- Contraindications: (Ref. Table 8.1 for full list).

  (a) Recent major surgery or trauma.
  (b) Active internal bleeding or known bleeding disorders.

S. B. Mishra et al., *Mastering ICU Care*,
https://doi.org/10.1007/978-981-95-0179-3_8

Table 8.1 Contraindications

Contraindications
Severe head trauma in previous 3 months
Symptoms suggestive of subarachnoid hemorrhage
Previous ICH
Intracranial/spinal surgery in previous 3 months
Intracerebral neoplasm
Infective endocarditis
Aortic arch dissection
Elevated blood pressure (systolic >185 mm hg or diastolic >110 mm hg) that cannot be lowered safely
Active internal bleeding
Acute bleeding diathesis, including but not limited to:
Platelet count <100,000/mm^3
Heparin received within 48 h with an elevated aPTT (>40 s)
Current use of treatment doses of low-molecular-weight heparin within the previous 24 h (not applicable to DVT prophylactic dosages of low-molecular-weight heparin)
Current use of anticoagulant with INR > 1.7 or PT > 15 s
Current use of direct thrombin inhibitors or direct factor Xa inhibitors
CT demonstrates infarction (hypodensity) >1/3 cerebral hemisphere
CT demonstrates an acute ICH
Relative contraindications
Mild and nondisabling or rapidly improving stroke symptoms
Very severe neurology deficits (NIHSS score > 25) within the 3 to 4.5 h window
Pregnancy
Seizure at onset (consider alteplase if neurologic deficits are thought to be caused by a stroke)
Arterial puncture at noncompressible site in previous 7 days
Untreated intracranial arteriovenous malformation
Untreated giant intracranial aneurysm
Recent major surgery or serious trauma (within previous 14 days)
Recent gastrointestinal or urinary tract hemorrhage (within previous 21 days)
Ischemic stroke within previous 3 months
Recent ST-elevation acute myocardial infarction (within previous 3 months)
Blood glucose concentration < 50 mg/dL (2.7 mmol/L) (consider IV alteplase if deficits still present after glucose normalization)

(c) Severe uncontrolled hypertension (systolic BP > 185 mmHg or diastolic BP > 110 mmHg).
(d) History of intracranial hemorrhage.

- Monitoring: Continuous neurological assessments and monitoring for signs of hemorrhagic transformation (e.g., worsening headache, acute hypertension, nausea/vomiting, or sudden neurological deterioration).

Time to Symptoms—4.5–6 H

- IV thrombolysis is not indicated. Proceed to Step 2 for further evaluation.

Time to Symptoms—6–24 H

- Mechanical Thrombectomy:

- Indications: Large vessel occlusions (LVOs, middle cerebral artery and internal carotid artery) within 6–24 h of symptom onset, pre-stroke mRS (modified Rankin score) score 0–1, NIHSS Score ≥ 6, and Alberta Stroke Program Early CT Score ASPECTS ≥6.

Thrombectomy for Posterior Circulation Stroke: Mechanical thrombectomy is recommended for vertebrobasilar artery occlusions up to 12 h from symptom onset.

2. **Medical Management**

Antiplatelet Therapy: Start Aspirin (160-300 mg) within 24–48 h of stroke onset if no thrombolysis.

Start dual antiplatelet therapy with aspirin (160–300 mg) and clopidogrel or ticagrelor within 24–48 h for minor stroke or transient ischemic attack (TIA), particularly when thrombolysis has not been performed.

Statins: Initiate high-intensity statin therapy to manage hyperlipidemia and reduce the risk of recurrent stroke.

Risk Factor Management: Control hypertension, diabetes, and encourage smoking cessation. Implement lifestyle changes and secondary prevention strategies to minimize future stroke risk.

3. **Blood Pressure Management**

Pre-thrombolysis: Target systolic blood pressure (SBP) < 185 mmHg and diastolic blood pressure (DBP) < 110 mmHg to minimize the risk of hemorrhagic transformation during thrombolysis.

Post-Thrombolysis: Maintain SBP < 180 mmHg and DBP < 105 mmHg for 24 h following thrombolysis to prevent complications and ensure optimal cerebral perfusion.

4. **Imaging and ASPECTS**

ASPECTS (Alberta Stroke Program Early CT Score)

- ASPECTS Overview: ASPECTS is a standardized scoring system to assess early ischemic changes in the brain and guide treatment decisions, particularly for thrombolysis and thrombectomy.
- Scoring:
- ASPECTS starts with a perfect score of 10. One point is subtracted for each region showing ischemic changes (focal swelling, hypodensity, or loss of gray-white differentiation).
- A score of 7–10 suggests a favorable prognosis, whereas a score of 0–3 indicates extensive ischemic changes and poorer outcomes.

Role of Imaging

- Advanced imaging modalities such as CT perfusion or MRI with diffusion-weighted imaging (DWI) and FLAIR mismatch help assess tissue salvage potential in patients presenting 6–24 h after symptom onset.

5. **Consider Decompressive Craniectomy**
   Indications: Decompressive craniectomy should be considered for malignant middle cerebral artery (MCA) infarction with significant brain swelling.

- Criteria:
  - Large infarct size.
  - Neurological deterioration.
  - Signs of herniation.
- Timing: Perform within 48 h of stroke onset for the best outcomes.

6. **Multidisciplinary Stroke Team and Continuum of Care**
   Pre-hospital and Acute Management: It is essential to establish pre-hospital stroke systems, including public awareness programs, EMS stroke assessment tools, and protocols for rapid hospital transport. Stroke teams should be ready to mobilize before the patient's arrival.

   Rehabilitation and Recovery: Post-stroke rehabilitation begins early and continues after discharge. Stroke patients should have access to multidisciplinary care, including physical therapy, occupational therapy, and psychological support. Telerehabilitation and early supported discharge play key roles in post-stroke care.

8.2 Conclusion

Managing ischemic stroke requires a dynamic and systematic approach based on the time of symptom onset, clinical status, and imaging findings. The integration of thrombolysis, mechanical thrombectomy, medical management, and early rehabilitation can significantly improve patient outcomes. Close adherence to the most recent guidelines and individualized patient care will optimize stroke recovery and reduce complications.

Algorithm 8.1: Management of ischemic stroke in the ICU

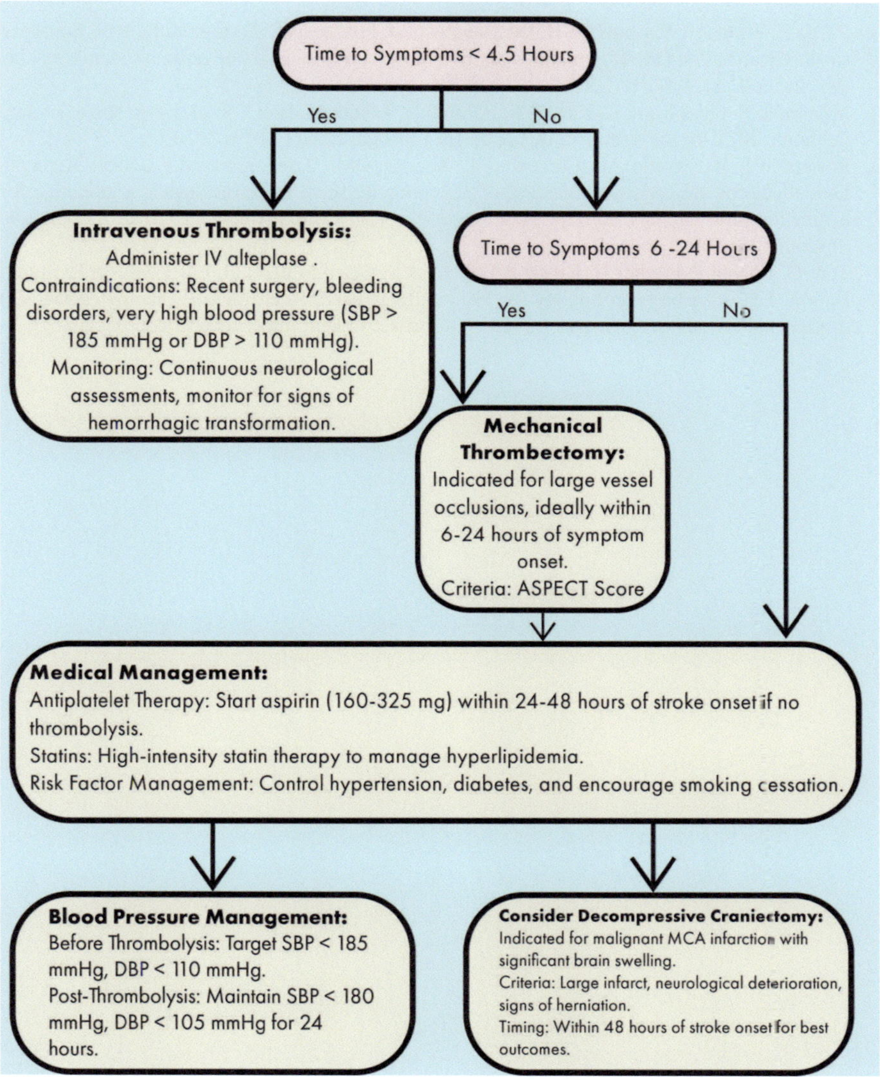

Bibliography

1. Berge E, Whiteley W, Audebert H, De Marchis GM, Fonseca AC, Padiglioni C, et al. European stroke organisation (ESO) guidelines on intravenous thrombolysis for acute ischaemic stroke. Eur Stroke J. 2021;6(1):I–LXII.
2. Miyamoto S, Ogasawara K, Kuroda S, Itabashi R, Toyoda K, Itoh Y, et al. Japan stroke society guideline 2021 for the treatment of stroke. Int J Stroke. 2022;17(9):1039–49.
3. Powers WJ, Rabinstein AA, Ackerson T, Adeoye OM, Bambakidis NC, Becker K, et al. Guidelines for the early management of patients with acute ischemic stroke: a guideline for healthcare professionals from the American Heart Association/American Stroke Association. Stroke. 2018;49(3):e46–e110.
4. Turc G, Bhogal P, Fischer U, Khatri P, Lobotesis K, Mazighi M, et al. European stroke organisation (ESO) – European Society for Minimally Invasive Neurological Therapy (ESMINT) mechanical Thrombectomy in acute ischemic stroke. J Neurointerv Surg 2023;15(8):e8.

Chapter 9
Management of Aneurysmal Subarachnoid Hemorrhage (aSAH) in the ICU

9.1 Introduction

Aneurysmal subarachnoid hemorrhage (aSAH) is a life-threatening condition resulting from the rupture of an intracranial aneurysm, leading to bleeding into the subarachnoid space. It carries significant mortality and morbidity and prompt, comprehensive management in the intensive care unit (ICU) is crucial to improve patient outcomes. A multidisciplinary approach involving neurologists, neurosurgeons, interventional neuroradiologists, and critical care specialists is essential. The general management strategy includes prompt diagnosis, stabilization, early aneurysm treatment, vigilant monitoring for complications, and planning for long-term recovery [1] (Ref. Algorithm 9.1).

9.2 Management Algorithm

1. **Initial Assessment and Grading**

Neurological Examination

- Thorough Neurological Assessment: Evaluate the patient's level of consciousness, motor and sensory functions, and cranial nerve integrity to determine the neurological status [2].

Grading Scales

- Hunt and Hess Scale: Assesses the clinical severity of aSAH.
  - Grade I: Asymptomatic or mild headache and slight nuchal rigidity.
  - Grade II: Moderate to severe headache, nuchal rigidity, no neurological deficit except cranial nerve palsy.
  - Grade III: Drowsiness, confusion, or mild focal deficit.

S. B. Mishra et al., *Mastering ICU Care*,
https://doi.org/10.1007/978-981-95-0179-3_9

  - Grade IV: Stupor, moderate to severe hemiparesis, early decerebrate rigidity.
  - Grade V: Deep coma, decerebrate rigidity, moribund appearance.

- World Federation of Neurological Societies (WFNS) Scale: Based on the Glasgow Coma Scale (GCS) score and presence of focal neurological deficits.

  - Grade I: GCS 15, no motor deficit.
  - Grade II: GCS 13–14, no motor deficit.
  - Grade III: GCS 13–14, with motor deficit.
  - Grade IV: GCS 7–12, with or without motor deficit.
  - Grade V: GCS 3–6, with or without motor deficit.

- Modified Fisher Scale: Radiologic grading based on the amount and distribution of subarachnoid blood on CT scans, useful for predicting the risk of cerebral vasospasm and delayed cerebral ischemia (DCI).

  - Grade 0: No blood detected.
  - Grade 1: Minimal thin layer of blood (<1 mm).
  - Grade 2: Thick layer of blood (>1 mm) without ventricular blood.
  - Grade 3: Thin layer of blood with ventricular hemorrhage.
  - Grade 4: Thick layer of blood with ventricular hemorrhage.

Blood Volume Estimation

- ABC/2 Method: A simplified quantitative method for estimating the volume of subarachnoid hemorrhage using CT scans. A = width/thickness, B = length, C = vertical extension) on head non-contrast computed tomography in five major SAH cisternal compartment. This estimation correlates with patient outcomes and the risk of DCI, especially useful in settings lacking advanced imaging modalities [3].

2. **Initial Management**

Blood Pressure (BP) Control

- Maintain Optimal BP: Keep systolic BP below 160 mm Hg or mean arterial pressure (MAP) below 110 mm Hg using short-acting intravenous medications to prevent rebleeding [4].
- Avoid Large BP Fluctuations: Stabilize BP to prevent sudden increases or decreases, which can contribute to poor outcomes.

Reverse Anticoagulation

- Anticoagulant Reversal: If the patient is on anticoagulants, administer appropriate reversal agents promptly to reduce the risk of further bleeding.

Administer Analgesics and Antiemetics

- Pain and Nausea Management: Use analgesics and antiemetics to improve patient comfort and prevent complications like increased intracranial pressure (ICP) due to vomiting.

Seizure Prophylaxis

- Avoid Routine Prophylactic Antiseizure Medications: Do not administer antiseizure medications prophylactically unless the patient has risk factors such as high-grade aSAH (Hunt and Hess Grades IV–V) or intraparenchymal hemorrhage.
- Treat New-Onset Seizures: If seizures occur, initiate antiepileptic drugs (AEDs) and continue for a duration guided by neurology consultation.

3. **Early Aneurysm Treatment (within 24 H)**

Endovascular Coiling

- Preferred Method: Especially for aneurysms in the posterior circulation or those amenable to coiling. Involves inserting detachable coils into the aneurysm to promote thrombosis and prevent rebleeding.

Surgical Clipping

- Alternative Option: Considered for younger patients (<40 years) or when coiling is not feasible. Involves placing a clip at the aneurysm neck during open surgery to exclude it from circulation.

Specialist Evaluation

- Multidisciplinary Assessment: Aneurysm evaluation by both endovascular and surgical specialists to determine the most appropriate treatment modality.

Partial Obliteration

- Interim Measures: If complete obliteration is not immediately feasible, partial obliteration may secure the rupture site, with plans for definitive treatment later.

4. **Preventing Rebleeding**

Frequent BP Monitoring and Maintenance

- Continuous Monitoring: Use arterial lines for real-time BP measurements to maintain BP within target ranges.

Avoid Large BP Fluctuations

- Stable Hemodynamics: Use vasoactive medications judiciously to prevent sudden changes in BP.

Avoid Routine Antifibrinolytic Therapy

- Risk of Complications: Routine use is not recommended due to increased risks of thromboembolic events and ischemia.

5. **Monitoring and Managing Complications**

9.3 Cerebral Vasospasm and Delayed Cerebral Ischemia

Early Identification

- Advanced Monitoring Techniques: Utilize transcranial Doppler ultrasonography, CT angiography (CTA), CT perfusion (CTP), or digital subtraction angiography (DSA) to detect cerebral vasospasm [5].
- Risk Stratification: Use grading scales (Hunt and Hess, WFNS, Modified Fisher) to predict the risk of vasospasm and DCI.

Nimodipine Administration

- Start Early: Initiate oral nimodipine (60 mg every 4 h) as soon as possible to reduce the risk of DCI and improve functional outcomes and continue for 21 days.

DCI Management

- Maintain Euvolemia: Ensure adequate fluid balance to optimize cerebral perfusion.
- Induced Hypertension: If signs of DCI develop, consider induced hypertension to improve cerebral blood flow under careful monitoring.

9.4 Cerebral Edema and Intracranial Pressure Control

Hyperosmolar Therapy

- Mannitol or Hypertonic Saline: Administer as needed to reduce cerebral edema and lower ICP.

ICP Monitoring

- Continuous Monitoring: Use ICP monitors in patients at risk of elevated ICP to guide therapy.

Additional Measures

- Hyperventilation: Temporarily reduce ICP in acute settings by lowering $PaCO_2$ levels.
- CSF Diversion: Utilize external ventricular drainage (EVD) to remove cerebrospinal fluid (CSF) and reduce ICP.
- Avoid Hypotonic Fluids: Prevent fluid shifts that can worsen cerebral edema.

9.5 Hydrocephalus Management

Early Detection

- Routine CT Scans: Perform serial imaging to monitor ventricular size and detect hydrocephalus promptly [6].

External Ventricular Drainage

- Acute Management: Place an EVD to relieve increased intracranial pressure and manage acute hydrocephalus effectively.

Seizure Management

- Treatment of Seizures: Initiate AEDs for patients who experience seizures, tailoring the duration and choice of medication to individual risk factors and consulting neurology services.

6. **Multidisciplinary Approach**

   - Comprehensive Stroke Centers: Manage patients in facilities equipped with dedicated neurocritical care units.
   - Team Collaboration: Involve neurosurgeons, neurologists, interventional neuroradiologists, critical care specialists, rehabilitation therapists, and nursing staff in patient care to improve outcomes.

7. **Long-Term Recovery**

Rehabilitation

- Cognitive and Behavioral Therapy: Address cognitive deficits through specialized rehabilitation programs.
- Physical Therapy: Implement physiotherapy to improve motor function and reduce disability.
- Screening Tools: Use validated instruments to assess post-discharge deficits and plan ongoing care.

Follow-Up Care

- Outpatient Services: Arrange for continued neurological assessments and support services after discharge.
- Patient and Family Education: Provide education on lifestyle modifications and adherence to follow-up appointments.

9.6 Conclusion

Effective management of aneurysmal subarachnoid hemorrhage in the ICU requires a comprehensive, multidisciplinary approach. Early assessment using clinical and radiological grading scales aids in risk stratification and guides management decisions. Prompt control of blood pressure, reversal of anticoagulation, and early aneurysm repair are critical to prevent rebleeding. Vigilant monitoring for complications such as cerebral vasospasm, DCI, cerebral edema, elevated ICP, hydrocephalus, and seizures is essential. Implementing advanced monitoring techniques and evidence-based interventions like nimodipine administration can improve outcomes. Addressing long-term recovery needs through rehabilitation and follow-up care is vital for enhancing quality of life in survivors. Managing patients in specialized centers with multidisciplinary teams further optimizes outcomes, emphasizing the importance of collaborative care in aSAH management.

Algorithm 9.1: Management of aneurysmal subarachnoid hemorrhage (aSAH) in the ICU

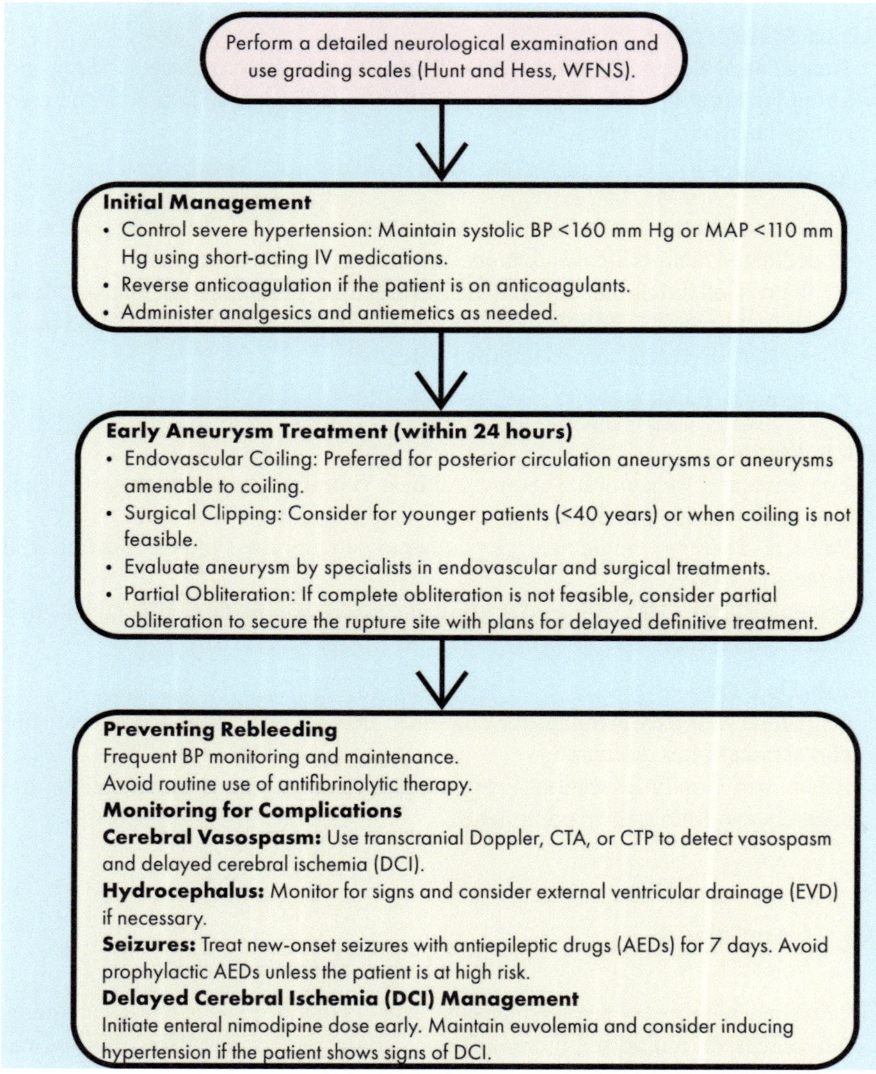

Bibliography

1. National Institute for health and care excellence: guidelines. Subarachnoid haemorrhage caused by a ruptured aneurysm: diagnosis and management. London: National Institute for Health and care excellence (NICE) Copyright © NICE 2022.; 2022.
2. Hoh BL, Ko NU, Amin-Hanjani S, Chou SH-Y, Cruz-Flores S, Dangayach NS, et al. 2023 guideline for the management of patients with aneurysmal subarachnoid hemorrhage: a guideline from the American Heart Association/American Stroke Association. Stroke. 2023;54(7):e314–e70.
3. Föttinger F, Sharma R, Salman SD, Weston AD, Erickson BJ, Huynh T, et al. The ABCs of subarachnoid hemorrhage blood volume measurement: a simplified quantitative method predicts outcomes and delayed cerebral ischemia. J Am Heart Assoc. 2024;13(20):e032195.
4. Solter VV, Breitenfeld T, Roje-Bedeković M, Supanc V, Lovrencić-Huzjan A, Serić V, et al. General recommendations for the management of aneurysmal subarachnoid hemorrhage. Acta Clin Croat. 2014;53(1):139–52.
5. Xiao ZK, Wang B, Liu J, Yang Y, Jie N, Mao X, et al. Risk factors for the development of delayed cerebral ischemia after aneurysmal subarachnoid hemorrhage: a systematic review and meta-analysis. World Neurosurg. 2024;193:427.
6. Cook AM, Morgan Jones G, Hawryluk GWJ, Mailloux P, McLaughlin D, Papangelou A, et al. Guidelines for the acute treatment of cerebral edema in Neurocritical care patients. Neurocrit Care. 2020;32(3):647–66.

Chapter 10
Hydrocephalus Management in the ICU

10.1 Introduction

Hydrocephalus is characterized by the abnormal accumulation of cerebrospinal fluid (CSF) within the brain's ventricles, leading to increased intracranial pressure (ICP). This condition can arise from various etiologies, including congenital malformations, infections, hemorrhage, tumors, and idiopathic causes. Effective management in the ICU requires a multidisciplinary approach encompassing clinical evaluation, neuroimaging, intracranial pressure monitoring, medical and surgical interventions, and rigorous postoperative care [1, 2].

A critical aspect of hydrocephalus management is differentiating between idiopathic normal pressure hydrocephalus (iNPH) and other forms such as secondary NPH and obstructive hydrocephalus. This distinction guides specific management decisions, including the consideration of shunting or surgical options. (Ref. Algorithm 10.1).

1. **Initial Assessment**

Clinical Evaluation

- Symptoms Indicative of Elevated ICP: Common symptoms include headache, nausea, vomiting, altered consciousness, and papilledema.
- Gait Disturbance: A hallmark feature of iNPH. Assess using specific tests like the iNPH grading scale and the Timed Up and Go (TUG) test to quantify gait impairment.
- Cognitive and Urinary Symptoms: Evaluate for cognitive decline and urinary incontinence, which, along with gait disturbance, constitute the classic triad of iNPH.
- Focal Neurological Deficits: Assess motor and sensory deficits to determine the extent and impact of hydrocephalus.

S. B. Mishra et al., *Mastering ICU Care*,
https://doi.org/10.1007/978-981-95-0179-3_10

Neuroimaging
Computed Tomography (CT) and Magnetic Resonance Imaging (MRI):

- Confirm Diagnosis: Identify ventricular enlargement and assess the extent of hydrocephalus.

Differentiate Types:

- Communicating vs. Noncommunicating Hydrocephalus: Determine if CSF flow is obstructed within the ventricular system.

Idiopathic Normal Pressure Hydrocephalus (iNPH):

- Disproportionately Enlarged Subarachnoid Space Hydrocephalus (DESH): Look for ventricular enlargement with disproportionately enlarged subarachnoid spaces.
- Evans Index: Calculate the ratio of the maximum width of the frontal horns to the maximum internal diameter of the skull (>0.3 suggests ventricular enlargement).
- Flow Void Signs: Identify hyperintensities in CSF flow areas on MRI indicative of altered dynamics.

Intracranial Pressure Monitoring
Consider ICP Monitoring:

- Indications: Suspected cases of elevated ICP or when clinical symptoms do not correlate with imaging findings.

External Ventricular Drain (EVD) Placement:

- Purpose: Monitor ICP and allow for therapeutic CSF drainage.

CSF Dynamics Investigation:

- Infusion Studies: Measure CSF outflow resistance and compliance.
- Tap Tests: Remove a volume of CSF to assess symptom improvement, particularly useful in diagnosing iNPH.

2. **Management Pathway**

Decision Point: Elevated ICP
If ICP is Elevated:

- Initiate medical management to reduce ICP.
- Consider CSF diversion procedures if ICP remains persistently elevated.

If ICP is Not Elevated:

- Continue monitoring the patient.
- Reassess if symptoms progress or new signs develop.

3. **Medical Management**

Osmotherapy
- Mannitol or Hypertonic Saline: Administered to reduce ICP through osmotic diuresis.

Acetazolamide

- Mechanism: Decreases CSF production by inhibiting carbonic anhydrase.

Maintaining Cerebral Perfusion Pressure (CPP)

- Blood Pressure and Fluid Management: Ensure adequate CPP and oxygen delivery to the brain.

Sedation and Analgesia

- Purpose: Reduce metabolic demand and control agitation to prevent further increases in ICP.

4. **Persistently Elevated ICP**

- Intervention: Proceed to CSF diversion procedures if ICP remains elevated despite medical management.

5. **CSF Diversion Procedures**

External Ventricular Drainage (EVD)

- Indications: Acute management and temporary CSF drainage.
- Management: Adjust drainage based on ICP readings and clinical status.
- Monitoring: Vigilant for complications such as infection or hemorrhage.

Ventriculoperitoneal (VP) Shunt

- Indications: Chronic or recurrent hydrocephalus, especially in communicating hydrocephalus and iNPH.

Shunt Management Considerations:

- Programmable Valves: Recommended for optimizing CSF drainage and allowing noninvasive postoperative adjustments.
- Overdrainage Prevention: Use anti-siphon devices or gravitational units to prevent complications like subdural hematomas.

Surgical Interventions

Endoscopic Third Ventriculostomy (ETV):

- Suitable for: Patients with obstructive hydrocephalus (e.g., aqueductal stenosis).
- Procedure: Create an opening in the floor of the third ventricle to divert CSF flow.

Cranioplasty:

- Purpose: Restore normal cranial anatomy and improve CSF dynamics after craniectomy.

6. **Postoperative Care**

Monitoring for Complications

- Infection: Watch for signs of meningitis or ventriculitis.

- Shunt Malfunction: Assess for recurrence of hydrocephalus symptoms, indicating possible obstruction or disconnection.
- Overdrainage: Monitor for headaches, nausea, or subdural hematomas due to excessive CSF drainage.

Regular Follow-Up Imaging

Serial Neuroimaging:

- Assess: Ventricular size, shunt position, and detect any new lesions or complications.

Adjust Shunt Settings

Programmable Valve Adjustments:

- Optimize CSF Drainage: Based on clinical response and imaging findings.
- Noninvasive Adjustments: Allow individualized patient management without additional surgeries.

Long-Term Follow-Up

Clinical Assessments:

- Neurological Status: Monitor gait, cognition, and urinary function using standardized scales like the iNPH grading scale.

Interdisciplinary Approach:

- Collaboration: Neurosurgeons, neurologists, physiotherapists, and rehabilitation specialists.

Complication Management:

- Prompt Intervention: Address shunt infections, obstructions, and mechanical failures swiftly.

7. **Advanced Monitoring and Management**

CSF Dynamics Studies

- Infusion Studies: Evaluate CSF outflow resistance to assess absorption capacity.
- Pressure-Volume Index (PVI): Determine brain compliance and compensatory reserve.
- Resistance-Area Product (RAP) Index: Analyze the relationship between ICP amplitude and mean ICP to assess intracranial compliance.
- B-Waves Analysis: Identify ICP waveform patterns indicative of impaired CSF dynamics.

Management of Associated Conditions

- Underlying Etiologies: Treat conditions such as subarachnoid hemorrhage (SAH), traumatic brain injury (TBI), or infections contributing to hydrocephalus.
- Rehabilitation Services: Provide physical therapy for gait disturbance and occupational therapy for cognitive deficits.

Interdisciplinary Approach

- Collaborative Care.
- Team Meetings: Regularly review and update the treatment plan based on patient responses.
- Family Involvement: Educate and involve caregivers in decision-making processes.

10.1.1 Interpretation of CSF Dynamics Studies and Appropriate Interventions

Normal CSF Dynamics

Parameters:

- CSF Outflow Resistance (R): 13–18 $mmHg·ml^{-1}·min^{-1}$
- Pressure-Volume Index (PVI): >26 ml
- Elasticity (E): <0.18 ml^{-1}
- RAP Index: <0.6
- B-Waves: Minimal or absent
- Interpretation: No significant obstruction or impaired absorption.
- Intervention: Routine monitoring and supportive care; no immediate CSF diversion required.

Increased CSF Outflow Resistance

Parameters:

- R: >18 $mmHg·ml^{-1}·min^{-1}$
- PVI: <13 ml
- E: >0.18 ml^{-1}
- RAP Index: ≈1
- B-Waves: Frequent and high amplitude
- Interpretation: Impaired CSF absorption or obstruction with poor compensatory reserve.
- Intervention: Surgical CSF diversion via VP shunt or ETV; close ICP monitoring and treatment adjustments.

Communicating Hydrocephalus

Parameters:

- Increased R, variable PVI, increased E, RAP Index ≈1, significant B-Waves.
- Interpretation: Impaired absorption at arachnoid granulations or other CSF pathways.
- Intervention: Long-term CSF diversion strategies like VP shunt placement; perform lumbar drainage or tap tests to assess symptom improvement before permanent shunting.

Obstructive Hydrocephalus
Parameters:

- Markedly increased R, low PVI, high E, high RAP Index, significant B-Waves.
- Interpretation: Blockage of CSF pathways (e.g., aqueductal stenosis).
- Intervention: Immediate surgical intervention (ETV or shunt placement) to relieve obstruction.

Brain Atrophy with Normal CSF Dynamics
Parameters:

- Low R, high PVI, low E, RAP Index <0.6, minimal or absent B-Waves.
- Interpretation: Normal CSF dynamics with evidence of brain atrophy; no significant hydrocephalus.
- Intervention: CSF diversion not required; focus on managing underlying conditions causing atrophy.

10.2 Conclusion

Management of hydrocephalus in the ICU is complex and requires careful assessment, timely intervention, and ongoing monitoring. Differentiating between types of hydrocephalus, particularly iNPH, is essential for tailoring management strategies. Incorporating advanced diagnostic tools like CSF dynamics studies and specific neuroimaging features enhances diagnostic precision. Postoperative care with long-term follow-up ensures optimal outcomes by promptly addressing complications and adjusting treatments as necessary. A structured, interdisciplinary approach enables clinicians to provide comprehensive care for patients with this challenging conditions.

Algorithm 10.1: Hydrocephalus management in the ICU

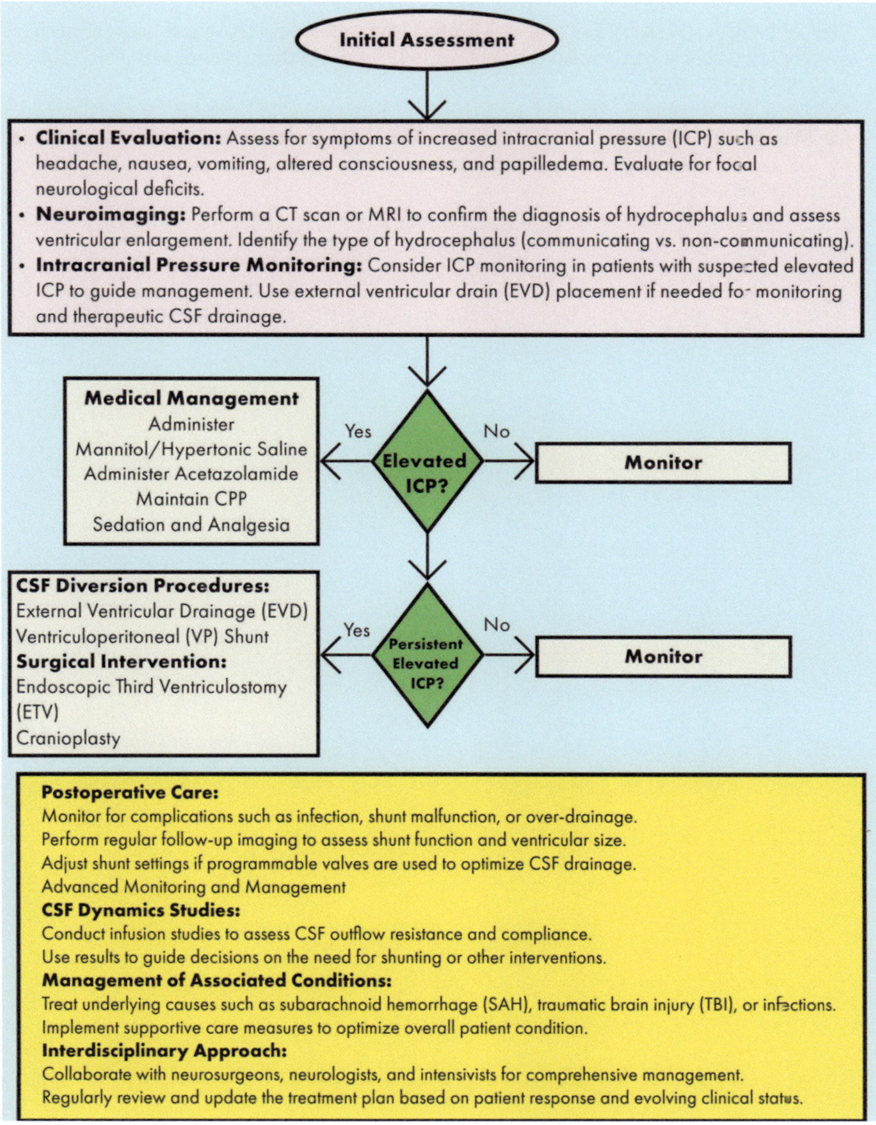

Bibliography

1. Mori E, Ishikawa M, Kato T, Kazui H, Miyake H, Miyajima M, et al. Guidelines for management of idiopathic normal pressure hydrocephalus: second edition. Neurol Med Chir (Tokyo). 2012;52(11):775–809.
2. Nakajima M, Yamada S, Miyajima M, Ishii K, Kuriyama N, Kazui H, et al. Guidelines for Management of Idiopathic Normal Pressure Hydrocephalus (third edition): endorsed by the Japanese Society of Normal Pressure Hydrocephalus. Neurol Med Chir (Tokyo). 2021;61(2):63–97.

Chapter 11
Management of Brain Abscess and Metastases in the ICU

11.1 Introduction

Brain abscesses and brain metastases are critical neurological conditions that require prompt diagnosis and management in the intensive care unit (ICU). A brain abscess is a localized collection of pus within the brain tissue, resulting from infections that may spread from nearby structures (like the sinuses or ears), through the bloodstream from other body parts, or following head injuries or neurosurgical procedures. Brain metastases, on the other hand, are cancerous tumors that have spread to the brain from primary tumors located elsewhere in the body.

Managing these conditions necessitates a multidisciplinary approach involving neurosurgeons, infectious disease specialists, oncologists, and critical care physicians. Rapid and accurate diagnosis, along with effective treatment strategies, are crucial to improve patient outcomes and minimize complications [1] (Ref. Algorithm 11.1).

11.2 Initial Assessment

A thorough initial assessment is vital for both brain abscesses and metastases.

For Brain Abscesses:

- Symptoms: Common symptoms include headaches, fever, focal neurological deficits (such as weakness or numbness in specific body parts), confusion, seizures, and signs of increased intracranial pressure (like nausea, vomiting, or altered consciousness).
- Medical History: Obtain details about recent infections (dental, sinus, or ear), immunosuppressive conditions (e.g., HIV/AIDS, diabetes), previous neurosurgical procedures, head injuries, or intravenous drug use.

S. B. Mishra et al., *Mastering ICU Care*,
https://doi.org/10.1007/978-981-95-0179-3_11

For Brain Metastases:

- Symptoms: Patients may present with headaches, seizures, cognitive or behavioral changes, and neurological deficits depending on the tumor location.
- Medical History: Assess for known primary cancers, symptoms suggestive of malignancy (unexplained weight loss, fatigue), and risk factors like smoking [2].

11.3 Imaging Modalities

Magnetic Resonance Imaging (MRI):

- Action: Perform MRI with diffusion-weighted imaging (DWI) and apparent diffusion coefficient (ADC) sequences, using gadolinium contrast.
- Rationale: MRI is the preferred modality for diagnosing both brain abscesses and metastases. For brain abscesses, MRI with DWI/ADC sequences has a sensitivity of 92% and specificity of 91%, aiding in differentiating abscesses from tumors [3].

If MRI Is Unavailable:

- Action: Perform contrast-enhanced computed tomography (CT) scan.

Differentiating Between Abscesses and Tumors

- MR Spectroscopy: Helps analyze the chemical composition of lesions, distinguishing abscesses (which may show amino acid peaks) from tumors (which often show elevated choline levels).
- DWI/ADC Imaging: Abscesses typically exhibit restricted diffusion due to thick pus, whereas tumors do not.

11.4 Severity of Disease

In Severe Cases:

- Action: Proceed with surgical intervention for abscess aspiration or excision. Collect samples for microbiological analysis.

In Patients Without Severe Disease:

- Action: Withhold antimicrobials until after aspiration or excision.

11.5 Empirical Antimicrobial Therapy

For Community-Acquired Brain Abscesses

- Action: Initiate intravenous ceftriaxone (a third-generation cephalosporin) combined with metronidazole [4, 5]. This combination covers common causative organisms like streptococci and anaerobes.

For Post-Neurosurgical Brain Abscesses

- Action: Use a combination of meropenem and vancomycin or linezolid [6]. This therapy targets a broad spectrum of pathogens, including Gram-negative bacilli and methicillin-resistant *Staphylococcus aureus* (MRSA).

Duration of Therapy

Complete Abscess Removal:

- Action: Consider a shorter duration of intravenous antibiotics (e.g., 4 weeks).
- Rationale: Surgical excision reduces bacterial load, potentially allowing for a reduced course of antibiotics.

Partial Removal or No Surgery:

- Action: Continue intravenous antibiotics for 6–8 weeks.
- Rationale: Ensures thorough eradication of the infection to prevent recurrence.

Definitive Antimicrobial Therapy

- Action: Adjust antibiotics based on culture and sensitivity results from aspirated material.

Management of Brain Metastases

Diagnosis:

- Neuroimaging: MRI with contrast is the standard for detecting brain metastases, focusing on identifying solid or ring-enhancing lesions. CT scans are alternatives if MRI is not feasible.

Treatment Options:
Surgical Resection:

- Action: Recommended for patients with a single accessible brain metastasis and controlled systemic disease.

Whole-Brain Radiation Therapy (WBRT):

- Action: Often used after surgery to treat microscopic disease.

Stereotactic Radiosurgery (SRS):

- Action: An alternative to surgery for solitary or few metastases, especially in eloquent brain areas.

Seizure Management
In Brain Abscesses:

- Action: Monitor for seizures but do not routinely prescribe antiepileptic drugs prophylactically. Prophylactic antiepileptics are not generally recommended unless the patient has experienced seizures.

In Brain Metastases:

- Action: Consider antiepileptic prophylaxis, especially if lesions are near the cerebral cortex as cortical involvement increases the risk of seizures; prophylaxis may prevent seizure occurrence.

Supportive Care
Corticosteroids:

- Action: Administer dexamethasone to reduce cerebral edema in patients with significant mass effect (metastases/malignancy).

Intracranial Pressure Management:

- Action: Employ measures like head elevation, osmotherapy, and hyperventilation when indicated.

Monitoring and Follow-Up
For Both Conditions:
Neurological Assessments:

- Action: Regularly evaluate neurological status and vital signs.

Imaging Studies:

- Action: Schedule follow-up MRIs to monitor treatment response and detect recurrence.

Specific to Brain Metastases:
Regular Surveillance:

- Action: Adhere to EANO-ESMO guidelines recommending periodic neuroimaging.

Rehabilitation and Long-Term Care
Early Rehabilitation:

- Action: Initiate physical, occupational, and speech therapy as needed.

Outpatient Follow-Up:

- Action: Arrange regular follow-up appointments with neurology, oncology, and rehabilitation services.

11.6 Prognosis and Survival

Brain Abscesses

- Improved Outcomes: Advances in imaging, surgical techniques, and antimicrobial therapy have significantly reduced mortality rates [7].
- Recovery Rates: Full recovery rates have increased from approximately 33% to 70%, reflecting better overall management.

Brain Metastases

- Survival Factors: Prognosis depends on factors like the number of metastases, control of the primary tumor, patient's performance status, and treatment modalities used.
- Best Survival Rates: Achieved with combined surgical resection and WBRT in patients with single brain metastases.

11.7 Conclusion

The management of brain abscesses and brain metastases in the ICU setting is complex and demands a rapid, coordinated, and evidence-based approach. Accurate diagnosis through advanced imaging techniques is essential for distinguishing between abscesses and tumors, which directly influences treatment strategies. Adherence to updated guidelines ensures optimal antimicrobial selection, surgical intervention, and supportive care.

Early intervention, tailored therapy, diligent monitoring, and comprehensive rehabilitation are pivotal in improving patient outcomes. With modern medical advancements, patients with these serious neurological conditions have a significantly better chance of recovery and improved quality of life.

Algorithm 11.1: Management of brain abscess and metastases in the ICU

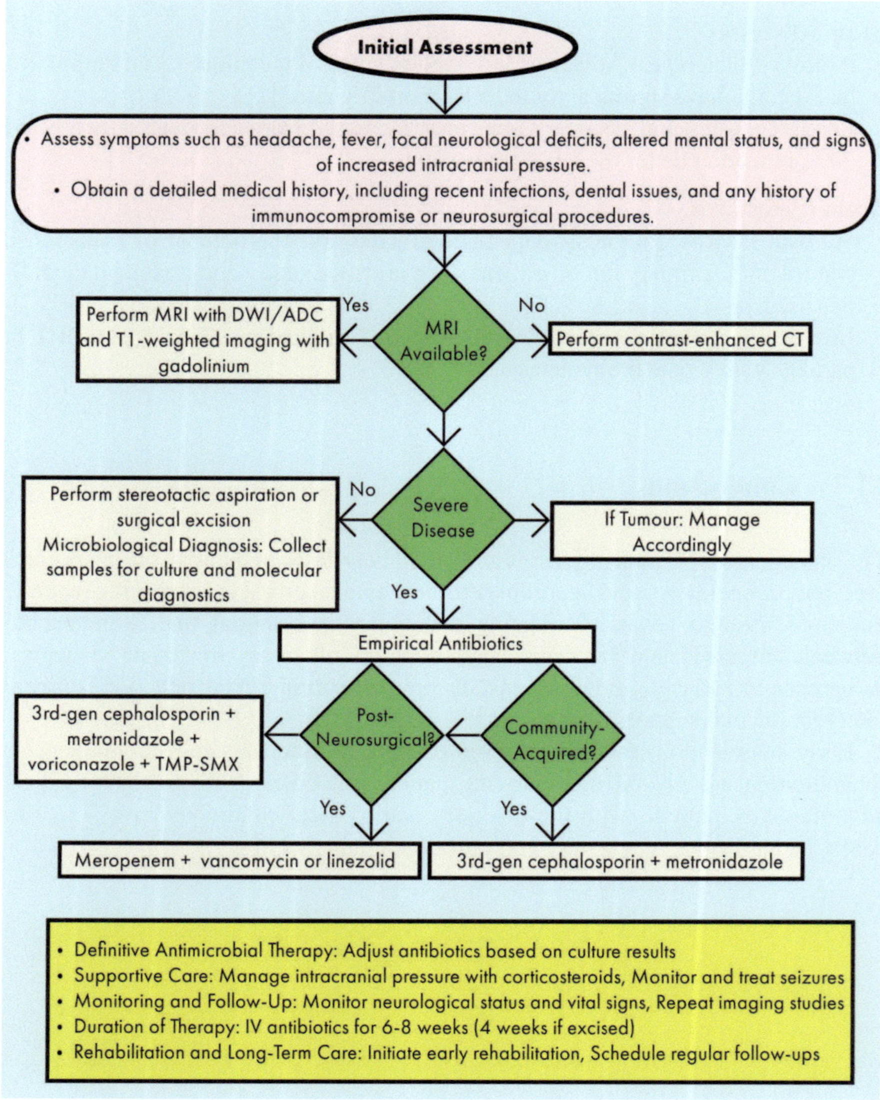

Bibliography

1. Bodilsen J, D'Alessandris QG, Humphreys H, Iro MA, Klein M, Last K, et al. European society of clinical microbiology and infectious diseases guidelines on diagnosis and treatment of brain abscess in children and adults. Clin Microbiol Infect. 2024;30(1):66–89.
2. Le Rhun E, Guckenberger M, Smits M, Dummer R, Bachelot T, Sahm F, et al. EANO-ESMO clinical practice guidelines for diagnosis, treatment and follow-up of patients with brain metastasis from solid tumours. Ann Oncol. 2021;32(11):1332–47.
3. Rock JP, Haines S, Recht L, Bernstein M, Sawaya R, Mikkelsen T, et al. Practice parameters for the management of single brain metastasis. Neurosurg Focus. 2000;9(6):ecp2.
4. The rational use of antibiotics in the treatment of brain abscess. Br J Neurosurg. 2000;14(6):525–30.
5. Omland LH, Nielsen H, Bodilsen J. Update and approach to patients with brain abscess. Curr Opin Infect Dis. 2024;37(3):211–9.
6. Thy M, Gaudemer A, d'Humières C, Sonneville R. Brain abscess in immunocompetent patients: recent findings. Curr Opin Infect Dis. 2022;35(3):238–45.
7. Brouwer MC, Coutinho JM, van de Beek D. Clinical characteristics and outcome of brain abscess: systematic review and meta-analysis. Neurology. 2014;82(9):806–13.

Chapter 12
Approach to Weakness in the ICU

12.1 Introduction

Weakness in the intensive care unit (ICU) is a critical symptom with a broad differential diagnosis. It can manifest as generalized weakness due to systemic illness or as focal neurological deficits indicative of significant underlying pathology. Weakness may be episodic or persistent, and distinguishing between these patterns is crucial for early diagnostic considerations. Episodic weakness can result from causes such as electrolyte imbalances, periodic paralyses, or myasthenia gravis, while persistent weakness may indicate ongoing neuromuscular or systemic issues.

Proper evaluation and management are vital to improve patient outcomes. This chapter outlines a systematic approach for assessing and managing weakness in ICU patients, integrating clinical assessment, diagnostic testing, and tailored therapeutic strategies. We will explore various etiologies, including central and peripheral causes, neuromuscular junction disorders like myasthenia gravis and Lambert-Eaton syndrome, metabolic myopathies such as mitochondrial disorders, and ICU-acquired conditions like critical illness polyneuropathy (CIP) and critical illness myopathy (CIM) [1, 2]. [Ref. Algorithm 12.1].

12.2 Patient History and Physical Examination

History

Document Onset, Pattern, and Progression

- Onset and Evolution: Understanding when the weakness began, its pattern (episodic vs. persistent), and how it has evolved provides clues about its etiology. Acute onset might suggest a stroke or acute inflammatory demyelinating

S. B. Mishra et al., *Mastering ICU Care*,
https://doi.org/10.1007/978-981-95-0179-3_12

polyradiculoneuropathy (AIDP), whereas a gradual onset could indicate a metabolic disorder or progressive neuromuscular disease (Table 12.1).

- Associated Symptoms: Inquire about symptoms such as fatigue, muscle pain, sensory changes, autonomic symptoms, or fluctuations in weakness.

Table 12.1 Causes of episodic generalized weakness

Electrolyte disturbances	Electrolyte imbalances: Low potassium levels (hypokalemia) High potassium levels (hyperkalemia) Low sodium levels (hyponatremia) High sodium levels (hypernatremia) Low phosphate levels (hypophosphatemia) High calcium levels (hypercalcemia) Low magnesium levels (hypomagnesemia) High magnesium levels (hypermagnesemia)
Neuromuscular junction disorders	Autoimmune conditions: Myasthenia gravis Lambert-Eaton myasthenic syndrome
	Toxin-mediated blockade: Botulism Exposure to certain pesticides (organophosphate poisoning)
	N,M: Medications like aminoglycoside antibiotics affecting neuromuscular transmission
Muscle ion channel disorders (channelopathies)	Periodic paralysis syndromes: Hypokalemic periodic paralysis Hyperkalemic periodic paralysis Andersen-Tawil syndrome
	Other channelopathies: Paramyotonia congenita Congenital myotonia
Central nervous system events	Transient ischemic attacks (TIAs): Brief episodes of neurological dysfunction due to temporary cerebral ischemia
	Migraine with aura: Neurological symptoms preceding headache, including weakness
	Multiple sclerosis relapses: Demyelinating events causing transient neurological deficits
	Seizure activity: Postictal weakness (Todd's paralysis) following a seizure

(continued)

Table 12.1 (continued)

Metabolic and endocrine disorders	Hypoglycemia Hypothyroidism Hyperthyroidism Hyperparathyroidism Addison's disease Acute intermittent porphyria Severe cases leading to muscle weakness
Toxic and drug-related causes	Substance abuse: Alcohol-induced hypoglycemia or electrolyte disturbances
	Medication side effects: Corticosteroid-induced myopathy Statin-associated muscle symptoms
	Environmental exposures: Heavy metal poisoning (e.g., lead, arsenic)
Psychogenic and functional disorders	Functional neurological symptom disorder (conversion disorder): Neurological symptoms not explained by medical Conditions
	Psychological factors: Anxiety or panic attacks leading to subjective weakness
	Chronic fatigue syndrome/myalgic encephalomyelitis: Persistent fatigue with episodes of worsened weakness
Others	Sleep disorders: Sleep paralysis causing transient inability to move upon Waking
	Periodic hypokalemic paralysis associated with thyrotoxicosis: Often seen in Asian populations with hyperthyroidism
	Neurological conditions: Narcolepsy with cataplexy causing sudden muscle weakness triggered by emotions

Medical and Surgical History

- Previous Conditions: Prior neurological disorders, endocrine dysfunctions, or autoimmune diseases.
- Recent Infections: Can suggest Guillain-Barré syndrome (GBS) or post-infectious myelitis [3].
- Surgeries and ICU Stays: Recent surgery or prolonged immobilization might hint at ICU-acquired weakness or postoperative complications.

Medications

- Drug-Induced Weakness: Certain drugs can induce muscle weakness or neuropathy, such as corticosteroids, neuromuscular blockers, aminoglycoside antibiotics, or chemotherapy agents.
- Exposure to Toxins: Organophosphates, botulinum toxin.

Family History

- Genetic Disorders: Predispositions to neuromuscular disorders, such as muscular dystrophy or hereditary metabolic myopathies.
- Periodic Paralysis: Family history of episodic weakness.

12.3 Examination

Neurological Examination

- Mental Status: Assess for delirium, encephalopathy, or focal neurological deficits.
- Cranial Nerve Function: Determine if there is involvement of cranial nerves, which may suggest central or peripheral etiologies.
- Motor Strength: Evaluate for differences between proximal vs. distal and symmetrical vs. asymmetrical weakness. Use the Medical Research Council (MRC) scale for grading muscle strength [4–6].
- Sensory Function: Loss of sensation may point toward peripheral neuropathy or spinal cord involvement.
- Reflexes: Hyperreflexia can indicate a central cause, while diminished reflexes might suggest a peripheral process.
- Muscle Tone and Bulk: Assess for atrophy, fasciculations, or changes in muscle tone, which could indicate chronic neuromuscular disease or recent immobilization.

Clinical Pearl

- Fluctuating Weakness: Suggests a neuromuscular junction disorder like myasthenia gravis.
- Descending Paralysis: Consider botulism or tick paralysis.
- Symmetrical Distal Weakness with Sensory Loss: Points toward peripheral neuropathy.

12.4 Algorithmic Approach to Weakness

A systematic, stepwise approach is essential for diagnosing the cause of weakness in ICU patients. By integrating clinical findings with diagnostic studies, clinicians can efficiently narrow down potential etiologies.

1. Assess Mental Status and Cranial Nerves
   - Altered mental status or cranial nerve involvement may indicate a central nervous system (CNS) cause.
2. Evaluate Motor and Sensory Function
   - Motor Weakness Pattern: Proximal vs. distal, symmetrical vs. asymmetrical.
   - Sensory Involvement: Presence suggests peripheral neuropathy or spinal cord pathology.
3. Examine Reflexes and Muscle Tone
   - Hyperreflexia and Spasticity: Suggest upper motor neuron (UMN) lesion.
   - Hyporeflexia and Flaccidity: Indicate lower motor neuron (LMN) involvement.
4. Early Neurophysiological Testing
   - EMG and NCS: Critical for differentiating between neuropathies, myopathies, and neuromuscular junction disorders.
5. Imaging Studies
   - MRI/CT: To identify central lesions or structural abnormalities.
6. Laboratory Tests
   - Basic and Specific Tests: To detect metabolic, infectious, or autoimmune causes.

12.5 Determining Central vs. Peripheral Causes (Table 12.2)

Central Causes
Brain Lesions

Table 12.2 Differentiate central vs. peripheral causes

Feature	Central causes	Peripheral causes
Mental status	Altered (encephalopathy)	Normal
Cranial nerves	May be involved (e.g., facial droop)	Usually spared
Weakness pattern	Unilateral, proximal, spasticity	Bilateral, distal, flaccid
Reflexes	Hyperreflexia, Babinski sign	Hyporeflexia, absent reflexes
Sensory loss	Localized (cortical pattern)	Diffuse (glove-and-stocking)
Muscle tone	Increased (spasticity)	Decreased (flaccid)
Fasciculations	Absent	Present (in lower motor neuron diseases)
Muscle atrophy	Rare (early stages)	Common (early onset in neuropathy)

- Stroke: Sudden onset weakness, often unilateral, with UMN signs.
- Tumors: Gradual onset, may present with headaches, seizures.
- Infections: Encephalitis or abscesses causing focal deficits.

Spinal Cord Disorders

- Compression: Due to tumors, abscesses, or herniated discs causing weakness below the lesion level.
- Inflammatory Conditions: Transverse myelitis, multiple sclerosis.

Peripheral Causes
Peripheral Neuropathy

- Guillain-Barré Syndrome (GBS): Acute, symmetrical ascending weakness, areflexia, often following infection.
- Diabetic Neuropathy: Chronic distal symmetric polyneuropathy with sensory loss.

Neuromuscular Junction Disorders
Myasthenia Gravis (MG)

- Etiology: Autoimmune antibodies against acetylcholine receptors.
- Clinical Features: Fluctuating weakness, ptosis, diplopia, dysphagia, proximal muscle weakness, worsens with activity.

Diagnostic Tests:

- Acetylcholine Receptor Antibodies: Elevated in most patients.
- Single-Fiber EMG: Shows increased jitter.
- Repetitive Nerve Stimulation: Decremental response.

Treatment Options:

- Acetylcholinesterase Inhibitors: Pyridostigmine.
- Immunosuppressive Therapy: Corticosteroids, azathioprine.
- Plasmapheresis and IVIg: For rapid improvement.
- Thymectomy: Considered in certain cases [7].

Lambert-Eaton Myasthenic Syndrome (LEMS)

- Etiology: Autoimmune antibodies against presynaptic voltage-gated calcium channels.
- Clinical Features: Proximal muscle weakness, autonomic symptoms, hyporeflexia, strength may improve with activity.

Diagnostic Tests:

- Voltage-Gated Calcium Channel Antibodies: Elevated levels.
- EMG: Incremental response on high-frequency stimulation.

Treatment Options:

- 3,4-Diaminopyridine: Enhances acetylcholine release.
- Immunotherapy: Similar to MG.
- Cancer Screening: Often associated with small-cell lung carcinoma [8].

Myopathies

- Critical Illness Myopathy (CIM): Proximal muscle weakness, difficulty weaning from ventilation.
- Metabolic Myopathies: Mitochondrial disorders causing exercise intolerance, muscle pain.

ICU-Acquired Weakness (ICU-AW)
Critical Illness Polyneuropathy (CIP):

- Features: Distal weakness, reduced reflexes, sensory deficits.
- NCS Findings: Reduced amplitude of SNAPs and CMAPs.

Critical Illness Myopathy (CIM):

- Features: Proximal weakness, preserved sensation.
- EMG Findings: Myopathic changes, early recruitment.

Critical Illness Neuromyopathy (CINM):

- Combination: Features of both CIP and CIM.

Management:

- Early Mobilization: Physical therapy initiation.
- Minimizing Sedation: Reduce neuromuscular blockers and corticosteroids.
- Optimizing Glycemic Control: Prevent hyperglycemia-induced nerve damage [4, 5].

Clinical Pearl

- ICU-AW is common in patients with sepsis, multi-organ failure, or prolonged immobilization. Early recognition and intervention can improve outcomes.

12.6 Neurophysiological Studies and Imaging

12.6.1 Neurophysiological Studies

Nerve Conduction Studies (NCS)

- Purpose: Evaluate the integrity and function of peripheral nerves.

Findings:

- Axonal Neuropathies: Reduced amplitude of CMAPs and SNAPs.
- Demyelinating Neuropathies: Prolonged latencies, slowed conduction velocities.

Conditions Diagnosed:

- GBS: Demyelinating patterns.
- CIP: Axonalloss.

Electromyography (EMG)

- Purpose: Differentiate between neuropathic and myopathic processes.

Findings:

- Neuropathic Changes: Fibrillations, positive sharp waves, large-amplitude motor units.
- Myopathic Changes: Small-amplitude, short-duration motor units, early recruitment.

Conditions Diagnosed:

- Myasthenia Gravis: Increased jitter on single-fiber EMG.
- CIM: Myopathic pattern.

Importance of Early Testing

- Guiding Diagnosis and Management: Early EMG and NCS can distinguish between various neuromuscular disorders, enabling prompt and appropriate interventions.

12.6.2 Imaging

MRI/CT Scan of Brain and Spine

- Purpose: Rule out central causes such as stroke, tumors, demyelinating lesions, or spinal cord compression.

Specific MRI Patterns:

- Inflammatory Myopathies: Muscle edema.
- GBS: Nerve root enhancement.
- Compressive Lesions: Epidural abscesses, hematomas.

Ultrasound

- Purpose: Assess muscles and peripheral nerves for structural abnormalities.
- Advantages: Bedside availability, real-time assessment.

Applications:

- Nerve Enlargement: Seen in chronic inflammatory demyelinating polyneuropathy (CIDP).
- Muscle Atrophy: Evaluation in prolonged ICU stays.

Clinical Pearl
- Spinal Imaging is crucial in patients with sudden onset weakness and sensory level to exclude compressive myelopathy, which is a neurosurgical emergency.

12.7 Laboratory Tests

Basic Metabolic Panel
- Electrolyte Imbalances: Hypokalemia, hyperkalemia, hypophosphatemia can cause weakness.
- Renal and Liver Function: Assess for metabolic encephalopathies.

Complete Blood Count (CBC)
- Infection Indicators: Leukocytosis or leukopenia.
- Anemia: Can contribute to fatigue and weakness.

12.7.1 Specific Tests

Creatine Kinase (CK)
- Elevated Levels: Indicate muscle damage, common in myopathies.

Blood Glucose Levels
- Hyperglycemia: Can cause neuropathy.
- Hypoglycemia: Can cause episodic weakness.

Thyroid Function Tests
- Hypothyroidism: Can cause proximal muscle weakness.
- Hyperthyroidism: Associated with thyrotoxic periodic paralysis.

Blood Cultures
- Sepsis Evaluation: In suspected infection-related weakness.

Autoantibodies
- Myasthenia Gravis: Acetylcholine receptor antibodies.
- Lambert-Eaton Syndrome: Voltage-gated calcium channel antibodies.
- Autoimmune Myopathies: ANA, anti-Jo-1 antibodies.

Clinical Pearl
- Electrolyte Corrections: Simple interventions like correcting potassium or phosphate levels can rapidly reverse episodic weakness.

12.8 Management Strategy

12.8.1 Supportive Care

Nutritional Support

- High-Protein Diet: Supports muscle mass and metabolic needs.
- Caloric Adequacy: Prevents catabolism and promotes healing.

Optimizing Physiological Status

- Fluid and Electrolyte Balance: Correct imbalances promptly.
- Oxygenation and Perfusion: Ensure adequate delivery to tissues.
- Glycemic Control: Prevent hyperglycemia-induced complications.

12.8.2 Pulmonary Rehabilitation

Respiratory Muscle Training

- Techniques: Incentive spirometry, inspiratory muscle training.
- Benefits: Improves weaning success from mechanical ventilation.

Noninvasive Ventilation (NIV)

- Indications: Respiratory muscle weakness, COPD exacerbations.
- Advantages: Reduces need for intubation, preserves airway defenses.

Weaning Strategies

- Gradual Reduction: Taper ventilatory support as strength improves.
- Multidisciplinary Approach: Involving respiratory therapists, nurses, physicians.

12.8.3 Physical Therapy and Early Mobilization

Evidence-Based Practice

- Improved Outcomes: Early mobilization reduces ICU stay, mechanical ventilation duration.

Studies:

- Early physiotherapy/occupational therapy led to better functional outcomes.
- ABCDEF Bundle: Incorporates early mobility and minimal sedation.

Sedation Management

- Minimizing Sedatives: Reduces delirium, facilitates participation in therapy.
- Protocols: Daily sedation interruption, sedation scales.

12.8.4 Immunotherapies

Guillain-Barré Syndrome (GBS)

- IVIg and Plasmapheresis: Reduce autoimmune attack on nerves.
- Early Initiation: Improves recovery time [3, 9–11].

Myasthenia Gravis (MG)

- Acetylcholinesterase Inhibitors: Symptomatic relief.
- Immunosuppressive Therapy: Corticosteroids, azathioprine.
- Plasmapheresis and IVIg: For myasthenic crisis.
- Thymectomy: Surgical option in certain patients.

12.8.5 Targeted Treatments

Metabolic Disorders

- Supplementation: Correct deficiencies (e.g., thiamine in Wernicke's encephalopathy).
- Dietary Modifications: For mitochondrial disorders.

Infections

- Antimicrobial Therapy: Based on culture and sensitivity.

Clinical Pearl

- Early Immunotherapy in autoimmune neuromuscular disorders can significantly improve outcomes and reduce morbidity.

12.9 Risk Factor Minimization

12.9.1 Preventative Measures

Physical Therapy

- Early Mobilization: Prevents deconditioning, reduces ICU-acquired weakness.
- Customized Programs: Tailored to patient's condition and tolerance.

Sedation Management

- Minimizing Neuromuscular Blockers: Avoid prolonged use to prevent CIM.
- Sedation Protocols: Use the lowest effective dose.

Nutritional Support

- Adequate Intake: Prevents muscle wasting.
- High-Protein Diets: Supports muscle repair.

Clinical Pearl

- Interdisciplinary Approach: Collaboration among healthcare professionals enhances patient recovery and reduces complications.

12.10 Stepwise Diagnostic Pathway

A structured approach ensures efficient identification of the underlying cause of weakness.

12.10.1 Initial Assessment

- Detailed Clinical History: Onset, pattern, progression, associated symptoms.
- Basic Laboratory Tests: Electrolytes, glucose, CBC, renal and liver function tests.

12.10.2 Focused Examination

- Neurological Examination: Localize the lesion and assess severity.

12.10.3 Initial Diagnostics

Episodic Weakness:

- Electrolyte Evaluation: Correct imbalances.
- ECG: Rule out cardiac arrhythmias.
- Persistent Weakness.
- Neurophysiological Studies: EMG and NCS to differentiate disorders.

12.10.4 Advanced Diagnostics

- Autoimmune Testing: Antibody panels for MG, LEMS, autoimmune myopathies.
- Imaging: MRI of brain and spine for central causes.
- Lumbar Puncture: CSF analysis in suspected GBS.

12.10.5 *Tailored Diagnostics*

- Muscle Biopsy: In metabolic or inflammatory myopathies.
- Genetic Testing: For hereditary neuromuscular disorders.

Medical Research Council (MRC) Scale for Muscle Strength Assessment
The MRC scale is a standardized tool for evaluating muscle strength in ICU patients, assessing six muscle groups bilaterally. Each muscle group is graded from 0 (no contraction) to 5 (normal strength), with a total score ranging from 0 to 60.

Muscle Groups Assessed
- Shoulder abductors.
- Elbow flexors.
- Wrist extensors.
- Hipflexors.
- Knee extensors.
- Foot dorsiflexors.

Each muscle group is examined on both the left and right sides, and a score is assigned based on the following scale:

MRC Scoring Guide
- Grade 5: Full strength, normal muscle function.
- Grade 4: Movement against gravity and resistance.
- Grade 3: Movement against gravity only.
- Grade 2: Movement of the limb without overcoming gravity.
- Grade 1: Visible muscle contraction without any limb movement.
- Grade 0: No visible contraction.

At the Bedside
1. Evaluate muscle strength bilaterally for each of the six muscle groups listed above.
2. Assign a score from 0 to 5 based on the patient's ability to move against gravity and resistance.
3. Sum the total MRC score out of 60. A score close to 60 indicates normal strength, while lower scores suggest varying degrees of muscle weakness.
4. Interpretation:

    - Score < 48: This indicates significant muscle weakness and may suggest critical illness-related myopathy.
    - Score $\leq$ 36: Suggests severe weakness, often seen in conditions like ICU-acquired weakness (ICUAW).

This bedside assessment helps in identifying and monitoring muscle strength, aiding in treatment decisions and rehabilitation planning for ICU patients.

12.11 Conclusion

Managing weakness in the ICU involves a comprehensive approach that integrates detailed clinical assessment, diagnostic testing, and individualized therapeutic strategies. Early identification and intervention are key to mitigating the impacts of ICU-acquired weakness and other neuromuscular complications.

Algorithm 12.1: Approach to weakness in the ICU

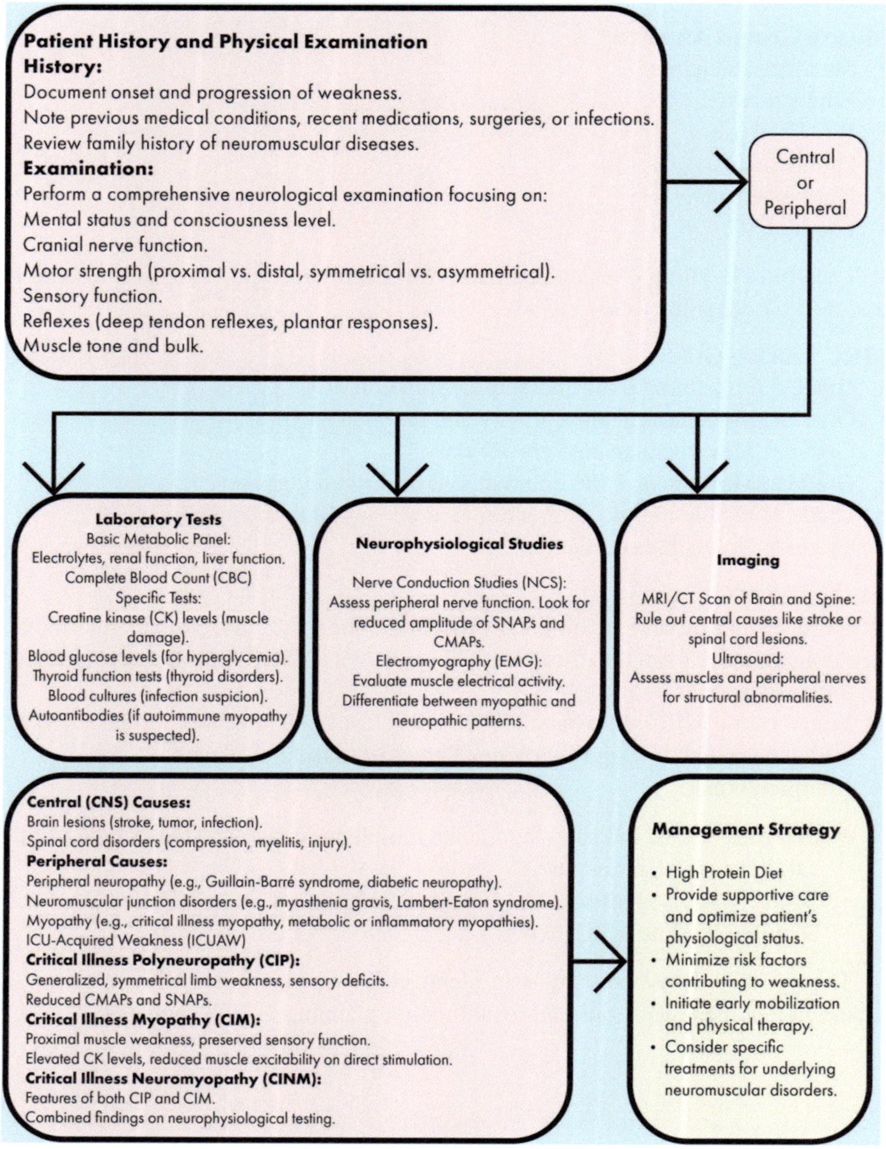

Bibliography

1. Latronico N, Gosselink R. A guided approach to diagnose severe muscle weakness in the intensive care unit. Rev Bras Ter Intensiva. 2015;27(3):199–201.
2. Larson ST, Wilbur J. Muscle Weakness in Adults: Evaluation and Differential Diagnosis. Am Fam Physician. 2020;101(2):95–108.
3. Hughes RA, Wijdicks EF, Benson E, Cornblath DR, Hahn AF, Meythaler JM, et al. Supportive care for patients with Guillain-Barré syndrome. Arch Neurol. 2005;62(8):1194–8.
4. Kress JP, Hall JB. ICU-Acquired Weakness and Recovery From Critical Illness. N Engl J Med. 2014;370(17):1626–35.
5. Jolley SE, Bunnell AE, Hough CL. ICU-Acquired Weakness. Chest J. 2016;150(5):1129–40.
6. Sumar AHS, Sousa TR, Sarmento T. Methods of Assessment of Muscle Weakness Acquired in ICU: A Narrative Description / Métodos De Avaliação Da Fraqueza Muscular Adquirida Na ICU: Uma Descrição Narrativa. Brazilian J Health Rev. 2022;5(2):4306–15.
7. Gronseth GS, Barohn R, Narayanaswami P. Practice advisory: Thymectomy for myasthenia gravis (practice parameter update): Report of the Guideline Development, Dissemination, and Implementation Subcommittee of the American Academy of Neurology. Neurology. 2020;94(16):705–9.
8. Legriel S, Azoulay E, Resche-Rigon M, Lemiale V, Mourvillier B, Kouatchet A, et al. Functional outcome after convulsive status epilepticus. Crit Care Med. 2010;38(12):2295–303.
9. Hughes RA, Wijdicks EF, Barohn R, Benson E, Cornblath DR, Hahn AF, et al. Practice parameter: immunotherapy for Guillain-Barré syndrome: report of the Quality Standards Subcommittee of the American Academy of Neurology. Neurology. 2003;61(6):736–40.
10. Racca F, Vianello A, Mongini T, Ruggeri P, Versaci A, Vita GL, et al. Practical approach to respiratory emergencies in neurological diseases. Neurol Sci. 2020;41(3):497–508.
11. Busl KM, Fried H, Muehlschlegel S, Wartenberg KE, Rajajee V, Alexander SA, et al. Guidelines for Neuroprognostication in Adults with Guillain-Barré Syndrome. Neurocrit Care. 2023;38(3):564–83.

Chapter 13
Management of Sedation in the ICU

13.1 Introduction

Sedation management in the intensive care unit (ICU) is a critical component of patient care, aimed at ensuring comfort, reducing anxiety, and facilitating the performance of necessary medical interventions. Proper sedation helps prevent complications such as delirium and prolonged mechanical ventilation [1] (Ref. Algorithm 13.1).

1. **Assessing Sedation Needs**
   - **Determine the Patient's Baseline:** Establishing the patient's baseline level of consciousness and responsiveness is crucial. This involves understanding the patient's usual mental status, which serves as a reference point to tailor sedation needs. It includes assessing their ability to respond to verbal commands or physical stimulation without sedation.
   - **Gather Information:** Detailed medical history is essential to identify conditions that may influence sedation requirements or responses. Conditions such as neurological disorders, psychiatric conditions, or a history of substance use can significantly impact how a patient tolerates and reacts to sedatives.
2. **Plan for Extubation?**
   - **Yes (Stop Sedation and Monitor):** If the patient is considered ready for extubation, sedation should be reduced or stopped to evaluate their ability to maintain adequate respiration without mechanical assistance. Monitoring involves assessing the patient's respiratory function and consciousness level to ensure safety post-extubation.

S. B. Mishra et al., *Mastering ICU Care*,
https://doi.org/10.1007/978-981-95-0179-3_13

- **No (Continue with Sedation Management):** If extubation is not planned, proceed with a detailed assessment of the sedation level to maintain patient comfort and safety during continued ICU care.

3. **Assessment of Sedation Score**

- **Using RASS or SAS:** The Richmond Agitation-Sedation Scale (RASS) and the Sedation-Agitation Scale (SAS) are tools used to measure the patient's level of sedation. The RASS ranges from +4 (combative) to −5 (unarousable), while SAS ranges from 1 (unarousable) to 7 (dangerously agitated). These scales help in setting appropriate sedation targets based on the patient's condition and treatment goals.

4. **Setting Sedation Levels**

- **Light Sedation (RASS -1 to − 2):** Light sedation is preferred for most patients to facilitate early mobility and maintain communication abilities. This level of sedation uses agents like propofol or dexmedetomidine, which allow patients to be arousable and interactive, aiding in quicker recovery and reducing ICU stays [2].
- **Moderate to Deep Sedation (RASS -3 to − 5):** In cases of severe agitation or during specific procedures, deeper sedation might be required. This involves using higher doses of sedatives like propofol or midazolam. Continuous monitoring is essential to ensure that the patient's respiratory function remains stable and to adjust sedation as needed to prevent complications.

5. **Daily Sedation Interruption**

- **Assessing Readiness for Extubation:** Implementing daily sedation interruptions helps in evaluating the patient's readiness for extubation and reducing unnecessary sedation. During these interruptions, patients are assessed for their ability to maintain respiratory function and cognitive awareness, which can inform decisions on reducing sedation or preparing for extubation.

6. **Continuous Reassessment**

- **Ongoing Evaluation:** Regular reassessment of sedation levels ensures that the patient's sedation is adjusted based on their current clinical status and treatment goals. This includes monitoring RASS/SAS scores, evaluating patient comfort, and assessing the need for ongoing sedation. Adjustments are made to align with the patient's evolving condition and to minimize the risks of oversedation or undersedation.

13.2 Sedation Scores

In the ICU, sedation levels are systematically assessed using scales like the Richmond Agitation-Sedation Scale (RASS) and the Sedation-Agitation Scale (SAS). These tools provide a standardized approach to gauge a patient's level of consciousness and agitation, guiding appropriate sedation management. Here's an elaborate breakdown of each score within these scales:

13.3 Richmond Agitation-Sedation Scale (RASS)

The RASS ranges from +4 (highly agitated) to −5 (deeply sedated), capturing the spectrum from severe agitation to deep sedation:

- **+4 (Combative):** Patients are overtly combative, violent, or pose an immediate danger to staff or themselves. This extreme agitation requires urgent intervention to ensure safety and may necessitate rapid sedation or physical restraints.
- **+3 (Very Agitated):** Patients are demonstrating aggressive behavior or exhibiting severe restlessness. They may attempt to remove catheters or other medical devices. This level often calls for immediate sedative administration to prevent self-harm and manage behavior.
- **+2 (Agitated):** Patients experience frequent movements that are purposeful but can be disruptive or unsafe, such as pulling on tubes. While they are not aggressive, they exhibit significant discomfort and unease, indicating a need for increased sedation to alleviate distress.
- **+1 (Restless):** Patients are anxious or restless but not aggressively so. They are capable of making movements or vocalizing concerns that are controlled. This stage might prompt consideration for mild sedation to promote relaxation and cooperation.
- **0 (Alert and Calm):** The ideal sedation level for many ICU patients, where they are fully awake, calm, and cooperative. Patients at this level can interact meaningfully with caregivers, facilitating communication and potentially speeding recovery.
- **−1 (Drowsy):** Patients are not fully awake but can be easily roused to full consciousness with verbal stimulation. They respond to commands but may appear slightly sluggish. This is often the target sedation level for patients who require minimal sedation while retaining the ability to respond.

- **−2 (Light Sedation):** Patients can be awakened briefly with mild verbal or tactile stimulation. They are responsive but not fully engaged or alert. This level balances patient comfort and the ability to follow commands when necessary.
- **−3 (Moderate Sedation):** Patients respond to loud verbal commands or gentle physical stimulation but do not stay awake or alert spontaneously. This deeper level of sedation may be used in patients requiring more intensive sedation for comfort or procedure tolerance.
- **−4 (Deep Sedation):** Patients are difficult to rouse and only respond to repeated or painful stimulation. They are not aware of their surroundings and do not follow commands. This level is reserved for patients needing profound sedation, such as those undergoing certain invasive procedures or those with severe agitation that requires intensive management.
- **−5 (Unarousable):** Patients are unresponsive to any verbal or physical stimulation, including pain. This level represents the deepest sedation and is typically only used in situations where the patient must be completely unconscious, such as during major surgery or in the case of severe refractory agitation.

13.4 Sedation-Agitation Scale (SAS)

The SAS ranges from 1 (unarousable) to 7 (dangerously agitated), capturing patient sedation and agitation across a similar spectrum:

- **1 (Unarousable):** Patients do not respond to any stimulation, including pain. This profound level of sedation is generally avoided unless absolutely necessary, as it indicates the patient is deeply unconscious and potentially at risk for complications.
- **2 (Very Sedated):** Patients are arousable only to physical stimulation and quickly drift back to sleep without significant interaction. This level is used in cases requiring deep sedation but where some level of responsiveness is still monitored.
- **3 (Sedated):** Patients can be roused to verbal commands or light tactile stimulation but may fall back asleep if left unstimulated. This level is common in ICU patients who need to be sedated for comfort but still require some monitoring for responsiveness.
- **4 (Calm and Cooperative):** Patients are calm, easily aroused, and able to follow commands. This is the goal for many ICU patients as it balances comfort with the ability to engage in their care.
- **5 (Agitated):** Patients are anxious or mildly agitated. They may be restless and attempt to adjust their position or interact more frequently, suggesting a need for mild sedation to maintain comfort and safety.

- **6 (Very Agitated):** Patients exhibit behaviors such as pulling at tubes or attempting to climb out of bed. They are visibly distressed and may need more intensive sedation to ensure safety and prevent self-harm.
- **7 (Dangerously Agitated):** Patients are in a state of severe agitation, potentially posing immediate danger to themselves or others. This extreme level of agitation necessitates immediate and robust sedation interventions to stabilize the patient and maintain a safe environment.

13.5 Practical Application of Sedation Scores

1. **Assess Regularly:** Sedation levels should be assessed frequently using the chosen scale, especially after changes in sedation dosage or when there is a change in the patient's condition.
2. **Tailor Sedation:** Target sedation levels should be individualized based on the patient's clinical status, medical history, and treatment goals. For instance, lighter sedation (RASS -1 to −2 or SAS 3–4) is often preferred for promoting patient engagement and early mobilization, whereas deeper sedation (RASS -3 to −5 or SAS 1–2) may be necessary for patients with severe agitation or those undergoing specific procedures.
3. **Document and Communicate:** Consistent documentation of sedation levels using these scales and clear communication with the ICU team are crucial for coordinated care. This helps in tracking trends and making informed decisions about sedation management.

By utilizing the RASS and SAS scales effectively, healthcare professionals can optimize sedation practices, enhance patient comfort, and improve overall outcomes in the ICU.

13.6 Conclusion

Effective sedation management in the ICU involves a dynamic approach tailored to each patient's unique needs and conditions. Regular assessment and adjustment of sedation levels using structured scales and protocols can enhance patient outcomes, reduce ICU stays, and improve overall patient safety. Adherence to the outlined algorithm helps in balancing sedation with patient responsiveness, leading to better management of critically ill patients.

Algorithm 13.1: Management of sedation in the ICU

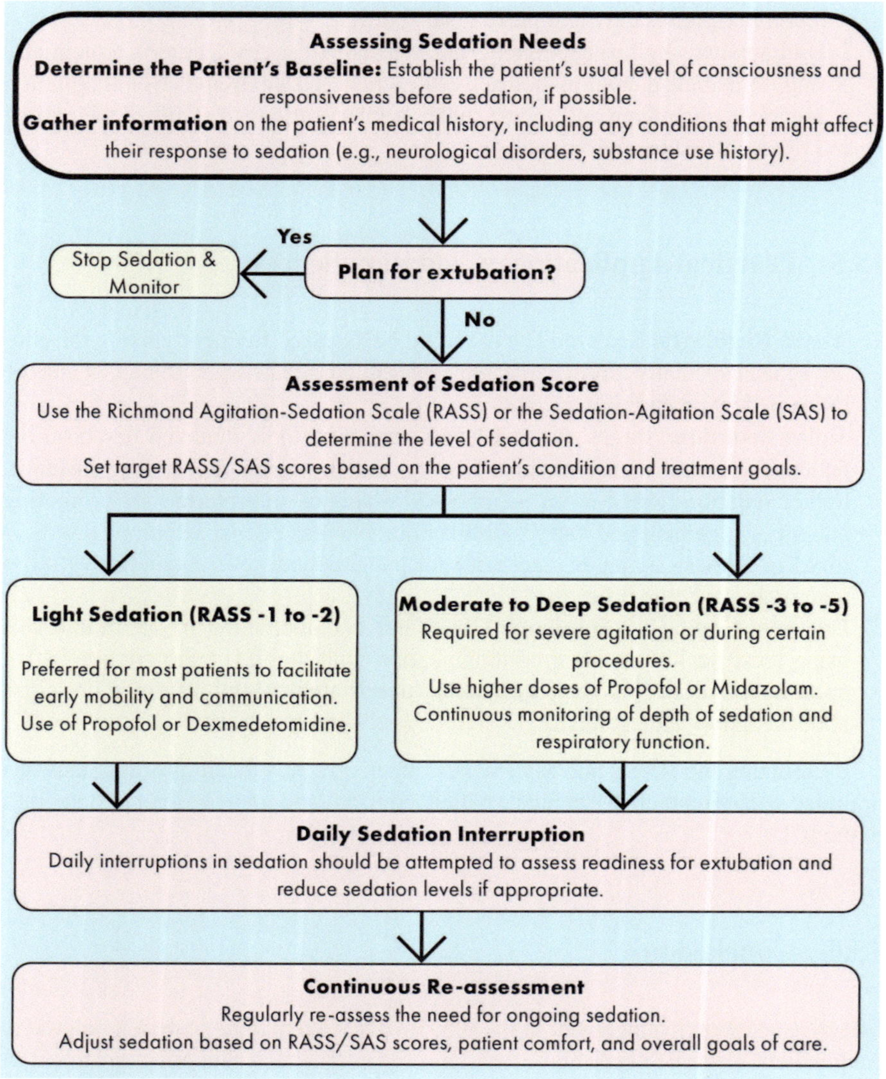

Bibliography

1. Devlin JW, Skrobik Y, Gélinas C, Needham DM, Slooter AJC, Pandharipande PP, et al. Clinical practice guidelines for the prevention and Management of Pain, agitation/sedation, delirium, immobility, and sleep disruption in adult patients in the ICU. Crit Care Med. 2018;46(9):e825–e73.
2. Lewis K, Alshamsi F, Carayannopoulos KL, Granholm A, Piticaru J, Al Duhailib Z, et al. Dexmedetomidine vs other sedatives in critically ill mechanically ventilated adults: a systematic review and meta-analysis of randomized trials. Intensive Care Med. 2022;48(7):811–40.

Chapter 14
Management of Pain in the ICU

14.1 Introduction

Pain management is a critical component of care in the intensive care unit (ICU). Critically ill patients often experience pain from various sources, including surgical procedures, trauma, mechanical ventilation, and invasive monitoring devices. Uncontrolled pain can lead to adverse outcomes such as increased stress responses, hemodynamic instability, impaired wound healing, prolonged mechanical ventilation, and the development of chronic pain syndromes. This chapter outlines a systematic approach to pain assessment and management in the ICU, emphasizing the use of appropriate assessment tools, differentiation of pain types, and implementation of multimodal analgesia strategies to optimize patient comfort while minimizing opioid-related side effects [1] (Ref. Algorithm 14.1).

1. **Assess the Patient's Ability to Communicate**
   - Clinical Considerations: Determine if the patient can self-report pain. Factors such as sedation, mechanical ventilation, delirium, or cognitive impairment may hinder communication.
   - Action: If the patient is able to communicate, utilize self-reporting tools like the Numeric Rating Scale (NRS), where the patient rates their pain on a scale from 0 (no pain) to 10 (worst possible pain).
2. **Use Behavioral Pain Assessment Tools for Noncommunicative Patients**
   - Clinical Considerations: For patients unable to self-report, employ validated behavioral pain assessment tools such as the Behavioral Pain Scale (BPS) or the Critical-Care Pain Observation Tool (CPOT) [2].

S. B. Mishra et al., *Mastering ICU Care*,
https://doi.org/10.1007/978-981-95-0179-3_14

Description of Tools:

- BPS: Assesses facial expression, upper limb movements, and compliance with mechanical ventilation, with scores ranging from 3 (no pain) to 12 (maximum pain).
- CPOT: Evaluates facial expressions, body movements, muscle tension, and compliance with the ventilator or vocalization, with scores ranging from 0 to 8.
- Action: Train staff on the proper use of these tools to ensure accurate and consistent pain assessment.

3. **Identify the Type and Source of Pain**
   Types of Pain:

   - Acute Pain: Typically arises from recent injury, surgery, or acute illness.
   - Chronic Pain: Persistent pain existing before ICU admission, such as due to arthritis or neuropathy.
   - Neuropathic Pain: Results from nerve injury, characterized by burning or tingling sensations.
   - Clinical Considerations: Identifying the pain type guides the selection of appropriate analgesic agents. Neuropathic pain may require adjunctive medications not typically used for nociceptive pain.

4. **Manage Mild Pain (NRS 1–3, BPS 3–4, CPOT 0–2)**
   Pharmacological Interventions:

   - Administer non-opioid analgesics such as acetaminophen or nonsteroidal anti-inflammatory drugs (NSAIDs), provided there are no contraindications (e.g., liver dysfunction for acetaminophen, renal impairment or bleeding risk for NSAIDs) [3].

   Non-pharmacological interventions:

   - Reposition the patient to alleviate discomfort.
   - Apply ice or heat packs as appropriate.
   - Ensure optimal body alignment and supportive devices.

   Drug doses and side effects are given in Table 14.1.

Note

- **Acetaminophen:** IV formulation should be used cautiously in patients with liver dysfunction. Oral and rectal routes may have variable absorption, especially in critically ill patients.
- **NSAIDs (Ibuprofen, Ketorolac):** Should be used cautiously in patients with renal impairment or those at risk for gastrointestinal bleeding. Limit the duration of Ketorolac to 5 days to minimize risk of adverse effects.

Table 14.1 Pharmacotherapy in pain

Drug class	Drug	Initial dose	Max dose	Duration of action	Monitoring for side effects
Non-opioid	Acetaminophen	650 mg orally/rectally q6h; 1 g IV q6h	4 g/day (oral/rectal); 4 g/day (IV)	4–6 h	Monitor for liver toxicity, especially in liver disease patients
NSAID	Ibuprofen	400–800 mg orally q6h	3200 mg/day	4–6 h	Monitor for GI bleeding, renal impairment, and cardiovascular events
NSAID	Ketorolac	15–30 mg IV/IM q6h	120 mg/day (IV/IM) for 5 days	4–6 h	Monitor for GI bleeding, renal impairment, and increased risk of bleeding
NSAID	Celecoxib	100–200 mg orally q12h	400 mg/day	12–24 h	Monitor for cardiovascular events and renal function
Opioid	Morphine	2–4 mg IV q1-2h	No max dose, titrate to effect	3–4 h	Monitor for respiratory depression, hypotension and constipation
Opioid	Fentanyl	25–100 mcg IV q1-2h	No max dose, titrate to effect	1–2 h (IV bolus)	Monitor for respiratory depression and bradycardia
Opioid	Hydromorphone	0.2–0.6 mg IV q2-3h	No max dose, titrate to effect	3–4 h	Monitor for respiratory depression, hypotension, and sedation
Opioid	Remifentanil	0.5–1 mcg/kg/min IV infusion	No max dose, titrate to effect	5–10 mins (infusion)	Monitor for rapid onset and offset respiratory depression
Opioid adjunct	Ketamine	0.1–0.3 mg/kg IV bolus, then 0.1–0.2 mg/kg/hr. infusion	No max dose, titrate to effect	5–10 mins (bolus); 30 min (infusion)	Monitor for dissociative reactions, hypertension, and tachycardia

(continued)

Table 14.1 (continued)

Drug class	Drug	Initial dose	Max dose	Duration of action	Monitoring for side effects
Neuropathic	Gabapentin	100–300 mg orally q8h	3600 mg/day	6–8 h	Monitor for sedation, dizziness, and renal function
Neuropathic	Pregabalin	50–150 mg orally q12h	600 mg/day	6–8 h	Monitor for sedation, dizziness, and peripheral edema
Local anesthetic	Lidocaine IV	1.5 mg/kg IV bolus, then 1–2 mg/min infusion	3 mg/kg/hr. infusion	10–20 mins (bolus)	Monitor for cardiac arrhythmias and CNS toxicity
Opioid adjunct	Dexmedetomidine	0.2–1 mcg/kg/hr. IV infusion	1.5 mcg/kg/hr	1–2 hours	Monitor for bradycardia, hypotension, and sedation

- **Opioids (Morphine, Fentanyl, Hydromorphone, Remifentanil):** Titrate to patient response while monitoring closely for respiratory depression, sedation, and gastrointestinal side effects. Remifentanil's short duration makes it suitable for procedures requiring rapid recovery.
- **Ketamine:** Useful for pain management in patients who are at risk of opioid side effects. Monitor for potential psychological side effects.
- **Gabapentin and Pregabalin:** Primarily used for neuropathic pain. Adjust doses in patients with renal impairment and monitor for CNS side effects.
- **Lidocaine IV:** Continuous monitoring is necessary due to potential for cardiac and CNS toxicity, especially with prolonged infusions.
- **Dexmedetomidine:** Provides sedative and analgesic effects without significant respiratory depression. Monitor for bradycardia and hypotension, especially at higher doses.

5. **Manage Moderate Pain (NRS 4–6, BPS 5–6, CPOT 3–5)**
   Pharmacological Interventions:

   - Continue non-opioid analgesics.
   - Add low-dose opioids such as intravenous morphine, fentanyl, or hydromorphone.
   - Consider adjunctive agents like low-dose ketamine, especially in patients with opioid tolerance or neuropathic pain components.

   Clinical Considerations:

   - Ketamine, an NMDA receptor antagonist, provides analgesia with minimal respiratory depression at sub-anesthetic doses.
   - Regional anesthesia techniques (e.g., nerve blocks, epidurals) may be considered when feasible.

6. **Manage Severe Pain (NRS 7–10, BPS 7–12, CPOT 6–8)**
   Pharmacological Interventions:

   - Administer higher doses of opioids, titrating to effect while monitoring for side effects.

   Use multimodal analgesia by adding adjunctive medications such as:

   - Gabapentinoids (gabapentin or pregabalin) for neuropathic pain.
   - Ketamine for opioid-sparing effects.
   - Lidocaine infusions (with caution and monitoring) in select patients.

   Clinical Considerations:

   - Monitor for opioid-induced adverse effects: respiratory depression, sedation, gastrointestinal dysmotility.
   - Frequent reassessment is essential to balance analgesia with safety.

7. **Reassess Pain Regularly and Adjust Treatment**
   Clinical Practice:

   - Reassess pain at regular intervals, such as every 30–60 mins after initiating or adjusting therapy, and before and after procedures known to cause pain.
   - Use the same pain assessment tool consistently to monitor trends.

   Action:

   - Adjust analgesic regimens based on reassessment findings.
   - Implement preemptive analgesia before painful procedures (e.g., dressing changes, repositioning) to reduce procedural pain.

8. **Implement Multimodal Analgesia**

   - Principle: Utilize a combination of medications and techniques that act on different pain pathways to enhance analgesia and reduce reliance on opioids.

   Components:

   - Non-opioid analgesics: Acetaminophen, NSAIDs.
   - Adjuvant medications: Gabapentinoids, ketamine, alpha-2 agonists (e.g., dexmedetomidine).
   - Regional anesthesia: Nerve blocks, epidural analgesia where appropriate.

   Benefits:

   - Improved pain control.
   - Reduction in opioid consumption and associated side effects.

9. **Address Special Considerations**
   Delirium and Sedation:

   - Avoid over-sedation, which can mask pain and delay recovery.
   - Use sedation protocols that prioritize analgesia-first approaches (analgosedation).

   Communication Barriers:

   - Employ alternative communication methods (e.g., communication boards) to facilitate self-reporting in patients with speech impairments.

   Patient-Specific Factors:

   - Adjust analgesic choices based on organ function (e.g., renal or hepatic impairment), allergy history, and potential drug interactions.

14.2 Conclusion

Effective pain management in the ICU requires a systematic approach that includes accurate assessment, identification of pain type, and implementation of individualized treatment plans. Utilizing validated assessment tools like NRS, BPS, and CPOT ensures consistent and reliable pain evaluation. A multimodal analgesia strategy, incorporating non-opioid analgesics and adjuvant therapies alongside opioids when necessary, optimizes pain control while minimizing adverse effects. Regular reassessment and adjustment of the analgesic regimen are crucial, as is the use of preemptive analgesia for painful procedures. By prioritizing pain management, ICU clinicians can improve patient comfort, facilitate recovery, and enhance overall outcomes.

Algorithm 14.1: Management of pain in the ICU

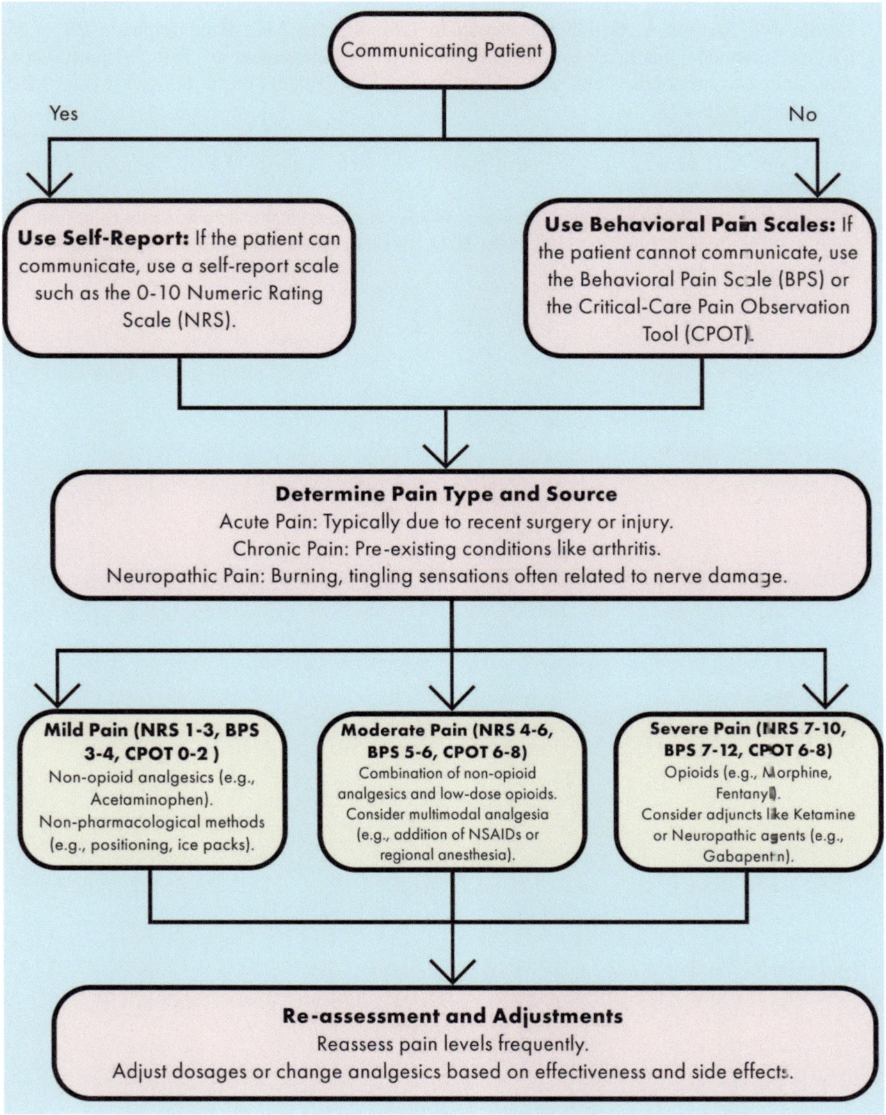

Bibliography

1. Devlin JW, Skrobik Y, Gélinas C, Needham DM, Slooter AJC, Pandharipande PP, et al. Clinical practice guidelines for the prevention and Management of Pain, agitation/sedation, delirium, immobility, and sleep disruption in adult patients in the ICU. Crit Care Med. 2018;46(9):e825–e73.
2. Zhai Y, Cai S, Zhang Y. The diagnostic accuracy of critical care pain observation tool (CPOT) in ICU patients: a systematic review and meta-analysis. J Pain Symptom Manag. 2020;60(4):847–56.e13.
3. Zhao H, Yang S, Wang H, Zhang H, An Y. Non-opioid analgesics as adjuvants to opioid for pain management in adult patients in the ICU: a systematic review and meta-analysis. J Crit Care. 2019;54:136–44.

Chapter 15
Management of Delirium in the ICU

15.1 Introduction

Delirium is a frequent and severe condition in the intensive care unit (ICU), marked by sudden disturbances in attention and cognition. It significantly worsens patient outcomes, including extended ICU stays, higher mortality, and potential long-term cognitive impairment. Delirium management in the ICU requires a comprehensive strategy that incorporates early detection, addressing reversible causes, and the judicious use of both non-pharmacologic and pharmacologic treatments [1, 2] (Ref. Algorithm 15.1).

15.2 Delirium Screening

Purpose: Early identification is essential to mitigate the effects of delirium.
Tools:

- Confusion Assessment Method for the ICU (CAM-ICU): Detects delirium by evaluating acute onset, inattention, altered consciousness, and disorganized thinking.
- Intensive Care Delirium Screening Checklist (ICDSC): A detailed checklist scoring of eight symptoms to assess delirium.

Frequency: Daily screening is recommended for prompt intervention.

S. B. Mishra et al., *Mastering ICU Care*,
https://doi.org/10.1007/978-981-95-0179-3_15

15.3 Identify and Address Underlying Causes

Comprehensive evaluation should target correctable factors:

- Hypoxia: Ensure proper oxygenation to avoid cognitive disturbances.
- Electrolyte and Metabolic Imbalances: Correct abnormal sodium, magnesium, calcium, urea levels. Also optimize blood sugar levels. Check for thyroid function test, thiamine deficiency, and hepatic encephalopathy.
- Infections: Treat systemic or localized infections, like sepsis or pneumonia.
- Withdrawal: Manage symptoms of alcohol or drug withdrawal carefully.
- Medication Side Effects: Adjust medications that may contribute to delirium, particularly anticholinergics or sedatives.

15.4 Non-pharmacologic Interventions [3]

- Reorientation: Reorient the patient regularly with clocks, calendars, and clear communication.
- Sleep Hygiene: Minimize nighttime noise and light, optimize comfort, and encourage consistent sleep schedules.
- Early Mobility: Promote physical activity early to reduce delirium duration and improve recovery.
- Family Involvement: Engaging family members can provide emotional support and reduce confusion.

15.5 Incorporate Sleep-Promoting Protocol

A sleep-promoting strategy is vital for managing PADIS (pain, agitation/sedation, delirium, immobility, sleep disturbance) in ICU patients. This includes minimizing disruptions during the night and scheduling procedures to allow for prolonged, uninterrupted sleep.

15.6 Multicomponent Intervention Strategy (ABCDEF Bundle)

Adopt the ABCDEF bundle, a proven strategy to reduce delirium duration, ICU stay, and mortality. It focuses on awakening, breathing coordination, sedation choice, delirium monitoring, early mobility, and family involvement.

15.7 Pharmacologic Management

Criteria for Use: Consider pharmacologic interventions only when non-pharmacologic measures fail, and the patient is at risk due to severe agitation or psychosis.

- Haloperidol: For short-term management of severe agitation.
- Atypical Antipsychotics (e.g., Quetiapine): Preferred for longer management with fewer side effects.
- Avoid Benzodiazepines: Except in cases of alcohol or benzodiazepine withdrawal, benzodiazepines should be avoided as they can worsen delirium.

15.8 Ongoing Pharmacologic Therapy Caution

Use haloperidol, atypical antipsychotics, or dexmedetomidine sparingly, ensuring they are reserved for when delirium poses a risk of harm. Monitor closely and reassess treatment regularly.

Delirium Risk Factors

Incorporate risk prediction models like PRE-DELIRIC and E-PRE-DELIRIC to anticipate delirium onset, focusing on modifiable factors such as benzodiazepine use and deep sedation.

1. **PRE-DELIRIC Model**

The PRE-DELIRIC model is a delirium risk prediction tool developed to estimate the likelihood of ICU patients developing delirium within the first 24 h of admission. It uses 10 clinical variables such as age, APACHE-II score, infection, coma, and the use of sedatives like benzodiazepines. The model's aim is to help clinicians identify patients at high risk of delirium early on, allowing for timely preventive measures.

2. **E-PRE-DELIRIC Model**

An updated version of the PRE-DELIRIC model, the E-PRE-DELIRIC (early prediction) model enhances prediction accuracy by incorporating dynamic variables, including changes in vital signs and clinical condition over the initial 24 hours of ICU admission. This model refines risk prediction by continuously monitoring and updating risk factors like sedation depth and benzodiazepine use, offering a more precise prediction of delirium onset during the ICU stay.

Reassessment and Adjustment

- Ongoing Monitoring: Reassess the patient's condition regularly to evaluate progress and adapt the treatment plan accordingly.
- Adjustment of Treatment: Taper or discontinue pharmacologic treatments as the patient's delirium improves, avoiding unnecessary side effects.

15.9 Detailed Overview of ICDSC and CAM-ICU for Delirium Screening

Delirium screening in the ICU is crucial for early identification and management. Two widely used tools for this purpose are the Intensive Care Delirium Screening Checklist (ICDSC) and the Confusion Assessment Method for the ICU (CAM-ICU). Each has unique features and criteria that help clinicians systematically assess and diagnose delirium in critically ill patients.

15.10 Intensive Care Delirium Screening Checklist (ICDSC)

The ICDSC is a checklist-based tool that quantifies delirium symptoms over an assessment period. It is designed to be user-friendly and can be administered by bedside nurses or other healthcare providers.

Components of the ICDSC The ICDSC consists of eight items, each reflecting common features of delirium. Each item is scored based on the presence or absence of the symptom within the past 24 hours.

1. **Altered Level of Consciousness**
   - Any change in consciousness, such as decreased alertness or hyperalert states, should be noted. The Richmond Agitation-Sedation Scale (RASS) is often used to evaluate this.
   - **Score 1 if present**.
2. **Inattention**
   - Difficulty in focusing, maintaining attention, or shifting attention. This may be assessed by tasks like counting backward or spelling a word.
   - **Score 1 if present**.
3. **Disorientation**
   - The patient's lack of awareness of their surroundings, including confusion about time, place, or person.
   - **Score 1 if present**.
4. **Hallucinations or Delusions**
   - The presence of perceptual disturbances such as seeing or hearing things that are not there, or having false beliefs.
   - **Score 1 if present**.

5. **Psychomotor Agitation or Retardation**
   - Changes in activity levels, either increased (agitation) or decreased (retardation).
   - **Score 1 if present**.
6. **Inappropriate Speech or Mood**
   - Incoherent, irrelevant, or illogical speech, or emotional disturbances that are inappropriate to the context.
   - **Score 1 if present**.
7. **Sleep/Wake Cycle Disturbances**
   - Irregular sleep patterns, such as daytime sleepiness or nighttime wakefulness.
   - **Score 1 if present**.
8. **Symptom Fluctuation**
   - Rapid changes in the severity or presence of delirium symptoms over time.
   - **Score 1 if present**.

Scoring
- Each item is scored 0 (absent) or 1 (present).
- A total score is calculated by summing the scores of all items.
- **Interpretation**:
  - A score of 0–3 suggests no or subsyndromal delirium.
  - A score of 4 or more indicates the presence of delirium.

Advantages
- Captures a broad range of delirium symptoms.
- Can be integrated into routine patient care by bedside staff.
- Useful for continuous monitoring and documentation.

15.11 Confusion Assessment Method for the ICU (CAM-ICU)

The CAM-ICU is a structured tool specifically adapted for use in the ICU, where patients may not be able to communicate effectively. It focuses on key diagnostic features of delirium and provides a quick and reliable assessment.

Components of the CAM-ICU The CAM-ICU consists of four features that are evaluated to determine the presence of delirium.

1. **Feature 1: Acute Onset or Fluctuating Course**
   - **Assessment**: Observe for evidence of an acute change in mental status from baseline or fluctuating course of symptoms over the past 24 hours.
   - **Criteria**: This can be established through direct observation, chart review, or communication with the healthcare team.
   - **Result**: No evidence of an acute change in mental status➔ No delirium.

   - If positive, check for feature 2.
2. **Feature 2: Inattention**
   - **Assessment**: Evaluate the patient's ability to focus and maintain attention.
   - **Task**: Ask the patient to squeeze your hand when they hear the letter "A" in a sequence of random letters (e.g., "SAVEAHAART").
   - **Criteria**: An error rate of more than 2 errors in 10 letters indicates inattention.
   - **Result**: 0–2 errors➔ No delirium.

   - >2 errors➔ Check for feature 3.
3. **Feature 3: Altered Level of Consciousness**
   - **Assessment**: Use the RASS to assess the patient's level of consciousness.
   - **Criteria**: Any level other than "alert and calm" (RASS 0) suggests altered consciousness.
   - **Result**: RAAS other than zero➔ Delirium present.

   - RAAS zero ➔Check for feature 4.
4. **Feature 4: Disorganized Thinking**
   - **Assessment**: Ask simple yes/no questions to evaluate the patient's coherence and logical thought processes (e.g., "Will a stone float on water?").
   - **Criteria**: Incorrect answers or the inability to engage coherently indicate disorganized thinking.
   - **Result**: 0–1 error➔ No delirium.

   - >1 error➔ Delirium present.

Diagnostic Algorithm
- **Delirium Diagnosis**: Requires the presence of Features 1 and 2 and either Feature 3 or 4.

Advantages
- Quick and easy to administer, often taking just a few minutes.
- High sensitivity and specificity for diagnosing delirium.
- Does not require verbal responses, making it suitable for nonverbal or intubated patients.

15.12 Conclusion

Managing delirium in the ICU demands a multifaceted approach involving early and regular screening, addressing modifiable causes, and implementing both non-pharmacologic and pharmacologic treatments when necessary. Incorporating sleep-promoting protocols, multicomponent interventions like the ABCDEF bundle, and judicious pharmacologic use, supported by continuous reassessment, ensures comprehensive care and better outcomes for critically ill patients.

Algorithm 15.1: Management of delirium in the ICU

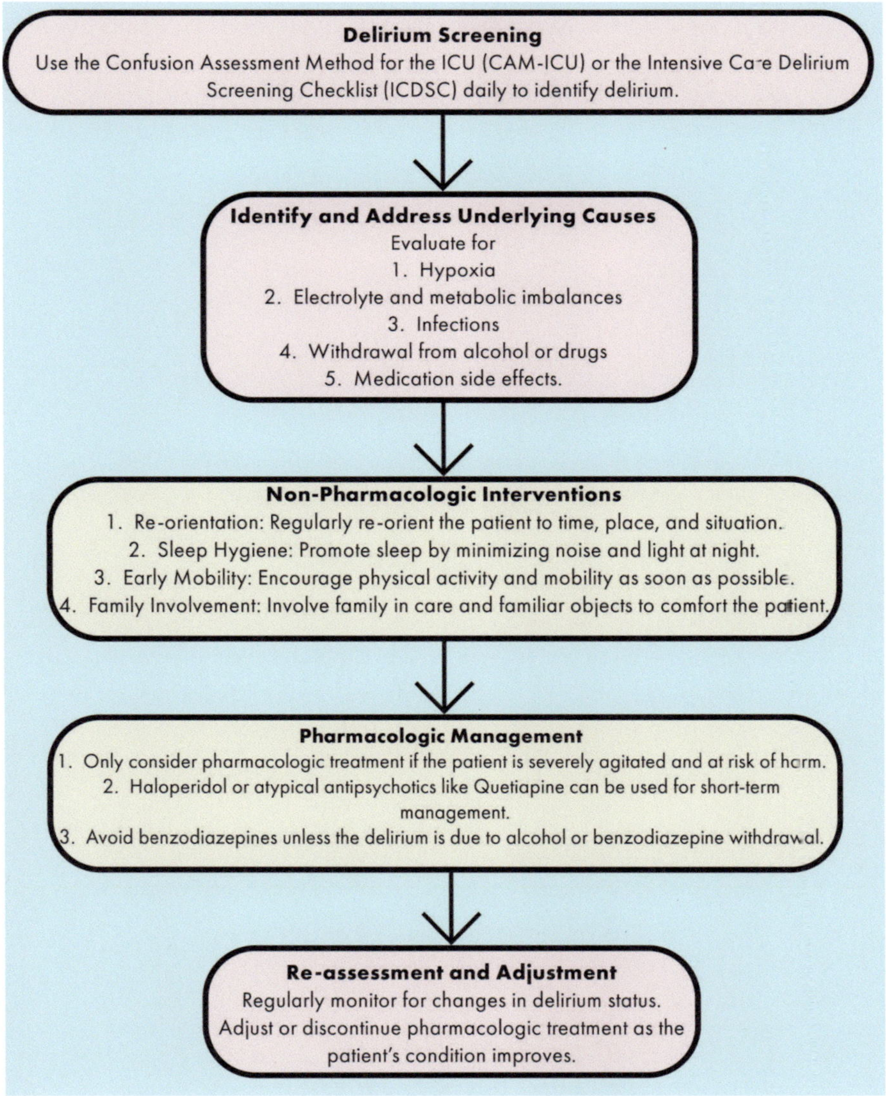

Bibliography

1. Devlin JW, Skrobik Y, Gélinas C, Needham DM, Slooter AJC, Pandharipande PP, et al. Clinical practice guidelines for the prevention and Management of Pain, agitation/sedation, delirium, immobility, and sleep disruption in adult patients in the ICU. Crit Care Med. 2018;46(9):e825–e73.
2. Kim SH, Kim KM, Lim YH, Yoo BH, Cho J, Jun IJ. Psychogenic coma after general anesthesia with remimazolam and remifentanil -a case report. Korean J Anesthesiol. 2022;75(5):449–52.
3. Celis-Rodríguez E, Díaz Cortés JC, Cárdenas Bolívar YR, Carrizosa González JA, Pinilla DI, Ferrer Záccaro LE, et al. Evidence-based clinical practice guidelines for the management of sedoanalgesia and delirium in critically ill adult patients. Med Intensiva (Engl Ed). 2020;44(3):171–84.

Part II
Nephrology

Chapter 16
Approach to Blood Gas Interpretation in the ICU

16.1 Introduction

Blood gas analysis is an essential tool in the intensive care unit (ICU) for assessing and managing patients with respiratory and metabolic disorders. It involves measuring the partial pressures of oxygen (PaO_2) and carbon dioxide ($PaCO_2$), as well as the pH and bicarbonate (HCO_3^-) levels in the blood. Accurate interpretation of these values aids in diagnosing acid-base imbalances, monitoring treatment responses, and guiding therapeutic interventions. A comprehensive understanding of the physiological principles, potential pitfalls, and advanced interpretation methods enhances clinical decision-making [1, 2] [Ref: Algorithm 16.1].

16.2 Pre-analytic Considerations

Proper collection and handling of blood gas samples are crucial to avoid pre-analytic errors that can lead to erroneous results. Key considerations include:

- Syringe Material: Use the appropriate syringe material—glass syringes are preferred for longer storage times, while plastic syringes are suitable for immediate analysis.
- Storage Conditions: Avoid storing plastic syringes on ice, as this can cause diffusion of gases through the plastic and alter the gas measurements.
- Rapid Analysis: Analyze samples promptly to prevent metabolic alterations that can change pH, $PaCO_2$, and PaO_2 values.
- Avoiding Air Bubbles: Ensure no air bubbles are present in the sample to prevent inaccurate PaO_2 readings.

S. B. Mishra et al., *Mastering ICU Care*,
https://doi.org/10.1007/978-981-95-0179-3_16

- Recognizing Spurious Results: Be aware of conditions like leukocytosis or thrombocytosis that can consume oxygen in the sample, leading to falsely low PaO_2 readings (spurious hypoxemia) [3].

16.3 Sampling Techniques

Arterial vs. Venous Blood Gas Analysis

While arterial blood gas (ABG) analysis is the gold standard for assessing oxygenation and acid-base status, central venous blood gas (VBG) analysis can sometimes serve as a less invasive alternative:

- VBG Utility: Central VBG can reliably reflect pH, bicarbonate, and $PaCO_2$ values, making it useful for monitoring acid-base status [4].
- Limitations for Oxygenation: VBG is unreliable for assessing oxygenation (PaO_2) due to significant differences between arterial and venous oxygen content.
- Clinical Implications: Utilizing VBG can reduce patient discomfort and risks associated with arterial puncture when oxygenation status does not need assessment [5].

16.4 Physiological Basis of Acid-Base Balance

Understanding the physiological mechanisms underlying acid-base balance is essential:

- Traditional Bicarbonate-Centered Approach: Focuses on the interplay between $PaCO_2$ and HCO_3^- in maintaining pH balance [1].
- Stewart Approach: Considers the roles of strong ion difference (SID), total weak acids (like albumin), and $PaCO_2$ in determining pH [2].
- Compensatory Responses: The body compensates for primary acid-base disturbances through respiratory or metabolic mechanisms, which can be predicted using empirical equations [6].

16.5 Stepwise Algorithm for Blood Gas Interpretation

A structured approach ensures accurate and efficient interpretation:

First validate the ABG. And then proceed to step-by-step analysis of the ABG.

$$\text{H+} = 24^{*}\left(\text{PaCO2}\right)/\text{HCO3}$$

If the pH and H+ values are not corroborative, then probably the ABG cannot be validated.
Validation:

pH	H+ (in nanomol/L)
6.90	125
7.00	100
7.10	79 ≡ 80
7.20	63 ≡ 60
7.30	50
7.40	**40**
7.50	31 ≡ 30
7.60	25
7.70	20

1. Assess pH
   - Normal Range: 7.38–7.42.
   - Acidemia: pH < 7.38.
   - Alkalemia: pH > 7.42.
2. Determine Primary Disorder

   Take proper history of the patient to determine or have an idea about the primary disorder.
   Evaluate $PaCO_2$ (Normal: 35–45 mm Hg).
   Respiratory Component: Changes in $PaCO_2$ indicate respiratory disorders.
   Metabolic Component: Changes in HCO_3^- indicate metabolic disorders.
3. Assess Compensation
   - Metabolic Acidosis Compensation:

$$\text{Expected PaCO}_2 = \left(1.5 \times \left[\text{HCO}_3^-\right]\right) + 8 \pm 2\,\text{mm Hg}\left(\text{Winters Formula}\right)$$

- Metabolic Alkalosis Compensation:

$$\text{Expected PaCO}_2 = 0.7 \times \left(\left[\text{HCO}_3^-\right] - 24\right) + 40 \pm 2\,\text{mm Hg}$$

- Respiratory Acidosis Compensation:

  Acute: HCO_3^- increases by 1 mmol/L per 10 mm Hg $PaCO_2$ above 40 mm Hg.
  Chronic: HCO_3^- increases by 4–5 mmol/L per 10 mm Hg $PaCO_2$ above 40 mm Hg.
- Respiratory Alkalosis Compensation:

Acute: HCO_3^- decreases by 2 mmol/L per 10 mm Hg $PaCO_2$ below 40 mm Hg.
Chronic: HCO_3^- decreases by 4–5 mmol/L per 10 mm Hg $PaCO_2$ below 40 mm Hg.

4. Calculate Anion Gap (if primary disorder is metabolic acidosis).

   - Formula: Anion Gap (AG) = $[Na^+]$—($[Cl^-]$ + $[HCO_3^-]$).
   - Normal Range: 8–12 mmol/L.
   - Adjusted Anion Gap: Correct for hypoalbuminemia (every 1 g/dL decrease in albumin increases the anion gap by ~2.5 mmol/L).

     Adjusted Anion Gap = AG + 2.5 * (4—measured albumin in g/dl).

   - Interpretation:

     Elevated Anion Gap Metabolic Acidosis: Indicates unmeasured anions (e.g., lactate, ketones).
     Normal Anion Gap Metabolic Acidosis: Suggests loss of bicarbonate or renal tubular acidosis.

5. Assess Oxygenation Status.

   - PaO_2 Levels: Evaluate in context of patient's age, FiO_2, and clinical condition.
   - PaO_2/FiO_2 Ratio:

     Normal: > 300 mm Hg.
     Mild ARDS: 200–300 mm Hg.
     Moderate ARDS: 100–200 mm Hg.
     Severe ARDS: < 100 mm Hg.

   - Pulse Oximetry:

     Useful for continuous monitoring but has limitations (e.g., cannot detect dyshemoglobins like carboxyhemoglobin or methemoglobin, incorrect readings in severe shock/high vasopressors, nail paint) [3].
     Multi-Wavelength Oximeters: Can detect dyshemoglobins, providing a more accurate assessment.

6. Consider V/Q Mismatch: From A-a gradient (Alveolar-arterial oxygen gradient); For details refer to Chap. 17/Algorithm 17.1.

   - Understanding V/Q Mismatch: Imbalance between ventilation and perfusion leading to gas exchange abnormalities [7].
   - Clinical Relevance: Common in conditions like pulmonary embolism, pneumonia, or ARDS.
   - Assessment Techniques:

     Imaging (CT scans, V/Q scans).
     Advanced methods (inert gas elimination studies).

16.6 Advanced Interpretation of Acid-Base Disorders

Beyond the basics, consider: (Stewarts Approach)—Chap. 18/Algorithm 18.1

Strong Ion Difference (SID):

- Definition: Difference between fully dissociated (strong) cations and anions.
- Role in Acid-Base Balance: Changes in SID affect plasma pH.

Unmeasured Ions:

- Examples: Lactate, ketones, toxins.
- Impact: Accumulation leads to metabolic acidosis with an elevated anion gap.

Albumin and Phosphate:

- Weak Acids: Contribute to buffering capacity.
- Hypoalbuminemia: Can mask the presence of an elevated anion gap acidosis.

16.7 Common Misinterpretations and Errors

Awareness of potential pitfalls is crucial:

Pre-analytic Errors:

- Improper sample collection or handling can lead to inaccurate results.
- Analyzer calibration issues can produce erroneous values.

Spurious Results:

- Leukocytosis can consume oxygen in the sample, causing falsely low PaO_2.
- Air bubbles can increase PaO_2 and decrease $PaCO_2$ readings [8].

Recalculations:

- Using the Henderson-Hasselbalch equation can help verify reported values and detect inconsistencies.

16.8 Conclusion

A comprehensive and methodical approach to blood gas interpretation enhances patient care in the ICU. By integrating traditional and advanced methods, clinicians can accurately diagnose acid-base disturbances, understand compensatory mechanisms, and identify underlying causes. Awareness of pre-analytic factors and potential errors ensures reliability of results. This structured algorithm serves as a valuable tool for clinicians, promoting effective diagnosis and timely, targeted interventions.

Algorithm 16.1: Approach to blood gas interpretation in the ICU

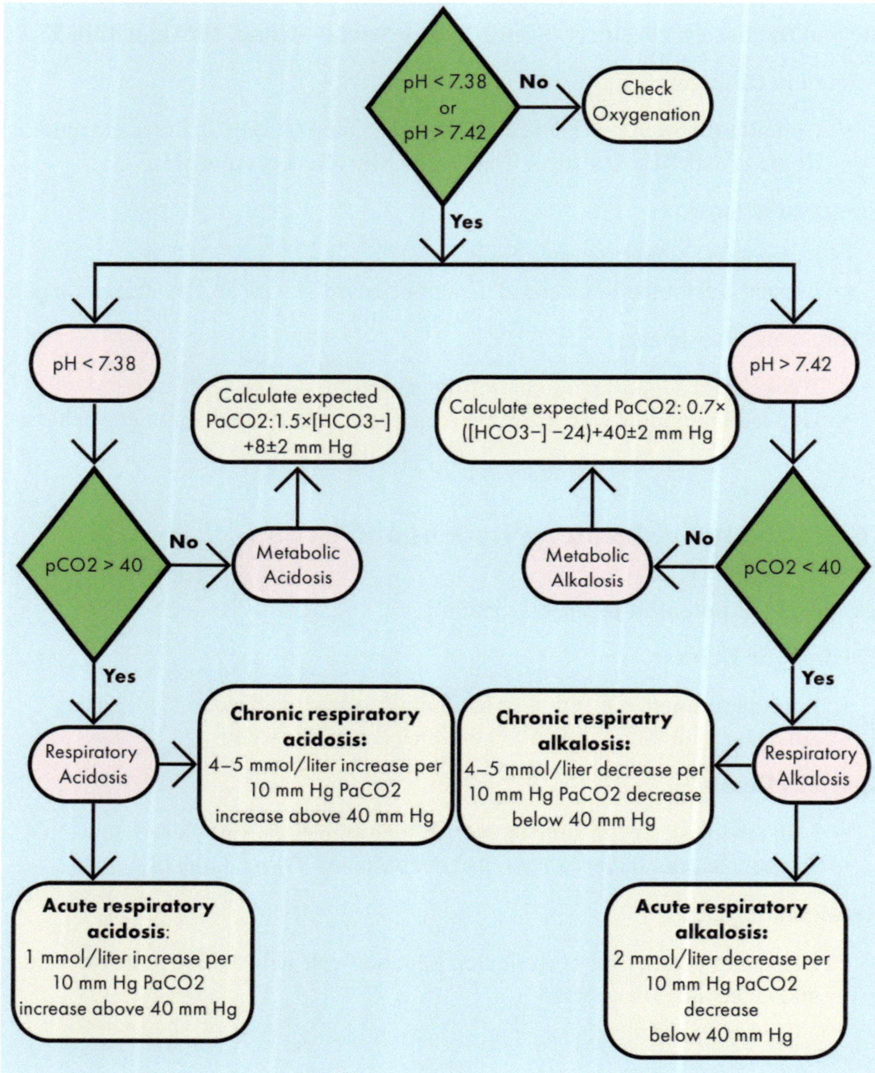

Bibliography

1. Berend K, de Vries AP, Gans RO. Physiological approach to assessment of acid-base disturbances. N Engl J Med. 2014;371(15):1434–45.
2. Seifter JL. Integration of acid-base and electrolyte disorders. N Engl J Med. 2014;371(19):1821–31.
3. Jubran A. Pulse oximetry. Crit Care. 2015;19(1):272.
4. Malatesha G, Singh NK, Bharija A, Rehani B, Goel A. Comparison of arterial and venous pH, bicarbonate, PCO2 and PO2 in initial emergency department assessment. Emerg Med J. 2007;24(8):569–71.
5. AARC clinical practice guideline. Sampling for arterial blood gas analysis. American Association for Respiratory Care. Respir Care. 1992;37(8):913–7.
6. Gattinoni L, Pesenti A, Matthay M. Understanding blood gas analysis. Intensive Care Med. 2018;44(1):91–3.
7. Hopkins SR. Ventilation/perfusion relationships and gas exchange: measurement approaches. Compr Physiol. 2020;10(3):1155–205.
8. Albert TJ, Swenson ER. Circumstances when arterial blood gas analysis can Lead us astray. Respir Care. 2016;61(1):119–21.

Chapter 17
Approach to Respiratory Abnormalities on Blood Gas in the ICU

17.1 Introduction

Respiratory abnormalities are prevalent in critically ill patients and are often unveiled through arterial blood gas (ABG) analysis. Accurate interpretation of ABGs is essential for diagnosing and managing a variety of respiratory conditions. This chapter provides a comprehensive approach to assessing respiratory acidosis and alkalosis, emphasizing the alveolar-arterial (A–a) gradient to differentiate underlying causes and guide appropriate management. Understanding the physiological mechanisms, compensation processes, and clinical implications enhances the clinician's ability to make informed decisions [1, 2]. [Ref: Algorithm 17.1].

17.2 Physiological Basis of Respiratory Acid-Base Disorders

The respiratory system plays a pivotal role in maintaining acid-base balance by regulating carbon dioxide (CO_2) levels through ventilation. CO_2 is a volatile acid; its accumulation leads to respiratory acidosis, while excessive elimination results in respiratory alkalosis.

- Respiratory Acidosis: Occurs when alveolar hypoventilation leads to CO_2 retention. Causes include impaired respiratory drive, neuromuscular dysfunction, or obstructive lung diseases.
- Respiratory Alkalosis: Results from alveolar hyperventilation causing excessive CO_2 elimination. Common triggers are hypoxemia-induced hyperventilation, central nervous system stimulation, or mechanical overventilation.

S. B. Mishra et al., *Mastering ICU Care*,
https://doi.org/10.1007/978-981-95-0179-3_17

17.3 Initial Classification: Acidosis vs. Alkalosis

Begin by evaluating the arterial pH:

- Acidosis: pH < 7.38
- Alkalosis: pH > 7.42

Determine whether the abnormality is acute or chronic from patient history:

Acute respiratory acidosis: Change in pH = 0.008*(40-$PaCO_2$).
Chronic respiratory acidosis: Change in pH = 0.003*(40-$PaCO_2$).
Acute respiratory alkalosis: Change in pH = 0.008*(40-$PaCO_2$).
Chronic respiratory alkalosis: Change in pH = 0.02*(40-$PaCO_2$).

Assess $PaCO_2$ to determine if the primary disorder is respiratory:

- Respiratory Acidosis: Elevated $PaCO_2$ (>45 mm Hg)
- Respiratory Alkalosis: Decreased $PaCO_2$ (<35 mm Hg)

17.4 Compensation Mechanisms

The body attempts to restore normal pH through compensatory mechanisms:

- Acute Respiratory Disorders: Limited renal compensation occurs over hours, with minimal changes in bicarbonate (HCO_3^-).
- Chronic Respiratory Disorders: Renal adaptation over days increases or decreases HCO_3^- reabsorption to buffer pH changes.

Compensatory Changes:

- Respiratory Acidosis:
  - Acute: HCO_3^- increases by ~1 mEq/L for every 10 mm Hg rise in $PaCO_2$.
  - Chronic: HCO_3^- increases by ~3.5 mEq/L for every 10 mm Hg rise in $PaCO_2$.
- Respiratory Alkalosis:
  - Acute: HCO_3^- decreases by ~2 mEq/L for every 10 mm Hg drop in $PaCO_2$.
  - Chronic: HCO_3^- decreases by ~5 mEq/L for every 10 mm Hg drop in $PaCO_2$.

17.5 Calculating the A–a Gradient

The A–a gradient assesses the efficiency of gas exchange:

$$PaO_2 = FiO2^* \left[\left(Patm - PH_2O \right) \right] - PaCO_2 / RQ$$

$$A - agradient = PaO_2 - PaO_2$$

Where:

At sea level on room air:

- PaO_2: Measured arterial oxygen tension
- FiO_2: Fraction of inspired oxygen (0.21 on room air)
- Patm: Atmospheric pressure (760 mm Hg at sea level)
- PH_2O: Water vapor pressure (47 mm Hg)
- RQ: Respiratory quotient (~0.8)

17.6 Key Clinical Considerations

Age-Related Changes in A–a Gradient

- The A–a O_2 tension difference increases by approximately 2 mm Hg per decade of life.
- Alternative formula: A–a O_2 difference = (Age/4) + 4.

Normal A–a Gradient

Increases with age:

- Young adults: <10 mm Hg
- Elderly (>60 years): <20 mm Hg

An elevated A–a gradient indicates impaired oxygen transfer due to ventilation-perfusion mismatch, diffusion defects, or shunting.

17.7 Diagnostic Algorithm

Step 1: Determine Primary Disorder

- Acidosis or Alkalosis: Based on arterial pH.
- Respiratory or Metabolic: Analyze $PaCO_2$ and HCO_3^-.

Step 2: Calculate Expected Compensation

- Use formulas for compensatory changes to assess if the compensation is appropriate.
- Inappropriate compensation suggests a mixed disorder.

Step 3: Calculate the A–a Gradient

- Determine if the gradient is normal or elevated.

Step 4: Analyze Causes Based on A–a Gradient

Respiratory Acidosis

- **Normal A–a Gradient**
  - **Acute Causes:**
    - Depression of the central respiratory center (e.g., drugs, stroke)
    - Cerebral disease (e.g., encephalitis or trauma)
    - Drugs (e.g., narcotics, barbiturates, benzodiazepines)
  - **Chronic Causes:**
    - Neuromuscular diseases (e.g., myasthenia gravis, amyotrophic lateral sclerosis, Guillain-Barré syndrome, muscular dystrophy)
    - Kyphoscoliosis
- **High A–a Gradient**

  Acute Causes:

  - Airway obstruction (e.g., asthma exacerbation, pneumonia)

  Chronic Causes:

  - Chronic obstructive pulmonary disease (COPD)

Respiratory Alkalosis

- **Normal A–a Gradient**
  - **Acute Causes:**
    - Pain, anxiety, fever
    - Stroke, meningitis, trauma
    - Severe anemia, salicylate toxicity
  - **Chronic Causes:**
    - Pregnancy, hyperthyroidism, hepatic failure
- **High A–a Gradient**
- **Acute Causes:**
  - Pneumonia, pulmonary edema, pulmonary embolism, aspiration, congestive heart failure, sepsis
- **Chronic Causes:**
  - Pulmonary embolism in pregnancy, liver failure with aspiration pneumonia

17.8 Clinical Case Examples

Case 1: Respiratory Acidosis with Elevated A–a Gradient
Presentation: A 68-year-old male with a history of COPD presents with increasing dyspnea and confusion.

ABG Results:

- pH: 7.25
- $PaCO_2$: 60 mm Hg
- PaO_2: 55 mm Hg
- HCO_3^-: 26 mEq/L

Analysis:

- Acidosis: pH <7.35
- $PaCO_2$ Elevated: Indicates respiratory acidosis.
- Compensation: HCO_3^- slightly elevated, suggesting partial renal compensation.
- A–a Gradient: Elevated, indicating impaired gas exchange.

Diagnosis
Acute-on-chronic respiratory acidosis due to COPD exacerbation.

Case 2: Respiratory Alkalosis with Normal A–a Gradient
Presentation: A 25-year-old female experiences palpitations and tingling in her fingers after a panic attack.

ABG Results:

- pH: 7.55
- $PaCO_2$: 28 mm Hg
- PaO_2: 95 mm Hg
- HCO_3^-: 22 mEq/L

Analysis:

- Alkalosis: pH >7.45

$PaCO_2$ Decreased: Indicates respiratory alkalosis.
Compensation: Minimal change in HCO_3^- suggests acute condition.
A–a Gradient: Normal.

Diagnosis
Acute respiratory alkalosis due to hyperventilation from anxiety.

17.9 Addressing Mixed Acid-Base Disorders

Mixed disorders occur when more than one primary acid-base disturbance is present. Indicators include:

- Inappropriate Compensation: The expected compensatory response is absent or exaggerated.
- Normal pH with Abnormal $PaCO_2$ and HCO_3^-: Suggests opposing disorders balancing pH.

  Example:

- pH: 7.40 (normal)
- $PaCO_2$: 60 mm Hg (elevated)
- HCO_3^-: 36 mEq/L (elevated)

  Interpretation:

- Elevated $PaCO_2$: Respiratory acidosis
- Elevated HCO_3^-: Metabolic alkalosis
- Normal pH: Mixed disorder.

17.10 Conclusion

A systematic approach to interpreting ABGs enhances the clinician's ability to diagnose and manage respiratory abnormalities effectively. By understanding the underlying pathophysiology, compensation mechanisms, and clinical presentations, clinicians can identify the causes of acidosis and alkalosis, recognize mixed disorders, and implement appropriate interventions. Utilizing tools like the A–a gradient and diagnostic algorithms streamlines the decision-making process, ultimately improving patient outcomes.

Algorithm 17.1: Approach to respiratory abnormalities on blood gas in the ICU

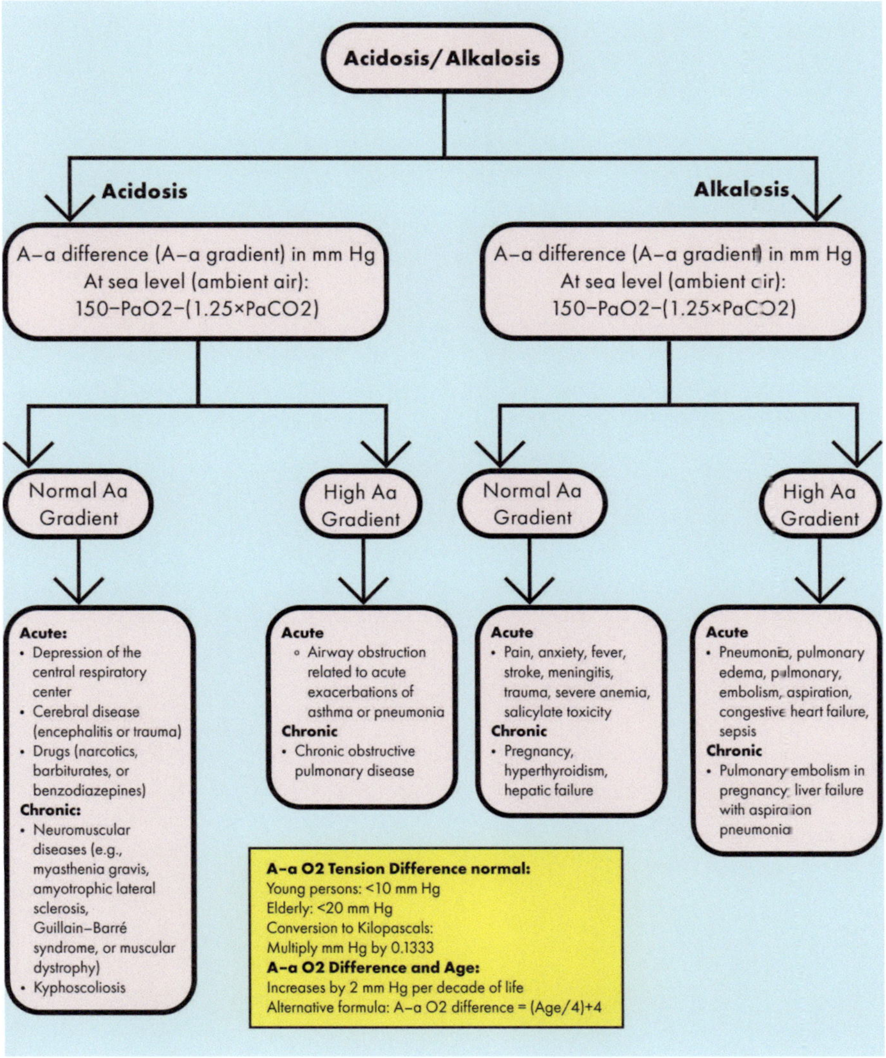

Bibliography

1. Berend K, de Vries AP, Gans RO. Physiological approach to assessment of acid-base disturbances. N Engl J Med. 2014;371(15):1434–45.
2. Blum F, Lund ET, Hall H, Tachauer A, Chedrawy EG, Zilberstein J. Reevaluation of the utilization of arterial blood gas analysis in the intensive care unit: effects on patient safety and patient outcome. J Crit Care. 2015;30(2):438.e1-.e5.

Chapter 18
Approach to Metabolic Acidosis in the ICU

18.1 Introduction

Metabolic acidosis is a common acid-base disturbance in critically ill patients, characterized by a decrease in blood pH due to an accumulation of hydrogen ions (H^+) or a loss of bicarbonate (HCO_3^-). Understanding its pathophysiology, diagnosis, and management is crucial in the Intensive Care Unit (ICU) setting, as it can significantly impact cellular function and overall metabolism [1, 2] [Ref: Algorithm 18.1].

18.2 Pathophysiology

18.2.1 Acid-Base Regulation

The body's acid-base balance is tightly regulated through the interplay between hydrogen ions (H^+), bicarbonate (HCO_3^-), and carbon dioxide (CO_2), as described by the Henderson-Hasselbalch equation:

$$pH = 6.1 + \log\left(\left[HCO_3^-\right] / \left(0.03 \times PaCO_2\right)\right)$$

This equation illustrates how pH is influenced by the ratio of bicarbonate to carbon dioxide. Metabolic acidosis occurs when there is a decrease in bicarbonate or an increase in hydrogen ions, shifting the equilibrium and lowering the pH.

S. B. Mishra et al., *Mastering ICU Care*,
https://doi.org/10.1007/978-981-95-0179-3_18

18.3 Traditional vs. Strong Ion Difference Model

18.3.1 Traditional Bicarbonate-Centered Model

This model focuses on the balance between bicarbonate and carbon dioxide in regulating pH. It emphasizes the role of the kidneys in reabsorbing bicarbonate and the lungs in excreting CO_2.

18.3.2 Strong Ion Difference (SID) Model

The SID model, proposed by Stewart, considers the role of strong ions (fully dissociated ions like Na^+, K^+, and Cl^-) in acid-base balance. According to this model, metabolic acidosis results from a decrease in SID due to an increase in strong anions (e.g., Cl^-) or a decrease in strong cations (e.g., Na^+).

Understanding both models provides a comprehensive view of acid-base regulation and aids in diagnosing complex acid-base disorders.

18.4 Compensation Mechanisms

18.4.1 Respiratory Compensation

The body responds to metabolic acidosis by increasing alveolar ventilation to reduce $PaCO_2$, a process known as respiratory compensation. This hyperventilation helps to normalize pH by shifting the equilibrium of the bicarbonate buffer system.

Winter's Formula is used to predict the expected respiratory compensation:

$$\text{Expected PaCO}_2 = \left(1.5 \times \left[\text{HCO}_3^-\right]\right) + 8 \pm 2$$

- Acute Compensation: Occurs within minutes to hours.
- Chronic Compensation: May take several days to reach maximal effect.

Clinical Application:

- Appropriate Compensation: Measured $PaCO_2$ matches the expected value from Winter's formula.
- Inadequate Compensation: Suggests concurrent respiratory acidosis.
- Excessive Compensation: Indicates a superimposed respiratory alkalosis.

18.5 Diagnostic Approach

1. **Check Compensation**

Before delving into the specifics of metabolic acidosis, it is crucial to assess whether the body is compensating for the acidosis. Compensation can be evaluated using the following formula:

$$\text{Expected PaCO2} = 1.5 \times \left[HCO_3^-\right] + 8 \pm 2$$

This equation helps determine if the respiratory system is compensating appropriately for the metabolic acidosis by reducing PaCO2 through hyperventilation.

2. **Anion Gap Calculation**

The next step is to calculate the anion gap (AG), which helps differentiate between different types of metabolic acidosis. The anion gap is calculated using the formula:

$$AG = [Na+] - ([Cl-] + [HCO_3^-])$$

- **Normal Anion Gap Metabolic Acidosis (NAGMA):** An anion gap within the normal range suggests a non-gap metabolic acidosis.
- **High Anion Gap Metabolic Acidosis (HAGMA):** An increased anion gap indicates the presence of unmeasured anions and suggests conditions like lactic acidosis or ketoacidosis.

Corrected anion gap should be calculated in case of hypoalbuminemia using the following formula cAG = AG + 0.25 × (normalalbumin − measuredalbumin(g/L)).

3. **Normal Anion Gap Pathway**

If the anion gap is normal, further evaluation is required to pinpoint the cause of the metabolic acidosis.

18.6 Purpose of the Urinary Anion Gap (UAG)

The urinary anion gap (UAG) is used to estimate the urinary ammonium (NH4+) excretion, which is important in diagnosing the cause of metabolic acidosis, particularly in differentiating between renal and nonrenal causes of normal anion gap metabolic acidosis (NAGMA). Ammonium excretion plays a crucial role in maintaining acid-base balance by facilitating the removal of excess hydrogen ions (H+).

18.7 Calculation of Urinary Anion Gap

The UAG is calculated using the formula:

$$UAG = ([Na+] + [K+]) - [Cl-]$$

Where:

- [Na+] = Sodium concentration in urine
- [K+] = Potassium concentration in urine
- [Cl−] = Chloride concentration in urine

18.8 Interpretation of the UAG

1. **Negative UAG:**
   - A negative UAG indicates high levels of urinary ammonium excretion. This is typical in cases where the kidneys are functioning normally and can excrete excess acid effectively. Common causes include gastrointestinal bicarbonate loss (e.g., diarrhea) where the kidneys respond appropriately by increasing ammonium excretion.
2. **Positive UAG:**
   - A positive UAG suggests impaired ammonium excretion, indicating a renal cause of metabolic acidosis. This is seen in conditions like renal tubular acidosis (RTA), where the kidneys are unable to adequately excrete hydrogen ions and ammonium.

18.9 Mechanism and Clinical Relevance

Ammonium Excretion

- The kidneys help maintain acid-base balance by excreting hydrogen ions in the form of ammonium (NH4+). In states of acidosis, the kidneys increase ammonium excretion to remove excess H+ from the body.
- Ammonium is generated in the renal tubules through the metabolism of glutamine to glutamate, which produces NH4+ and bicarbonate (HCO_3^-). The bicarbonate is reabsorbed into the blood to buffer excess H+, while NH4+ is excreted in the urine.

Clinical Application

- Measuring the UAG provides an indirect estimate of urinary ammonium excretion, as direct measurement is not commonly available in routine clinical practice.

- By interpreting the UAG, clinicians can determine whether the kidneys are responding appropriately to metabolic acidosis. A negative UAG confirms that the kidneys are excreting adequate amounts of ammonium, thus pointing toward a nonrenal cause of acidosis. Conversely, a positive UAG indicates inadequate ammonium excretion, suggesting a renal cause of acidosis.

18.10 Limitations of the Urinary Anion Gap (UAG)

While the urinary anion gap (UAG) is a valuable tool for assessing ammonium excretion and differentiating causes of normal anion gap metabolic acidosis (NAGMA), there are several conditions and factors where its reliability and accuracy are compromised. Here is why the UAG might not be applicable or reliable in certain situations:

1. **Polyuria**
    - **Description:** Polyuria is the production of abnormally large volumes of dilute urine.
    - **Issue:** In polyuria, the concentrations of sodium, potassium, and chloride in urine may be significantly diluted, leading to inaccuracies in the calculation of the UAG. The diluted urine may not reflect the actual excretion rates of these electrolytes, thereby misleading the estimation of ammonium excretion.
2. **High Urine pH (>6.5)**
    - **Description:** Urine pH above 6.5 indicates a more alkaline urine.
    - **Issue:** At high urine pH levels, ammonium (NH4+) is converted to ammonia (NH3), which is a gas and can diffuse back into the bloodstream. This conversion reduces the amount of NH4+ excreted in the urine, making the UAG less reliable as it no longer accurately reflects ammonium excretion.
3. **Presence of Non-chloride Anions in Urine**
    - **Description:** Conditions where significant amounts of non-chloride anions (e.g., ketoacids, salicylates) are present in the urine.
    - **Issue:** The UAG assumes that chloride is the primary anion accompanying ammonium in the urine. When non-chloride anions are present, they can alter the balance of the equation, leading to a positive or less negative UAG that does not accurately indicate ammonium excretion. For example:
        - **Ketoacidosis:** The presence of ketoacids like beta-hydroxybutyrate can result in an inaccurate UAG.
        - **Salicylate Toxicity:** Salicylates and their metabolites can also affect the UAG calculation.

4. **Low Urinary Sodium Concentration (<20 mmol/L)**
    - **Description:** Low levels of sodium in the urine, often seen in conditions of sodium depletion or dehydration.
    - **Issue:** Adequate distal delivery of sodium to the renal tubules is necessary for proper acidification of urine and ammonium excretion. When urinary sodium levels are low, the ability to accurately use the UAG to estimate ammonium excretion is compromised.
5. **Use of Diuretics**
    - **Description:** Diuretics can alter the excretion of electrolytes in the urine.
    - **Issue:** Diuretics can increase urinary excretion of sodium and potassium, which can lead to a positive UAG even in the presence of adequate ammonium excretion. This makes the UAG unreliable for assessing renal ammonium excretion in patients on diuretics.

18.11 Urinary Osmolal Gap: Explanation and Interpretation

18.11.1 Purpose of the Urinary Osmolal Gap

The urinary osmolal gap is used to estimate the presence and concentration of unmeasured osmoles in the urine, primarily ammonium (NH4+), which is crucial in the assessment of renal function and the diagnosis of metabolic acidosis. It is particularly useful when the urinary anion gap (UAG) is unreliable, such as in conditions of polyuria, high urine pH, and the presence of non-chloride anions.

18.11.2 Calculation of the Urinary Osmolal Gap

The urinary osmolal gap (UOG) is calculated as the difference between the measured urine osmolality and the calculated urine osmolality:

$$\text{Urinary Osmolal Gap} = \text{Measured Urine Osmolality} - \text{Calculated Urine Osmolality}$$

The calculated urine osmolality is determined using the formula:

$$\text{Calculated Urine Osmolality} = 2 \times \left(\left[\text{Na}+\right] + \left[\text{K}+\right]\right) + \text{Urine Urea Nitrogen} / 2.8 + \text{Urine Glucose} / 18$$

Where:

- [Na+] = Sodium concentration in urine (mmol/L)
- [K+] = Potassium concentration in urine (mmol/L)
- Urine urea nitrogen is often given in mg/dL and converted using the factor 2.8.

- Urine glucose is often given in mg/dL and converted using the factor 18.

In practice, glucose is often omitted from the calculation unless the patient is diabetic.

18.11.3 Interpretation of the Urinary Osmolal Gap

1. **Low or Normal Urinary Osmolal Gap (<10 mOsm/kg):**
    - A low or normal UOG suggests that there are few unmeasured osmoles in the urine. This can occur in cases where the kidney is effectively excreting ammonium or in conditions not associated with significant production of unmeasured osmoles.
    - It indicates that the kidney's ability to excrete ammonium is likely intact, and the metabolic acidosis is not due to a renal tubular defect.
    - **Nonrenal Causes:** Elevated UOG in metabolic acidosis typically indicates that the acidosis is due to extrarenal factors such as diarrhea, where the kidneys compensate by increasing ammonium excretion.
2. **Elevated Urinary Osmolal Gap (>10 mOsm/kg):**
    - An elevated UOG indicates the presence of significant unmeasured osmoles in the urine, most commonly ammonium (NH4+). This suggests that the kidneys are responding to metabolic acidosis by increasing ammonium excretion.
    - **Renal Causes:** In conditions like distal renal tubular acidosis (RTA), where there is impaired ammonium excretion, the UOG will be low despite metabolic acidosis.

18.11.4 Clinical Significance

- **Differentiating Causes of Metabolic Acidosis:**
    - The urinary osmolal gap helps differentiate between renal and nonrenal causes of normal anion gap metabolic acidosis. A high UOG supports a diagnosis of nonrenal causes (e.g., gastrointestinal bicarbonate loss), whereas a low UOG suggests renal causes (e.g., renal tubular acidosis).
- **Assessment of Renal Ammonium Excretion:**
    - A high UOG indicates effective renal excretion of ammonium, which is an appropriate response to metabolic acidosis. Conversely, a low UOG suggests inadequate ammonium excretion, pointing to a renal tubular defect.

3. **High Anion Gap Pathway**

    If the anion gap is high, further calculations and assessments are needed.

18.12 Delta-Delta (Δ-Δ) Calculation and Interpretation

18.12.1 Purpose of Delta-Delta Calculation

The Delta-Delta (Δ-Δ) calculation is used to assess mixed acid-base disorders, specifically to identify the presence of concurrent metabolic acidosis and metabolic alkalosis or to distinguish between different types of metabolic acidosis. It compares the changes in the anion gap and bicarbonate levels to provide insight into the underlying metabolic disturbances.

18.12.2 Calculation of Delta-Delta

The Δ-Δ is calculated using the following formulas:

$$\Delta AG = \text{Measured AG} - \text{Normal AG}$$
$$\Delta \text{HCO}_3^- = \text{Normal HCO}_3^- - \text{Measured HCO}_3^-$$

The normal values commonly used are:

- Normal AG: 12 mmol/L (may vary slightly depending on the lab reference range).
- Normal HCO_3^-: 24 mmol/L.

The Δ-Δ can be interpreted as:

$$\Delta\Delta = \Delta AG - \Delta \text{HCO}_3^-$$

For lactic acidosis:

$$\Delta\Delta = [0.6 \times \Delta AG] - \Delta \text{HCO}_3^-$$

18.12.3 Interpretation of Delta-Delta

1. **Δ-Δ = −5 to + 5 mmol/L:**
   - Indicates a pure high anion gap metabolic acidosis (HAGMA) without additional metabolic disturbances.
2. **Δ-Δ > +5 mmol/L:**
   - Suggests the presence of both HAGMA and metabolic alkalosis. This means that the increase in the anion gap is greater than the decrease in bicarbonate, indicating an additional metabolic alkalosis.

3. **Δ-Δ < −5 mmol/L:**
    - Suggests the presence of HAGMA and normal anion gap metabolic acidosis (NAGMA). This means that the decrease in bicarbonate is greater than the increase in the anion gap, indicating an additional NAGMA.

18.13 Specific Formula for Lactic Acidosis

Reason for the Different Formula

- In lactic acidosis, the relationship between the increase in the anion gap and the decrease in bicarbonate is not strictly 1:1. This is because lactic acid metabolism and renal handling differ from other causes of HAGMA.
- Studies have shown that in lactic acidosis, the decrease in bicarbonate is typically 0.6 times the increase in the anion gap. This reflects the body's partial compensation for the increased $\Delta\Delta(\text{Lactic Acidosis}) = [0.6 \times \Delta AG] - \Delta \text{HCO}_3^-$.

Clinical Relevance

- This adjusted formula accounts for the partial renal and cellular buffering that occurs in lactic acidosis.
- Using the standard 1:1 Δ-Δ formula in lactic acidosis can lead to underestimating the severity of the bicarbonate decrease or missing concurrent metabolic disturbances.

18.14 Osmolar Gap: Explanation and Interpretation

18.14.1 Purpose of the Osmolar Gap

The osmolar gap is used to detect the presence of unmeasured osmoles in the blood, which can indicate the ingestion of toxic substances or other metabolic disturbances. It is particularly useful in cases of suspected poisoning or unexplained high anion gap metabolic acidosis.

18.14.2 Calculation of the Osmolar Gap

The osmolar gap is calculated as the difference between the measured serum osmolality and the calculated serum osmolality:

$$\text{Osmolar Gap} = \text{Measured Serum Osmolality} - \text{Calculated Serum Osmolality}$$

Measured Serum Osmolality

- This is determined directly using an osmometer.

Calculated Serum Osmolality

- The calculated serum osmolality is derived from the concentrations of the main solutes in the serum, typically sodium, glucose, and blood urea nitrogen (BUN).

  The formula for calculated serum osmolality is:

$$\text{Calculated Serum Osmolality} = 2 \times [\text{Na}+] + \text{Glucose} / 18 + \text{BUN} / 2.8$$

  Where:

- [Na+] = Sodium concentration in mmol/L.
- Glucose is in mg/dL (divide by 18 to convert to mmol/L).
- BUN is in mg/dL (divide by 2.8 to convert to mmol/L).

18.14.3 Interpretation of the Osmolar Gap

1. **Normal Osmolar Gap:**
   - A normal osmolar gap is typically within the range of −10 to +10 mOsm/kg.
   - This indicates that the measured and calculated serum osmolalities are in close agreement, suggesting no significant presence of unmeasured osmoles.
2. **Elevated Osmolar Gap (>10 mOsm/kg):**
   - An elevated osmolar gap indicates the presence of unmeasured osmoles in the blood.
   - Common causes include the ingestion of toxic alcohols (e.g., methanol, ethylene glycol, isopropanol, propylene glycol), which are not accounted for in the calculated osmolality formula.

18.14.4 Clinical Relevance

Toxic Alcohol Ingestion

- **Methanol and Ethylene Glycol:** Both can cause severe metabolic acidosis and elevated osmolar gap. These substances are metabolized into toxic metabolites (formic acid from methanol and glycolic/oxalic acids from ethylene glycol), leading to an increased anion gap metabolic acidosis and elevated osmolar gap.
- **Isopropanol:** Leads to elevated osmolar gap but typically does not cause metabolic acidosis because it is metabolized to acetone, which is less acidic.

Case of Unexplained Metabolic Acidosis

- When a patient presents with high anion gap metabolic acidosis and the cause is not immediately apparent, measuring the osmolar gap can help identify the presence of unmeasured toxic substances.

18.15 Conclusion

The management of metabolic acidosis in the ICU involves a structured approach to diagnose the underlying cause. By calculating the anion gap, urinary anion gap, and delta-delta, clinicians can narrow down potential etiologies and tailor treatment accordingly. Recognizing and addressing the root cause is paramount to effective management and improving patient outcomes.

Algorithm 18.1: Approach to metabolic acidosis in the ICU

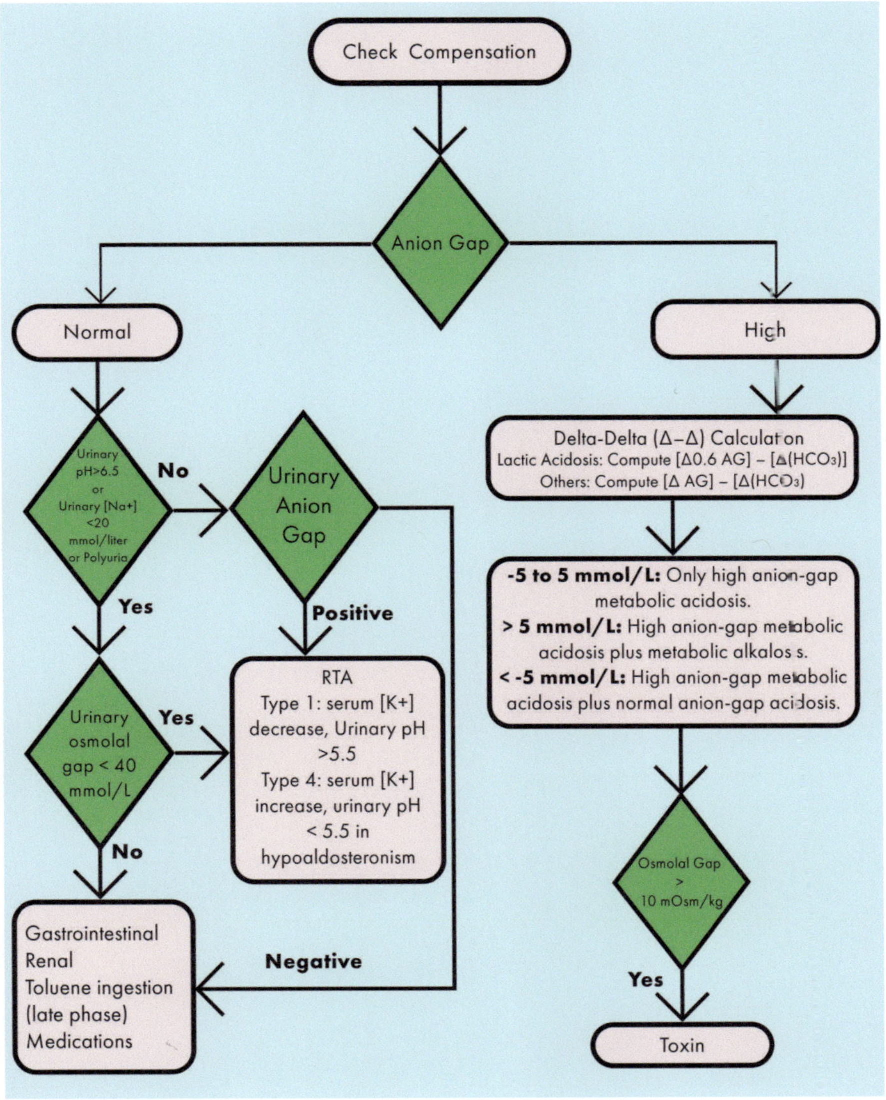

Bibliography

1. Berend K, de Vries AP, Gans RO. Physiological approach to assessment of acid-base disturbances. N Engl J Med. 2014;371(15):1434–45.
2. Seifter JL. Integration of acid-base and electrolyte disorders. N Engl J Med. 2014;371(19):1821–31.

Chapter 19
Approach to Metabolic Alkalosis in the ICU

19.1 Introduction

Metabolic alkalosis is a condition characterized by an increase in blood pH due to an excess of bicarbonate (HCO_3^-) or a loss of hydrogen ions (H^+). It involves two phases: the generation phase, where the initial disturbance occurs, and the maintenance phase, where the alkalosis is sustained. The generation phase often results from a loss of acid via gastrointestinal (GI) or renal routes or an excessive gain of bicarbonate, while the maintenance phase is typically due to impaired renal excretion of bicarbonate.

Sustained metabolic alkalosis usually requires both a generating factor and a maintenance factor. The kidneys play a crucial role in excreting excess bicarbonate; thus, impaired renal function or factors that reduce bicarbonate excretion are essential in maintaining alkalosis. Severe metabolic alkalosis is associated with significant mortality risks. Studies have shown that mortality increases markedly when the arterial pH exceeds 7.55, reaching as high as 80% with pH levels above 7.65. This underscores the critical nature of timely diagnosis and intervention [1] [Ref: Algorithm 19.1].

19.2 Pathophysiology

19.2.1 Generation Phase

- Loss of Acid: Common causes include vomiting or nasogastric suction, leading to the loss of gastric hydrochloric acid (HCl). Renal losses can occur due to diuretic use, which increases the excretion of sodium and chloride, indirectly causing bicarbonate retention.

S. B. Mishra et al., *Mastering ICU Care*,
https://doi.org/10.1007/978-981-95-0179-3_19

- Gain of Bicarbonate: Excessive ingestion of bicarbonate or antacids, often seen in conditions like milk-alkali syndrome, can elevate serum bicarbonate levels [2].

19.2.2 Maintenance Phase

- Impaired Bicarbonate Excretion: The kidneys are central to maintaining acid-base balance. Under normal circumstances, the kidneys can excrete excess bicarbonate to correct alkalosis. However, factors such as volume depletion, hypokalemia, and decreased chloride availability impair the kidney's ability to excrete bicarbonate, thus maintaining the alkalosis.

19.2.3 Role of Chloride Depletion

Chloride depletion plays a pivotal role in driving metabolic alkalosis, often referred to as "chloride depletion alkalosis." In conditions like vomiting, diuretic use, or Bartter and Gitelman syndromes, there is a significant loss of chloride. Chloride is essential for bicarbonate excretion in the distal nephron; its depletion impairs the kidney's ability to excrete bicarbonate, thereby maintaining alkalosis [3].

19.2.4 Role of Potassium Depletion

Potassium depletion exacerbates metabolic alkalosis by several mechanisms:

- Increased Hydrogen Ion Secretion: Hypokalemia stimulates the renal secretion of hydrogen ions to conserve potassium, leading to increased bicarbonate reabsorption.
- Enhanced Ammonia (NH_3) Generation: Hypokalemia increases renal ammonia production, which combines with secreted hydrogen ions to form ammonium (NH_4^+), facilitating further acid loss.

19.3 Renal Mechanisms in Acid-Base Regulation

- Proximal Tubule: The Na^+-H^+ exchanger plays a significant role in bicarbonate reabsorption. Hydrogen ions are secreted in exchange for sodium, facilitating the reabsorption of filtered bicarbonate.

- Collecting Ducts: In the distal nephron, specifically the alpha-intercalated cells, hydrogen ions are secreted via H^+-ATPase and H^+-K^+-ATPase pumps. This secretion is vital for acid excretion and bicarbonate reabsorption.
- Distal Nephron Segments: Both bicarbonate reabsorption and secretion occur here, and their regulation is crucial in the maintenance phase of metabolic alkalosis [4].

19.4 Diagnostic Approach

1. **Confirm Compensation**
   - Arterial Blood Gases (ABG): Review ABG to assess respiratory compensation. In metabolic alkalosis, the body hypoventilates to retain CO_2, which combines with water to form carbonic acid, partially offsetting the alkalosis. Assessing compensation ensures that concurrent acid-base disorders are not overlooked [5].
2. **Evaluate Clinical History**
   - Vomiting or Nasogastric Suction: Indicates loss of gastric acid.
   - Diuretic Use: Loop and thiazide diuretics cause loss of sodium and chloride.
   - Recent Surgery: May cause fluid shifts and electrolyte imbalances.
   - Mineralocorticoid Excess: Conditions like hyperaldosteronism increase sodium retention and potassium loss.
3. **Serum Calcium Assessment**
   - Serum Calcium >14 mg/dL (3.5 mmol/L): Suggests milk-alkali syndrome or hypercalcemia of malignancy, both of which can contribute to metabolic alkalosis.
4. **Assess Chloride Responsiveness via Urine Chloride**
   - Urine Chloride <10 mmol/L: Indicates chloride-responsive metabolic alkalosis, commonly due to volume depletion from vomiting or diuretic use. The low urine chloride reflects the kidneys' attempt to conserve chloride.
   - Management: Administration of isotonic saline replenishes chloride and volume, allowing the kidneys to excrete excess bicarbonate.
   - Urine Chloride >30 mmol/L: Suggests chloride-resistant metabolic alkalosis, often due to mineralocorticoid excess or severe potassium depletion.
5. **Assess Potassium Status**
   - Hypokalemia: Further exacerbates alkalosis and is common in both chloride-responsive and resistant forms. Measurement of serum and urine potassium can help in identifying the cause.

6. **Blood Pressure Measurement**

   - Low or Normal Blood Pressure:

     – Bartter Syndrome: Characterized by hypokalemia, metabolic alkalosis, normal to low blood pressure, and high urinary calcium excretion.
     – Gitelman Syndrome: Similar to Bartter syndrome but with low urinary calcium excretion.

   - High Blood Pressure:

     – Mineralocorticoid Excess: Conditions like primary hyperaldosteronism cause sodium retention (leading to hypertension), potassium loss, and metabolic alkalosis.

19.5 Mortality Risks

Severe metabolic alkalosis is associated with increased mortality rates. An arterial pH greater than 7.55 significantly elevates the risk of cardiac arrhythmias, neuromuscular instability, and decreased cerebral blood flow. Mortality rates can reach up to 80% when pH exceeds 7.65, emphasizing the urgency of prompt diagnosis and management [6].

19.6 Treatment Modalities

Address Underlying Causes
- Vomiting: Use antiemetics to control nausea and vomiting.
- Diuretic Use: Discontinue or adjust dosage under medical supervision.
- Mineralocorticoid Excess: Treat underlying endocrine disorders.

Chloride Repletion
- Intravenous Saline Infusion: Restores volume and chloride levels in chloride-responsive alkalosis, promoting renal bicarbonate excretion.

Potassium Repletion
- Oral or Intravenous Potassium Chloride: Corrects hypokalemia, reduces renal hydrogen ion secretion, and aids in correcting alkalosis.

Acetazolamide
- Carbonic Anhydrase Inhibitor: Promotes renal bicarbonate excretion by inhibiting bicarbonate reabsorption in the proximal tubule. Useful in patients who cannot tolerate volume repletion.

Supportive Care
- Monitor Electrolytes and ABGs: Regular monitoring to guide therapy.
- Dialysis: In severe cases or when conservative measures fail, especially in patients with renal failure.

19.7 Conclusion

Effective management of metabolic alkalosis requires a systematic approach that includes understanding the pathophysiological mechanisms, accurately diagnosing the underlying cause, and implementing appropriate treatment strategies. Recognizing the roles of chloride and potassium depletion, renal function, and hormonal imbalances is crucial. Prompt intervention not only corrects the biochemical abnormalities but also reduces the associated mortality risks.

Algorithm 19.1: Approach to metabolic alkalosis in the ICU

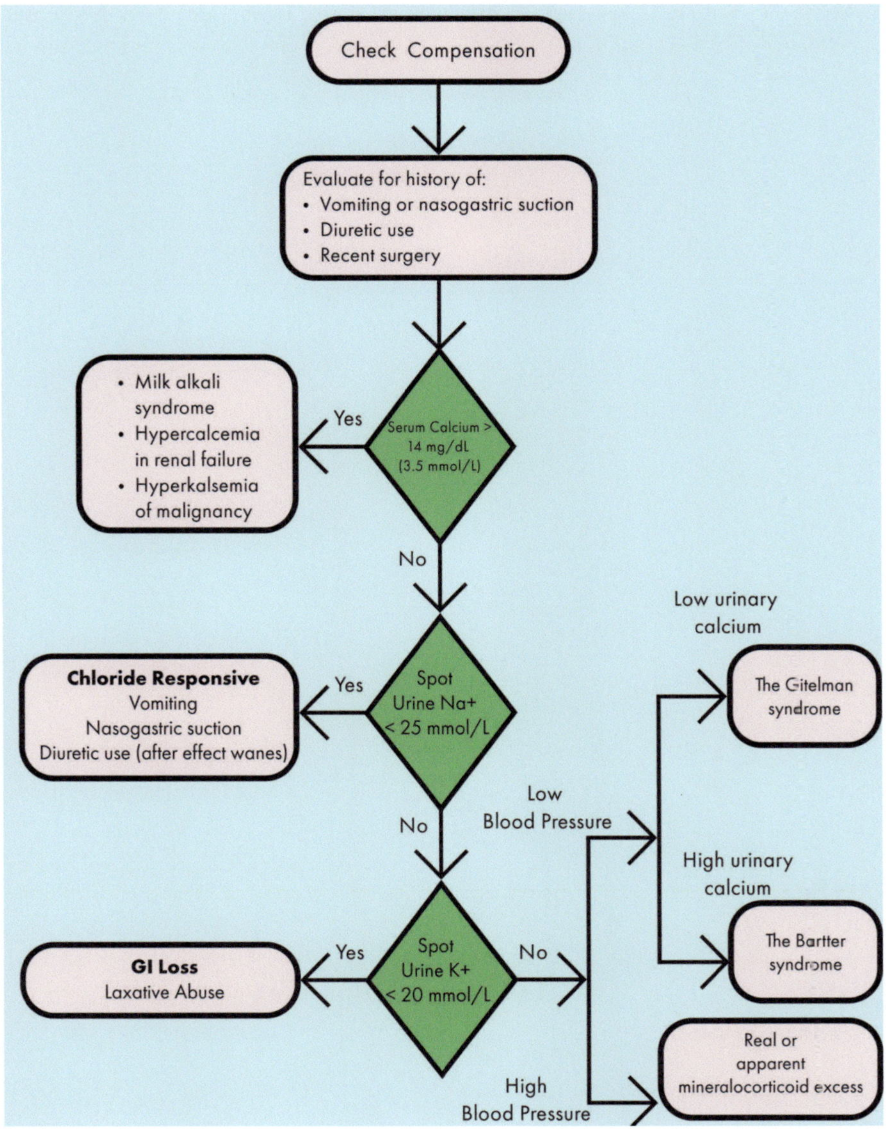

Bibliography

1. Do C, Vasquez PC, Soleimani M. Metabolic alkalosis pathogenesis, diagnosis, and treatment: core curriculum 2022. Am J Kidney Dis. 2022;80(4):536–51.
2. Emmett M. Metabolic alkalosis: a brief pathophysiologic review. Clin J Am Soc Nephrol. 2020;15(12):1848–56.
3. Gennari FJ. Pathophysiology of metabolic alkalosis: a new classification based on the centrality of stimulated collecting duct ion transport. Am J Kidney Dis. 2011;58(4):626–36.
4. Pahari DK, Kazmi W, Raman G, Biswas S. Diagnosis and management of metabolic alkalosis. J Indian Med Assoc. 2006;104(11):630–4, 6.
5. Tinawi M. Pathophysiology, evaluation, and management of metabolic alkalosis. Cureus. 2021;13(1):e12841.
6. Soifer JT, Kim HT. Approach to metabolic alkalosis. Emerg Med Clin North Am. 2014;32(2):453–63.

Chapter 20
Approach to Oliguria in the ICU

20.1 Introduction

Oliguria, commonly defined as a urine output (UO) of less than 0.5 mL/kg/h over a period of 6 h, is a frequent clinical concern in the intensive care unit (ICU). However, recent evidence suggests that lower thresholds, such as UO less than 0.3 mL/kg/h, may be more predictive of acute kidney injury (AKI) in perioperative and critically ill patients. Oliguria can represent either a physiological response to various stimuli or a pathological process indicating decreased renal perfusion or injury. Distinguishing between physiological and pathological oliguria is essential to guide appropriate interventions and avoid potential harm from unnecessary treatments. This chapter provides a comprehensive approach to assessing and managing oliguria in the ICU, incorporating current guidelines and evidence-based practices [1] [Ref: Algorithm 20.1].

20.2 Initial Assessment

20.2.1 Confirm Oliguria and Assess Urine Output Trends

Rationale: Accurate diagnosis of oliguria requires confirmation of reduced urine output over a specific period. While traditionally defined as UO less than 0.5 mL/kg/h for 6 h, recent studies suggest that thresholds such as less than 0.3 mL/kg/h may be more reliable indicators of impending AKI in critically ill patients [1].

Clinical Considerations: Document urine output meticulously using an indwelling Foley catheter, ensuring consistent readings over the specified period. Evaluate trends in urine output rather than isolated measurements to identify persistent oliguria [2].

S. B. Mishra et al., *Mastering ICU Care*,
https://doi.org/10.1007/978-981-95-0179-3_20

20.2.2 Check for Mechanical Issues

Rationale: Mechanical problems associated with urinary catheters can falsely indicate oliguria.
Clinical Considerations: Inspect the catheter for kinks, obstructions, or dislodgement, and ensure proper placement.

20.2.3 Evaluate Hemodynamics and Renal Perfusion Pressure

Rationale: Hemodynamic instability, such as hypotension and tachycardia, can lead to decreased renal perfusion and oliguria.
Clinical Considerations: Measure mean arterial pressure (MAP) and heart rate, and assess for signs of poor perfusion like cool extremities or altered mental status. In cases of vasodilatory hypotension, vasopressors may be necessary to maintain adequate renal perfusion pressure.
Intervention: Administer isotonic fluids judiciously and simultaneously start vasopressors as needed to achieve target MAP (usually ≥65 mm Hg) and improve renal perfusion. Watch out for patients in fluid overload status. Monitor the response of urine output to fluid and vasopressor therapy, as improvements may indicate restoration of renal perfusion [3].

20.3 Diagnostic Work-Up

20.3.1 Distinguish Physiological from Pathological Oliguria

Rationale: Oliguria may be a physiological response to factors such as pain, stress, or the release of antidiuretic hormone (ADH), rather than an indicator of AKI or decreased renal perfusion.
Intervention: Address the underlying causes of physiological oliguria, such as providing adequate analgesia or adjusting medications. Avoid unnecessary fluid administration to prevent fluid overload [4].

20.3.2 Check Volume Status and Fluid Responsiveness

Rationale: Determining a patient's fluid status is critical for deciding appropriate interventions. Dynamic assessments can help identify whether a patient is likely to respond to fluid administration.

Clinical Considerations: Evaluate fluid balance over the last 24–72 h, check for signs of hypovolemia (e.g., dry mucous membranes, hypotension) or fluid overload (e.g., edema, jugular venous distension). Use tools such as the Venous Excess UltraSound (VExUS) score and lung ultrasound to assess volume status.

Diagnostic Tests: Perform dynamic assessments like passive leg raising (PLR) or administer a small-volume fluid challenge while monitoring hemodynamic parameters (e.g., stroke volume, cardiac output) to assess fluid responsiveness.

20.3.3 Consider Intra-abdominal Pressure

Rationale: Increased intra-abdominal pressure (IAP), as seen in conditions like abdominal compartment syndrome or after laparoscopic surgery, can reduce renal perfusion and lead to oliguria that is not responsive to fluid administration.

Clinical Considerations: Assess for risk factors of increased IAP, such as recent abdominal surgery, trauma, or ascites. Measure bladder pressure as a surrogate for IAP if increased pressure is suspected.

Intervention: Manage elevated IAP through decompression techniques, optimizing ventilator settings, or surgical intervention if necessary.

20.3.4 Consider Furosemide Stress Test (FST)

Rationale: The Furosemide Stress Test can assess tubular function and help predict progression to severe AKI in oliguric patients.

Clinical Considerations: In patients with suspected AKI, administer a single dose of furosemide (1.0 mg/kg for loop diuretic naïve patients and 1.5 mg/kg for those with prior loop diuretic exposure) intravenously and observe the urine output response over the next 2 h.

Diagnostic Implications: A poor diuretic response (urine output less than 200 ml over 2 h) may indicate severe tubular injury and a higher risk of progression to severe AKI, potentially prompting earlier intervention or renal replacement therapy.

20.4 Management Based on Volume Status

Hypovolemia: Administer isotonic fluids judiciously to restore intravascular volume and improve renal perfusion, guided by dynamic assessments of fluid responsiveness.

20.5 Euvolemia with Oliguria (Permissive Oliguria)

Rationale: In some hemodynamically stable patients who are not fluid responsive, tolerating lower urine outputs (permissive oliguria) may be safe and can prevent the risks associated with fluid overload.

Clinical Considerations: Consider the overall clinical context, and monitor for signs of worsening renal function or fluid overload. Recognize that aggressive fluid resuscitation to increase urine output may not improve outcomes and can be harmful.

Intervention: Avoid unnecessary fluid administration. Focus on optimizing hemodynamics and treating underlying conditions without overloading the patient with fluids.

20.6 Fluid Overload (Congestion)

Rationale: Fluid overload can cause oliguria due to increased venous pressures, leading to decreased renal perfusion and increased intra-abdominal pressure.

Clinical Considerations: Look for signs of fluid overload, such as peripheral edema, jugular venous distension, pulmonary crackles, and positive fluid balance.

Intervention: Use diuretics to remove excess fluid and reduce congestion. In cases where diuretics are ineffective, consider renal replacement therapy for fluid removal.

20.7 Monitoring and Follow-Up

20.7.1 Continuous Monitoring

Rationale: Ongoing assessment is crucial for detecting changes in renal function and response to therapy.

Clinical Considerations: Monitor urine output hourly, and regularly measure serum creatinine, blood urea nitrogen (BUN), fractional excretion of Sodium (FeNa), and electrolytes. Reassess hemodynamic parameters and volume status frequently.

20.7.2 Advanced Biomarkers for AKI

Rationale: Biomarkers such as neutrophil gelatinase-associated lipocalin (NGAL), cystatin C, and TIMP-2 × IGFBP7 can provide early detection of AKI and assist in risk stratification.

Clinical Considerations: Utilize these biomarkers in patients at high risk of AKI or when early detection is critical for management decisions.

Diagnostic Tests: Measure serum or urinary levels of NGAL, cystatin C, or TIMP-2 × IGFBP7 as adjuncts to traditional markers.

20.8 Medication Management

Rationale: Adjusting medication doses based on renal function is essential to avoid further renal impairment.

Clinical Considerations: Discontinue nephrotoxic drugs if possible, and adjust doses of essential medications. Consider the renal clearance of all medications prescribed.

20.9 Conclusion

Managing oliguria in the ICU requires a systematic and nuanced approach to distinguish between physiological and pathological causes. Early and accurate diagnosis, appropriate use of dynamic hemodynamic assessments, judicious fluid management—including the concept of permissive oliguria—and timely interventions are crucial for effective management. Monitoring advanced biomarkers can aid in early detection of AKI and guide therapeutic decisions. Continuous reassessment helps optimize treatment strategies and improve outcomes for critically ill patients.

Algorithm 20.1: Approach to oliguria in the ICU

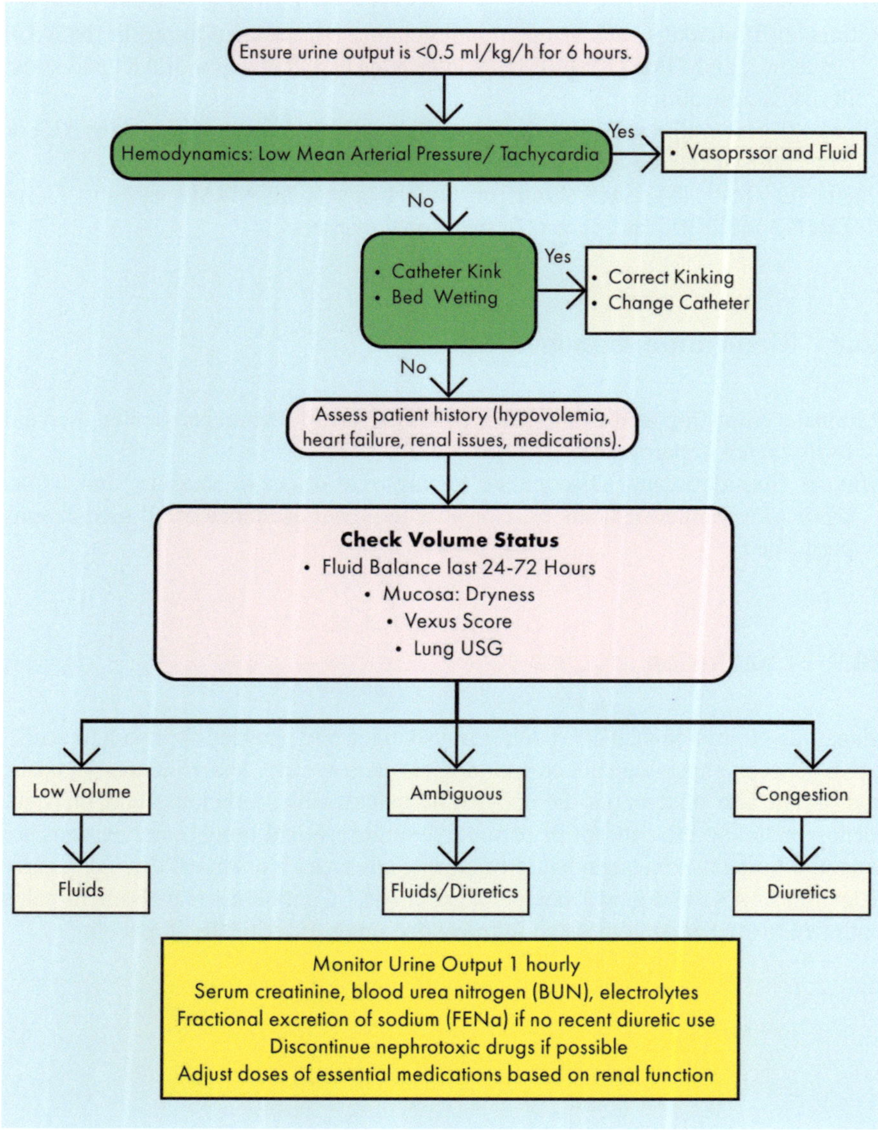

Bibliography

1. Ostermann M, Shaw AD, Joannidis M. Management of oliguria. Intensive Care Med. 2023;49(1):103–6.
2. Klein SJ, Lehner GF, Forni LG, Joannidis M. Oliguria in critically ill patients: a narrative review. J Nephrol. 2018;31(6):855–62.
3. Schetz M, Hoste E. Understanding oliguria in the critically ill. Intensive Care Med. 2017;43(6):914–6.
4. Schortgen F, Schetz M. Does this critically ill patient with oliguria need more fluids, a vasopressor, or neither? Intensive Care Med. 2017;43(6):907–10.

Chapter 21
Approach to Polyuria in the ICU

21.1 Introduction

Polyuria, defined as urine output exceeding 3 L per day in adults, is a significant concern in critically ill patients. It can lead to dehydration, electrolyte imbalances, and hemodynamic instability, complicating the management of patients in the Intensive Care Unit (ICU). Polyuria may result from various etiologies, including endocrine disorders, renal dysfunction, fluid imbalances, or as an adverse effect of medications.

A systematic approach to diagnosing and managing polyuria is essential to prevent complications and improve patient outcomes. A critical aspect of this evaluation is classifying polyuria based on urine osmolality, which helps differentiate between water diuresis, solute diuresis, and mixed diuresis. This classification guides further diagnostic testing and management strategies [1, 2] [Ref: Algorithm 21.1].

21.2 Classification of Polyuria Based on Urine Osmolality

1. Water Diuresis (Urine Osmolality<150 mOsm/kg)
2. Solute Diuresis (Urine Osmolality>300 mOsm/kg)
3. Mixed Diuresis (Urine Osmolality 150–300 mOsm/kg)

Diagnostic Approach

1. **Initial Assessment**

- Hemodynamic Stability:
- Assessment: Check for signs of hypotension, tachycardia, or hypovolemia.
- If Unstable:
- Initiate immediate resuscitation with isotonic intravenous fluids (e.g., 0.9% normal saline).

S. B. Mishra et al., *Mastering ICU Care*,
https://doi.org/10.1007/978-981-95-0179-3_21

- Monitor serum sodium and osmolality closely to prevent rapid shifts that can lead to osmotic demyelination or cerebral edema.
- If Stable:
- Proceed with a detailed evaluation of urine output and laboratory investigations.

2. **Quantify Urine Output**

   - Urine Output >250 mL/h:
   - Confirm polyuria by measuring urine output over several hours.
   - Rule out common causes such as excessive fluid administration or diuretic use.

3. **Immediate Laboratory Tests**

   - Urine Osmolality:
   - <150 mOsm/kg: Suggests water diuresis.
   - 150–300 mOsm/kg: Indicates mixed diuresis.
   - >300 mOsm/kg: Consistent with solute diuresis.
   - Serum Osmolality and Electrolytes:
   - Evaluate serum sodium, potassium, calcium, glucose, blood urea nitrogen (BUN), and creatinine.
   - Assess plasma osmolality to determine the gradient driving water movement.
   - Serum and Urine Glucose:
   - Rule out hyperglycemia-induced osmotic diuresis.
   - Serum Copeptin Levels:
   - Copeptin is a stable surrogate marker for vasopressin (antidiuretic hormone, ADH) and aids in differentiating between CDI and NDI.

4. **Interpretation Based on Urine Osmolality**

   A. **Water Diuresis (<150 mOsm/kg).**
   Possible Causes:

   - Central Diabetes Insipidus (CDI): Deficiency in ADH production.
   - Nephrogenic Diabetes Insipidus (NDI): Renal resistance to ADH.
   - Primary Polydipsia: Excessive water intake suppressing ADH secretion.

   Diagnostic Approach:

   - Water Deprivation Test: Gradual water restriction under close monitoring to assess the ability to concentrate urine.

     CDI: Inability to concentrate urine; significant (>50%) increase in urine osmolality after desmopressin administration.
     NDI: Little to no change in urine osmolality after desmopressin.
     Primary Polydipsia: Gradual increase in urine osmolality during deprivation; partial response to desmopressin.

   - Copeptin Measurement:

     Low Copeptin Levels: Suggest CDI.
     High Copeptin Levels: Suggest NDI.

- MRI Imaging:

  Perform MRI of the brain to identify structural abnormalities in the hypothalamic-pituitary axis in suspected CDI.

B. **Solute Diuresis (>300 mOsm/kg)**
   Possible Causes:

- Hyperglycemia: Uncontrolled diabetes mellitus leading to glucose-induced osmotic diuresis.
- Mannitol Administration: Osmotic diuretic used in cases of increased intracranial pressure.
- High-Protein Diets/Urea Diuresis: Common in ICU patients receiving enteral or parenteral nutrition.
- Radiocontrast Agents: Can cause osmotic diuresis post-imaging studies.

Diagnostic Approach:

- Measure Serum Glucose:

  Hyperglycemia requires prompt insulin therapy to reduce glucose levels and osmotic diuresis.

- Medication Review:

  Identify and adjust medications like mannitol or diuretics contributing to solute diuresis.

- Electrolyte-Free Water Clearance:

Calculation:

Osmolar Clearance (Cosm) : $C = UV/P$
Free Water Clearance (C) : $CH2O = V \times [1 - (Uosm/Posm)]$
Electrolyte − Free Water Clearance : $E — Ch2O = VE — Cosm$
V—Total urinary volume per unit time, U—Urinary concentration of the substance, P—plasma concentration of the substance, Uosm—Urine osmolality, Posm—Plasma osmolality.

Clinical Application:

- Guides fluid management in patients with hypernatremia due to osmotic diuresis.
- Aids in preventing rapid correction of sodium levels, which can be harmful.

Management of Iatrogenic Causes:

- Adjust nutritional support to prevent excessive protein intake.
- Limit use of osmotic agents when possible.

C. **Mixed Diuresis (150–300 mOsm/kg).**
   Possible Causes:

- Partial Diabetes Insipidus: Partial deficiency or resistance to ADH.

- Concurrent Solute Overload with Water Diuresis: Combination of factors causing both solute and water loss.

Diagnostic Approach:

- Detailed History and Examination:
- Assess for conditions that may cause partial DI or solute overload.

Laboratory Evaluation:

- Evaluate serum and urine electrolytes, glucose, and other solutes.
- Assess for medications or conditions contributing to mixed diuresis.

Water Deprivation Test and Copeptin Levels:

- May help identify partial CDI or NDI.

5. **Common ICU Causes of Polyuria**

- Resolving Acute Tubular Necrosis (ATN):
  - Description: During the diuretic phase of ATN recovery, patients may have high urine output.
  - Management: Careful fluid and electrolyte replacement to match losses.
- Post-Obstructive Diuresis:
  - Description: Significant diuresis following relief of urinary tract obstruction.
  - Management: Monitor and replace fluid and electrolyte losses to prevent hypovolemia.
- Medication-Induced Diuresis:
  - Description: Use of diuretics or other medications leading to increased urine output.
  - Management: Review and adjust medications as necessary.

6. **Further Diagnostic Tests**

- Hypertonic Saline Infusion Test:
  - Purpose: Assesses arginine vasopressin (AVP) release in response to increased plasma osmolality.
  - Usefulness: Helps distinguish between CDI and NDI when the water deprivation test is inconclusive.
- MRI Imaging:
  - Purpose: Detects structural abnormalities in the hypothalamus or pituitary gland in suspected CDI.
- Renal Function Tests:
  - Purpose: Evaluate for intrinsic renal diseases contributing to polyuria.

7. **Management Tailored to the ICU Setting**

- Fluid Balance:
  - Monitoring: Accurate recording of intake and output is essential.
  - Adjustment: Modify fluid administration to match losses, prevent dehydration, and maintain hemodynamic stability.
- Medication Adjustments:
  - Review: Identify and modify medications contributing to polyuria.
  - Desmopressin Administration:
  - Indication: Used in CDI to reduce urine output.
- Dosage:
  - IV or SC: 1–2 μg every 12 h.
  - Intranasal: 10–20 μg every 12 h.
  - Monitoring: Observe for response and monitor for hyponatremia.
  - Electrolyte and Osmolality Monitoring:
  - Frequency: Regular checks of serum electrolytes and osmolality.
  - Goal: Detect and correct imbalances promptly; avoid rapid sodium correction.
- Nutritional Support:
  - Adjustment: Modify protein intake to prevent urea-induced osmotic diuresis.
  - Balance: Ensure appropriate caloric and electrolyte intake.
- Patient Safety:
  - Prevent Complications: Implement measures to avoid hypotension, acute kidney injury, and electrolyte disturbances.
  - Education: Inform the healthcare team about the importance of monitoring and timely intervention.

21.3 Conclusion

Managing polyuria in the ICU requires a thorough and systematic approach to diagnose and treat underlying causes promptly. Classifying polyuria based on urine osmolality into water diuresis, solute diuresis, or mixed diuresis is fundamental in guiding further investigations and management. Essential diagnostic tools include urine and serum osmolality measurements, water deprivation tests, copeptin levels, and imaging studies.

Tailored management strategies in the ICU emphasize fluid balance, careful monitoring of electrolytes and osmolality, medication adjustments, and addressing the underlying cause. Early recognition and appropriate intervention are crucial to prevent complications such as dehydration, electrolyte imbalances, and hemodynamic instability, ultimately improving patient outcomes in the critical care environment.

Algorithm 21.1 Approach to polyuria in the ICU

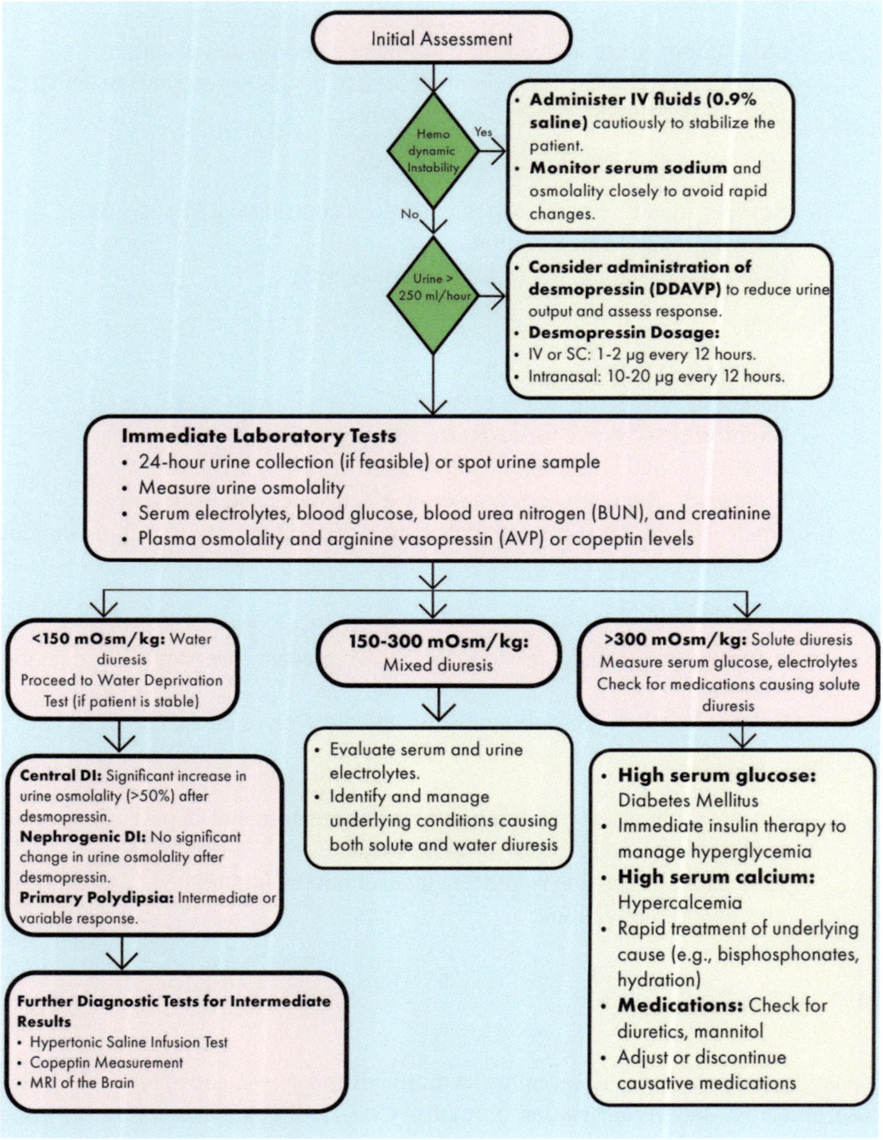

Bibliography

1. Lamas C, del Pozo C, Villabona C. Clinical guidelines for management of diabetes insipidus and syndrome of inappropriate antidiuretic hormone secretion after pituitary surgery. Endocrinol Nutr. 2014;61(4):e15–24.
2. Ramírez-Guerrero G, Müller-Ortiz H, Pedreros-Rosales C. Polyuria in adults. A diagnostic approach based on pathophysiology. Rev Clin Esp (Barc). 2022;222(5):301–8.

Chapter 22
Approach to Hyponatremia

22.1 Introduction

Hyponatremia, defined as a serum sodium concentration below 135 mmol/L, is the most common electrolyte disturbance encountered in clinical practice, particularly in the intensive care unit (ICU). It is associated with a spectrum of clinical manifestations, ranging from mild, nonspecific symptoms to severe, life-threatening neurological complications. Even mild hyponatremia (serum sodium 130–134 mmol/L) has been linked to increased mortality, falls, and cognitive impairments, especially in the elderly. Effective management requires a comprehensive understanding of the underlying pathophysiological mechanisms, careful assessment, and prompt, appropriate treatment to prevent complications such as cerebral edema and osmotic demyelination syndrome [1, 2] [Ref: Algorithm 22.1].

22.2 Pathophysiological Mechanisms

Hyponatremia results from an imbalance between water intake and excretion relative to sodium [3].

22.2.1 Classification by Serum Osmolality

- Hypotonic Hyponatremia: Most common form; reflects true excess of water relative to sodium.
- Isotonic Hyponatremia: Often a laboratory artifact (pseudohyponatremia) due to hyperlipidemia or hyperproteinemia.

S. B. Mishra et al., *Mastering ICU Care*,
https://doi.org/10.1007/978-981-95-0179-3_22

- Hypertonic Hyponatremia: Caused by the presence of osmotically active substances (e.g., hyperglycemia, mannitol) that draw water into the extracellular space, diluting serum sodium.
- Hyperglycemia-Induced Hyponatremia: Elevated glucose increases plasma osmolality, causing water shift from intracellular to extracellular space, diluting serum sodium.
- **Pseudohyponatremia:** Hyperlipidemia or Hyperproteinemia: Excess lipids or proteins can interfere with laboratory measurements, falsely lowering serum sodium concentration without affecting osmolality.

22.3 Clinical Presentation

22.3.1 Initial Assessment

22.3.1.1 Rule Out Non-hypotonic Causes

- The first step in managing hyponatremia is to rule out other causes of low sodium that are not due to hypotonicity, such as hyperglycemia or the presence of other osmoles (e.g., mannitol). These conditions do not require the same treatment as true hypotonic hyponatremia, and correcting them often resolves the hyponatremia.

22.3.1.2 Severe Symptoms of Hyponatremia

Severe symptoms of hyponatremia typically arise from the effects of acute cerebral edema caused by a rapid decline in serum sodium levels. These symptoms include:

- **Seizures**: Hyponatremia can lead to neuronal swelling, which disrupts normal brain function, resulting in seizures. Seizures in hyponatremia are an emergency and indicate a critical imbalance of electrolytes in the brain.
- **Coma**: When the brain swells due to fluid shifts from the extracellular to the intracellular space, consciousness can be profoundly impaired, leading to coma. This is a life-threatening condition and requires immediate intervention.
- **Respiratory Arrest**: In extreme cases, the brainstem can be affected by the swelling, leading to respiratory arrest due to impaired autonomic control. This represents the most severe manifestation of hyponatremia.
- **Profound Confusion or Agitation**: Severe hyponatremia can cause a significant alteration in mental status, leading to agitation or severe confusion, which can progress to coma.
  - If the patient presents with severe symptoms (e.g., seizures, altered mental status), immediate treatment is required. Administer a 100 mL bolus of 3% normal saline (NS) intravenously over 10 min. This can be repeated up to two

additional times if severe symptoms persist. The goal here is rapid correction of serum sodium to alleviate life-threatening symptoms, with careful monitoring to avoid overly rapid correction, which could lead to osmotic demyelination syndrome.

22.3.1.3 Moderately Severe Symptoms of Hyponatremia

Moderately severe symptoms are less dramatic but still require prompt attention to prevent progression to more severe states:

- **Nausea and Vomiting**: These symptoms are often the first indicators of hyponatremia and result from cerebral edema.
- **Headache**: As cerebral edema progresses, intracranial pressure increases, leading to headaches. This is an early sign that the brain is being affected by the hyponatremia.
- **Confusion**: This can range from mild disorientation to severe confusion. It reflects the impact of sodium imbalance on brain function.
  - For patients with moderately severe symptoms (e.g., nausea, headache, confusion), a less aggressive approach is recommended. Administer a 100 mL bolus of 3% NS intravenously over 20 min. This approach aims to stabilize the patient while avoiding the risks associated with rapid sodium correction.

22.4 Method of Estimating Volume Status

Assessing volume status is critical in determining the etiology of hyponatremia and guiding treatment. This involves a combination of clinical examination and laboratory tests:

- **Physical Examination**: Look for signs of hypovolemia such as low blood pressure, tachycardia, dry mucous membranes, poor skin turgor, and reduced urine output. Conversely, hypervolemia may present with signs like jugular venous distension, peripheral edema, and ascites.
- **Laboratory Tests**:
  - **Blood Urea Nitrogen (BUN) and Creatinine**: These can indicate kidney function and help in assessing volume status. Elevated BUN/creatinine ratios are often seen in hypovolemic states.
  - **Hematocrit**: Hematocrit levels can rise in hypovolemia due to hemoconcentration.
  - Once immediate symptoms are managed, the next step is to assess the patient's volume status. This is a critical decision point, as the management of hyponatremia varies significantly based on whether the patient is hypovolemic, euvolemic, or hypervolemic.

- **Hypovolemic Hyponatremia:**
  - In cases of hypovolemia, where there is a deficit of both sodium and water, the cause is often due to gastrointestinal losses (e.g., vomiting, diarrhea), transdermal losses (e.g., sweating), or third-spacing (e.g., burns, pancreatitis). Urine sodium will be low (<30 mmol/L) if nonrenal causes predominate. If renal causes are responsible (e.g., diuretic use, adrenal insufficiency), urine sodium will be higher (>30 mmol/L). Treatment involves fluid resuscitation, typically with isotonic saline, to restore intravascular volume and inhibit further vasopressin release.
- **Hypervolemic Hyponatremia:**
  - Hypervolemia, characterized by fluid overload, is usually associated with conditions like heart failure, cirrhosis, or nephrotic syndrome. These patients will also have low urine sodium (<30 mmol/L) as the body attempts to retain sodium. Management includes fluid restriction, diuretics, and addressing the underlying condition.
- **Euvolemic Hyponatremia:**
  - In euvolemia, the patient appears to have normal fluid volume, but there is an inappropriate retention of water relative to sodium. This is often due to the syndrome of inappropriate antidiuretic hormone secretion (SIADH). Urine osmolality will be high (>100 mOsm/kg) and urine sodium will be elevated (>30 mmol/L). Treatment involves fluid restriction, addressing the underlying cause of SIADH, and in some cases, pharmacological agents like vasopressin receptor antagonists.

- **Role of Antidiuretic Hormone (ADH)/Arginine Vasopressin (AVP)**
- AVP plays a pivotal role in water reabsorption in the kidneys. Inappropriate secretion or action of AVP can lead to water retention and hyponatremia:
  - Euvolemic Hyponatremia: Often due to the syndrome of inappropriate antidiuretic hormone secretion (SIADH), where AVP is secreted despite normal or low plasma osmolality.
  - SIADH: Characterized by euvolemia, hyponatremia, high urine osmolality (>100 mOsm/kg), and elevated urine sodium (>30 mmol/L).

22.5 Osmolarity

Osmolarity is a measure of solute concentration in the blood and urine and is essential in understanding the type of hyponatremia:

- **Serum Osmolality**: This helps differentiate between hypotonic, isotonic, and hypertonic hyponatremia.

  - **Hypotonic Hyponatremia**: Most common and often due to excessive water retention relative to sodium. It reflects true water intoxication or sodium deficiency.
  - **Isotonic Hyponatremia**: Often a laboratory artifact, like pseudohyponatremia, where the sodium concentration appears low, but the osmolarity is normal due to high levels of lipids or proteins.
  - **Hypertonic Hyponatremia**: Occurs when other solutes like glucose or mannitol are present in high concentrations, pulling water from the intracellular space and diluting serum sodium.

- **Urine Osmolality**: This helps assess the kidneys' ability to dilute or concentrate urine.
  - **High Urine Osmolality (>100 mOsm/kg)**: Indicates that ADH (antidiuretic hormone) is being secreted and the kidneys are retaining water, which is inappropriate in cases like SIADH.
  - **Low Urine Osmolality (<100 mOsm/kg)**: Suggests that ADH is not active and points towards conditions like primary polydipsia or low solute intake.
  - **SIADH:**
    - If urine osmolality is high (>100 mOsm/kg) and urine sodium is elevated (>30 mmol/L) with a normal or low serum osmolality, SIADH is likely. Treatment focuses on fluid restriction and addressing the underlying cause.
  - **Primary Polydipsia or Low Solute Intake:**
    - If urine osmolality is low (<100 mOsm/kg), it suggests conditions like primary polydipsia or low solute intake (e.g., beer potomania). The management is primarily fluid restriction and dietary changes to increase solute intake.

22.6 Urine Sodium: Its Measurement and Interpretation

Urine sodium concentration is critical for identifying the underlying cause of hyponatremia:

- **High Urine Sodium (>30 mmol/L)**: Indicates that the kidneys are excreting sodium appropriately, which can occur in euvolemic hyponatremia (e.g., SIADH) or renal causes of sodium loss.
- **Low Urine Sodium (<30 mmol/L)**: Suggests that the kidneys are conserving sodium, which is seen in hypovolemic states due to nonrenal causes like gastrointestinal losses.

22.7 Renal Causes of Hyponatremia

Renal causes of hyponatremia are associated with impaired sodium handling by the kidneys:

1. **Diuretics (Thiazides)**
   - Thiazide diuretics impair the kidneys' ability to dilute urine by inhibiting sodium reabsorption in the distal tubules, leading to hyponatremia. This effect is more pronounced in the elderly and those with low baseline sodium intake.
2. **Renal Failure**
   - In advanced chronic kidney disease, the kidneys' ability to excrete free water is impaired, leading to dilutional hyponatremia. This is compounded by factors such as overuse of diuretics or excessive fluid intake.
3. **Adrenal Insufficiency**
   - Primary adrenal insufficiency (Addison's disease) can lead to hyponatremia due to aldosterone deficiency, which impairs sodium reabsorption in the kidneys and leads to volume depletion.
4. **Cerebral Salt Wasting**
   - This is a condition where renal sodium loss occurs due to a brain injury or neurosurgical procedure, leading to hyponatremia and hypovolemia. It is often confused with SIADH but requires volume replacement instead of fluid restriction.

22.8 Nonrenal Causes of Hyponatremia

Nonrenal causes typically involve extrarenal sodium loss or conditions that impair the body's ability to excrete water:

1. **Gastrointestinal Losses**
   - Vomiting, diarrhea, or nasogastric suctioning can lead to significant sodium loss. The kidneys respond by retaining sodium, leading to low urine sodium concentrations.
2. **Transdermal Losses**
   - Conditions such as excessive sweating, cystic fibrosis, or burns can lead to sodium loss through the skin. This is particularly significant in hot climates or during vigorous exercise without adequate sodium replacement.

3. **Third Spacing**
    - Conditions like sepsis, pancreatitis, or trauma can cause fluid to shift into nonfunctional spaces (third spacing), leading to hypovolemia and hyponatremia. This triggers the body to conserve sodium, reflected in low urine sodium levels.
4. **Primary Polydipsia**
    - Excessive water intake, often due to psychiatric conditions, overwhelms the kidneys' ability to excrete water, leading to dilutional hyponatremia. Urine osmolality is typically low due to the large volume of dilute urine.
5. **Syndrome of Inappropriate Antidiuretic Hormone Secretion (SIADH)**
    - SIADH is characterized by inappropriate secretion of ADH, leading to water retention and dilutional hyponatremia. This condition is often associated with lung diseases, CNS disorders, or certain medications.
6. **Hypothyroidism**
    - Severe hypothyroidism can lead to decreased cardiac output and renal blood flow, triggering non-osmotic release of ADH and leading to hyponatremia. However, this is a rare cause and typically only seen in severe cases.

22.9 Risk of Overcorrection

Osmotic Demyelination Syndrome (ODS)
- Mechanism: Rapid rise in serum sodium leads to demyelination in the central pontine region [4].
- Prevention:
- Correction Rate: Do not exceed 8–10 mmol/L increase in serum sodium over 24 h.
- High-Risk Patients: Lower target correction rates in patients with chronic hyponatremia or risk factors.

Use of Desmopressin
- Mechanism: Synthetic AVP analog; prevents rapid water diuresis.
- Indications: Patients at risk of overcorrection or when overcorrection has occurred.
- Dosage: Administer as per institutional protocols, with close monitoring.

22.10 Special Considerations

Hyponatremia in Oncology Patients

- Etiology:
- SIADH: Paraneoplastic syndromes (e.g., small cell lung carcinoma).
- Chemotherapy-Induced SIADH: Agents like vincristine, cyclophosphamide.
- Management:
- Fluid Restriction and Pharmacotherapy: Similar to SIADH management.
- Treat Underlying Malignancy: May resolve hyponatremia.
- Monitor for Recurrence: Regular assessment due to risk of SIADH relapse.

Mortality and Morbidity Data

- Elderly Patients: Increased susceptibility to hyponatremia-induced complications.
- Falls and Fractures: Hyponatremia-associated gait disturbances.
- Cognitive Impairment: Subtle neurological deficits even in mild hyponatremia.

22.11 Conclusion

The approach to hyponatremia in the ICU is a systematic process that begins with ruling out non-hypotonic causes, followed by the assessment and treatment of the severity of symptoms. Subsequent steps involve careful evaluation of the patient's volume status and targeted management of the underlying cause. The key to successful management is the balance between correcting sodium levels rapidly enough to prevent or treat severe symptoms while avoiding the risks of overly rapid correction, which can result in serious complications such as osmotic demyelination syndrome.

Algorithm 22.1: Approach to hyponatremia

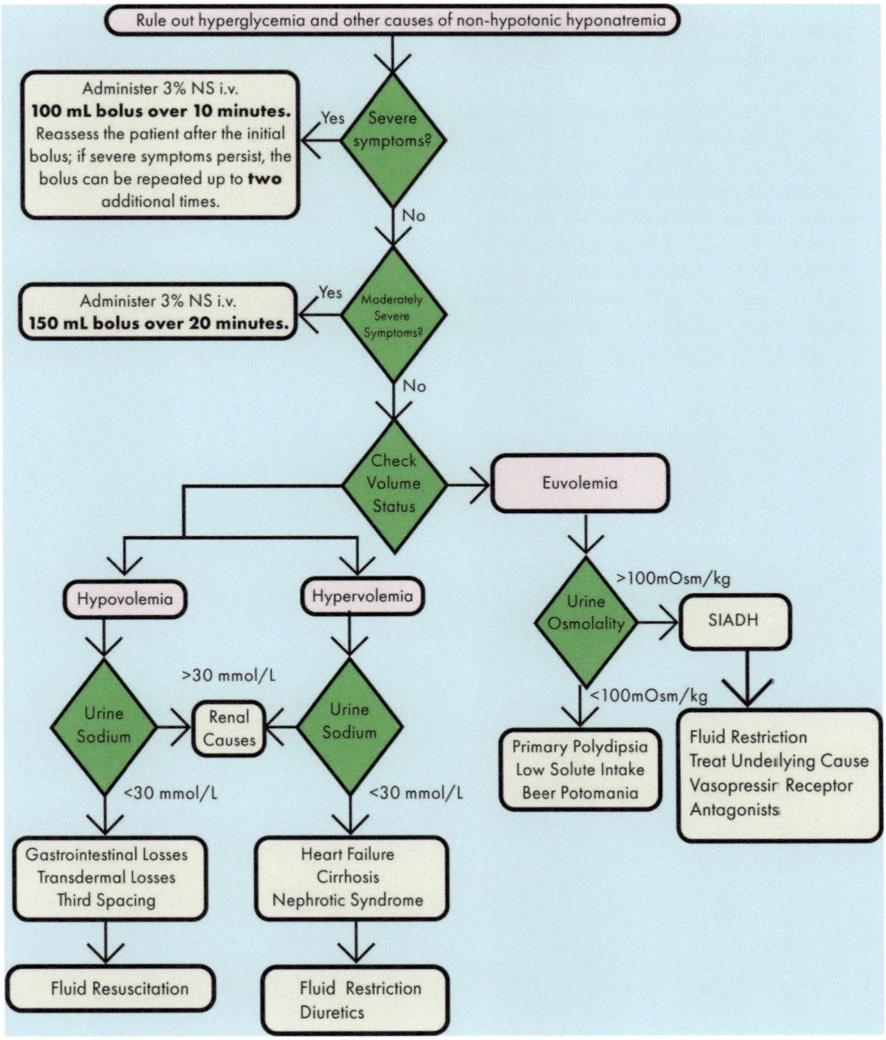

Bibliography

1. Spasovski G, Vanholder R, Allolio B, Annane D, Ball S, Bichet D, et al. Clinical practice guideline on diagnosis and treatment of hyponatraemia. Nephrol Dial Transplant. 2014;29(Suppl 2):i1–i39.
2. Spasovski G. Hyponatraemia—treatment standard 2024. Nephrol Dial Transplant. 2024;39(10):1583–92.
3. Sbardella E, Isidori AM, Arnaldi G, Arosio M, Barone C, Benso A, et al. Approach to hyponatremia according to the clinical setting: consensus statement from the Italian Society of Endocrinology (SIE), Italian Society of Nephrology (SIN), and Italian Association of Medical Oncology (AIOM). J Endocrinol Investig. 2018;41(1):3–19.
4. Barajas Galindo DE, Ruiz-Sánchez JG, Fernández Martínez A, de la Vega IR, Ferrer García JC, Ropero-Luis G, et al. Consensus document on the management of hyponatraemia of the Acqua Group of the Spanish Society of Endocrinology and Nutrition. Endocrinol Diabetes Nutr (Engl Ed). 2023;70(Suppl 1):7–26.

Chapter 23
Approach to Hypernatremia in the ICU

23.1 Introduction

Hypernatremia, defined as a serum sodium concentration greater than 145 mEq/L, represents a hyperosmolar condition where there is a deficit of free water relative to sodium. This electrolyte imbalance is critical in the ICU due to its association with high morbidity and mortality, particularly in vulnerable populations such as the elderly and those with impaired thirst mechanisms or altered mental status. The clinical management of hypernatremia requires a nuanced understanding of its etiology, the patient's volume status, and the timing of the onset [1, 2] [Ref: Algorithm 23.1].

23.2 Initial Assessment

23.2.1 Differentiate Between Acute and Chronic Hypernatremia

- The initial step in managing hypernatremia is to determine whether the condition is acute (developed within 48 h) or chronic (developed over more than 48 h or timing unknown). Acute hypernatremia poses a greater risk of neurological sequelae due to the brain's inability to adapt quickly to rapid changes in osmolarity. Conversely, chronic hypernatremia allows for some degree of cerebral adaptation, and rapid correction can lead to cerebral edema. Acute hypernatremia may result from recent administration of hypertonic fluids or massive water loss. Chronic cases are often seen in patients with impaired thirst mechanisms or those with long-standing underlying conditions.

S. B. Mishra et al., *Mastering ICU Care*,
https://doi.org/10.1007/978-981-95-0179-3_23

23.3 Volume Status Assessment

In the context of hypernatremia, assessing the patient's extracellular fluid (ECF) volume is a pivotal step in identifying the underlying cause and guiding treatment.

Increased ECF volume often points toward hypernatremia resulting from excessive sodium intake rather than from water loss. Sodium is an osmotically active ion that drives water retention in the extracellular compartment, which can manifest clinically in several ways:

1. **Positive Fluid Balance**: This is determined by comparing fluid intake and output. A positive fluid balance occurs when fluid intake exceeds fluid losses, resulting in fluid accumulation in the body. In the setting of hypernatremia, a positive fluid balance indicates that the excess sodium intake is causing water retention, leading to expanded ECF volume.
2. **Elevated Jugular Venous Pressure (JVP)**: Elevated JVP is a clinical sign of increased central venous pressure, reflecting fluid overload in the venous system. This can be assessed by observing the height of the venous column in the neck when the patient is positioned at a 45-degree angle. An elevated JVP often correlates with conditions such as heart failure or excessive intravenous sodium administration.
3. **Peripheral Edema**: The presence of swelling, particularly in the lower extremities, is another hallmark of fluid overload. Edema occurs when excess fluid leaks from the capillaries into the interstitial tissues due to elevated hydrostatic pressure in the veins. This is frequently observed in conditions of sodium and water retention.
4. **Ultrasound Findings (VExUS Grade 2–3)**: VExUS, or venous excess ultrasound grading system, is a relatively newer and noninvasive method used to assess fluid overload. A VExUS Grade 2–3 indicates significant venous congestion, seen in major veins such as the inferior vena cava and hepatic veins, which is consistent with a substantial increase in ECF volume. This finding supports the diagnosis of hypernatremia due to excessive sodium administration.

The VExUS (Venous Excess Ultrasound) grading system assesses venous congestion based on Doppler ultrasound findings in the inferior vena cava (IVC), hepatic veins, portal vein, and intrarenal veins. Here's a detailed description of the criteria for classifying congestion into mild, moderate, and severe categories, including relevant numerical cutoffs:

1. **Inferior Vena Cava (IVC) Findings:** If IVC diameter is >2.0 cm, then measure the hepatic vein, portal vein, and intra-renal vein Doppler pattern.
2. **Hepatic Vein Doppler Patterns:**

   - **Mild Congestion:**

     – **Waveform**: Slight reduction in the normal triphasic waveform, with a possible increase in A wave amplitude and a slight decrease in S wave amplitude.

- **Moderate Congestion:**
  - **Waveform**: Biphasic waveform, indicating significant increase in right atrial pressure.
- **Severe Congestion:**
  - **Waveform**: Monophasic waveform or systolic flow reversal, where the S wave is either absent or reversed, indicating critically elevated right atrial pressure.

3. **Portal Vein Doppler Patterns:**
   - **Mild Congestion:**
     - **Pulsatility**: Slight increase in pulsatility, but still predominantly continuous flow (less than 30% pulsatility index).
   - **Moderate Congestion:**
     - **Pulsatility**: Moderate pulsatility, often between 30% and 50% pulsatility index.
   - **Severe Congestion:**
     - **Pulsatility**: High pulsatility, greater than 50%, often with biphasic flow or even flow reversal.
4. **Intrarenal Vein Doppler Patterns:**
   - **Mild Congestion:**
     - **Waveform**: Continuous monophasic flow below the baseline, with minor pulsatility.
   - **Moderate Congestion:**
     - **Waveform**: Interrupted biphasic flow, corresponding to the S and D waves, indicating moderate congestion.
   - **Severe Congestion:**
     - **Waveform**: Discontinuous monophasic flow, often only showing diastolic phase flow, indicating severe congestion.
5. **VExUS Grading Summary:**
   - **VExUS Grade 0 (No Congestion):** Normal findings across all evaluated vessels.
   - **VExUS Grade 1 (Mild Congestion):** Mild congestion findings, indicated by an IVC diameter of more than 2 cm and any combination of normal or mildly abnormal flow patterns.

- **VExUS Grade 2 (Moderate Congestion):** Moderate congestion, indicated by an IVC diameter of more than 2 cm and one severely abnormal flow pattern.
- **VExUS Grade 3 (Severe Congestion):** Severe congestion, indicated by an IVC diameter of more than 2 cm and two or more severely abnormal flow patterns.

Management
Once increased ECF volume is confirmed, the immediate clinical priority is to halt any further sodium administration to prevent exacerbating the hypernatremia and fluid overload. The subsequent management strategy involves:

1. **Cessation of Hypertonic Solutions**: Any ongoing administration of hypertonic sodium solutions (such as hypertonic saline or sodium bicarbonate) should be stopped immediately. Continued administration would only increase the sodium load and worsen the hypernatremia.
2. **Diuretic Therapy**: Diuretics may be employed to promote the excretion of excess sodium and water. The choice of diuretic depends on the patient's overall condition:

   - **Loop diuretics** (e.g., furosemide) are often preferred as they are potent and act quickly by inhibiting sodium and chloride reabsorption in the loop of Henle. This leads to significant sodium and water excretion, which can help reduce both sodium levels and ECF volume.
   - **Thiazidediuretics** can also be considered, especially if the patient has a mild degree of fluid overload and requires a gentler diuretic effect.

3. **Monitoring Electrolyte Levels**: Careful monitoring of serum sodium and other electrolytes is crucial during diuretic therapy to avoid overly rapid changes in sodium levels, which could lead to complications such as cerebral edema. The correction of hypernatremia should be gradual, especially in chronic cases, to avoid iatrogenic harm.
4. **Fluid Management**: In some cases, it may be necessary to administer hypotonic fluids to aid in the correction of hypernatremia. However, this must be done cautiously to avoid rapid shifts in osmolality. Hypotonic fluids help to dilute the sodium concentration, but the infusion rate should be controlled to align with the target sodium correction rate.
5. **Addressing Underlying Causes**: If hypernatremia and increased ECF volume are secondary to underlying conditions such as heart failure or renal dysfunction, these should be concurrently managed. This might include optimizing heart failure therapy, adjusting other medications, or addressing renal insufficiency.
6. **Ongoing Assessment**: Continuous monitoring of the patient's fluid status, including daily weight, fluid balance charts, and regular physical examinations, is essential. Serial measurements of JVP, edema assessment, and repeat ultrasound examinations can help track the effectiveness of the management plan and guide further adjustments.

23.4 Evaluate for Water Loss

In cases where hypernatremia is present without an increase in extracellular fluid (ECF) volume, the condition is typically secondary to water loss rather than sodium gain. Identifying the source of water loss is crucial for accurate diagnosis and effective treatment. Water loss can occur through various mechanisms:

1. **Insensible Losses**: These include losses through the skin and respiratory tract. Increased insensible water loss can occur in conditions such as fever, high environmental temperature, or hyperventilation.
2. **Gastrointestinal Losses**: Diarrhea, vomiting, or the use of osmotic laxatives can lead to significant water loss. Gastrointestinal losses often present with signs of dehydration and can lead to electrolyte imbalances.
3. **Renal Losses**: This includes water loss due to renal pathologies like diabetes insipidus (central or nephrogenic), osmotic diuresis (as seen in uncontrolled diabetes mellitus), or the use of diuretics. These conditions result in the inability of the kidneys to concentrate urine, leading to excessive water loss.

Identifying the source of water loss is essential as it directs the specific management approach. For instance, treating hypernatremia due to insensible losses would differ significantly from managing hypernatremia due to renal causes.

23.5 Clinical Considerations

When evaluating for water loss, a thorough clinical assessment is necessary:

1. **Patient History**: Investigate any history of conditions or factors that could contribute to water loss, such as recent infections, gastrointestinal symptoms, or medication use (e.g., diuretics).
2. **Physical Examination**: Assess signs of dehydration, including dry mucous membranes, decreased skin turgor, tachycardia, and hypotension. These signs can indicate significant fluid loss.
3. **Urine Output**: A critical component of the evaluation is assessing urine output, which can provide insights into the underlying cause of hypernatremia.

23.6 Urine Output and Osmolality Assessment

1. **Assess Urine Output and Osmolarity**

Minimal Urine Output (<0.5 mL/kg/h)

- **Clinical Implication**: Minimal urine output is concerning and often suggests a state of prerenal azotemia, which may result from volume depletion due to dehydration or renal injury. The kidneys, in response to decreased perfusion, attempt to conserve fluid, leading to reduced urine output.

- **Management**: The primary approach to managing hypernatremia in this context involves cautious fluid replacement. Hypotonic solutions such as 0.45% saline or 5% dextrose in water (D5W) are typically used to correct the free water deficit. The correction rate should be carefully controlled, generally not exceeding 0.5 mEq/L/h, to prevent complications such as cerebral edema. Frequent monitoring of serum sodium levels and patient status is essential to guide the rate of correction.

Urine Osmole Excretion Rate (>750 mOsm/Day)

- **Clinical Implication**: A high urine osmole excretion rate indicates that the kidneys are actively trying to conserve water by concentrating urine. This condition is often seen in osmotic diuresis, where substances like glucose (in uncontrolled diabetes) or mannitol draw water into the urine, leading to high osmolarity and significant water loss. Diuretic use can also lead to high urine osmolarity.
- **Management**: Management in this scenario involves addressing the underlying cause of the osmotic diuresis. For instance, in diabetes mellitus, controlling blood glucose levels is crucial. In the case of diuretic-induced hypernatremia, adjusting or discontinuing the diuretic may be necessary. Fluid replacement should be carefully calculated to replace the free water deficit without causing rapid shifts in sodium levels.

23.7 Urine Osmole Excretion Rate (<750 mOsm/Day)

23.7.1 Renal Response to Desmopressin (DDAVP) in Hypernatremia

Rationale

In patients with hypernatremia and minimal urine output accompanied by low urine osmolality, it is essential to differentiate between central and nephrogenic diabetes insipidus (DI). Both conditions result in the inability to concentrate urine, leading to significant water loss and subsequent hypernatremia. The desmopressin (DDAVP) challenge test is a diagnostic tool used to distinguish between these two forms of DI:

- **Central Diabetes Insipidus (CDI)**: Caused by a deficiency in the production or release of antidiuretic hormone (ADH), also known as vasopressin.
- **Nephrogenic Diabetes Insipidus (NDI)**: Caused by renal resistance to the action of ADH, despite normal or elevated levels of the hormone.

The DDAVP challenge test involves administering desmopressin, a synthetic analogue of ADH, and then measuring urine osmolality before and after the administration. The response of urine osmolality to DDAVP helps to distinguish between CDI and NDI.

Interpretation of the DDAVP Challenge Test

1. **Increased Urine Osmolality (Positive Response to DDAVP):**
   - **Mechanism**: In CDI, the kidneys are still capable of responding to ADH, but there is a deficiency in ADH production or release. When desmopressin is administered, it binds to V2 receptors in the renal collecting ducts, promoting water reabsorption and leading to an increase in urine osmolality.
   - **Clinical Implication**: A significant increase in urine osmolality following DDAVP administration (typically by more than 50%) confirms a diagnosis of central diabetes insipidus.
   - **Management**: Treatment for CDI includes ongoing administration of desmopressin to replace the deficient ADH. Fluid replacement should be carefully monitored to correct hypernatremia without causing rapid shifts in serum sodium levels, which could result in cerebral edema.

2. **Unchanged Urine Osmolality (No Response to DDAVP):**
   - **Mechanism**: In NDI, the kidneys are resistant to the action of ADH due to defects in the V2 receptors, signaling pathways, or aquaporin channels in the renal collecting ducts. Therefore, even when desmopressin is administered, the kidneys are unable to increase water reabsorption, resulting in little to no change in urine osmolality.
   - **Clinical Implication**: A lack of increase in urine osmolality after DDAVP administration indicates nephrogenic diabetes insipidus.
   - **Management**: The treatment of NDI focuses on addressing the underlying cause, which may include discontinuing causative drugs (e.g., lithium, certain antibiotics) or correcting electrolyte imbalances such as hypercalcemia or hypokalemia. Pharmacologic treatments like thiazide diuretics or amiloride may also be employed. Thiazides reduce urine output by promoting mild volume depletion, leading to increased proximal tubule reabsorption of sodium and water. Amiloride is particularly useful in lithium-induced NDI, as it blocks lithium uptake in the renal tubules.

23.8 Hypernatremia in Neurosurgical Patients

Hypernatremia is particularly concerning in neurosurgical patients, where it is an independent predictor of poor outcomes, especially in those with severe elevations of sodium (>160 mmol/L). In such patients, the risk of secondary brain injury increases due to the exacerbation of cerebral ischemia. Hypernatremia in neurosurgical cases requires prompt management, including free-water replacement and addressing any volume abnormalities, to prevent complications such as cerebral edema.

23.9 Monitoring and Preventing Overcorrection

A critical aspect of hypernatremia management is avoiding overcorrection, which can lead to cerebral edema. To prevent this, sodium correction should not exceed 12 mmol/L per day, and diuresis should be carefully monitored. Desmopressin may be used to control rapid water excretion if brisk diuresis occurs during treatment. Regular monitoring of serum sodium, electrolytes, and patient fluid status is essential to ensure safe and effective correction.

23.10 Conclusion

The management of hypernatremia in the ICU requires careful consideration of the patient's volume status, underlying etiology, and the timing of onset. Acute hypernatremia demands prompt but cautious correction to avoid complications, while chronic hypernatremia requires a more gradual approach. By following a structured approach as outlined in this guide, clinicians can effectively address hypernatremia and minimize associated risks.

Algorithm 23.1: Approach to hypernatremia in the ICU

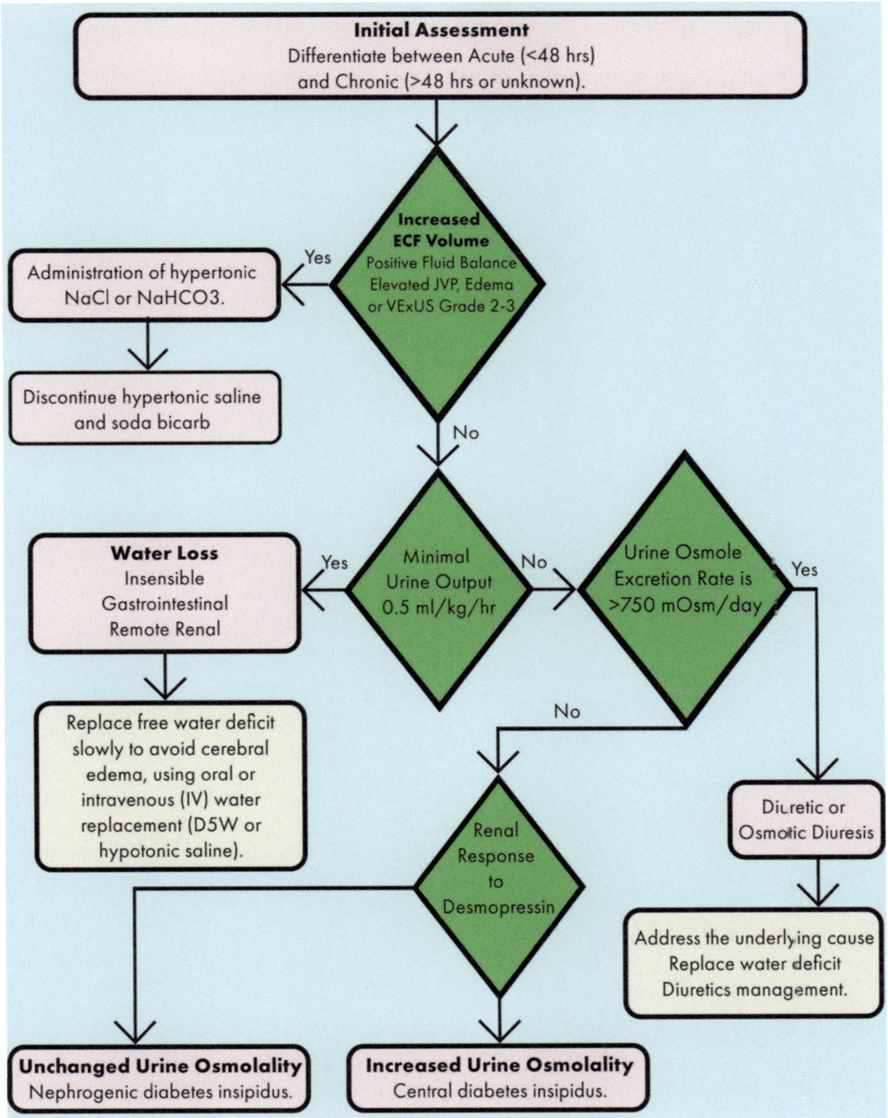

Bibliography

1. Overgaard-Steensen C, Ring T. Clinical review: practical approach to hyponatraemia and hypernatraemia in critically ill patients. Crit Care. 2013;17(1):206.
2. Castle-Kirszbaum M, Kyi M, Wright C, Goldschlager T, Danks RA, Parkin WG. Hyponatraemia and hypernatraemia: disorders of water balance in neurosurgery. Neurosurg Rev. 2021;44(5):2433–58.

Chapter 24
Approach to Hypokalemia

24.1 Introduction

Hypokalemia, defined as a serum potassium level below 3.5 mmol/L, is a common electrolyte disturbance encountered in clinical practice, particularly in the ICU setting. Potassium plays a crucial role in maintaining cellular function, particularly in the heart, muscles, and nerves. A significant deficit can lead to serious complications, including arrhythmias, muscle weakness, and even paralysis [1] [Ref: Algorithm 24.1].

24.2 Initial Assessment (History)

The management of hypokalemia begins with a thorough initial assessment to identify the underlying cause.

Every 1 mEq/L decrease in serum potassium levels represents a potassium deficit of approximately 200–400 mEq.

Key areas to investigate include:

1. **Gastrointestinal (GI) Losses**: Common causes of potassium loss include diarrhea, vomiting, and nasogastric suctioning. These conditions lead to significant potassium depletion, often exacerbated by concurrent sodium and fluid loss.
2. **Diuretic Use**: Certain diuretics, particularly loop (e.g., furosemide) and thiazide diuretics, promote potassium excretion in the urine. It is crucial to evaluate the patient's medication history to determine if these drugs are contributing to hypokalemia.

S. B. Mishra et al., *Mastering ICU Care*,
https://doi.org/10.1007/978-981-95-0179-3_24

3. **Other Medications**: Medications such as cisplatin (a chemotherapy agent), amphotericin B (an antifungal), and licorice (which can act similarly to aldosterone) can also cause potassium loss.
4. **Acute Intracellular Shifts**: Conditions that drive potassium into cells, such as insulin administration (often in diabetic ketoacidosis) or catecholamine excess (e.g., stress, pheochromocytoma), should be considered. These shifts can lead to transient hypokalemia without actual depletion of total body potassium [2].

24.3 Potassium Level Assessment and Initial Management

Clinical Features: Muscle weakness and cramps, arrhythmia, abdominal discomfort, and constipation.

ECG Findings: Prolonged PR, QT interval; decreased amplitude of T or T inversion, ST depression, appearance of U wave.

The next step is to assess the serum potassium level:

- **Potassium <2.5 mmol/L**: This is a critical threshold where aggressive intervention is required. Patients with potassium levels below 2.5 mmol/L are at high risk for life-threatening arrhythmias. Immediate management includes:
  - **IV Potassium Infusion**: Administer potassium at a rate of 20–40 meq/h depending on the severity of symptoms and ECG changes.
  - **ECG Monitoring**: Continuous cardiac monitoring is necessary due to the risk of arrhythmias.
  - **Consider ENaC Blockers**: In cases where hypokalemia is refractory to standard therapy, ENaC blockers like amiloride may be considered to reduce renal potassium loss.
- **Potassium ≥2.5 mmol/L**: For patients with potassium levels above this threshold, the approach is slightly less urgent but still requires prompt correction:
  - **IV Potassium Infusion**: Typically, 60 mmol over 6 h is administered.
  - **Oral Replacement**: Where appropriate, oral potassium supplementation can be considered as part of the management plan.

24.4 Further Evaluation and Management

If hypokalemia persists despite initial treatment, further evaluation is necessary:

- **Urinary Potassium Excretion**:

When managing a patient with hypokalemia, one of the critical steps is to assess whether the kidneys are responsible for the loss of potassium. This is particularly important if the serum potassium levels do not improve with initial replacement therapy. The presence of **urinary potassium levels greater than 20 mEq/L** or a **Transtubular Potassium Gradient (TTKG) greater than 7** indicates that the kidneys are actively excreting potassium. This finding suggests renal potassium loss, and further investigation is necessary to pinpoint the exact cause.

What Does Urinary Potassium >20 mEq/L or TTKG >7 Mean?

- **Urinary Potassium >20 mEq/L**: Normally, when the body is potassium-depleted, the kidneys should conserve potassium by reducing its excretion to below 20 mEq/L. However, if the urinary potassium level remains above 20 mEq/L in the setting of hypokalemia, it suggests that the kidneys are losing potassium despite the body's need to retain it. This is a sign that the renal tubules are unable to reabsorb potassium efficiently, or that there is a factor driving increased potassium excretion.
- **TTKG >7**: The TTKG is a calculation used to estimate the activity of potassium secretion in the cortical collecting duct of the kidneys. A TTKG above 7 suggests that the kidneys are inappropriately secreting potassium into the urine, even when serum potassium is low. This can occur in various conditions where potassium wasting is a feature.

24.5 Transtubular Potassium Gradient (TTKG): Detailed Explanation

The **Transtubular Potassium Gradient (TTKG)** is a clinical calculation used to assess potassium secretion in the cortical collecting duct (CCD) of the kidneys. It is particularly useful in evaluating the kidneys' response to hypokalemia (low potassium levels) or hyperkalemia (high potassium levels). Understanding TTKG is essential for residents as it provides insight into whether the kidneys are appropriately conserving or excreting potassium based on the body's needs [3].

24.5.1 What Is TTKG?

TTKG is an indirect measurement of the ratio of potassium concentration between the urine in the CCD and the plasma, corrected for the amount of water reabsorption that occurs in the medullary collecting duct. In simpler terms, it helps us understand how much potassium is being secreted into the urine relative to the plasma potassium concentration, while accounting for the concentration effects due to water reabsorption.

24.5.2 *The Formula*

TTKG is calculated using the following formula:

$$\text{TTKG} = \{[\text{K}+]\text{urine})/[\text{K}]+\text{plasma}\}/\{(\text{Osmurine}/\text{Osmplasma})\}$$

Where:

- [K+]urine is the potassium concentration in the urine.
- [K+]plasma is the potassium concentration in the plasma.
- Osmplasma is the osmolality of the plasma.
- Osmurine is the osmolality of the urine.

24.5.3 *How to Interpret TTKG*

TTKG helps clinicians determine whether the kidneys are responding appropriately to the body's potassium needs:

- **TTKG >7**: This suggests that the kidneys are secreting potassium into the urine, which is expected in conditions of hyperkalemia (high plasma potassium). In hypokalemia, a TTKG greater than 7 indicates inappropriate renal potassium loss, meaning the kidneys are excreting potassium when they should be conserving it.
- **TTKG < 3**: This indicates that the kidneys are conserving potassium by reducing its secretion into the urine. This response is expected in hypokalemia, where the body needs to retain as much potassium as possible to correct the deficiency.

24.5.4 *Clinical Utility of TTKG*

TTKG is particularly useful in the following scenarios:

1. **Evaluating Hypokalemia**: When a patient presents with hypokalemia, calculating the TTKG can help determine if the kidneys are contributing to the potassium loss. If TTKG is greater than 7 in a hypokalemic patient, it suggests that the

kidneys are inappropriately excreting potassium, which may be due to conditions like hyperaldosteronism, diuretic use, or other renal tubular defects.
2. **Assessing Hyperkalemia**: Details in Hyperkalemia Chap. 25/Algorithm 25.1.
3. **Guiding Treatment Decisions**: TTKG can also help guide treatment decisions, particularly in determining the effectiveness of treatments aimed at modifying potassium balance. For example, if a patient with hypokalemia has a high TTKG despite adequate potassium replacement, it may indicate the need to address underlying causes of renal potassium loss, such as discontinuing a potassium-wasting diuretic or treating hyperaldosteronism.

24.6 Causes of Renal Potassium Loss

Once it is established that the kidneys are responsible for the ongoing potassium loss, the next step is to determine the underlying cause. This often involves reviewing the patient's medication history and evaluating for conditions that might promote potassium excretion.

1. **Diuretic Use**

- **Loop and Thiazide Diuretics**: These are common causes of renal potassium loss. Loop diuretics (e.g., furosemide) act on the loop of Henle, while thiazide diuretics act on the distal convoluted tubule. Both classes of diuretics increase the excretion of sodium and water, which leads to increased flow through the distal nephron where potassium is secreted. The increased flow and sodium delivery to the distal tubules promote the secretion of potassium into the urine, leading to hypokalemia.
- **Patient Medication Chart Review**: For residents, it is crucial to review the patient's medication list carefully. Diuretics, especially if not recently discontinued, could be the primary driver of hypokalemia. It's important to consider the dose and duration of diuretic therapy and whether the hypokalemia corresponds with the start or intensification of diuretic use.

2. **Osmotic Diuresis**

- **High Sodium Intake**: Excessive sodium intake can contribute to potassium loss in patients, especially when the kidneys are under the influence of diuretics or osmotic agents. High sodium intake increases the amount of sodium delivered to the distal nephron, thereby increasing potassium excretion.
- **Presence of Osmoles**: Conditions that cause osmotic diuresis, such as hyperglycemia (high blood glucose) in uncontrolled diabetes or the use of mannitol, or high levels of urea also lead to increased urinary potassium loss. Osmotic diuresis occurs when non-reabsorbed solutes (osmoles) in the renal

tubules attract water, increasing urine flow. This increased flow washes potassium out of the distal nephron, leading to its loss in the urine.

- **Hypertension Present**: If the patient is hypertensive, the likely etiology involves conditions associated with enhanced sodium reabsorption, leading to increased potassium excretion:
  - **Primary Hyperaldosteronism**: This condition leads to excessive aldosterone production, driving potassium excretion in exchange for sodium reabsorption.
  - **Apparent Mineralocorticoid Excess (AME)**: Conditions mimicking the effects of aldosterone due to genetic mutations or the use of certain substances.
  - **Liddle's Syndrome**: A rare genetic disorder causing increased sodium reabsorption and potassium loss due to a mutation in the epithelial sodium channel (ENaC).
  - **Glucocorticoid-Remediable Aldosteronism**: Another genetic condition leading to excess aldosterone activity.
- **No Hypertension**: In the absence of hypertension, the focus shifts to conditions causing slower chloride reabsorption:
  - **Bartter's Syndrome and Gitelman's Syndrome**: These are genetic disorders leading to impaired chloride reabsorption in the renal tubules, causing hypokalemia.
  - **Magnesium Depletion**: Hypomagnesemia often accompanies and exacerbates hypokalemia by promoting renal potassium loss.
  - **Bicarbonaturia**: Conditions leading to increased bicarbonate excretion can also result in potassium loss.

24.7 Conclusion

The management of hypokalemia requires a methodical approach, starting with identifying the underlying cause through history and initial investigations, followed by appropriate correction of potassium levels and further diagnostic evaluation. Close monitoring, particularly with severe hypokalemia, is crucial to avoid complications such as arrhythmias. Understanding the interplay of various factors influencing potassium balance is essential for effective management.

Algorithm 24.1: Approach to Hypokalemia

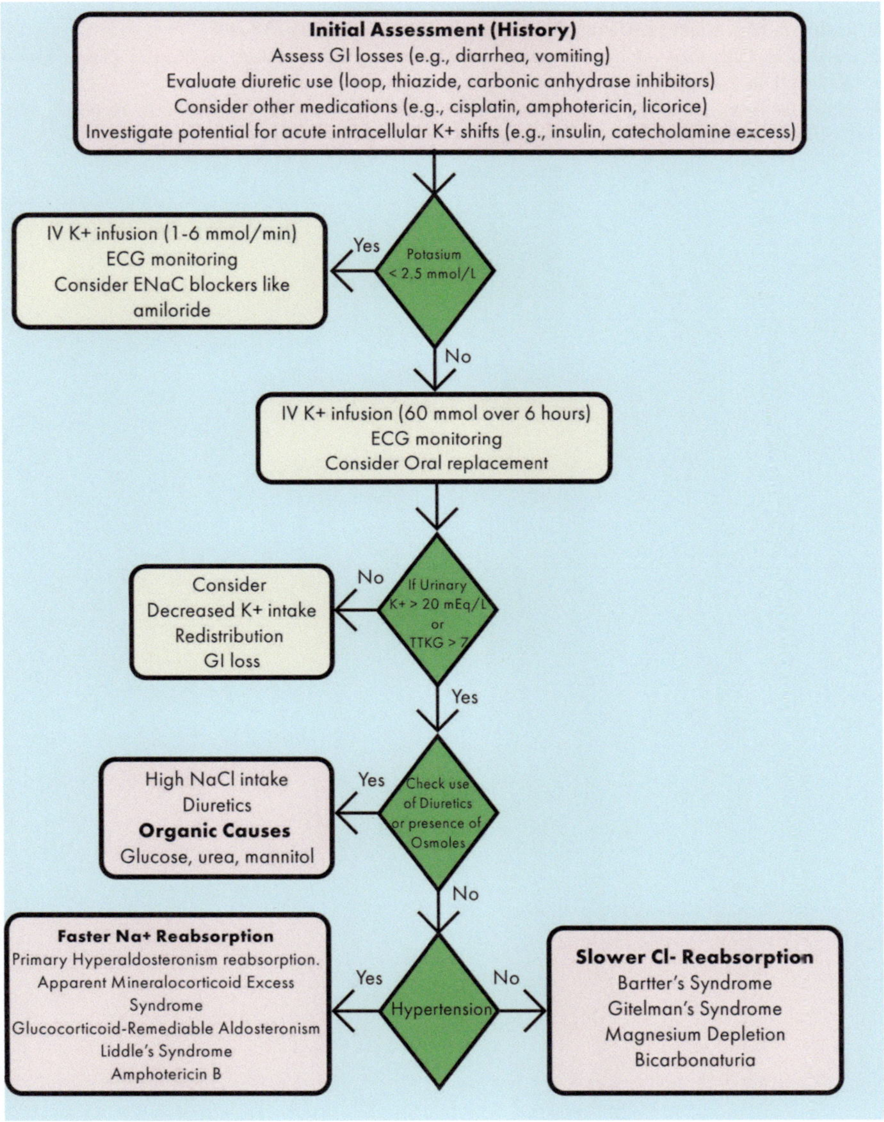

Bibliography

1. Halperin ML, Kamel KS. Potassium. Lancet. 1998;352(9122):135–40.
2. Assadi F. Diagnosis of hypokalemia: a problem-solving approach to clinical cases. Iran J Kidney Dis. 2008;2(3):115–22.
3. Kardalas E, Paschou SA, Anagnostis P, Muscogiuri G, Siasos G, Vryonidou A. Hypokalemia: a clinical update. Endocr Connect. 2018;7(4):R135–R46.

Chapter 25
Approach to Hyperkalemia in the ICU

25.1 Introduction

Hyperkalemia, defined as a serum potassium level greater than 5.0 mmol/L, is a potentially life-threatening condition that requires prompt assessment and management. Potassium plays a crucial role in maintaining cellular membrane potential, particularly in cardiac and neuromuscular tissues. Severe hyperkalemia can lead to dangerous cardiac arrhythmias and muscle weakness, making it critical to quickly identify and treat the underlying cause.

This approach to hyperkalemia is structured to guide healthcare providers through a systematic evaluation and management process. The initial step is to differentiate between acute and chronic hyperkalemia, as the management strategies may differ. Subsequent steps focus on immediate stabilization, diagnosis, and long-term treatment strategies [1] [Ref: Algorithm 25.1].

A. **Initial Assessment: Differentiating Between Acute and Chronic Hyperkalemia**

- The first step in managing hyperkalemia is determining whether the hyperkalemia is acute (less than 48 h) or chronic (more than 48 hours or unknown duration). This differentiation is important because acute hyperkalemia is more likely to cause severe cardiac arrhythmias due to the rapid rise in potassium levels, while chronic hyperkalemia might allow time for some adaptation in the body.

Pseudohyperkalemia

Pseudohyperkalemia refers to a falsely elevated serum potassium level that does not reflect the actual in vivo potassium concentration. This condition often arises due to the release of potassium from cells during or after blood sample collection,

S. B. Mishra et al., *Mastering ICU Care*,
https://doi.org/10.1007/978-981-95-0179-3_25

particularly if there is hemolysis, thrombocytosis, or leukocytosis. It is essential to distinguish pseudohyperkalemia from true hyperkalemia because the management of true hyperkalemia involves urgent therapeutic interventions to prevent life-threatening complications. In contrast, pseudohyperkalemia requires no specific treatment. Clinicians should suspect pseudohyperkalemia if there are elevated potassium levels without corresponding clinical symptoms or ECG changes indicative of hyperkalemia. Confirmation can be achieved by rechecking the serum potassium level using plasma rather than serum and ensuring proper sample handling techniques.

Clinical features: Muscle weakness and cramps and arrhythmias are the most common features. Gastrointestinal disturbances may also be seen. Involvement of respiratory muscles can lead to hypoventilation and apnea.

ECG changes: PR interval prolonged, P wave flattening, shortening of QT interval, Pointed T waves, Wide QRS complex.

B. **Immediate Stabilization: Administering Calcium (presence of ECG changes)**

- **Calcium Gluconate**: Administer 10 mL of 10% solution intravenously over 2–3 min. Calcium gluconate is preferred for peripheral administration because it is less irritating to veins compared to calcium chloride.
- **Calcium Chloride**: Administer 5–10 mL of 10% solution intravenously. This option provides more potent calcium but is generally administered through a central line due to the risk of tissue necrosis if extravasation occurs.
- **Rationale**: Calcium does not lower serum potassium levels but stabilizes the cardiac membrane, reducing the risk of arrhythmias associated with hyperkalemia [2].

C. **Lowering Potassium levels:**

Shifting Potassium Intracellularly

- **Insulin and Dextrose**: Administer 10 units of regular insulin IV followed by 50 mL of 50% dextrose. Insulin promotes the uptake of potassium into cells, temporarily lowering serum potassium levels. Onset of time: 20 min.
- **Beta-2 Agonist (Albuterol)**: Administer 20 mg via nebulization in 4 mL of saline as an adjunct to insulin. This can also drive potassium into cells. Onset of time: 30 to 60 min.
- **Sodium Bicarbonate**: Consider this if there is metabolic acidosis. Sodium bicarbonate can help shift potassium into cells, particularly in patients with acidosis. Onset of time: 30 to 60 min.
- Potassium elimination: Potassium binding agents, loop diuretics, and hemodialysis.

D. **Electrocardiogram (ECG) Evaluation**

- An ECG should be performed immediately to assess for signs of hyperkalemia, such as tall peaked T waves, widened QRS complex (seen with potassium level greater than 6 mmol/L). These findings necessitate urgent treatment.

E. **Identifying the Cause: History and Assessment**

- Gather a detailed history to identify potential causes of hyperkalemia, including increased potassium intake, decreased renal excretion, or transcellular shifts (e.g., acidosis, tissue breakdown).
- Assess for conditions that could contribute to a transcellular shift of potassium or an increased potassium load.

F. **Transtubular Potassium Gradient (TTKG)**

- **TTKG Calculation**: This is calculated to assess the kidney's ability to excrete potassium. A TTKG greater than 8 suggests appropriate renal excretion in the presence of hyperkalemia.

TTKG >8:

When the Transtubular Potassium Gradient (TTKG) is greater than 8, it typically indicates that the kidneys are appropriately excreting potassium in response to hyperkalemia, suggesting that the tubular function is intact. However, the high TTKG in the presence of persistent hyperkalemia may indicate reduced tubular flow, which can result from advanced kidney failure or reduced extracellular volume (ECV) [3].

1. **Advanced Kidney Failure**:

- In the context of chronic kidney disease (CKD) or acute kidney injury (AKI), the kidney's ability to filter blood is severely compromised. Even though the renal tubules may still be responding to aldosterone by excreting potassium effectively (reflected by a high TTKG), the overall decrease in glomerular filtration rate (GFR) means that the total amount of potassium excreted in the urine is insufficient to balance intake, leading to hyperkalemia.
- Management in this scenario focuses on addressing the underlying renal failure. This may include optimizing volume status, managing comorbid conditions like hypertension or diabetes, and considering dialysis in cases of severe kidney dysfunction.

2. **Reduced Extracellular Volume (ECV)**:
- Reduced ECV can occur in conditions such as dehydration, heart failure, or cirrhosis. In these situations, the body perceives a low blood volume, leading to increased aldosterone secretion and enhanced renal potassium excretion

(reflected by a high TTKG). However, the reduced overall urine flow due to the low volume status results in insufficient potassium clearance, contributing to hyperkalemia.

- Management in these cases focuses on restoring the ECV. This might involve administering intravenous fluids to correct dehydration; optimizing heart failure management (e.g., with diuretics, vasodilators), or addressing underlying liver disease. Care must be taken to balance fluid replacement with the risk of fluid overload, especially in patients with heart failure or cirrhosis.

In both scenarios, addressing the underlying cause is crucial to restoring normal potassium balance. While acute measures to lower serum potassium levels (e.g., using insulin, beta-agonists) may be necessary, long-term management must focus on improving kidney function or correcting volume status to prevent recurrent hyperkalemia. Additionally, careful monitoring and adjustment of medications that affect potassium levels (e.g., RAAS inhibitors, potassium-sparing diuretics) are essential in the management plan.

TTKG ≤5: Suggests inadequate aldosterone (resistance) activity or tubular dysfunction, and indicates the need for further investigation.

Administering 9α-Fludrocortisone.

- If TTKG is less than 5, consider the administration of 9α-Fludrocortisone to promote renal potassium excretion by enhancing the effects of aldosterone.
- **Rationale**: 9α-Fludrocortisone is a synthetic mineralocorticoid that helps in cases where aldosterone deficiency or resistance is suspected.

TTKG ≥8: Low Aldosterone

A TTKG (Transtubular Potassium Gradient) greater than or equal to 8, along with low aldosterone levels, suggests that the kidney's ability to excrete potassium is intact, but the issue lies in the regulation of aldosterone itself. Aldosterone is a hormone that plays a crucial role in regulating potassium and sodium balance in the body. When aldosterone levels are low, potassium excretion is reduced, leading to hyperkalemia. The evaluation of renin levels, which regulates aldosterone production, can further help determine the underlying cause of low aldosterone.

25.2 High Renin Levels: Causes and Implications

When renin levels are high in the setting of low aldosterone and hyperkalemia, it usually indicates a problem with the adrenal glands or a blockade in the pathway that produces aldosterone:

1. **Primary Adrenal Insufficiency**:
   - Also known as Addison's disease; this condition results in the destruction or dysfunction of the adrenal cortex, leading to inadequate production of aldosterone (and cortisol). This insufficiency results in hyperkalemia due to the inability to excrete potassium properly.
2. **Isolated Aldosterone Deficiency**:
   - This rare condition involves a specific deficiency in aldosterone production, leading to hyperkalemia and sometimes hyponatremia, without affecting cortisol levels. It can be due to genetic mutations or acquired conditions affecting aldosterone synthesis.
3. **Heparin/Low Molecular Weight Heparin**:
   - These anticoagulants can cause hyperkalemia by reducing aldosterone production, particularly with long-term use. This effect is more pronounced in patients with underlying renal impairment or those on other medications that affect potassium balance.
4. **ACE Inhibitors/ARBs (Angiotensin-Converting Enzyme Inhibitors/ Angiotensin Receptor Blockers)**:
   - These drugs interfere with the renin-angiotensin-aldosterone system (RAAS) by blocking the conversion of angiotensin I to angiotensin II (in the case of ACE inhibitors) or by blocking angiotensin II receptors (in the case of ARBs). Both mechanisms reduce aldosterone production, leading to hyperkalemia.
5. **Ketoconazole**:
   - This antifungal agent inhibits adrenal steroidogenesis, including aldosterone synthesis, leading to hyperkalemia. The effect is dose-dependent and reversible upon discontinuation of the drug.

25.3 Low Renin Levels: Causes and Implications

Low renin levels, in the presence of low aldosterone and hyperkalemia, point to conditions where renin production is suppressed or where there is resistance to the action of renin:

1. **Diabetes Mellitus**:
   - Long-standing diabetes can lead to a state known as hyporeninemic hypoaldosteronism. This condition is characterized by low renin and aldosterone

levels, often leading to hyperkalemia. It is particularly common in diabetic nephropathy.

2. **Acute Glomerulonephritis (GN)**:
   - Inflammatory conditions of the glomeruli can reduce the kidneys' ability to excrete potassium. This reduction is often accompanied by a decrease in renin production due to altered renal function.
3. **Tubulointerstitial Diseases**:
   - Chronic kidney diseases affecting the renal tubules and interstitium can impair renin release and aldosterone synthesis, leading to hyperkalemia.
4. **Pseudo-hypoaldosteronism (PHA) Type II**:
   - Also known as Gordon's syndrome, this genetic condition is characterized by hypertension, hyperkalemia, and normal or low levels of renin and aldosterone. The disorder is caused by mutations that lead to increased sodium reabsorption and potassium retention in the distal nephron.
5. **Nonsteroidal Anti-inflammatory Drugs (NSAIDs)**:
   - These drugs reduce the production of prostaglandins, which are necessary for the release of renin. Chronic use of NSAIDs can therefore lead to decreased renin and aldosterone levels, contributing to hyperkalemia.
6. **Beta-Blockers**:
   - Beta-adrenergic blockers reduce renin secretion by inhibiting the sympathetic nervous system's stimulation of the juxtaglomerular cells in the kidney. This suppression can lead to reduced aldosterone production and subsequent hyperkalemia.

25.4 Management Strategies

The management of hyperkalemia in the context of low aldosterone and varying renin levels involves addressing the underlying cause:

- For conditions like primary adrenal insufficiency, hormone replacement therapy with fludrocortisone may be necessary.
- Adjusting or discontinuing medications like ACE inhibitors, ARBs, or NSAIDs may be required, particularly if these are contributing to hyperkalemia [4].

- In cases of drug-induced hyperkalemia (e.g., with heparin or ketoconazole), discontinuation or dose adjustment of the offending drug is the primary treatment.
- For patients with conditions like diabetes mellitus, careful management of blood glucose and monitoring of kidney function are critical to preventing and treating hyperkalemia.

I. **TTKG < 8: Tubular Resistance and Its Implications**
A Transtubular Potassium Gradient (TTKG) less than 8 in the setting of hyperkalemia suggests that the renal tubules are not responding appropriately to aldosterone. This condition is often referred to as **tubular resistance** to aldosterone. Several factors can lead to this resistance, including certain medications and underlying medical conditions.

25.5 Drugs Leading to Tubular Resistance

Several medications can impair the renal tubules' ability to respond to aldosterone, thereby reducing potassium excretion and contributing to hyperkalemia.

1. **Amiloride, Spironolactone, and Triamterene**: These are potassium-sparing diuretics that act on the distal nephron. They inhibit sodium reabsorption in exchange for potassium and hydrogen ion secretion, effectively reducing potassium excretion.
2. **Trimethoprim**: This antibiotic, often used in treating urinary tract infections, acts similarly to potassium-sparing diuretics and can cause hyperkalemia, particularly in patients with renal impairment.
3. **Pentamidine**: An antimicrobial agent used in the treatment of *Pneumocystis jirovecii* pneumonia, especially in immunocompromised patients, can cause renal potassium retention through a mechanism similar to that of potassium-sparing diuretics.
4. **Eplerenone**: Another potassium-sparing diuretic, it acts as an aldosterone antagonist and is used in the management of heart failure. Like spironolactone, it can impair potassium excretion.
5. **Drospirenone**: A synthetic progestin found in some oral contraceptives, it has antimineralocorticoid properties, which can lead to increased potassium retention.
6. **Calcineurin Inhibitors (e.g., cyclosporine, tacrolimus)**: These immunosuppressants, commonly used in organ transplantation, can cause hyperkalemia by reducing renal potassium excretion.

25.6 Other Causes of Tubular Resistance

1. **Tubulointerstitial Diseases**: Conditions affecting the renal interstitium, such as chronic interstitial nephritis, can impair the kidney's ability to respond to aldosterone, leading to reduced potassium excretion.
2. **Urinary Tract Obstruction**: Chronic obstruction can cause tubular dysfunction, leading to impaired potassium excretion and hyperkalemia.
3. **Pseudo-hypoaldosteronism (PHA) Types I**: These rare genetic disorders are characterized by a lack of response to aldosterone. In PHA type I, there is a mutation in the mineralocorticoid receptor or in the epithelial sodium channel (ENaC), leading to severe hyperkalemia and metabolic acidosis.
4. **Sickle Cell Disease**: Chronic sickle cell nephropathy can cause tubular damage and lead to aldosterone resistance, contributing to hyperkalemia.
5. **Renal Transplant**: Post-transplant patients may develop hyperkalemia due to calcineurin inhibitors, tubular damage from ischemia-reperfusion injury, or rejection episodes that impair tubular function.
6. **Systemic Lupus Erythematosus (SLE)**: Lupus nephritis can cause interstitial nephritis and other forms of renal damage that impair the kidney's ability to excrete potassium effectively.

25.7 Management Implications

When a low TTKG suggests tubular resistance, the management of hyperkalemia involves addressing the underlying causes, such as discontinuing or adjusting medications that contribute to hyperkalemia. Additionally, managing the underlying conditions like urinary tract obstruction or treating tubulointerstitial diseases is essential. In cases of genetic conditions like PHA, management may involve specific dietary modifications, and in some cases, medications that help enhance potassium excretion or bypass the defective pathway.

25.7.1 Consideration of Contemporary Pharmacotherapies

In addition to traditional therapies, newer pharmacological agents such as sodium zirconium cyclosilicate (SZC) and patiromer have emerged as effective options for managing chronic hyperkalemia. These agents work by binding potassium in the gastrointestinal tract, helping to lower serum potassium levels without significant systemic absorption. They offer an advantage in patients with chronic kidney disease (CKD) by reducing the risk of hyperkalemia without requiring discontinuation of renin-angiotensin-aldosterone system inhibitors (RAASi), which are crucial for managing CKD and heart failure.

Sodium-glucose cotransporter 2 (SGLT2) inhibitors have emerged as a valuable tool in managing hyperkalemia, particularly in patients who are on RAAS inhibitors. By promoting renal excretion of potassium and glucose, SGLT2 inhibitors allow patients to continue on RAAS inhibitors without significantly increasing the risk of hyperkalemia. This helps in managing patients with CKD or heart failure where RAAS inhibition is crucial for long-term outcomes [5].

25.7.2 Chronic Hyperkalemia Management

Chronic hyperkalemia, unlike its acute counterpart, develops over a longer period and is often seen in patients with CKD, diabetes, or heart failure. Management involves reviewing medications, particularly RAAS inhibitors, and ensuring effective diuretic therapy. When chronic hyperkalemia persists, newer agents such as SZC and patiromer can be introduced to maintain potassium homeostasis without discontinuing RAAS inhibitors. Dietary potassium restriction is another component of management, although recent evidence suggests that moderate, individualized adjustments may be more appropriate than severe restriction.

25.7.3 Dietary Considerations

In patients with CKD, dietary potassium intake can be managed without entirely restricting healthy foods like fruits and vegetables. Individualized and stepwise reduction in potassium intake is recommended, focusing on avoiding processed foods with hidden potassium sources and employing methods like soaking or boiling to reduce potassium content in foods. This approach allows for a more balanced diet while mitigating the risk of hyperkalemia.

25.8 Conclusion

Effective management of hyperkalemia requires a systematic approach, beginning with the differentiation between acute and chronic cases, immediate stabilization to prevent life-threatening complications, and a thorough investigation to identify and address the underlying cause. Using tools like the TTKG, ECG, and renin levels, clinicians can tailor treatment to the specific needs of the patient, ensuring the best possible outcomes.

Algorithm 25.1: Approach to hyperkalemia in the ICU

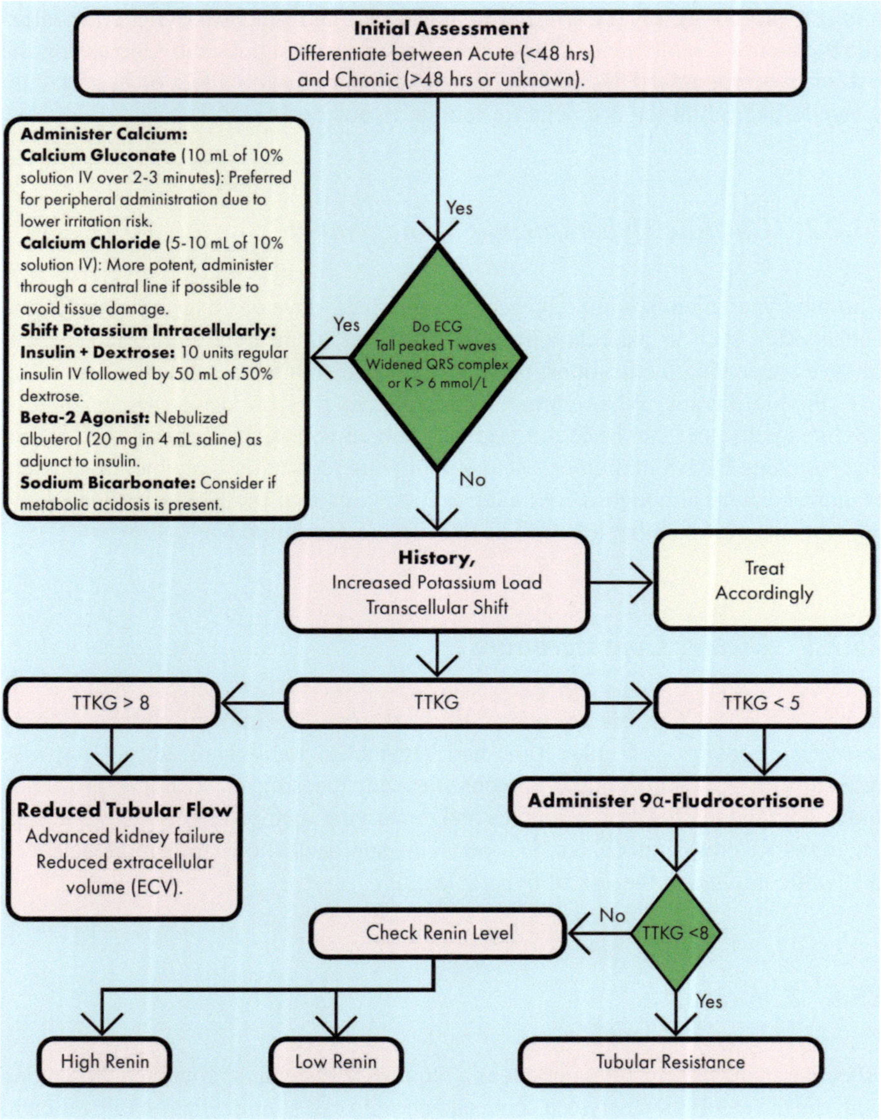

Bibliography

1. Emektar E. Acute hyperkalemia in adults. Turk J Emerg Med. 2023;23(2):75–81.
2. Massicotte-Azarniouch D, Canney M, Sood MM, Hundemer GL. Managing hyperkalemia in the modern era: a case-based approach. Kidney Int Rep. 2023;8(7):1290–300.
3. Palmer BF, Clegg DJ. Hyperkalemia treatment standard. Nephrol Dial Transplant. 2024;39(7):1097–104.
4. AlSahow A. Moderate stepwise restriction of potassium intake to reduce risk of hyperkalemia in chronic kidney disease: a literature review. World J Nephrol. 2023;12(4):73–81.
5. Sinnathamby ES, Banh KT, Barham WT, Hernandez TD, De Witt AJ, Wenger DM, et al. Hyperkalemia: pharmacotherapies and clinical considerations. Cureus. 2024;16(1):e52994.

Chapter 26
Approach to Hypocalcemia in the ICU

26.1 Introduction

Hypocalcemia, defined as an abnormally low level of calcium in the blood, is a critical condition that can have serious consequences if not managed promptly and effectively. Calcium plays a vital role in various physiological processes, including muscle contraction, nerve function, blood clotting, and cardiac rhythm regulation. The management of hypocalcemia in an intensive care setting requires a systematic approach, beginning with the confirmation of the condition and continuing through appropriate treatment based on the severity of symptoms and laboratory findings [1] [Ref: Algorithm 26.1].

1. **Initial Assessment**

   - **Confirm True Hypocalcemia**

     Begin by confirming hypocalcemia through laboratory tests. Total serum calcium levels can be affected by albumin levels and blood pH, so it is essential to adjust the calcium level for serum albumin and consider the effects of acid-base status on calcium binding.

   - Correcting for Albumin: Calcium binds to albumin; thus, hypoalbuminemia can lead to a falsely low total calcium level while ionized calcium remains normal. The corrected calcium can be calculated using the formula:

$$\text{Corrected Calcium}(\text{mg/dL}) = \text{Measured Total Calcium} + \left[0.8 \times \left(4.0 - \text{Serum Albumin}(\text{g/dL})\right)\right]$$

   - Effects of Blood pH: Alkalemia increases calcium binding to albumin, decreasing ionized calcium levels, while acidemia decreases binding, increasing ionized calcium levels. In ICU patients with frequent acid-base

S. B. Mishra et al., *Mastering ICU Care*,
https://doi.org/10.1007/978-981-95-0179-3_26

disturbances, these shifts can significantly impact ionized calcium levels, which is the biologically active form.

- **Measure Ionized Calcium**

  If available, measure ionized calcium directly, as it is the most accurate marker of biologically active calcium, especially in critically ill patients where albumin levels and pH can be significantly altered. Ionized calcium measurement is superior to total calcium in assessing true calcium status under these conditions [2].

2. **Clinical Manifestations**

   After confirming hypocalcemia, assess the severity based on clinical manifestations and the measured calcium level.

   A. **Mild Hypocalcemia (Calcium Level 7.5–8.5 mg/dL)**

   - Symptoms: Patients may be asymptomatic or present with mild symptoms, such as:
   - Paresthesias, particularly tingling around the mouth, hands, and feet.
   - Muscle cramps or mild muscle stiffness.
   - Fatigue, anxiety, or mild prolongation of the QT interval on an EKG.
   - Management:
   - Oral Calcium and Vitamin D Supplementation: First-line treatments to correct calcium levels.
   - Correct Magnesium Levels: Magnesium deficiency can impair PTH secretion and calcium absorption; correct if deficient.
   - Monitor Cardiac Rhythm: Even in mild cases, monitor for changes in cardiac rhythm due to potential QT prolongation.

   B. **Moderate Hypocalcemia (Calcium Level 6.0–7.5 mg/dL)**

   - Symptoms: More pronounced symptoms, including:
   - Intensified paresthesias.
   - Muscle spasms, particularly in the hands and feet (carpopedal spasm).
   - Positive Trousseau's sign (hand spasm induced by inflating a blood pressure cuff).
   - Positive Chvostek's sign (twitching of facial muscles when tapped).
   - More noticeable QT interval prolongation on EKG.
   - Psychological symptoms like irritability, confusion, or mood changes.
   - Management:
   - Higher Doses of Oral Calcium and Vitamin D: May be required to restore calcium levels.
   - Ensure Adequate Magnesium Levels: Correct any deficiencies.
   - Cardiac Monitoring: Monitor EKG for arrhythmias due to QT prolongation.

C. **Severe Hypocalcemia (Calcium Level <6.0 mg/dL or Ionized Calcium <1.0 mmol/L)**

- Symptoms: Severe hypocalcemia is a medical emergency characterized by:
- Neuromuscular: Tetany (severe, involuntary muscle contractions), seizures, laryngospasm leading to respiratory distress.
- Cardiac: Significant prolongation of the QT interval, potentially leading to life-threatening arrhythmias like Torsades de Pointes, heart failure, or hypotension.
- Neuropsychiatric: Severe irritability, psychosis, or altered mental status.
- Management:
- IV Calcium Administration:
- Calcium Gluconate: Preferred for peripheral IV administration due to lower risk of tissue necrosis if extravasation occurs. Administer 1–2 g (10–20 mL of 10% solution) over 10–20 min.
- Calcium Chloride: Contains three times more elemental calcium than calcium gluconate but poses a higher risk of tissue injury with extravasation. Reserved for central line administration in severe cases.
- Continuous Infusion: May be necessary for persistent symptoms or critically low calcium levels. Prepare an infusion of calcium gluconate diluted in 1000 mL of D5W, administered at a rate adjusted based on serial ionized calcium measurements.
- Correct Magnesium Levels: Essential to correct any concurrent magnesium deficiency to ensure effective treatment.
- Continuous Cardiac Monitoring: Due to the risk of arrhythmias, patients require close cardiac monitoring in an ICU setting.

3. **Diagnostic Evaluation**

After initial management, identify the underlying cause of hypocalcemia to guide long-term treatment.

1. **Measure Serum Parathyroid Hormone (PTH)**

A. **Low Parathyroid Hormone Levels (Hypoparathyroidism)**
Hypoparathyroidism occurs when there is insufficient production or action of PTH, leading to impaired regulation of calcium levels.

- Parathyroid Agenesis:
- Isolated: Congenital absence of parathyroid glands.
- DiGeorge's Syndrome: Genetic disorder with thymic aplasia/hypoplasia and absent or underdeveloped parathyroid glands.
- Parathyroid Destruction:
- Surgical: Accidental removal or damage during thyroid or neck surgeries.
- Radiation: Damage from neck radiation therapy.

- Infiltration: Metastases or systemic diseases like sarcoidosis infiltrating the glands.
- Autoimmune: Autoimmune destruction of parathyroid tissue.
- Reduced Parathyroid Function:
- Hypomagnesemia: Low magnesium impairs PTH secretion and action.
- Autosomal Dominant Hypocalcemia: Activating mutations in the calcium-sensing receptor suppress PTH secretion despite low calcium levels.

B. **High Parathyroid Hormone Levels (Secondary Hyperparathyroidism)** Elevated PTH in response to low calcium levels, often due to impaired calcium absorption or metabolism.

- Vitamin D Deficiency or Impaired Production/Action:
- Nutritional Deficiency: Poor intake or limited sunlight exposure.
- Renal Insufficiency: Impaired conversion to active 1,25-dihydroxyvitamin D.
- Vitamin D Resistance: Genetic defects in the vitamin D receptor.
- Parathyroid Hormone Resistance Syndromes:
- PTH Receptor Mutations: Resistance to PTH action.
- Pseudohypoparathyroidism: Genetic defect in the PTH signaling pathway.
- Drugs:
- Calcium Chelators: Citrate (in blood transfusions), EDTA.
- Inhibitors of Bone Resorption: Bisphosphonates, plicamycin.
- Altered Vitamin D Metabolism: Phenytoin, ketoconazole.
- Miscellaneous Causes:
- Acute Pancreatitis: Saponification binds calcium.
- Acute Rhabdomyolysis: Phosphate release precipitates calcium.
- Hungry Bone Syndrome: Post-parathyroidectomy increased bone uptake.
- Osteoblastic Metastases: Increased bone formation traps calcium.

2. **Measure Serum Phosphate**

- Role: Phosphate levels are closely linked to calcium metabolism, regulated by PTH and vitamin D.
- Interpretation:
- Elevated Phosphate Levels: Suggest hypoparathyroidism or renal failure.
- Low Phosphate Levels: May indicate vitamin D deficiency or impaired absorption.

3. **Measure Serum Vitamin D**

- Role: Essential for calcium absorption in the intestines.
- Interpretation:
- Low 25-Hydroxyvitamin D Levels: Indicate vitamin D deficiency.
- Low 1,25-Dihydroxyvitamin D Levels: Seen in renal insufficiency or vitamin D resistance.

4. **Calcium Reabsorption Mechanisms in the Kidneys**
   Understanding renal calcium handling helps contextualize why renal conditions can exacerbate hypocalcemia.

   - Proximal Tubules: Approximately 65% of filtered calcium is reabsorbed passively via paracellular transport, driven by sodium and water reabsorption.
   - Thick Ascending Limb: About 20% is reabsorbed here, also via paracellular pathways influenced by the lumen-positive voltage gradient.
   - Distal Convoluted Tubules: Fine-tuning of calcium reabsorption occurs here (~10%), regulated by PTH and vitamin D. Active transcellular transport mechanisms are involved [3].

   Renal conditions affecting these processes, such as acute kidney injury or chronic kidney disease, can impair calcium reabsorption, contributing to hypocalcemia.
5. **Detailed Guidelines on IV Calcium Administration**
   Indications for IV Calcium
   - Severe symptomatic hypocalcemia (e.g., tetany, seizures).
   - Critically low ionized calcium levels.
   - Presence of cardiac arrhythmias due to hypocalcemia.
   - In situations where rapid correction is necessary.

   Calcium Preparations

   - Calcium Gluconate:
   - Concentration: 10% solution contains 90 mg elemental calcium per 10 mL.
   - Advantages: Safer for peripheral administration, less irritating to veins.
   - Administration: 1–2 g (10–20 mL) diluted in 50–100 mL of 5% dextrose or normal saline, infused over 10–20 min.
   - Calcium Chloride:
   - Concentration: 10% solution contains 270 mg elemental calcium per 10 mL.
   - Advantages: Higher bioavailability of elemental calcium.
   - Disadvantages: Risk of severe tissue injury with extravasation; should be administered via central line.
   - Administration: 500–1000 mg (5–10 mL) administered cautiously over 10–20 min.

Administration Guidelines
- Monitoring:
- Cardiac Monitoring: Continuous EKG monitoring during administration due to the risk of arrhythmias.
- Serial Calcium Measurements: Check ionized calcium levels every 4–6 h to guide therapy.
- Infusion Rates:
- Bolus Dose: Provides immediate correction; effects last 1–2 h.

- Continuous Infusion: May follow bolus dose; typically 0.5–1.5 mg/kg/h of elemental calcium.
- Precautions:
- Avoid Rapid Administration: Can cause cardiac arrhythmias or vasodilation leading to hypotension.
- Extravasation Risk: Ensure secure IV access to prevent tissue necrosis.
- Drug Interactions: Do not mix with bicarbonate or phosphate-containing solutions to prevent precipitation.

26.2 Conclusion

Managing hypocalcemia in the ICU requires careful assessment and prompt treatment to prevent serious complications. A systematic approach includes confirming true hypocalcemia, understanding the patient's acid-base status, and recognizing the significance of ionized calcium levels. Clinical manifestations guide the urgency and aggressiveness of treatment, with severe cases necessitating immediate IV calcium administration and continuous cardiac monitoring due to the risk of life-threatening arrhythmias. Understanding the underlying mechanisms, including calcium reabsorption in the kidneys and the roles of PTH and vitamin D, is essential for identifying the cause and preventing recurrence. By following this comprehensive approach, healthcare providers can ensure that patients with hypocalcemia receive timely and effective care, optimizing outcomes in the ICU setting.

Algorithm 26.1: Approach to hypocalcemia in the ICU

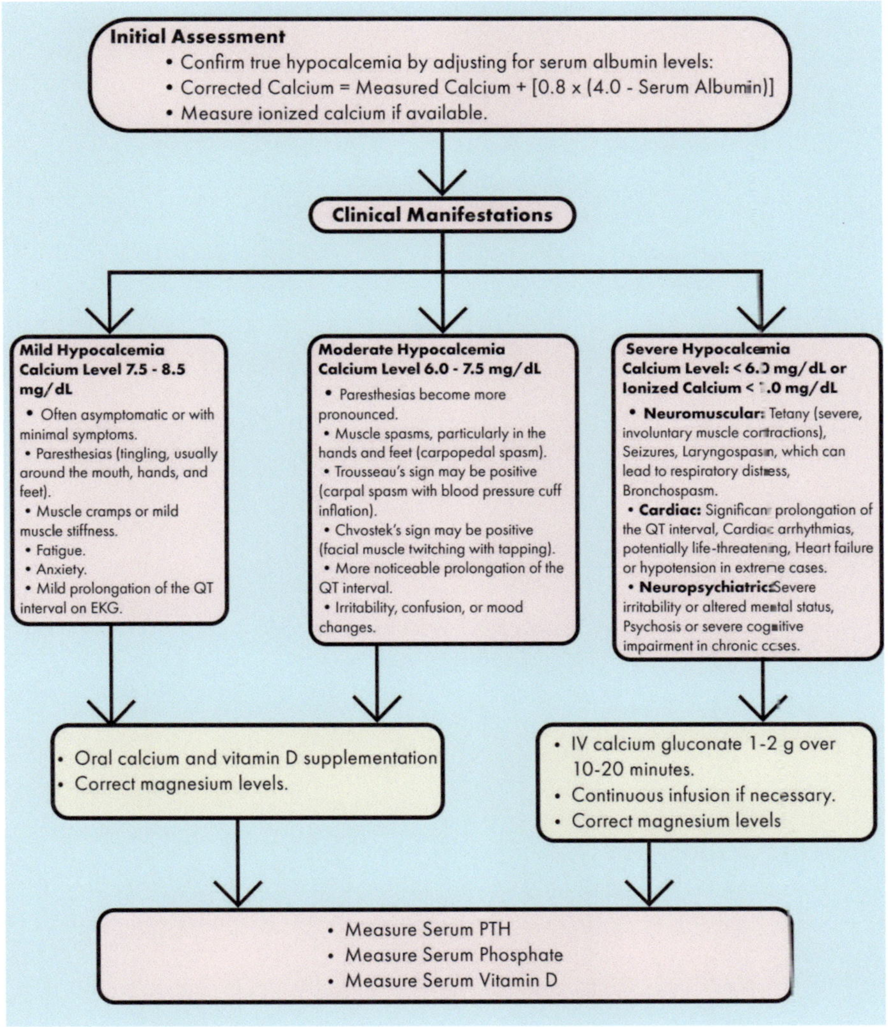

Bibliography

1. Murray SL, Wolf M. Calcium and phosphate disorders: core curriculum 2024. Am J Kidney Dis. 2024;83(2):241–56.
2. Bushinsky DA, Monk RD. Electrolyte quintet: calcium. Lancet. 1998;352(9124):306–11.
3. Guise TA, Wysolmerski JJ. Cancer-associated hypercalcemia. N Engl J Med. 2022;386(15):1443–51.

Chapter 27
Approach to Hypercalcemia in the ICU

27.1 Introduction

Hypercalcemia, defined as an abnormally elevated level of calcium in the blood, is a common electrolyte disorder with significant clinical consequences. Calcium plays a crucial role in various physiological processes, including neuromuscular function, blood coagulation, and bone metabolism. In the bloodstream, calcium exists in three distinct fractions: ionized calcium (approximately 50%), which is the biologically active form; protein-bound calcium, primarily attached to albumin (about 40%); and calcium complexed with anions like phosphate and citrate (around 10%). The management of hypercalcemia, especially in the intensive care unit (ICU), is critical because severe cases can lead to life-threatening complications such as cardiac arrhythmias, renal failure, and neurological impairments [1].

Calcium homeostasis is tightly regulated by a complex interplay of hormones, notably parathyroid hormone (PTH), 1,25-dihydroxyvitamin D [1,25(OH)_2D], and fibroblast growth factor 23 (FGF-23). Disruptions in this regulatory system can result from various conditions, including malignancies, primary hyperparathyroidism, granulomatous diseases, thyrotoxicosis, and prolonged immobilization. Effective management involves assessing the severity of hypercalcemia, identifying the underlying cause, and implementing appropriate treatment strategies to normalize calcium levels and prevent complications [2] [Ref: Algorithm 27.1].

27.2 Pathophysiology of Calcium Regulation

Understanding calcium regulation is essential for diagnosing and managing hypercalcemia. Calcium homeostasis is maintained through a balance of intestinal absorption, renal excretion, and bone remodeling. Key hormones involved include:

S. B. Mishra et al., *Mastering ICU Care*,
https://doi.org/10.1007/978-981-95-0179-3_27

- Parathyroid Hormone (PTH): Secreted by the parathyroid glands in response to low serum calcium levels, PTH increases calcium levels by stimulating osteoclast-mediated bone resorption, enhancing renal reabsorption of calcium, and promoting the activation of vitamin D to its active form.
- 1,25-Dihydroxyvitamin D [1,25(OH)_2D]: The active form of vitamin D enhances intestinal absorption of calcium and phosphate and works synergistically with PTH to regulate bone remodeling.
- Fibroblast Growth Factor 23 (FGF-23): Produced by osteocytes and osteoblasts, FGF-23 regulates phosphate metabolism and indirectly influences calcium levels by modulating vitamin D activity.

27.3 Ionized Calcium vs. Total Calcium

In clinical practice, measuring ionized calcium is preferable when available, as it reflects the biologically active fraction responsible for physiological effects. Total serum calcium measurements can be misleading, especially in patients with abnormal serum albumin levels or acid-base disturbances, as they do not accurately represent the ionized fraction. Although corrected calcium calculations attempt to adjust for albumin levels, they may not always be precise, particularly in critically ill patients. Therefore, relying on ionized calcium provides a more accurate assessment for diagnosis and treatment.

27.4 Clinical Manifestations

The symptoms of hypercalcemia correlate with both the absolute level of serum calcium and the rate at which it rises:

Mild Hypercalcemia (≤11.5 mg/dL):

- Often asymptomatic.
- May present with vague neuropsychiatric symptoms such as fatigue, depression, or mild cognitive impairment.

Moderate Hypercalcemia (11.5–14 mg/dL):

- Gastrointestinal Disturbances: Nausea, vomiting, constipation, and anorexia.
- Renal Impairment: Polyuria, polydipsia, and dehydration due to nephrogenic diabetes insipidus.
- Neuropsychiatric Symptoms: Confusion, irritability, or depression.
- Cardiovascular Effects: Hypertension and shortened QT interval.

Severe Hypercalcemia (>14 mg/dL):

- Neurological symptoms can progress from lethargy and stupor to coma.

- Severe gastrointestinal symptoms, including vomiting and pancreatitis.
- Cardiovascular Complications: Arrhythmias and possible cardiac arrest.
- Peptic ulcer disease due to increased gastrin secretion.

27.5 Causes of Hypercalcemia

Hypercalcemia arises from increased calcium entry into the circulation, decreased renal excretion, or a combination of both. The causes can be broadly categorized into PTH-dependent and PTH-independent mechanisms.

1. **PTH-Dependent Hypercalcemia:**
   Primary Hyperparathyroidism:

   - Most common cause in outpatients.
   - Usually due to a parathyroid adenoma leading to excessive PTH secretion.
   - Results in increased bone resorption, renal calcium reabsorption, and intestinal calcium absorption.

   Tertiary Hyperparathyroidism:

   - Occurs in patients with chronic renal insufficiency.
   - Prolonged secondary hyperparathyroidism leads to autonomous PTH secretion and hypercalcemia.

   Familial Hypocalciuric Hypercalcemia (FHH):

   - Genetic condition caused by mutations in the calcium-sensing receptor.
   - Characterized by mild hypercalcemia, low urinary calcium excretion, and inappropriately normal or slightly elevated PTH levels.

2. **PTH-Independent Hypercalcemia:**
   Malignancy-Associated Hypercalcemia:

   - Humoral Hypercalcemia of Malignancy (HHM):
   - Caused by secretion of PTH-related protein (PTHrP) by tumors such as squamous cell carcinomas, renal cell carcinoma, and breast cancer.
   - PTHrP mimics the effects of PTH, leading to increased bone resorption and renal calcium reabsorption.

   Local Osteolytic Hypercalcemia:

   - Seen in cancers with bone metastases, such as breast cancer and multiple myeloma.
   - Tumor cells produce cytokines that stimulate osteoclasts, leading to bone resorption and calcium release.

Granulomatous Diseases:

- Diseases like sarcoidosis and tuberculosis involve activated macrophages that increase extrarenal production of 1,25(OH)_2D.
- Leads to enhanced intestinal calcium absorption independent of PTH.

Thyrotoxicosis:

- Excess thyroid hormones stimulate bone turnover, increasing bone resorption and serum calcium levels.

Immobilization:

- Prolonged immobilization, particularly in individuals with high bone turnover (e.g., adolescents, Paget's disease), leads to increased osteoclastic activity and bone resorption.

Vitamin D Intoxication:

- Excessive intake of vitamin D supplements or overproduction due to granulomatous disease increases intestinal absorption of calcium.

Medications:

- Thiazide Diuretics: Reduce renal calcium excretion.
- Lithium: Increases PTH secretion.
- Vitamin A Excess: Stimulates osteoclast activity.

Milk-Alkali Syndrome:

- Results from excessive intake of calcium and absorbable alkali.
- Leads to hypercalcemia, metabolic alkalosis, and renal impairment.

Adrenal Insufficiency:

- May cause mild hypercalcemia due to hemoconcentration and increased bone resorption.

27.6 Diagnostic Approach

The evaluation of hypercalcemia involves confirming elevated calcium levels and determining the underlying cause.

1. **Confirm Hypercalcemia:**
   - Measure Ionized Calcium:
   - Preferred method as it reflects the biologically active fraction.
   - Avoids inaccuracies due to variations in albumin or pH levels.
   - Correct Total Calcium:
   - If ionized calcium is unavailable, adjust total calcium for serum albumin:

$$\text{Corrected Calcium}(\text{mg}/\text{dL}) = \text{Measured Total Calcium} + [0.8 \times (4.0 - \text{Serum Albumin}(\text{g}/\text{dL}))]$$

2. **Assess Parathyroid Hormone (PTH) Levels:**
   - Elevated or Inappropriately Normal PTH:
   - Suggests PTH-dependent causes like primary hyperparathyroidism or FHH.
   - Suppressed PTH:
   - Indicates PTH-independent hypercalcemia.
   - Prompts evaluation for malignancy, vitamin D intoxication, granulomatous disease, or other causes.
3. **Additional Investigations:**
   PTHrP Levels:
   - Elevated in humoral hypercalcemia of malignancy.
   - Order when malignancy is suspected.

   Vitamin D Metabolites:
   - 25(OH)D: Elevated in vitamin D intoxication.
   - 1,25(OH)_2D: Elevated in granulomatous diseases and some lymphomas.

   Thyroid Function Tests:
   - To assess for thyrotoxicosis.

   Bone Imaging:
   - If local osteolytic hypercalcemia is suspected.

   Urinary Calcium Excretion:
   - Low in FHH.
   - High in primary hyperparathyroidism.

27.7 Management by Severity

27.7.1 Mild Hypercalcemia

- Observation and Investigation:
- Focus on identifying and treating the underlying cause.
- Ensure adequate hydration.
- Avoid factors that can worsen hypercalcemia, such as thiazide diuretics and high calcium intake.

27.7.2 Moderate to Severe Hypercalcemia

Management aims to reduce serum calcium levels rapidly and address the underlying cause.

1. **Hydration and Renal Calcium Excretion:**
   - Intravenous Normal Saline:
   - Administer aggressively (e.g., 200–300 mL/h) to correct volume depletion.
   - Enhances glomerular filtration rate and promotes calciuresis.
   - Loop Diuretics:
   - Furosemide:
   - Used after rehydration to promote diuresis and calciuresis.
   - Monitor electrolytes to prevent hypokalemia and hypomagnesemia.
2. **Inhibition of Bone Resorption:**
   - Bisphosphonates:
   - Zoledronic Acid: 4 mg IV over 15 min.
   - Pamidronate: 60–90 mg IV over 2–4 h.
   - Inhibit osteoclast-mediated bone resorption.
   - Onset of action is 48–72 h.
   - Denosumab:
   - Monoclonal antibody against RANKL.
   - Effective in patients resistant or intolerant to bisphosphonates.
   - Particularly useful in malignancy-associated hypercalcemia.
3. **Calcitonin:**
   - Mechanism:
   - Rapidly reduces serum calcium by inhibiting osteoclast activity and increasing renal calcium excretion.
   - Administration:
   - Given subcutaneously or intramuscularly.
   - Tachyphylaxis develops within 48 h, limiting long-term use.
4. **Glucocorticoids:**
   - Indications:
   - Hypercalcemia due to vitamin D intoxication or granulomatous diseases.
   - Reduce intestinal calcium absorption and inhibit 1,25(OH)_2D production.
   - Dosage:
   - Prednisone 40–60 mg daily.

5. **Dialysis:**

- Indications:
- Severe, life-threatening hypercalcemia refractory to medical therapy.
- Patients with renal failure or contraindications to aggressive hydration.
- Procedure:
- Hemodialysis with low-calcium dialysate.

27.8 Prognosis and Complications

Malignancy-Associated Hypercalcemia:

- Carries a poor prognosis.
- Median survival ranges from 25 to 52 days in severe cases.
- Hypercalcemia often indicates advanced disease [3].

Renal Complications:

- Nephrocalcinosis and renal insufficiency due to prolonged hypercalcemia.
- Cardiovascular Effects:
- Risk of arrhythmias and hypertension due to shortened QT interval.

Neurological Effects:

- Cognitive dysfunction, neuromuscular weakness, and, in severe cases, coma.

27.9 Conclusion

Effective management of hypercalcemia requires a comprehensive understanding of calcium homeostasis and a methodical diagnostic approach to identify the underlying cause. Early recognition and prompt treatment are vital, particularly in severe cases, to prevent life-threatening complications. Clinicians should focus on stabilizing the patient through hydration and medications that reduce serum calcium levels while addressing the primary etiology to prevent recurrence.

Algorithm 27.1: Approach to hypercalcemia in the ICU

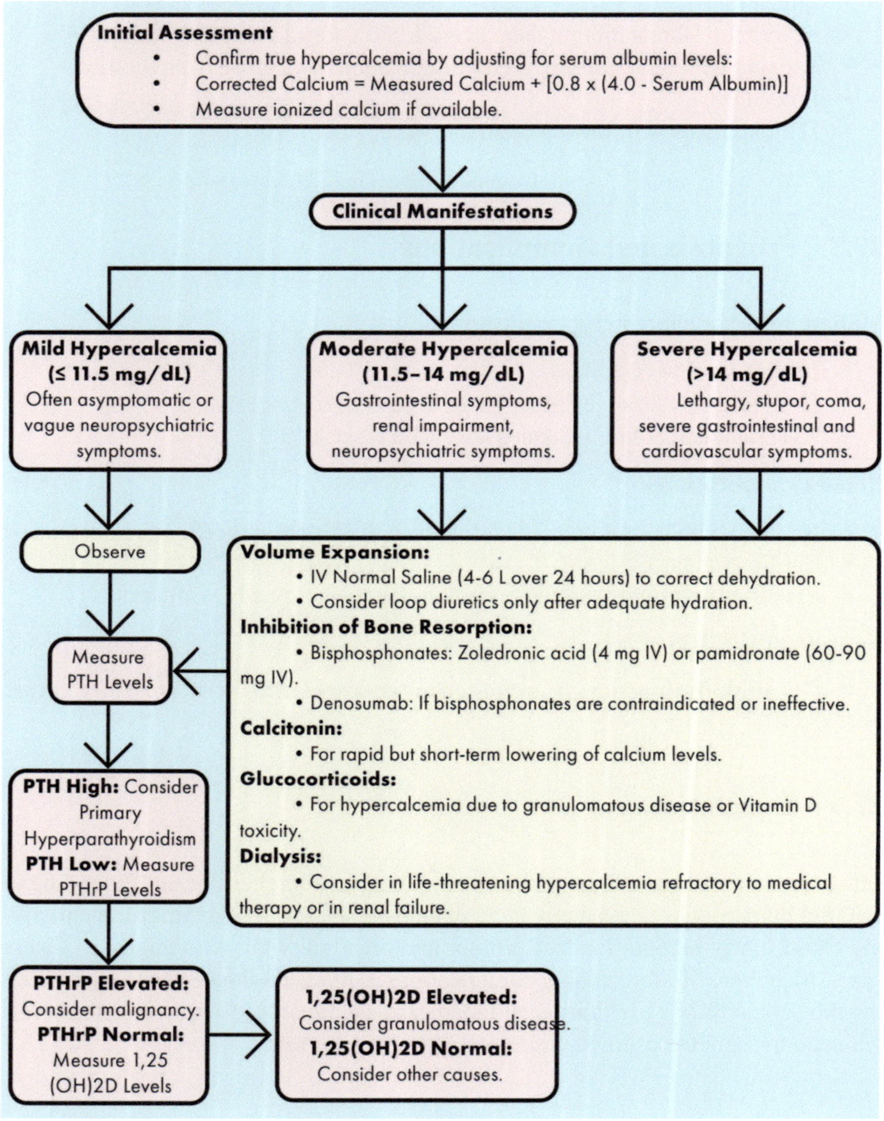

Bibliography

1. Murray SL, Wolf M. Calcium and phosphate disorders: core curriculum 2024. Am J Kidney Dis. 2024;83(2):241–56.
2. Bushinsky DA, Monk RD. Electrolyte quintet: calcium. Lancet. 1998;352(9124):306–11.
3. Guise TA, Wysolmerski JJ. Cancer-associated hypercalcemia. N Engl J Med. 2022;386(15):1443–51.

Chapter 28
Approach to Hypophosphatemia in the ICU

28.1 Introduction

Hypophosphatemia is a common electrolyte disturbance in critically ill patients and can have significant clinical consequences if not properly managed. Phosphate plays a crucial role in cellular energy metabolism, membrane integrity, bone mineralization, and the function of the muscular and nervous systems. Phosphate homeostasis is tightly regulated by hormones such as parathyroid hormone (PTH), fibroblast growth factor 23 (FGF-23), and 1,25-dihydroxyvitamin D. These hormones manage phosphate balance through their actions on the kidneys, intestines, and bones, ensuring adequate phosphate availability for physiological processes.

Hypophosphatemia is typically defined as a serum phosphate level of less than 0.8 mmol/L (or <2.5 mg/dL). The approach to managing hypophosphatemia involves initial assessment, classification based on severity, and addressing underlying causes. This detailed guide will walk through each step outlined in the flowchart for the management of hypophosphatemia [1, 2] [Ref: Algorithm 28.1].

28.2 Phosphate Homeostasis Mechanisms

Understanding phosphate homeostasis is essential for effective management of hypophosphatemia. PTH is secreted by the parathyroid glands in response to low calcium levels and increases renal excretion of phosphate while promoting calcium reabsorption. FGF-23, produced by osteocytes and osteoblasts, inhibits renal phosphate reabsorption and suppresses 1,25-dihydroxyvitamin D synthesis, leading to decreased intestinal phosphate absorption. Conversely, 1,25-dihydroxyvitamin D

S. B. Mishra et al., *Mastering ICU Care*,
https://doi.org/10.1007/978-981-95-0179-3_28

enhances intestinal absorption of both calcium and phosphate and promotes bone mineralization. The interplay among these hormones maintains serum phosphate levels within a narrow range.

28.2.1 Initial Assessment

28.2.1.1 Confirm Diagnosis

The first step in managing hypophosphatemia is to confirm the diagnosis through accurate measurement of serum phosphate levels. It is important to recognize that phosphate levels can fluctuate with various physiological and pathological conditions, so repeated measurements may be necessary. Additionally, assessing levels of PTH, FGF-23, and 1,25-dihydroxyvitamin D can provide insights into the hormonal regulation contributing to hypophosphatemia.

28.2.1.2 Assess Severity

Once hypophosphatemia is confirmed, the next step is to assess the severity of the condition. The severity is classified into three categories:

1. **Mild Hypophosphatemia (1.86–2.48 mg/dL)**
   Mild hypophosphatemia is generally asymptomatic and may be detected incidentally. Patients with mild hypophosphatemia may not require aggressive treatment and can often be managed with dietary modifications and oral supplementation.
2. **Moderate Hypophosphatemia (0.93–1.86 mg/dL)**
   Moderate hypophosphatemia can present with symptoms such as muscle weakness, fatigue, or respiratory difficulty. It may necessitate more active intervention, including oral or intravenous phosphate supplementation, depending on the clinical context and the patient's ability to tolerate oral intake.
3. **Severe Hypophosphatemia (< 0.93 mg/dL)**
   Severe hypophosphatemia is a medical emergency that can lead to significant clinical complications, including rhabdomyolysis, hemolysis, impaired myocardial contractility, and respiratory failure. This level of severity requires prompt intravenous phosphate replacement and careful monitoring.

28.3 Impact of Hypophosphatemia on Organ Systems

Hypophosphatemia can affect multiple organ systems:

- Musculoskeletal System: Muscle weakness, myalgia, and, in severe cases, rhabdomyolysis can occur due to decreased ATP production.

- Skeletal System: Chronic hypophosphatemia impairs bone mineralization, leading to osteomalacia in adults and rickets in children. Phosphate depletion affects the formation of hydroxyapatite crystals, essential for bone strength, increasing the risk of fractures.
- Cardiovascular System: Severe hypophosphatemia may impair myocardial contractility, potentially leading to arrhythmias and heart failure.
- Respiratory System: Weakness of the diaphragmatic and intercostal muscles can result in respiratory failure.
- Hematologic System: Decreased ATP in red blood cells can cause hemolytic anemia.
- Neurologic System: Patients may experience paresthesias, confusion, seizures, or coma in severe cases.

28.4 Management Based on Severity

28.4.1 Mild Hypophosphatemia

Patients with mild hypophosphatemia should be managed with oral phosphate supplementation. This approach includes encouraging the intake of dietary phosphate-rich foods such as dairy products, meat, poultry, fish, nuts, and whole grains. Oral phosphate supplements may be prescribed if dietary measures alone are insufficient.

28.4.2 Moderate Hypophosphatemia

For moderate hypophosphatemia, oral supplementation is typically the first-line treatment if the patient can tolerate it. The usual oral dose is 0.5–1 g of phosphate daily, divided into multiple doses to minimize gastrointestinal side effects. If the patient is unable to take oral supplements or has significant symptoms, intravenous phosphate may be administered. The dosage should be tailored to the patient's needs and adjusted based on serum phosphate levels.

28.4.3 Severe Hypophosphatemia

In cases of severe hypophosphatemia, intravenous phosphate replacement is the treatment of choice. The recommended starting dose is 0.08–0.16 mmol/kg of elemental phosphate, administered over 4–6 h. It is crucial to monitor serum phosphate, calcium, and magnesium levels closely during this period, as phosphate repletion can lead to shifts in other electrolytes, potentially causing hypocalcemia or hypomagnesemia. Continuous cardiac monitoring may be necessary due to the risk of arrhythmias.

28.5 Identifying Potential Causes of Hypophosphatemia

After initiating treatment for hypophosphatemia, it is imperative to investigate and identify the underlying causes to effectively manage the condition and prevent recurrence. The causes of hypophosphatemia can be broadly categorized into three groups: internal redistribution, increased renal excretion, and decreased intestinal absorption. Understanding these mechanisms will guide targeted therapeutic strategies.

1. **Internal Redistribution**

   - **Respiratory Alkalosis**
     Respiratory alkalosis, a condition where carbon dioxide levels drop due to hyperventilation, causes a shift of phosphate from the extracellular space into cells. This internal redistribution reduces serum phosphate levels without necessarily indicating a total body phosphate deficit. Management involves addressing the underlying cause of hyperventilation, such as pain, anxiety, or respiratory distress.
   - **Insulin Administration or Glucose Loading**
     Insulin therapy, especially when combined with glucose administration—as seen in the treatment of diabetic ketoacidosis or during refeeding—promotes cellular uptake of phosphate. Insulin facilitates the transport of phosphate along with glucose into cells, reducing serum phosphate levels. Monitoring and gradual correction of phosphate levels are crucial during intensive insulin therapy to avoid severe hypophosphatemia.
   - **Refeeding Syndrome**
     Refeeding syndrome is a metabolic disturbance that occurs when nutritional support is initiated in malnourished patients, particularly those with anorexia nervosa, chronic alcoholism, or prolonged fasting. The sudden increase in insulin secretion upon reintroduction of carbohydrates drives phosphate into cells, leading to a precipitous drop in serum phosphate levels. Preventative strategies include slow refeeding with gradual caloric increases and phosphate supplementation.

2. **Increased Renal Excretion**

   - **Diuretic Use (Especially Loop and Thiazide Diuretics)**
     Loop and thiazide diuretics increase renal phosphate excretion by reducing reabsorption in the proximal renal tubules. This mechanism is particularly pronounced in patients with concurrent conditions such as chronic kidney disease or hypomagnesemia. Management involves careful monitoring of electrolyte levels and adjusting diuretic therapy to minimize phosphate loss.
   - **Hyperparathyroidism**
     Hyperparathyroidism, characterized by excessive secretion of parathyroid hormone (PTH), increases renal excretion of phosphate. PTH enhances renal tubule phosphate clearance, leading to hypophosphatemia. Treating hyper-

parathyroidism, whether surgically or medically, is essential to correct this cause of hypophosphatemia.

- **Fanconi Syndrome**

  Fanconi syndrome is a disorder of proximal renal tubular function leading to impaired reabsorption of glucose, amino acids, bicarbonate, and phosphate. This results in phosphate wasting and subsequent hypophosphatemia. Management focuses on treating the underlying cause and supplementing lost substances, including phosphate.
- **Fibroblast Growth Factor 23 (FGF-23)-Related Disorders**

  Elevated levels of FGF-23 can lead to increased renal phosphate excretion. Measurement of FGF-23 is useful in distinguishing renal causes of hypophosphatemia, especially in cases involving phosphate-wasting syndromes such as tumor-induced osteomalacia or genetic disorders like X-linked hypophosphatemic rickets. Targeted therapies may include treatments that reduce FGF-23 levels or its effects.

3. **Decreased Intestinal Absorption**

- **Chronic Alcoholism**

  Chronic alcohol use is associated with multiple mechanisms that contribute to hypophosphatemia, including poor dietary intake, malabsorption due to gastrointestinal mucosal damage, and increased renal excretion due to alcohol-induced diuresis. Alcoholism often coexists with malnutrition and liver disease, which exacerbate phosphate loss. Addressing alcohol use disorder, improving nutritional status, and supplementing phosphate are key management strategies.
- **Malnutrition and Malabsorption Syndromes**

  Conditions that impair nutrient absorption, such as celiac disease, inflammatory bowel disease, or pancreatic insufficiency, can lead to decreased phosphate absorption. Similarly, inadequate dietary intake in malnutrition reduces phosphate availability. Management involves treating the underlying malabsorption disorder and ensuring adequate nutritional support.
- **Chronic Diarrhea**

  Chronic diarrhea leads to significant losses of phosphate through the gastrointestinal tract. The loss of intestinal contents, including phosphate, contributes to hypophosphatemia. Treating the underlying cause of diarrhea and providing phosphate supplementation can help restore normal phosphate levels.
- **Use of Phosphate-Binding Antacids**

  Phosphate-binding antacids, such as aluminum or magnesium-containing compounds, can inadvertently cause hypophosphatemia if used excessively or inappropriately. These antacids bind dietary phosphate in the gut, reducing its absorption. Adjusting the use of phosphate binders and monitoring serum phosphate levels are essential to prevent and manage hypophosphatemia in these patients.

28.6 Diagnostic Testing

Differentiating between renal and nonrenal causes of hypophosphatemia is essential for targeted treatment. Measurement of urinary phosphate excretion, fractional excretion of phosphate ($FePO_4$), and levels of FGF-23 can aid in this distinction. Elevated urinary phosphate excretion suggests renal phosphate wasting, whereas low urinary phosphate indicates internal redistribution or decreased intake/absorption. Measuring FGF-23 is particularly useful in diagnosing conditions like tumor-induced osteomalacia or genetic phosphate-wasting disorders.

28.7 Bone Metabolism

Chronic hypophosphatemia adversely affects bone health. Phosphate is a critical component of hydroxyapatite crystals, which provide strength and rigidity to bones. Phosphate depletion impairs bone mineralization, leading to osteomalacia in adults—characterized by bone pain, fractures, and muscle weakness—and rickets in children, which presents with bone deformities and growth retardation. Early recognition and correction of hypophosphatemia are crucial to prevent these complications.

28.8 Management of Severe Cases

In managing severe hypophosphatemia, it is important to monitor not only phosphate levels but also calcium and magnesium levels during treatment. Rapid shifts in phosphate can lead to hypocalcemia due to precipitation of calcium-phosphate complexes, potentially causing tetany or cardiac arrhythmias. Hypomagnesemia can also occur, further complicating electrolyte balance. Regular monitoring and appropriate supplementation of these electrolytes are essential to ensure patient safety.

28.9 Conclusion

The management of hypophosphatemia requires a structured approach that begins with confirming the diagnosis and assessing the severity of the condition. Treatment strategies range from dietary and oral phosphate supplementation in mild cases to intravenous phosphate replacement in severe cases. Identifying and correcting underlying causes is crucial to prevent recurrence and complications. Understanding the mechanisms of phosphate homeostasis and the impact of hypophosphatemia on various organ systems enhances the clinician's ability to provide comprehensive care. By following this approach, healthcare providers can effectively manage hypophosphatemia and mitigate its potential impact on patient outcomes.

Algorithm 28.1: Approach to hypophosphatemia in the ICU

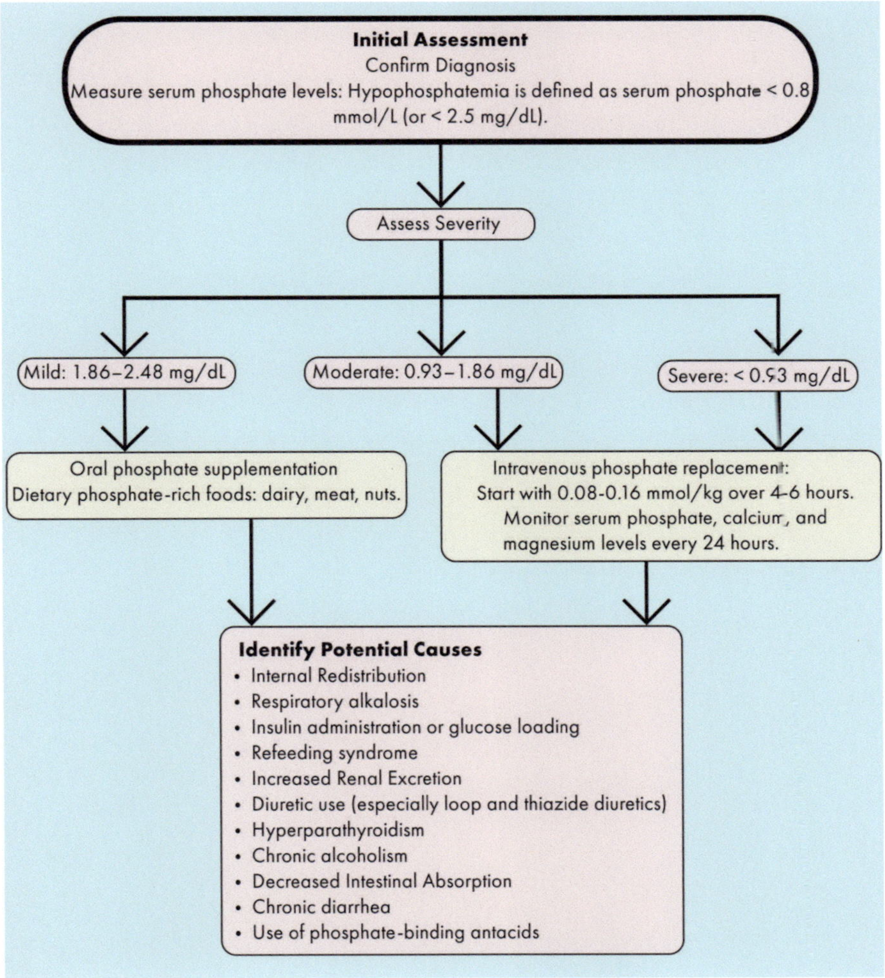

Bibliography

1. Imel EA, Econs MJ. Approach to the hypophosphatemic patient. J Clin Endocrinol Metab. 2012;97(3):696–706.
2. Murray SL, Wolf M. Calcium and phosphate disorders: core curriculum 2024. Am J Kidney Dis. 2024;83(2):241–56.

Chapter 29
Approach to Hyperphosphatemia in the ICU

29.1 Introduction

Hyperphosphatemia, an elevated level of phosphate in the blood, is a common electrolyte disturbance in critically ill patients. It can result from various underlying conditions such as renal failure, tumor lysis syndrome, or rhabdomyolysis, and may lead to significant complications if not managed appropriately. Phosphate homeostasis is tightly regulated by a complex interplay of hormones, including parathyroid hormone (PTH), fibroblast growth factor 23 (FGF-23), and 1,25-dihydroxyvitamin D (calcitriol). These hormones regulate calcium and phosphate levels through feedback mechanisms involving the kidneys, bones, and intestines. Understanding these physiological mechanisms is essential for effective management of hyperphosphatemia, particularly in patients with chronic kidney disease (CKD), where FGF-23 plays a crucial role in phosphate excretion [1] [Ref: Algorithm 29.1].

1. **Assess Severity**
   - Serum Phosphate Measurement: The first step in managing hyperphosphatemia is to assess the severity of the condition by measuring serum phosphate levels. Based on the results, hyperphosphatemia can be categorized as:
   - Mild: Serum phosphate levels between 4.5 and 5.6 mg/dL.
   - Moderate: Serum phosphate levels between 5.6 and 7.8 mg/dL.
   - Severe: Serum phosphate levels greater than 7.8 mg/dL.

2. **Mild Hyperphosphatemia (4.5–5.6 mg/dL)**

   Intervention:

   - Dietary Phosphate Restriction: Advise patients to reduce their intake of phosphate-rich foods, such as dairy products, nuts, and certain meats.

S. B. Mishra et al., *Mastering ICU Care*,
https://doi.org/10.1007/978-981-95-0179-3_29

- Discontinue Phosphate-Containing Medications: Substitute medications containing phosphate with alternatives that do not contribute to the phosphate load.

Rationale:

- Controlling the intake and absorption of phosphate is often sufficient to prevent further elevation of serum phosphate levels and maintain them within the normal range.

3. **Moderate Hyperphosphatemia (5.6–7.8 mg/dL)**

Intervention:

- Phosphate Binders: Administer phosphate binders such as calcium carbonate, calcium acetate, or sevelamer to reduce serum phosphate levels by binding dietary phosphate in the gastrointestinal tract and preventing its absorption.
- Intravenous (IV) Fluids and Diuretics: Use IV fluids and diuretics to promote renal excretion of phosphate.

Rationale:

- More aggressive management is required to prevent progression to severe hyperphosphatemia, which can lead to complications like calcium-phosphate precipitation and vascular calcification.

4. **Severe Hyperphosphatemia (> 7.8 mg/dL).**

Intervention:

- Phosphate Binders: Continue the use of phosphate binders to reduce phosphate absorption.
- IV Fluids and Diuretics: Maintain IV fluids and diuretics to enhance phosphate excretion.
- Dialysis: Initiate dialysis if serum phosphate levels are critically high and unresponsive to other interventions, to rapidly reduce phosphate levels.

Rationale:

- Severe hyperphosphatemia is a medical emergency requiring prompt intervention to prevent life-threatening complications such as cardiac arrhythmias or tissue calcifications.

5. **Identify Potential Causes of Hyperphosphatemia**

After initiating treatment based on the severity of hyperphosphatemia, it is crucial to identify and address the underlying cause(s) to prevent recurrence and tailor long-term management strategies effectively. Hyperphosphatemia can result from various etiologies, including decreased renal excretion, increased intake, cellular release, and pseudohyperphosphatemia. Understanding the underlying mechanisms of each cause is vital for effective management.

A. **Decreased Renal Excretion**

Chronic Kidney Disease (CKD) and Acute Kidney Injury (AKI):

- Mechanism: The kidneys are central in maintaining phosphate homeostasis by filtering and excreting excess phosphate. In CKD and AKI, impaired renal function leads to phosphate retention.

Pathophysiology:

- FGF-23 Role: Elevated phosphate levels stimulate the secretion of FGF-23 from osteocytes. FGF-23 increases renal phosphate excretion by reducing sodium-phosphate co-transporters in the renal proximal tubules.
- PTH Interaction: PTH is also elevated in response to hyperphosphatemia and hypocalcemia, promoting phosphate excretion and calcium reabsorption.
- Vitamin D Suppression: FGF-23 suppresses 1,25-dihydroxyvitamin D synthesis, leading to decreased intestinal absorption of calcium and phosphate.
- Feedback Loops: Despite elevated FGF-23 and PTH, the declining GFR in CKD limits phosphate excretion, leading to persistent hyperphosphatemia.
- Clinical Implications: Hyperphosphatemia contributes to secondary hyperparathyroidism and vascular calcification, increasing morbidity and mortality in CKD patients.

B. **Tumor Lysis Syndrome (TLS)**

Mechanism:

Cellular Release: TLS results from the massive lysis of tumor cells, releasing intracellular phosphate into the bloodstream.

- Renal Overload: The acute phosphate load overwhelms renal excretion capacity, especially in patients with preexisting renal impairment.

C. **Rhabdomyolysis**

Mechanism:

- Muscle Breakdown: Destruction of muscle tissue releases phosphate and other intracellular ions into the circulation.
- AKI Association: The released myoglobin can cause AKI, further impairing phosphate excretion.

D. **Increased Intake**

- Excessive Dietary Phosphate or Phosphate-Containing Medications:
- Mechanism: High intake of phosphate through diet or medications increases serum phosphate levels, particularly dangerous in patients with reduced renal function.

E. **Cellular Release**

- Conditions like Hemolysis or Severe Infection:

- Mechanism: Breakdown of cells releases intracellular phosphate, contributing to elevated serum levels.

F. **Pseudohyperphosphatemia**

- Lab Errors and Conditions Like Hyperlipidemia or Hyperproteinemia:
- Mechanism: Interference from lipids or proteins can falsely elevate phosphate levels in laboratory assays.

6. **Long-Term Management and the Role of FGF-23**

Understanding the hormonal regulation of phosphate is essential for long-term management, especially in CKD patients.

FGF-23 in Chronic Management

- Central Role: FGF-23 is crucial in regulating phosphate homeostasis by increasing renal excretion and decreasing intestinal absorption.
- CKD Implications: In CKD, elevated FGF-23 levels are a response to hyperphosphatemia but may lead to left ventricular hypertrophy and increased cardiovascular risk.
- Interplay with PTH and Vitamin D:
- PTH: Elevated phosphate and reduced calcium stimulate PTH secretion, leading to secondary hyperparathyroidism.
- Vitamin D: Suppressed 1,25-dihydroxyvitamin D levels reduce calcium absorption, exacerbating hypocalcemia.

Management Strategies

- Phosphate Binders: Long-term use helps control serum phosphate, reducing the stimulus for FGF-23 and PTH secretion.
- Vitamin D Analogues: Supplementation can suppress PTH levels and improve calcium absorption.
- Dietary Restrictions: Limiting phosphate intake reduces the burden on renal excretion mechanisms.
- Monitoring FGF-23 Levels: May provide insights into disease progression and guide therapy adjustments.

29.2 Conclusion

Effective management of hyperphosphatemia requires a comprehensive understanding of the physiological mechanisms regulating phosphate homeostasis, particularly the roles of FGF-23, PTH, and vitamin D. Assessing the severity of phosphate elevation and implementing appropriate interventions are essential steps. Addressing underlying causes, especially in CKD and AKI, is crucial for long-term management and preventing recurrence. Integrating knowledge of hormonal feedback loops and renal handling of phosphate enhances treatment strategies, ultimately improving patient outcomes.

Algorithm 29.1 Approach to hyperphosphatemia in the ICU

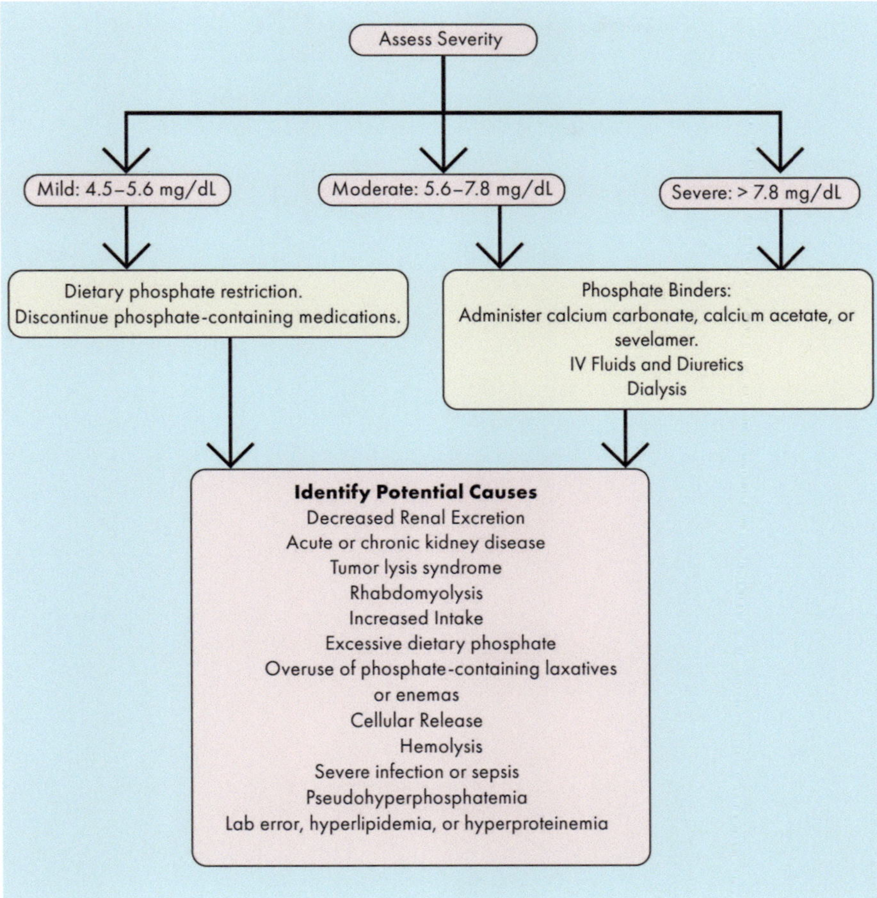

Bibliography

1. Murray SL, Wolf M. Calcium and phosphate disorders: core curriculum 2024. Am J Kidney Dis. 2024;83(2):241–56.

Chapter 30
Approach to Hypomagnesemia in the ICU

30.1 Introduction

Magnesium is an essential mineral that plays a pivotal role in numerous physiological processes. Serving as a cofactor in over 300 enzymatic reactions—including ATP synthesis and DNA replication—it is fundamental to energy production, muscle and nerve function, and the immune response. Magnesium's influence extends from cellular metabolism to the maintenance of normal heart rhythm and bone health. Hypomagnesemia, defined as low serum magnesium levels, is a common electrolyte disturbance not only in the intensive care unit (ICU) but also among patients with chronic illnesses such as diabetes, cardiovascular diseases, and gastrointestinal disorders.

Magnesium deficiency is prevalent in hospitalized patients and is associated with increased morbidity and mortality. Given its widespread impact and the potential severity of hypomagnesemia—including life-threatening conditions like seizures and arrhythmias—early recognition and appropriate management are crucial. This guide provides a structured approach to diagnosing and treating hypomagnesemia, emphasizing understanding the underlying causes, identifying risk factors, and implementing evidence-based treatment strategies to improve patient outcomes [1] [Ref: Algorithm 30.1].

30.2 Identify Symptoms and Risk Factors

The initial step in managing hypomagnesemia is to identify patients who are at risk or already symptomatic. Common symptoms include:

- Neuromuscular Symptoms: Lethargy, muscle cramps, muscle weakness, tremors, tetany, and seizures.
- Cardiovascular Symptoms: Arrhythmias (such as torsades de pointes), hypertension, and coronary vasospasm.

S. B. Mishra et al., *Mastering ICU Care*,
https://doi.org/10.1007/978-981-95-0179-3_30

- Electrolyte Imbalances: Refractory hypokalemia and hypocalcemia that do not respond to supplementation.

Hypomagnesemia often coexists with other electrolyte disturbances, including hypokalemia, hypocalcemia, and metabolic alkalosis. Magnesium deficiency can exacerbate these conditions, making treatment more complex. For example, hypokalemia may be refractory to potassium supplementation unless magnesium levels are corrected, due to magnesium's role in maintaining cellular potassium levels [2].

Risk Factors

- Chronic Illnesses: Diabetes mellitus, cardiovascular diseases, gastrointestinal disorders (e.g., Crohn's disease, celiac disease), and chronic kidney disease.
- Medications: Diuretics (loop and thiazide), proton-pump inhibitors (PPIs), aminoglycosides, amphotericin B, and certain chemotherapeutic agents like cisplatin.
- Lifestyle Factors: Chronic alcohol use, malnutrition, and prolonged hospitalization, especially in the ICU setting.
- Gastrointestinal Losses: Diarrhea, vomiting, and malabsorption syndromes.
- Endocrine Disorders: Hyperaldosteronism and hyperparathyroidism.

Identifying these symptoms and risk factors necessitates a high index of suspicion, particularly in at-risk populations, to facilitate early detection and proactive management.

2. **Evaluate Serum Magnesium Levels**

Once hypomagnesemia is suspected, the next step is to measure serum magnesium levels. However, it is important to note that serum magnesium may not accurately reflect total body magnesium stores, especially in critically ill patients. Continuous monitoring and clinical correlation are essential.

- Threshold Levels: A serum magnesium level below 1.7 mg/dL (0.7 mmol/L) indicates hypomagnesemia.
- Normal or High Levels: If serum magnesium is above this threshold but symptoms persist, evaluate other electrolyte imbalances such as calcium, potassium, or phosphate.
- Low Levels: Confirm hypomagnesemia and proceed with classification to guide treatment [3].

3. **Differentiate Between Mild and Moderate to Severe Hypomagnesemia**

Treatment is guided by the severity of hypomagnesemia and the presence of symptoms, following evidence-based guidelines.

Mild Hypomagnesemia (1.2–1.6 mg/dL) Without Symptoms

- Treatment: Oral magnesium supplementation.
- Options: Magnesium oxide, magnesium citrate, or magnesium glycinate.
- Dosage: 200–400 mg of elemental magnesium daily.
- Considerations: Monitor for diarrhea, a common side effect. Adjust the dose if necessary.

Moderate to Severe Hypomagnesemia (<1.2 mg/dL) or Symptomatic

- Treatment: Intravenous magnesium supplementation.
- Regimen: IV magnesium sulfate, 1–2 g over 1–2 h.
- Repetition: May need to repeat every 6–12 h based on serum levels and clinical response.
- Monitoring: Continuous cardiac monitoring is recommended due to the risk of arrhythmias. Recheck serum magnesium levels at least every 24 h to ensure adequate correction and prevent toxicity.

Studies have demonstrated the beneficial effects of intravenous magnesium replacement in severe cases, including the reduction of arrhythmias and improvement of neuromuscular function. Continuous monitoring is especially crucial in the ICU, where serum levels may not accurately reflect total body magnesium.

4. **Determine the Underlying Cause of Hypomagnesemia**

Identifying and addressing the underlying cause is essential for effective management and prevention of recurrence.

1. **Detailed Patient History**
   - Medication Review: Identify drugs that may cause renal magnesium loss.
   - Dietary Assessment: Evaluate for insufficient magnesium intake or malabsorption issues.
   - Renal Function: Assess for chronic kidney disease or tubular dysfunction.
   - Alcohol Use: Consider the multifactorial impact of chronic alcohol consumption.
   - Endocrine Evaluation: Screen for disorders like diabetes mellitus, hyperaldosteronism, and hyperparathyroidism.

   Magnesium deficiency contributes to chronic conditions such as osteoporosis, hypertension, and metabolic syndrome. Addressing these factors has implications not only for acute management but also for long-term health.
2. **Comprehensive Diagnostic Testing**
   - 24-h Urinary Magnesium Excretion:
   - Low Excretion (<10–20 mg/day): Suggests gastrointestinal losses or poor intake.
   - High Excretion (>20 mg/day): Indicates renal wasting.
   - Fractional Excretion of Magnesium (FEMg):
   - Calculation:

$$\text{FEMg} = (\text{Urine Mg} \times \text{Serum Creatinine}) / (\text{Serum Mg} \times \text{Urine Creatinine}) \times 100\%$$

   - Interpretation: FEMg >2% suggests renal magnesium wasting.
   - Serum Electrolytes and Additional Tests:

- Evaluate for coexisting electrolyte imbalances (e.g., hypokalemia, hypocalcemia).
- Consider tests for parathyroid function if hypocalcemia is present.
- Genetic Testing (if indicated):
- For familial hypomagnesemia or when other causes are excluded.
- Imaging and Specialized Tests:
- Renal ultrasound to assess structural abnormalities.
- Bone density studies in chronic cases [4].

30.3 Consequences of Mismanagement

Failure to properly manage hypomagnesemia can lead to severe, life-threatening complications:

- Cardiovascular Risks: Increased incidence of arrhythmias, including ventricular tachycardia and torsades de pointes.
- Prolonged Hospitalization: Extended ICU stays due to unresolved symptoms and complications.
- Increased Mortality: Higher risk of death in both acute and chronic settings.

These risks underscore the importance of early recognition, appropriate treatment, and continuous monitoring to improve patient outcomes.

30.4 Conclusion

Managing hypomagnesemia requires a systematic and comprehensive approach. Early identification is essential, with prompt recognition of symptoms and risk factors to initiate timely intervention. Accurate evaluation involves measuring serum magnesium levels, though it is important to acknowledge that these may not always reflect total body magnesium stores, especially in critically ill patients. Treatment should be guided by evidence-based protocols, adjusting supplementation based on the severity of the deficiency. Addressing underlying causes is crucial for preventing recurrence, necessitating a thorough patient assessment. Continuous monitoring of magnesium levels is necessary, with regular reassessment to ensure appropriate adjustment of treatment and to avoid complications.

Magnesium's role extends beyond the ICU, impacting public health and the prevention of chronic diseases like osteoporosis, diabetes, and cardiovascular disorders. Addressing magnesium deficiency is therefore crucial not only for immediate patient care but also for long-term health outcomes. By implementing evidence-based strategies and maintaining vigilance in monitoring, healthcare providers can effectively manage hypomagnesemia and mitigate its associated risks.

Algorithm 30.1 Approach to hypomagnesemia in the ICU

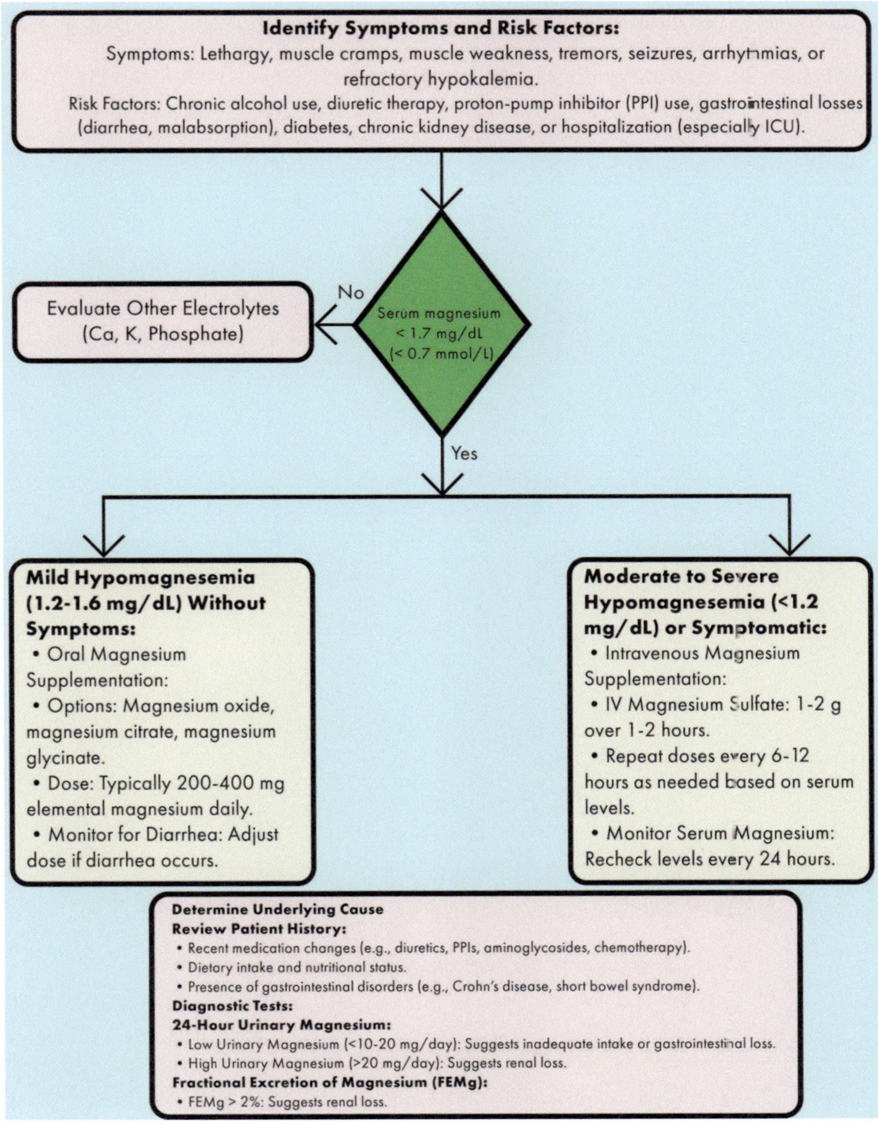

Bibliography

1. Adomako EA, Yu ASL. Magnesium disorders: core curriculum 2024. Am J Kidney Dis. 2024;83(6):803–15.
2. Al Alawi AM, Majoni SW, Falhammar H. Magnesium and human health: perspectives and research directions. Int J Endocrinol. 2018;2018:9041694.
3. Touyz RM, de Baaij JHF, Hoenderop JGJ. Magnesium disorders. N Engl J Med. 2024;390(21):1998–2009.
4. Weisinger JR, Bellorin-Font E. Magnesium and phosphorus. Lancet. 1998;352(9125):391–6.

Chapter 31
Approach to Hypermagnesemia

31.1 Introduction

Magnesium is a vital electrolyte integral to over 300 enzymatic reactions essential for normal physiological functions. These include ATP metabolism, nucleic acid synthesis, muscle contraction, and nerve function. Its crucial role in cellular energy production and stabilization of cellular processes underscores the importance of maintaining appropriate magnesium levels. Despite its significance, magnesium imbalance, particularly hypermagnesemia, is relatively rare but can have severe clinical implications, especially in critically ill patients.

Hypermagnesemia is characterized by elevated serum magnesium levels exceeding 2.5 mg/dL. This condition can lead to profound cardiovascular, neuromuscular, and respiratory complications. Effective management in the intensive care unit (ICU) necessitates prompt identification, assessment of severity, and implementation of appropriate interventions to mitigate adverse outcomes [1, 2] [Ref: Algorithm 31.1].

31.2 Magnesium Homeostasis and Regulation

31.2.1 Renal and Intestinal Regulation

Magnesium balance is tightly regulated through intestinal absorption and renal excretion. The kidneys play a pivotal role in maintaining magnesium homeostasis by filtering and reabsorbing magnesium primarily in the thick ascending loop of Henle and the distal convoluted tubule. Approximately 70% of filtered magnesium is reabsorbed in the loop of Henle, with another 10% reabsorbed in the distal tubule. Any impairment in renal function can significantly affect this balance, leading to elevated serum magnesium levels [3].

S. B. Mishra et al., *Mastering ICU Care*,
https://doi.org/10.1007/978-981-95-0179-3_31

31.3 Etiology and Pathophysiology

31.3.1 Renal Failure

Renal failure is the predominant cause of hypermagnesemia. Since the kidneys are responsible for excreting the majority of absorbed magnesium, impaired renal function can lead to accumulation. Patients with chronic kidney disease (CKD) or acute kidney injury (AKI) are particularly susceptible due to decreased glomerular filtration rate (GFR) and impaired tubular reabsorption processes.

31.3.2 Iatrogenic Causes

Excessive intake of magnesium-containing medications is a significant iatrogenic contributor. Antacids and laxatives containing magnesium hydroxide or magnesium citrate can lead to elevated serum levels, especially in patients with compromised renal function. Intravenous magnesium therapy, often used in obstetric care for conditions like severe preeclampsia with premonitory signs and eclampsia, can also result in hypermagnesemia if not carefully monitored.

31.3.3 Clinical Manifestations

Hypermagnesemia presents with a spectrum of clinical manifestations that correlate with serum magnesium levels:

- Neuromuscular Symptoms: Lethargy, muscle weakness, hyporeflexia, and, in severe cases, flaccid paralysis.
- Cardiovascular Symptoms: Hypotension due to vasodilation, bradycardia, and arrhythmias. High levels can lead to complete heart block or cardiac arrest.
- Respiratory Symptoms: Depressed respiratory drive and apnea in extreme cases.
- Effect on Calcium Homeostasis: Elevated magnesium levels can suppress PTH secretion, leading to hypocalcemia. This hypocalcemia exacerbates neuromuscular irritability and cardiac dysfunction, adding complexity to the clinical picture [3].

Understanding these manifestations is crucial for timely diagnosis and intervention.

31.4 Diagnostic Approach

Clinical Evaluation

1. History and Risk Factor Assessment:
   - Dietary and Medication History: Evaluate intake of magnesium-rich foods, supplements, antacids, and laxatives.
   - Renal Function: Assess for history of CKD or AKI.
   - Medication Use: Review any recent intravenous magnesium administration.
2. Physical Examination:
   - Vital Signs: Check for hypotension and bradycardia.
   - Neuromuscular Assessment: Test deep tendon reflexes, muscle strength, and consciousness level.
   - Respiratory Evaluation: Monitor for signs of respiratory depression.

Laboratory Tests

1. Serum Magnesium Levels:
   - Interpretation: Levels exceeding 2.5 mg/dL confirm hypermagnesemia, but serum levels may not accurately reflect total body magnesium stores.
2. Urinary Magnesium Excretion Tests:
   - Purpose: Differentiate between renal and nonrenal causes.
   - Interpretation: Low urinary magnesium suggests impaired renal excretion, while high levels indicate excessive intake or increased absorption.
3. Electrolyte Panel:
   - Calcium and Potassium Levels: Check for hypocalcemia due to suppressed PTH secretion and other electrolyte imbalances.
4. Renal Function Tests:
   - Serum Creatinine and BUN: Elevated levels indicate reduced renal clearance.

Electrocardiogram (ECG)

- ECG Changes: Look for prolonged PR intervals, widened QRS complexes, peaked T waves, and arrhythmias. These changes help assess the cardiac impact of elevated magnesium levels.

31.5 Management Based on Severity

31.5.1 Mild Hypermagnesemia (2.5–4.0 mg/dL)

Interventions

- Discontinue Magnesium Sources: Immediately halt all magnesium-containing medications and dietary supplements.
- Promote Renal Excretion:
- Intravenous Fluids: Administer isotonic saline (0.9% NaCl) to enhance glomerular filtration and magnesium excretion.
- Monitoring:
- Serum Magnesium Levels: Check levels every 24 hours until normalization.
- Renal Function Tests: Monitor to ensure adequate excretion.

31.5.2 Moderate Hypermagnesemia (4.1–6.0 mg/dL)

Interventions

- Discontinue Magnesium Sources: Stop all exogenous magnesium intake.
- Enhance Excretion:
- Loop Diuretics: Administer furosemide (20–40 mg IV) to inhibit magnesium reabsorption in the loop of Henle.
- Monitoring:
- Cardiac Monitoring: Continuous ECG to detect arrhythmias.
- Neurological Assessment: Regular checks for changes in reflexes and muscle strength.

31.5.3 Severe Hypermagnesemia (>6.0 mg/dL)

Interventions

- Immediate Actions:
- Discontinue Magnesium Sources: Eliminate all sources promptly.
- Intravenous Calcium Gluconate: Administer 1–2 g IV over 5–10 min.

- Mechanism: Acts as a physiological antagonist to magnesium, stabilizing cardiac membranes and restoring neuromuscular function.
- Aggressive Management:
- Hydration: Provide isotonic saline to promote diuresis.
- Diuretics: Use higher doses of furosemide (40–80 mg IV) to facilitate magnesium excretion.

31.5.4 Renal Replacement Therapy

Hemodialysis

- Indications: Renal failure patients or refractory cases.
- Effectiveness: Rapidly reduces serum magnesium levels.
- Monitoring:
- Vital Signs: Continuous monitoring of blood pressure, heart rate, and respiratory status.
- Electrolytes: Frequent checks to manage potential shifts and prevent hypocalcemia.

31.6 Conclusion

Hypermagnesemia is a serious electrolyte disturbance that demands prompt recognition and management, especially in the ICU setting. Understanding the physiological importance of magnesium and the mechanisms regulating its balance is essential. Clinicians must be vigilant for signs of hypermagnesemia in patients with renal dysfunction or those receiving magnesium-containing treatments.

Algorithm 31.1: Approach to hypermagnesemia

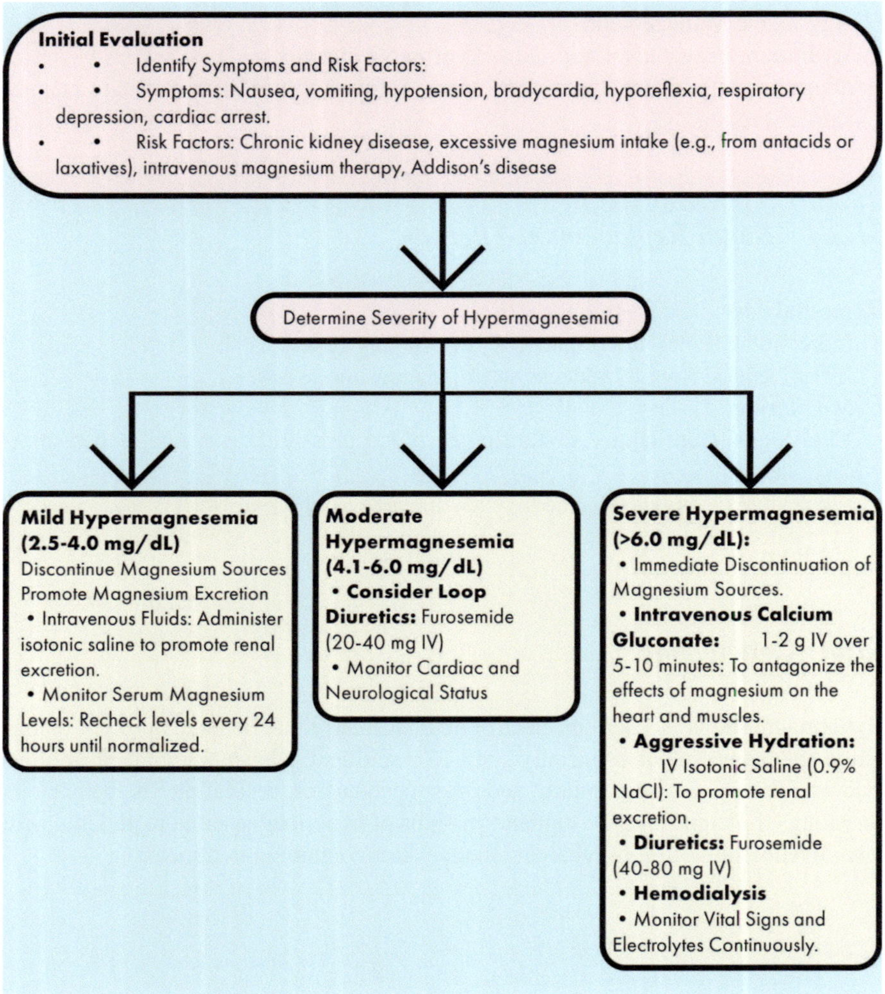

Bibliography

1. Touyz RM, de Baaij JHF, Hoenderop JGJ. Magnesium disorders. N Engl J Med. 2024;390(21):1998–2009.
2. Adomako EA, Yu ASL. Magnesium disorders: core curriculum 2024. Am J Kidney Dis. 2024;83(6):803–15.
3. Al Alawi AM, Majoni SW, Falhammar H. Magnesium and human health: perspectives and research directions. Int J Endocrinol. 2018;2018:9041694.

Chapter 32
Approach to Acute Kidney Injury (AKI) in Critically Ill Patients in the ICU

32.1 Introduction

32.1.1 Definition and Significance of AKI

Acute kidney injury (AKI) is a sudden decline in kidney function. This leads to the buildup of waste products like urea and creatinine in the blood and causes imbalances in fluids and electrolytes. In critically ill patients, AKI is a serious complication associated with high rates of illness and death. It is common in the intensive care unit (ICU) because patients there are exposed to multiple risk factors such as severe infections (sepsis), medications that can harm the kidneys (nephrotoxins), and unstable blood flow (hemodynamic instability). The KDIGO (Kidney Disease: Improving Global Outcomes) guidelines provide a standard definition of AKI based on increases in serum creatinine and decreases in urine output.

AKI is significant not only because it affects the kidneys but also because it can impact other organ systems. In critically ill patients, AKI often indicates underlying problems like septic shock or heart failure. It can worsen other organ failures due to mechanisms like fluid overload and increased urea levels. AKI also leads to longer ICU stays, higher healthcare costs, and can negatively affect long-term patient outcomes [1] [Ref: Algorithm 32.1].

32.2 Epidemiology: How Common Is AKI in the ICU?

AKI occurs in about 30% to 60% of ICU patients. This wide range is due to differences in patient populations and how AKI is diagnosed. The KDIGO criteria have helped standardize AKI diagnosis by emphasizing increases in serum creatinine and low urine output (oliguria) for early detection. However, in critically ill patients,

S. B. Mishra et al., *Mastering ICU Care*,
https://doi.org/10.1007/978-981-95-0179-3_32

factors like low blood volume (hypovolemia), fluid shifts, and muscle wasting can affect urine output and creatinine levels, making diagnosis challenging.

ICU patients are particularly prone to AKI because of the severity of their illnesses, exposure to multiple nephrotoxic drugs, and the invasive procedures they often undergo. AKI can also be part of multi-organ dysfunction syndrome, complicating the clinical picture. When AKI is present, it usually indicates a worse prognosis, including higher rates of needing mechanical ventilation and renal replacement therapy (RRT) [2].

32.3 Impact on Short- and Long-Term Health

In the short term, AKI increases the risk of longer ICU stays, the need for RRT, and higher in-hospital mortality rates. Mortality rates for ICU patients with AKI can exceed 50%, especially for those requiring RRT. AKI often leads to fluid overload, which can worsen heart function, lung mechanics, and overall blood flow. This increases the likelihood of multiple organ failure and the need for advanced life-support measures.

In the long term, many patients who survive AKI do not fully regain kidney function, leading to chronic kidney disease (CKD). Persistent AKI—kidney dysfunction lasting more than 48 h—has a particularly poor prognosis. Survivors are also at increased cardiac risk, recurrent AKI episodes, and eventually needing long-term dialysis. This underscores the importance of early recognition, prevention strategies, and long-term follow-up for patients with AKI during critical illness [3].

32.4 Pathophysiology of AKI

32.4.1 Different Types and How They Present

AKI is a complex condition with various causes and presentations, known as phenotypes. The main types are:

- **Prerenal AKI:** Caused by reduced blood flow to the kidneys without direct kidney damage. Common causes include dehydration, low blood volume, or low blood pressure due to sepsis. It is often reversible if treated promptly.
- **Intrinsic (Intrarenal) AKI:** Results from direct damage to the kidney tissues, such as acute tubular necrosis (ATN), inflammation of the kidney (nephritis), or diseases affecting the kidney's filtering units (glomerulonephritis). Causes include prolonged ischemia, sepsis, and exposure to nephrotoxins.
- **Post-renal AKI:** Occurs due to blockage in the urinary tract (e.g., kidney stones or tumors), causing backpressure and impairing kidney function.

In critically ill patients, these types can overlap. For example, a patient might have decreased kidney blood flow (prerenal) and also direct kidney damage from toxins (intrinsic) [4].

32.5 How AKI Happens: Key Mechanisms

1. **Ischemia (Lack of Blood Flow):** Reduced blood flow leads to oxygen deprivation in kidney cells, causing cell injury or death, especially in areas like the proximal tubules. This is common in shock, heart failure, or major surgeries.
2. **Sepsis:** Severe infections cause systemic inflammation, leading to endothelial dysfunction and altered renal blood flow. Inflammatory substances can directly damage kidney cells. AKI from sepsis can occur even without significant drops in blood pressure.
3. **Nephrotoxicity (Drug-Induced Damage):** Certain medications and substances can harm kidney cells by causing oxidative stress and cell death. Common nephrotoxins include some antibiotics (like aminoglycosides), contrast dyes used in imaging, and NSAIDs. Critically ill patients are at higher risk due to multiple medications and other factors like dehydration.
4. **Inflammation:** The body's immune response can contribute to kidney damage through the release of inflammatory substances, activation of white blood cells, and production of harmful free radicals. This can worsen kidney injury from other causes [5].

32.6 From AKI to Chronic Kidney Problems

The concept of acute kidney disease (AKD) bridges the gap between AKI and CKD. AKD refers to kidney dysfunction lasting between 7 and 90 days. Even if AKI seems to resolve, there may be ongoing damage leading to CKD.

Key factors in the progression from AKI to CKD include:

- Incomplete healing of kidney tissues.
- Persistent inflammation.
- Development of scar tissue (fibrosis).
- Loss of renal functional reserve.

Patients with persistent AKI are at higher risk for CKD. Risk factors for progression include preexisting kidney problems, repeated episodes of AKI, and ongoing exposure to factors that harm the kidneys.

32.7 Classification and Diagnosis

32.7.1 KDIGO Criteria: How AKI Is Staged

The KDIGO guidelines provide a standardized way to diagnose and stage AKI using two main measures:

1. Serum Creatinine:
   - An increase of ≥0.3 mg/dL (26.5 μmol/L) within 48 h.
   - Or an increase to ≥1.5 times the baseline level, occurring within the prior 7 days.
2. Urine Output:
   - Less than 0.5 mL/kg/h for 6 h.

32.7.2 Staging of AKI

Stage 1:

- Serum Creatinine: 1.5–1.9 times baseline or increase of ≥0.3 mg/dL.
- Urine Output: <0.5 mL/kg/h for 6–12 h.

Stage 2:

- Serum Creatinine: 2.0–2.9 times baseline.
- Urine Output: <0.5 mL/kg/h for ≥12 h.

Stage 3:

- Serum Creatinine: 3.0 times baseline or increase to ≥4.0 mg/dL.
- Urine Output: <0.3 mL/kg/h for ≥24 h or anuria for ≥12 h.
- Initiation of renal replacement therapy (RRT).

These criteria help identify patients at risk and guide treatment decisions.

32.7.3 Transient vs. Persistent AKI

- Transient AKI: Kidney dysfunction that resolves within 48 h. Often due to reversible factors like dehydration. Patients usually have a better prognosis if treated promptly.
- Persistent AKI: Lasts more than 48 h and often involves direct kidney damage. Associated with higher risks of complications, progression to AKD, and development of CKD.

Distinguishing between transient and persistent AKI is important because persistent AKI requires more intensive management and monitoring for long-term kidney health.

32.8 Challenges in Diagnosing AKI in the ICU

Diagnosing AKI in critically ill patients can be difficult due to limitations of traditional markers:

- **Serum Creatinine:**
  - Rises late in AKI—only after significant kidney damage.
  - Affected by factors like muscle mass (which may be low in ICU patients due to muscle wasting) and fluid status (dilution from fluid overload can lower creatinine levels).
- **Urine Output:**
  - Can be influenced by diuretics, fluid resuscitation, and other factors unrelated to kidney function.
  - Oliguria may not always reflect the severity of kidney injury.

32.9 Biomarkers and Early Detection

Established Biomarkers

- Neutrophil Gelatinase-Associated Lipocalin (NGAL):
  - Released by damaged kidney cells.
  - Detectable in blood and urine within a few hours of injury.
  - Helps distinguish between prerenal and intrinsic AKI.
- Tissue Inhibitor of Metalloproteinases-2 (TIMP-2) and Insulin-Like Growth Factor Binding Protein 7 (IGFBP-7):
  - Indicators of cell stress in the kidneys.
  - Combined as the [TIMP-2]*[IGFBP7] test.
  - Predict risk of developing severe AKI within 12 h.

Emerging Biomarkers

- Kidney Injury Molecule-1 (KIM-1):
  - Appears on kidney cells after injury.
  - Useful for detecting early tubular damage.

- Cystatin C:
  - A protein filtered by the kidneys, less affected by muscle mass.
  - May provide a more accurate estimate of kidney function in critically ill patients.
- Proenkephalin (PenKid):
  - Reflects real-time kidney function.
  - Less influenced by external factors like fluid status.

Others
Uromodulin, Calprotectin, IgG, Nephrin, Podocalyxin, Podocin, Transferrin, IL-18, Vanin 1, Galactin 3, PDGF.

Using Technology: Machine Learning and AI
- Machine learning (ML) and artificial intelligence (AI) can analyze large amounts of patient data to predict AKI risk.
- AI models use factors like vital signs, lab results, and patient history to generate risk scores.
- These tools can provide early warnings to clinicians, potentially improving patient outcomes.

32.10 Management Strategies

Preventing AKI
- Fluid Management: Balance is key—avoid both dehydration and fluid overload.
- Hemodynamic Monitoring: Use tools to assess and maintain adequate blood flow and pressure.
- Avoiding Nephrotoxins: Minimize exposure to harmful medications; monitor levels when use is necessary.

Optimizing Blood Flow to the Kidneys
- Maintain Adequate Blood Pressure: Aim for a mean arterial pressure (MAP) of at least 65 mmHg, adjusted based on individual patient needs.
- Use of Vasopressors and Inotropes: Medications that support blood pressure and heart function can help maintain kidney perfusion.

Fluid Management Approaches
- Restrictive Fluid Therapy: Limiting fluids to prevent overload, which can worsen outcomes.

- Liberal Fluid Therapy: More generous fluid administration; may be needed in cases of hypovolemia.
- Individualized Care: The best approach depends on the patient's condition; careful monitoring is essential.

Renal Replacement Therapy (RRT)

- When to Start: Indications include severe electrolyte imbalances, acid-base disturbances, fluid overload, and signs of uremia.
- Timing: Early initiation is debated; some studies suggest waiting until it is absolutely necessary, while others advocate for starting sooner.

32.11 Special Considerations in Critically Ill Patients

AKI in Sepsis

Mechanisms:

- Hemodynamic Changes: Sepsis can cause low blood pressure and poor kidney perfusion.
- Inflammation: Release of cytokines damages kidney tissues.
- Microcirculatory Dysfunction:
- Management Challenges:
- Fluid Resuscitation: Necessary but can lead to fluid overload.
- Vasopressors: Support blood pressure but may reduce kidney blood flow if overused.
- Balancing Treatments: Requires careful monitoring to support circulation without harming the kidneys.

Impact of Mechanical Ventilation and Blood Pressure Instability

Mechanical Ventilation:

- High PEEP Levels: intrathoracic pressure reducing venous return to the heart and kidney perfusion.
- Neurohormonal Activation: Triggers systems that can constrict blood vessels in the kidneys.
- Hemodynamic Instability:
- Hypotension: Low blood pressure reduces kidney perfusion.
- Vasopressors: Necessary to raise blood pressure but can cause renal vasoconstriction.
- Monitoring: Continuous assessment of blood pressure and kidney function is vital.

32.12 Outcomes and Follow-Up

Long-Term Consequences

- Chronic Kidney Disease (CKD): Up to 30% of AKI survivors develop CKD.
- Major Adverse Kidney Events (MAKE):
- Mortality: Increased risk of death even after discharge.
- Need for RRT: Some patients require long-term dialysis.
- Decline in Kidney Function: Significant loss of kidney performance over time.

Importance of Follow-Up Care

- Regular Monitoring: Check renal function tests periodically.
- Multidisciplinary Approach: Involvement of nephrologists, primary care physicians, and other specialists.
- Risk Factor Management:
- Control Blood Pressure: Helps prevent further kidney damage.
- Avoid Nephrotoxins: Be cautious with medications that can harm the kidneys.
- Lifestyle Changes: Healthy diet, exercise, and smoking cessation can improve outcomes.
- Patient Education: Inform patients about the risk of recurrent AKI and signs to watch for.

32.13 Conclusion

Acute kidney injury is a frequent and severe complication in critically ill patients, significantly increasing morbidity and mortality. Early detection through standardized criteria and the use of biomarkers is crucial for timely and effective management. Preventive strategies focus on maintaining optimal fluid balance, ensuring adequate hemodynamic support, and minimizing exposure to nephrotoxic agents. Since AKI can lead to long-term kidney damage, follow-up care is essential to monitor for complications such as CKD and mitigate its progression.

Algorithm 32.1: Approach to acute kidney injury in the ICU (AKI) in Critically Ill Patients in the ICU

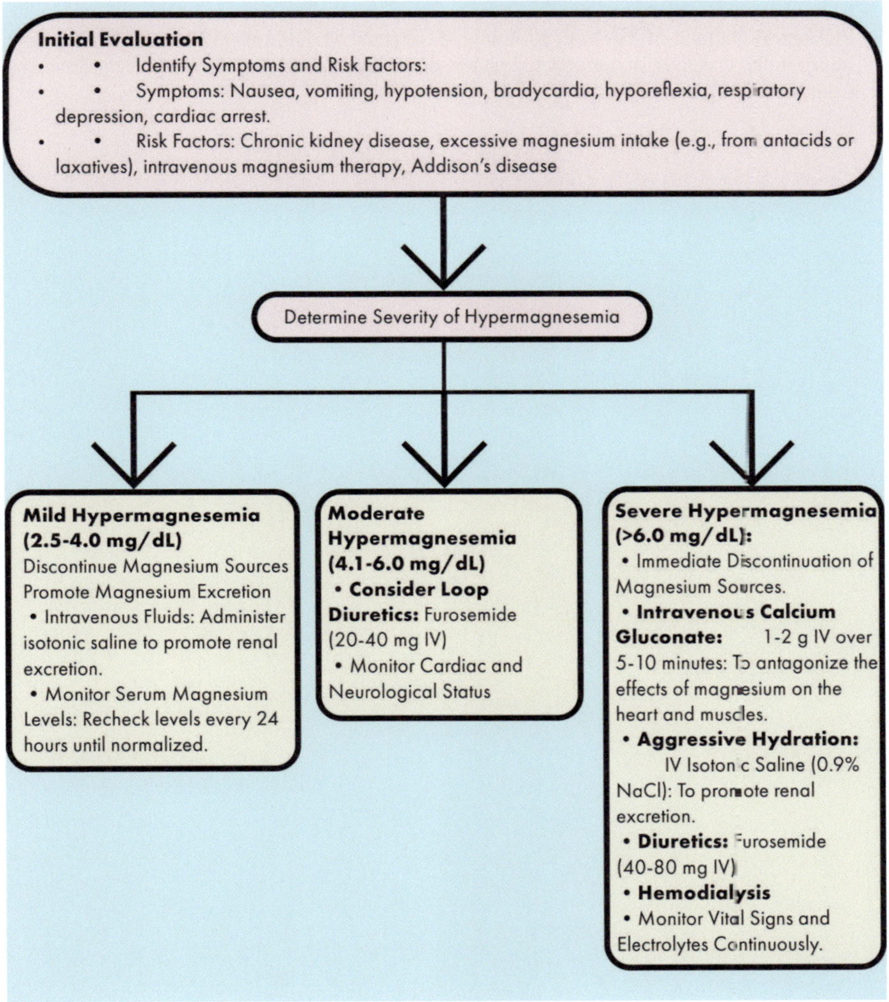

Bibliography

1. Joannidis M, Meersch-Dini M, Forni LG. Acute kidney injury. Intensive Care Med. 2023;49(6):665–8.
2. Barmpas P, Tasoulis S, Vrahatis AG, Georgakopoulos SV, Anagnostou P, Prina M, et al. A divisive hierarchical clustering methodology for enhancing the ensemble prediction power in large scale population studies: the ATHLOS project. Health Inf Sci Syst. 2022;10(1):6.

3. Andonovic M, Traynor JP, Shaw M, Sim MAB, Mark PB, Puxty KA. Short- and long-term outcomes of intensive care patients with acute kidney disease. EClinicalMedicine. 2022;44:101291.
4. Mohsenin V. Practical approach to detection and management of acute kidney injury in critically ill patient. J Intensive Care. 2017;5:57.
5. Pickkers P, Darmon M, Hoste E, Joannidis M, Legrand M, Ostermann M, et al. Acute kidney injury in the critically ill: an updated review on pathophysiology and management. Intensive Care Med. 2021;47(8):835–50.

Part III
Gastroenterology

Chapter 33
Approach to Acute Abdomen in the ICU

33.1 Introduction

Acute abdominal pain is a critical and challenging presentation in the ICU, requiring immediate and careful assessment to determine whether surgical intervention is necessary. It can stem from various causes, ranging from benign conditions to life-threatening surgical emergencies. ICU patients often have complicated health profiles, making diagnosis and treatment more difficult. Special populations, such as immunocompromised individuals, pregnant patients, and the elderly, add another layer of complexity to the diagnostic and therapeutic approach. Early identification and management are crucial to improving outcomes and preventing complications [1, 2] [Ref: Algorithm 33.1].

33.2 Initial Assessment and Stabilization

The first and most urgent step in managing acute abdomen is assessing the patient's hemodynamic stability.

- Hemodynamic Status: If the patient is not hemodynamically stable (e.g., hypotensive or tachycardic), immediate resuscitation is required, which may include:
- Intravenous fluids to stabilize circulatory volume.
- Vasopressors for septic or distributive shock.
- Blood transfusions if hemorrhage is suspected.

Rapid bedside assessments should be made for critical conditions such as a ruptured aortic aneurysm or exsanguinating intra-abdominal hemorrhage. If these are present, urgent surgical consultation is required.

For stable patients, a more methodical approach can be undertaken, including detailed history taking, physical examination, and diagnostic testing.

S. B. Mishra et al., *Mastering ICU Care*,
https://doi.org/10.1007/978-981-95-0179-3_33

33.3 History Taking and Physical Examination

History: After stabilizing the patient, gather a detailed history focusing on the acute onset and location of pain.

- The chronology, character, and associated symptoms such as vomiting, fever, or changes in bowel habits can provide important clues.
- Pain location helps narrow the differential diagnosis:
  - Right Upper Quadrant: Consider biliary disease (e.g., cholecystitis), hepatic pathology, or renal causes.
  - Left Upper Quadrant: Think of pancreatitis, splenic injury, or renal issues.
  - Lower Quadrants: Consider appendicitis, diverticulitis, gynecologic causes, or colitis.
  - Epigastric: Causes might include peptic ulcer disease, pancreatitis, or myocardial ischemia.

Physical Examination:

- Look for signs of peritonitis (rebound tenderness, guarding, or rigidity) as these indicate a likely surgical emergency.
- Absence of these signs necessitates further diagnostic evaluation.
- Perform pelvic and rectal exams in patients with lower abdominal or pelvic pain to assess for gynecological or colorectal pathology.

33.4 Diagnostic Evaluation

Laboratory Testing

Laboratory evaluation plays a key role in narrowing down potential diagnoses:

- Complete Blood Count (CBC): Leukocytosis can suggest infection or inflammation, while decreased hemoglobin suggests hemorrhage.
- Amylase/Lipase: Elevated levels suggest pancreatitis.
- Liver Function Tests: Useful for evaluating hepatic or biliary pathology.
- Electrolytes and Renal Function Tests: These help assess overall metabolic status and identify kidney involvement.

Imaging Studies

Imaging is a cornerstone of diagnosing acute abdomen. The choice of imaging modality depends on the clinical suspicion.

- CT with Contrast: This remains the gold standard for many causes of acute abdomen, especially in cases of suspected bowel perforation, obstruction, or vascular emergencies like mesenteric ischemia.
- Ultrasound: Can be used in cases where radiation exposure is a concern (e.g., pregnancy) or to evaluate biliary disease, free fluid, or appendicitis.

33.5 Special Considerations for Immunocompromised Patients

Immunocompromised patients present unique challenges in diagnosing and managing acute abdomen. Their symptoms may be atypical, and they are prone to delayed inflammatory responses, which can lead to missed or late diagnoses.

- High Index of Suspicion: Always maintain a heightened awareness for intra-abdominal infections or other surgical emergencies in immunocompromised patients. Misdiagnosis can significantly increase morbidity and mortality.
- Imaging: In this population, contrast-enhanced CT scans are the most reliable imaging modality. Ultrasound and plain radiographs may not provide sufficient sensitivity.
- Common Causes:
  - Neutropenic enterocolitis (typhlitis) is a frequent and life-threatening cause of acute abdomen in patients undergoing chemotherapy or with hematologic malignancies. It is usually managed conservatively unless there are signs of bowel perforation or ischemia.
  - Cytomegalovirus (CMV) colitis and *Clostridioides difficile* colitis are significant causes of abdominal pain in immunocompromised patients and require prompt diagnosis and treatment.

33.6 Diagnostic Approach: Expanding on Imaging and Laboratory Studies

The diagnostic approach should be tailored based on the patient's presentation, immunocompromised state, and likelihood of differential diagnoses.

- Laboratory Testing: In addition to the basic blood work, immunocompromised patients may need additional testing, such as C-reactive protein (CRP) to assess the degree of inflammation, and specific microbiological cultures depending on the clinical suspicion.
- Imaging: While CT with contrast remains the gold standard, ultrasound may be used in select populations, such as pregnant patients, or for specific conditions like biliary disease. However, CT should not be delayed in cases where life-threatening conditions are suspected.

33.7 Treatment Considerations in Special Populations

Special populations such as pregnant women and the elderly require unique considerations when managing acute abdomen.

- Pregnant Patients: Pregnancy alters normal anatomy and physiology, making the diagnosis more challenging. A multidisciplinary approach is critical, considering both obstetric and non-obstetric causes. Imaging decisions should balance the need for rapid diagnosis with minimizing fetal radiation exposure.
- Elderly Patients: The elderly often present with atypical symptoms and may have a higher incidence of serious complications like vascular diseases (e.g., aortic dissection, mesenteric ischemia) or bowel obstruction. They are at increased risk for poor outcomes, particularly in emergency surgery settings.

33.8 Expanded Treatment and Surgical Decision-Making

Surgical decision-making in ICU patients with acute abdomen, particularly those who are immunocompromised, requires careful judgment.

- Neutropenic Enterocolitis: Conservative management is preferred unless bowel perforation or ischemia is suspected. A damage-control approach may be necessary in severely ill patients.
- Immunocompromised Patients: Surgery is often delayed unless absolutely necessary. However, in cases of suspected perforation, ischemia, or uncontrolled sepsis, immediate surgery is indicated.
- Diverticulitis in Transplant Patients: These patients are at higher risk for complicated diverticulitis. Surgery should be considered promptly if medical management fails.

33.9 Conclusion

Managing acute abdomen in ICU patients requires a systematic approach that takes into account the patient's history, clinical findings, and diagnostic tests. This is especially true for immunocompromised, pregnant, and elderly populations. For immunocompromised patients, the absence of typical symptoms such as fever or leukocytosis necessitates a high index of suspicion, and imaging like contrast-enhanced CT scans should be used liberally. Early and accurate diagnosis combined with tailored treatment strategies, including conservative management where appropriate, can significantly improve patient outcomes.

Algorithm 33.1: Approach to acute abdomen in the ICU

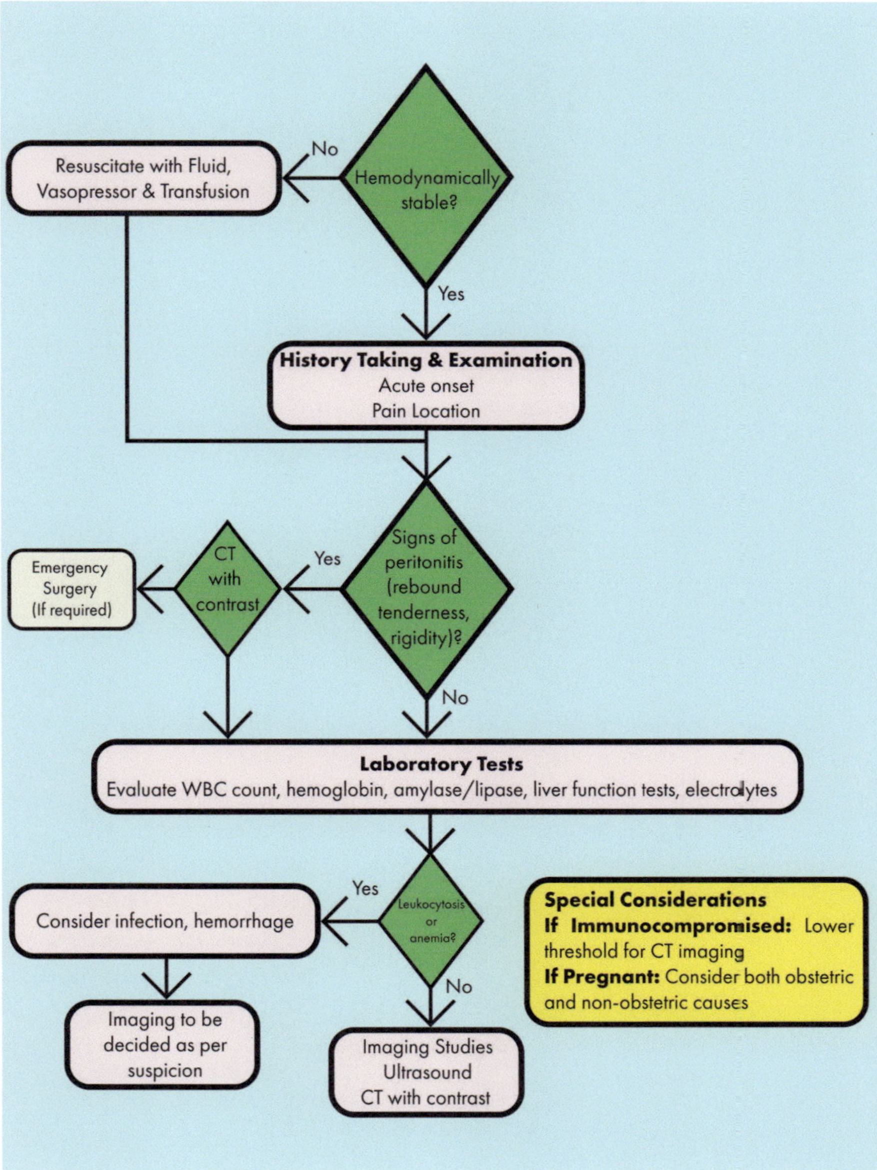

Bibliography

1. Mayumi T, Yoshida M, Tazuma S, Furukawa A, Nishii O, Shigematsu K, et al. The practice guidelines for primary care of acute abdomen 2015. Jpn J Radiol. 2016;34(1) 80–115.
2. Coccolini F, Improta M, Sartelli M, Rasa K, Sawyer R, Coimbra R, et al. Acute abdomen in the immunocompromised patient: WSES, SIS-E, WSIS, AAST, and GAIS guidelines. World J Emerg Surg. 2021;16(1):40.

Chapter 34
Approach to Acute and Chronic Pancreatitis in the ICU

34.1 Introduction

Acute pancreatitis (AP) is an inflammatory condition that varies in severity, from mild cases with rapid recovery to severe forms leading to necrosis, infection, and multi-organ failure. Chronic pancreatitis (CP), on the other hand, is a long-standing inflammation that results in fibrosis and the irreversible loss of pancreatic function, often requiring a different management strategy. Early intervention, appropriate diagnosis, and treatment in the ICU are essential to minimize morbidity and mortality. This chapter provides a structured, evidence-based approach for managing both acute and chronic pancreatitis, with an emphasis on ICU-level care and chronic management [1] [Ref: Algorithm 34.1].

34.2 Acute Pancreatitis Management

34.2.1 Initial Assessment and Diagnosis

Diagnostic Criteria: Acute pancreatitis is diagnosed based on ***at least two*** of the following criteria:

- Abdominal pain consistent with AP.
- Serum amylase or lipase levels elevated more than three times the upper limit of normal.
- Characteristic findings on imaging (CT or MRI). Ultrasonography may be used in resource limited settings or unstable patients.

Severity Assessment: The Revised Atlanta classification is used to classify AP into mild, moderately severe, or severe, based on the presence of organ failure and complications such as necrosis.

S. B. Mishra et al., *Mastering ICU Care*,
https://doi.org/10.1007/978-981-95-0179-3_34

Mild: No organ failure. No local or systemic complications.

Moderately Severe: Transient organ failure (resolves within 48 h) and/or local or systemic complications without persistent organ failure.

Severe: Persistent organ failure—single/multiple (> 48 h) and often associated with local complications.

- Scoring Systems: Utilize BISAP, APACHE II, and Modified Marshall Score to assess severity. A BISAP score ≥ 3 indicates a high risk for severe AP, while the Modified Marshall assesses organ dysfunction [1].

Types of pancreatitis	
Interstitial edematous pancreatitis	**< 4 weeks**
	Acute pancreatic fluid collection
	Sterile (< 2 weeks)
	Infected (> 2 weeks)
	>4 weeks
	Pancreatic pseudocyst
	Sterile (< 2 weeks)
	Infected (> 2 weeks)
Necrotizing pancreatitis	**< 4 weeks**
	Acute necrotizing collection
	Sterile (< 2 weeks)
	Infected (> 2 weeks)
	>4 weeks
	Walled off necrosis (WON)
	Sterile (< 2 weeks)
	Infected (> 2 weeks)

Etiology of AP:

Most common causes: Gallstones (40–70%) and alcohol (25–35%).

Other causes:

Medications—mercaptopurine, azathioprine, didanosine, valproic acid.
Infections—CMV, HIV, coxsackie, mumps.
Metabolic causes—hypercalcemia and hypertriglyceridemia.

34.2.2 Initial Stabilization and Supportive Care

Fluid Resuscitation:

- Initial Dose: Start with Lactated Ringer's solution at 250–500 mL/hour for the first 12–24 h.

- Monitoring: Adjust fluid administration based on hemodynamic parameters such as urine output ≥0.5 mL/kg/hour and mean arterial pressure (MAP) ≥65 mmHg. Frequent reassessment (every 6–12 h) is essential to avoid complications like abdominal compartment syndrome (ACS).

Pain Management:

- Analgesics: Use opioids like morphine, with careful monitoring to avoid respiratory depression. Adjunctive NSAIDs may be added to reduce opioid requirements.

Nutritional Support:

- Enteral Feeding: Start within 48 h to prevent gut barrier dysfunction and reduce infection risk. Oral feeding should be encouraged. If the patient is unable to tolerate oral feeds, nasogastric (NG) feeds can be initiated. However, on failure of both the above modalities, the nasojejunal route may be tried. Initial caloric goals are 20–25 kcal/kg/day, progressing as tolerated.
- Parenteral Nutrition: Reserved for cases where enteral feeding is not possible [2].

Role of ERCP:

In case of cholangitis or progressive cholestasis (rising bilirubin >3–5 mg/dL in the setting of severe or moderately severe AP), early ERCP within 24 h is indicated.

34.2.3 *Ongoing Monitoring and Complication Management*

Monitoring Clinical Response:

- Evaluate clinical response every 48–72 h through clinical, laboratory, and radiological markers. Persistent organ failure or clinical deterioration warrants imaging (CT or MRI) to assess for necrosis or complications.

34.2.4 *Management of Necrosis and Infection*

Management of necrosis and infection in acute pancreatitis is complex, requiring a strategic approach that minimizes invasiveness, limits infection risk, and supports optimal recovery.

Necrosis

Sterile vs. Infected Necrosis:

- Sterile Necrosis: In cases of sterile necrosis, conservative management is preferred, as sterile necrotic tissue does not generally benefit from invasive

procedures. Most patients with sterile necrosis improve with supportive care alone, including fluid resuscitation, nutritional support, and pain management.
- Infected Necrosis: When infection of necrotic pancreatic tissue occurs, it significantly increases the risk of morbidity and mortality. Infection is suspected when clinical signs worsen (fever, increased WBC count, persistent organ dysfunction) and can be confirmed by imaging (air in the necrotic tissue on CT) or fine-needle aspiration (FNA) if there is uncertainty [3].

Step-Up Approach

The step-up approach begins with the least invasive options, typically starting with percutaneous or endoscopic drainage for infected necrosis. This strategy reduces the need for open surgical intervention, thereby decreasing the risk of complications.

- Percutaneous Drainage: Image-guided percutaneous drainage is often the first step. This minimally invasive technique allows for effective drainage of infected collections with relatively low risk.
- Endoscopic Drainage: If percutaneous drainage is insufficient, endoscopic drainage is considered. Drainage is typically performed via a transgastric or transduodenal route, allowing access to peripancreatic collections without open surgery. This is especially useful for walled-off necrosis (WON), a mature collection with a well-defined capsule that develops 4 weeks or more after onset.
- Surgical Intervention: Surgical necrosectomy is reserved for cases where percutaneous and endoscopic drainage are unsuccessful, or in patients with large, complex necrotic areas that cannot be managed through minimally invasive methods. Delaying surgery until 4 weeks after onset is recommended to allow for encapsulation of necrotic tissue, which makes debridement safer and more effective.

Antibiotics

- Prophylactic Use: Prophylactic antibiotics for sterile necrosis are not recommended, as they do not improve outcomes and can contribute to antibiotic resistance. Antibiotic therapy should be withheld unless infection is suspected or confirmed.
- Indications for Antibiotics: Antibiotics are reserved for confirmed infected necrosis. Empirical broad-spectrum antibiotics may be started when infection is strongly suspected, with adjustments based on culture results. Agents with good tissue penetration, such as carbapenems, fluoroquinolones, or metronidazole, are preferred for treating infected necrosis.

Endoscopic Management

Endoscopic Ultrasound (EUS)-Guided Drainage for Walled-Off Necrosis:

- Indications: In patients with walled-off necrosis (WON), EUS-guided drainage has become the preferred approach due to its minimally invasive nature and effectiveness in accessing peripancreatic fluid collections. WON is typically mature and well-defined, with a fibrotic wall that allows safe drainage through endoscopic means.

- Procedure: EUS-guided drainage involves placing stents through the stomach or duodenum into the necrotic cavity. Self-expanding metal stents (LAMS) are often used, as they provide larger drainage channels compared to plastic stents, facilitating drainage and enabling direct endoscopic necrosectomy if required.
- Endoscopic Ultrasound (EUS)-Guided Drainage of pancreatic pseudocyst: Only if symptomatic.
- Direct Endoscopic Necrosectomy (DEN): If initial drainage is inadequate or if residual necrotic material remains, DEN can be performed through the previously placed stents. This technique allows for repeated debridement sessions without open surgery, which is beneficial for patients at high surgical risk [4].

34.3 Chronic Pancreatitis Management

34.3.1 Overview of Chronic Pancreatitis (CP)

Chronic pancreatitis (CP) is characterized by long-standing inflammation leading to irreversible fibrosis and functional impairment of the pancreas. It often presents with recurrent episodes of abdominal pain, exocrine insufficiency, and endocrine dysfunction (e.g., diabetes). CP management focuses on symptom control and preventing disease progression [5].

34.3.2 Diagnosis and Assessment

- Diagnosis: CP is diagnosed based on clinical presentation, imaging (CT, MRI, or EUS), and pancreatic function tests. It is important to differentiate CP from acute relapses of pancreatitis.
- Assessment Tools: Use imaging techniques like endoscopic ultrasonography (EUS) or CT scans to assess the degree of fibrosis and ductal abnormalities. Functional tests like fecal elastase can help assess exocrine insufficiency.

34.3.3 Treatment of Chronic Pancreatitis

Pain Management:

- Analgesia: Chronic pain in CP may require a multimodal approach, including opioids (e.g., morphine) and adjuncts like NSAIDs or tricyclic antidepressants for neuropathic pain.
- Endoscopic Treatment: Endoscopic interventions like EUS-guided drainage of pseudocysts or stenting of strictures can be useful for pain relief and management of complications.

Nutritional Management:

- Pancreatic Enzyme Replacement Therapy (PERT): Patients with exocrine pancreatic insufficiency (EPI) should receive PERT with meals to aid digestion and prevent malnutrition.
- Nutritional Screening: Regular screening for malnutrition, osteoporosis, and diabetes is recommended due to the high prevalence of these conditions in CP patients [5].

34.4 Multidisciplinary and Step-Up Approaches in Pancreatitis

Effective management of pancreatitis, particularly in severe cases or those with complications, benefits significantly from a multidisciplinary approach that incorporates early intervention, cross-specialty collaboration, and evidence-based bundled care protocols. This structured approach improves patient outcomes by coordinating timely interventions and comprehensive support.

Pancreatitis Bundles

- Overview: The Japanese guidelines emphasize the importance of a bundled care approach for severe acute pancreatitis, integrating key interventions like fluid resuscitation, pain management, and early nutritional support. The goal of these "Pancreatitis Bundles" is to standardize care in a way that minimizes complications and improves overall prognosis [6, 7].

Components

- *Fluid Resuscitation*: Start with controlled, isotonic fluid administration (e.g., Lactated Ringer's), monitoring closely to avoid under- or over-resuscitation. Adjust fluid rates based on parameters such as urine output, blood pressure, and hematocrit levels to maintain organ perfusion without risking complications like abdominal compartment syndrome.
- *Pain Control*: Effective pain management is essential to minimize patient distress and prevent respiratory complications from shallow breathing due to pain. Opioids are typically used, though carefully titrated, with adjunctive medications like NSAIDs if appropriate.
- *Early Enteral Nutrition*: Initiate enteral feeding within 48 hours to preserve gut integrity and prevent bacterial translocation. This component of the bundle is particularly emphasized in Japanese guidelines as it supports immune function and reduces infection risk. Nasogastric or nasojejunal feeding is preferred over parenteral nutrition, except in cases where enteral routes are contraindicated.
- *Outcome Improvement*: Implementing pancreatitis bundles has been associated with reduced mortality and shorter ICU stays by proactively addressing the fac-

tors that lead to complications in severe acute pancreatitis. Studies indicate that following these protocols can also reduce the need for intensive interventions by controlling inflammation and maintaining physiological stability early in the disease course.

Multidisciplinary Management

- Rationale: Given the complexity and variability in the progression of pancreatitis, particularly in cases involving necrosis, strictures, or pseudocysts, a multidisciplinary approach ensures that all potential complications are managed effectively. Complex cases often require expertise across gastroenterology, surgery, critical care, radiology, and nutrition.

  Specialist Involvement:

  - Gastroenterologists: Provide expertise in diagnostic and therapeutic endoscopy, including ERCP for biliary pancreatitis and endoscopic drainage of pseudocysts or walled-off necrosis (WON). Gastroenterologists play a central role in early intervention, particularly with minimally invasive procedures.
  - Surgeons: Reserved for cases where invasive intervention is unavoidable, such as when percutaneous or endoscopic drainage fails in infected necrosis. Surgeons are also involved in necrosectomy, either minimally invasive or open, particularly if the patient has developed complications that cannot be managed nonsurgically.
  - Radiologists: Essential for diagnostic imaging, including contrast-enhanced CT or MRI, to guide decisions on the timing and type of intervention for necrotic or infected pancreatic collections. Interventional radiologists can perform percutaneous drainage, which is often the first step in the step-up approach to managing infected necrosis.
  - Critical Care Specialists: Oversee the hemodynamic and respiratory support of patients with severe acute pancreatitis in the ICU. This includes monitoring for complications like systemic inflammatory response syndrome (SIRS) and managing any organ dysfunction.
  - Nutritionists: Essential for managing malnutrition risk, particularly in patients with severe or chronic pancreatitis. Nutritionists guide the implementation of early enteral feeding and adjust caloric and macronutrient intake to meet patient needs and prevent complications like infection and prolonged recovery time.

  - Collaborative Case Reviews: Regular, collaborative reviews of complex cases (e.g., severe acute pancreatitis with necrosis) enable a team-based approach to decision-making. This is particularly beneficial for optimizing the timing of invasive interventions and ensuring that all treatment avenues are considered before resorting to more invasive options [8].

34.5 Conclusion

The management of acute and chronic pancreatitis in the ICU requires a structured and multidisciplinary approach. Fluid resuscitation, pain management, and early nutritional support are cornerstones of care in acute pancreatitis, while chronic pancreatitis treatment focuses on symptom relief, nutritional support, and preventing complications. Close monitoring, the use of minimally invasive techniques for necrosis, and a focus on multidisciplinary team-based care are essential to improving patient outcomes.

Algorithm 34.1: Approach to acute and chronic pancreatitis in the ICU

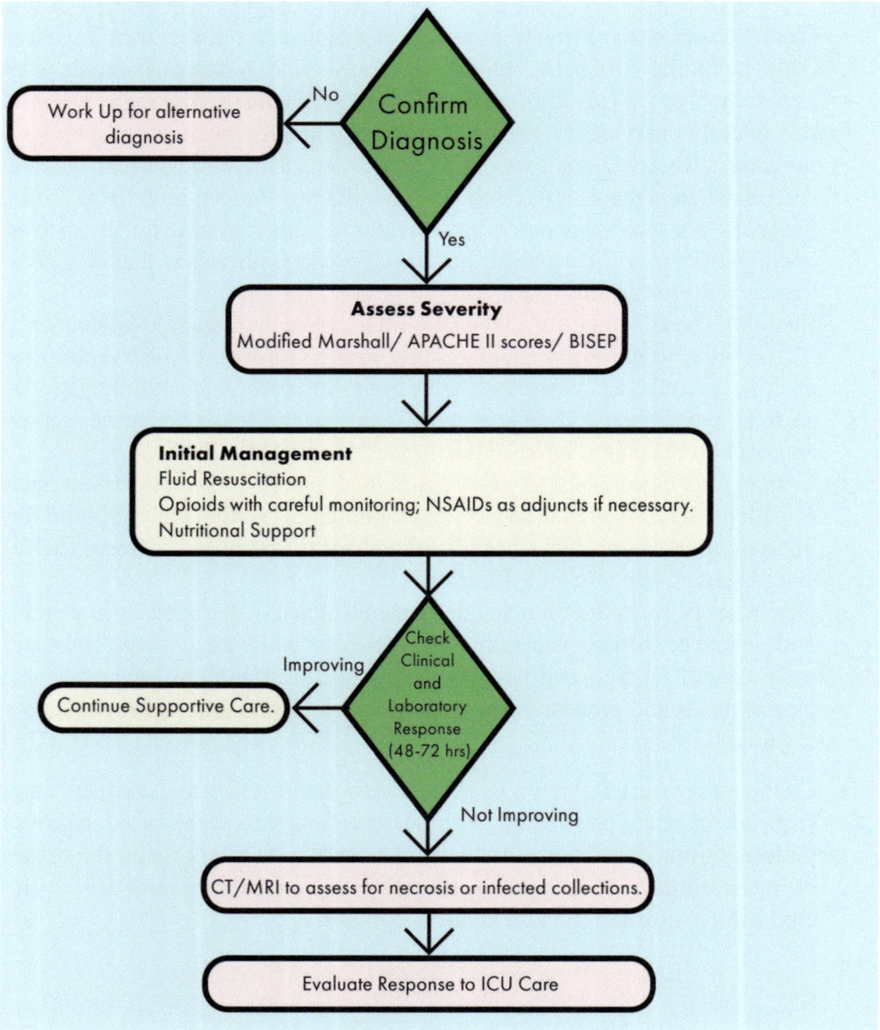

Bibliography

1. Tenner S, Vege SS, Sheth SG, Sauer B, Yang A, Conwell DL, et al. American College of Gastroenterology guidelines: management of acute pancreatitis. ACG. 2024;(3):119.
2. Arvanitakis M, Ockenga J, Bezmarevic M, Gianotti L, Krznarić Ž, Lobo DN, et al. ESPEN guideline on clinical nutrition in acute and chronic pancreatitis. Clin Nutr. 2020;39(3):612–31.
3. Leppäniemi A, Tolonen M, Tarasconi A, Segovia-Lohse H, Gamberini E, Kirkpatrick AW, et al. 2019 WSES guidelines for the management of severe acute pancreatitis. World J Emerg Surg. 2019;14(1):27.
4. González-Haba Ruiz M, Betés Ibáñez MT, Martínez Moreno B, Repiso Ortega A, de la Serna HC, Iglesias García J, et al. Endoscopic management of pancreatic collections. Endoscopic ultrasound group, Spanish Society of Digestive Endoscopy (GSEED-USE) clinical guidelines. Rev Esp Enferm Dig. 2024;116(8):423–37.
5. Gardner TB, Adler DG, Forsmark CE, Sauer BG, Taylor JR, Whitcomb DC. ACG clinical guideline: chronic pancreatitis. Am J Gastroenterol. 2020;115(3):322–39.
6. Liao WC, Tu TC, Lee KC, Tseng JH, Chen MJ, Sun CK, et al. Taiwanese consensus recommendations for acute pancreatitis. J Formos Med Assoc. 2020;119(9):1343–52.
7. Takada T, Isaji S, Mayumi T, Yoshida M, Takeyama Y, Itoi T, et al. JPN clinical practice guidelines 2021 with easy-to-understand explanations for the management of acute pancreatitis. J Hepatobiliary Pancreat Sci. 2022;29(10):1057–83.
8. Jaber S, Garnier M, Asehnoune K, Bounes F, Buscail L, Chevaux JB, et al. Guidelines for the management of patients with severe acute pancreatitis, 2021. Anaesth Crit Care Pain Med. 2022;41(3):101060.

Chapter 35
Approach to Cholangitis and Cholecystitis in the ICU

35.1 Introduction

Cholangitis and cholecystitis are acute biliary conditions commonly encountered in critically ill patients, requiring prompt diagnosis and intervention to prevent significant morbidity and mortality. Acute cholangitis results from an infection of the biliary system, typically secondary to obstruction by stones or strictures. Cholecystitis refers to the inflammation of the gallbladder, often caused by gallstones obstructing the cystic duct. Both conditions can lead to life-threatening complications, including sepsis, organ failure, and death if left untreated. This chapter outlines the evidence-based management of these conditions, incorporating recent guidelines such as the 2024 IDSA (Infectious Diseases Society of America) Guidelines and the ASGE (American Society of Gastrointestinal Endoscopy) Guidelines for cholangitis [1, 2] [Ref: Algorithm 35.1].

35.2 Initial Presentation and Resuscitation

Patients typically present with Charcot's Triad (fever, jaundice, right upper quadrant pain (RUQ)) for cholangitis and symptoms like RUQ pain, fever, nausea, and vomiting for cholecystitis. Early recognition and resuscitation are critical.

- Hemodynamic Instability: If the patient is hemodynamically unstable, the primary focus should be fluid resuscitation, antibiotics, and vasopressors. Patients with signs of sepsis must be stabilized with broad-spectrum antibiotics covering biliary pathogens, such as Gram-negative bacteria and anaerobes. The ASGE recommends starting antibiotics early as a bridge to definitive therapy.

S. B. Mishra et al., *Mastering ICU Care*,
https://doi.org/10.1007/978-981-95-0179-3_35

35.3 Diagnostic Approach and Imaging

First-Line Imaging

- Abdominal ultrasound (US) remains the first-line imaging modality, particularly in pregnant patients and those unable to tolerate contrast media. Ultrasound helps visualize biliary dilation, gallstones, and signs of cholecystitis, such as gallbladder wall thickening or pericholecystic fluid. For cholangitis, bile duct dilation is a critical finding [3, 4].

Advanced Imaging

- If the ultrasound is inconclusive, computed tomography (CT) scan or magnetic resonance cholangiopancreatography (MRCP) should be pursued. CT with intravenous contrast provides an excellent view of both the gallbladder and bile ducts, especially when MRCP is not available.
- MRCP is noninvasive and highly sensitive for detecting bile duct obstructions, stones, and biliary strictures, making it ideal for patients who cannot tolerate ERCP.
- In cases where acute cholangitis is suspected, early imaging and biliary decompression are vital to prevent worsening infection.

35.4 Assessing Severity: The Tokyo Guidelines

The Tokyo Guidelines provide a robust framework for assessing the severity of both cholangitis and cholecystitis, which informs treatment decisions.

- Mild Cholangitis: Characterized by a lack of organ dysfunction. These patients typically respond well to antibiotics and may not require immediate decompression.
- Moderate Cholangitis: Includes patients with a systemic inflammatory response or transient organ dysfunction. These patients require early biliary drainage.
- Severe Cholangitis: Involves organ failure, such as altered mental status, hypotension, or renal dysfunction. This is a medical emergency, requiring urgent drainage and intensive care.

In patients with cholecystitis, classification into mild, moderate, or severe guides treatment decisions, including the need for early surgery.

35.5 Treatment Strategies

35.5.1 Cholangitis Management

1. **ERCP Within 48 Hours:**
   - The ASGE guidelines emphasize performing endoscopic retrograde cholangiopancreatography (ERCP) within 48 hours of diagnosis in patients with confirmed cholangitis. ERCP serves as both a diagnostic and therapeutic tool, allowing for the removal of bile duct stones and biliary stent placement to relieve the obstruction.
   - In patients too unstable for a complete ERCP, biliary decompression alone (e.g., stent placement without stone removal) may be sufficient as an initial approach.
2. **Alternative Drainage Techniques:**
   - When ERCP is unavailable or delayed, or if the patient is too unstable to tolerate endoscopic procedures, percutaneous transhepatic biliary drainage (PTBD) offers a valuable alternative. PTBD is often used in ICU settings when surgical options are too risky or delayed, especially in critically ill patients.
   - Percutaneous biliary drainage involves placing a catheter into the bile ducts via the skin, which effectively decompresses the biliary system [5, 6].

35.5.2 Cholecystitis Management

1. **Early Laparoscopic Cholecystectomy:**
   - In stable patients diagnosed with cholecystitis, early laparoscopic cholecystectomy within 72 h is the treatment of choice. Early surgery reduces the risk of recurrent episodes and gallbladder perforation.
2. **Percutaneous Cholecystostomy:**
   - In patients who are poor surgical candidates due to severe comorbidities, percutaneous cholecystostomy is recommended as a bridging option. This procedure involves inserting a drainage catheter into the gallbladder to relieve pressure and infection, particularly in critically ill patients where immediate surgery poses a high risk.

Management in Special Populations

- Pregnancy: Ultrasound is the preferred imaging modality during pregnancy to avoid radiation exposure from CT. Surgery is generally deferred unless there is a risk of sepsis or gallbladder perforation.
- Elderly patients: Frail, elderly patients may not tolerate aggressive interventions. In these cases, conservative management with antibiotics and percutaneous drainage may be preferable.

Complications and Comorbidities

- Sepsis and Multiorgan Failure: Patients with cholangitis are at high risk for septic shock. In these cases, aggressive fluid resuscitation, broad-spectrum antibiotics, and early source control (via drainage or surgery) are paramount.
- Chronic Pancreatitis or Cholangiocarcinoma: These comorbidities complicate the management of biliary disease. If malignancy or chronic pancreatitis is suspected, referral for advanced imaging and possibly biopsy or additional surgical evaluation may be required [7].

35.6 Role of Antibiotics

Limiting systemic response and local inflammation and preventing hepatic abscess formation is the primary goal of antibiotics. Antibiotics can be given prophylactically in early, non-severe cases or therapeutic in severe cases or till the removal of the gall bladder. The most common pathogens involved in acute cholangitis are Gram-negative bacteria (especially *Escherichia coli*, *Klebsiella*, *Enterobacter*, and *Pseudomonas*), with some Gram-positive bacteria (e.g., *Enterococcus* species) and anaerobes also implicated in certain cases. Whereas Gram-negative organisms (e.g., *E. coli*), Gram-positive cocci (e.g., *Streptococcus* and *Enterococcus*), and anaerobes can complicate acute cholecystitis. Targeted organisms, local epidemiology and susceptibility data (antibiogram), alignment of in vitro activity (or spectrum) of the agents with these local data, characteristics of the agents such as pharmacokinetics and pharmacodynamics, and toxicities, renal and hepatic function, and any history of allergies and other adverse events with antimicrobial agent should guide the antimicrobial therapy.

Empiric antimicrobial therapy should target both Gram-negative organisms and anaerobes. Once culture results are available, antibiotic therapy should be adjusted to target the specific pathogens identified. If cholangitis is complicated (e.g., with sepsis, shock, or multi-organ failure), broader coverage may be required initially.

1. **Grade I and II Cholecystitis**:

   - **Therapy Duration**: Discontinue within 24 h after cholecystectomy.
   - **Extended Therapy**: If there are complications like perforation or necrosis, continue therapy for 4–7 days.

2. **Grade I and II Cholangitis**:
    - **Therapy Duration**: 4–7 days after infection source is controlled.
    - **Extended Therapy**: If bacteremia with Gram-positive cocci (*Enterococcus*, *Streptococcus*) is present, continue for a minimum of 2 weeks.
3. **Grade III Cholangitis and Cholecystitis**:
    - **Therapy Duration**: Minimum of 2 weeks if bacteremia with Gram-positive cocci is present.
    - **Extended Therapy**: Continue until any underlying issues (e.g., residual stones, bile duct obstruction, liver abscess) are resolved.
4. **Healthcare-Associated Cholangitis and Cholecystitis** (all grades):
    - **Therapy Duration**: Minimum of 2 weeks if bacteremia with Gram-positive cocci is present.
    - **Extended Therapy**: Continue until resolution of any anatomical issues or liver abscesses.

1. **Community-Acquired Biliary Infections:**
    - **Grade I (Mild)**:
        - **Penicillin-Based Therapy**: Not recommended if >20% resistance to *E. coli* (Ampicillin/sulbactam).
        - **Cephalosporin-Based Therapy**: Cefazolin, Cefuroxime, Ceftriaxone, Cefotaxime ± Metronidazole.
        - **Carbapenem-Based Therapy**: Ertapenem.
        - **Fluoroquinolone-Based Therapy**: Ciprofloxacin, Levofloxacin, Pazufloxacin ± Metronidazole.
    - **Grade II (Moderate)**:
        - **Penicillin-Based Therapy**: Piperacillin/tazobactam.
        - **Cephalosporin-Based Therapy**: Ceftriaxone, Cefotaxime, Cefepime, or Ceftazidime ± Metronidazole.
        - **Carbapenem-Based Therapy**: Ertapenem.
        - **Fluoroquinolone-Based Therapy**: Ciprofloxacin, Levofloxacin, or Pazufloxacin ± Metronidazole.
    - **Grade III (Severe)**:
        - **Penicillin-Based Therapy**: Piperacillin/tazobactam.
        - **Cephalosporin-Based Therapy**: Cefepime, Ceftazidime ± Metronidazole.
        - **Carbapenem-Based Therapy**: Imipenem/cilastatin, Meropenem, or Doripenem.
        - **Monobactam-Based Therapy**: Aztreonam± Metronidazole.
        - **Fluoroquinolone-Based Therapy**: Moxifloxacin, Ciprofloxacin, Levofloxacin with Metronidazole.

2. **Healthcare-Associated Biliary Infections (All Grades):**
   - **Penicillin-Based Therapy**: Piperacillin/tazobactam.
   - **Cephalosporin-Based Therapy**: Cefepime, Ceftazidime ± Metronidazole.
   - **Carbapenem-Based Therapy**: Imipenem/cilastatin, Meropenem, or Doripenem.
   - **Monobactam-Based Therapy**: Aztreonam ± Metronidazole.
   - **Vancomycin** is recommended for **Grade III** community-acquired and healthcare-associated infections to cover *Enterococcus* spp. If vancomycin resistance (VRE - Vancomycin resistant *Enterococcus*) is a concern, **Linezolid** or **Daptomycin** should be used.
   - **Anti-anerobic therapy** (e.g., Metronidazole, Tinidazole) is necessary if there is a biliary-enteric anastomosis.
   - **Fluoroquinolones** are recommended for patients with beta-lactam allergies or when the susceptibility of cultured isolates is known.

35.7 Outcomes and Mortality

The outcomes in cholangitis and cholecystitis depend heavily on early intervention. Mortality rates for severe cholangitis range from 10% to 40%, particularly in cases where biliary decompression is delayed. Early ERCP within 48 h significantly reduces mortality, morbidity, and the length of hospitalization compared to delayed intervention.

35.8 Conclusion

The management of cholangitis and cholecystitis in the ICU is guided by early recognition, appropriate imaging, and timely interventions such as ERCP or percutaneous drainage. The 2024 IDSA guidelines and ASGE guidelines provide a strong framework for diagnostic and therapeutic decision-making, while the Tokyo Guidelines help assess severity and guide treatment. Ultimately, early biliary decompression, whether through ERCP or percutaneous drainage, remains the cornerstone of managing these conditions and reducing mortality.

Algorithm 35.1: Approach to cholangitis and cholecystitis in the ICU

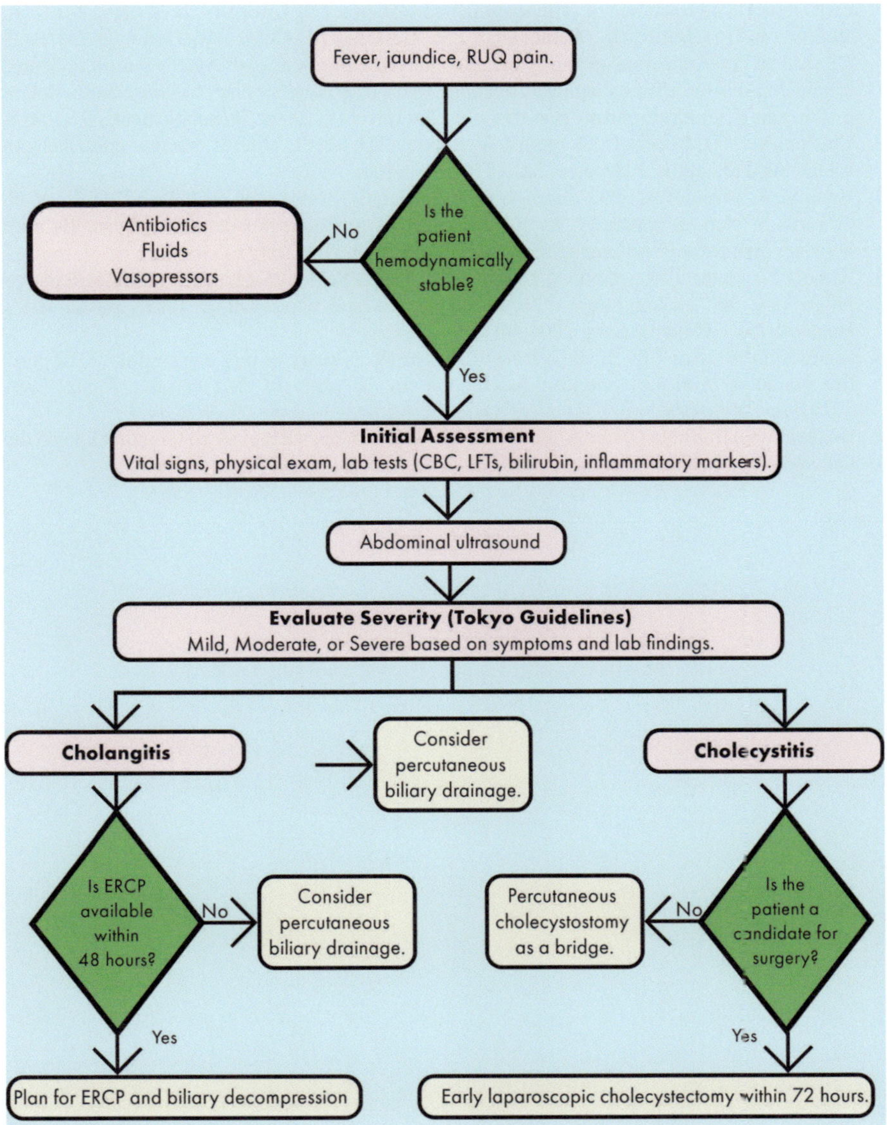

Bibliography

1. Carbone M, et al. Position paper of the Italian Association for the Study of the liver (AISF): management and treatment of primary biliary cholangitis. Dig Liver Dis. 2024;56(9):1461–74.
2. Bonomo RA, Edwards MS, Abrahamian FM, Bessesen M, Chow AW, Dellinger EP, et al. Clinical practice guideline update by the infectious diseases Society of America on complicated intraabdominal infections: diagnostic imaging of suspected acute cholecystitis and acute cholangitis in adults, children, and pregnant people. Clin Infect Dis. 2024;79(Supplement_3):S104–8.
3. Chazouilleres O, Beuers U, Bergquist A, Karlsen TH, EASL clinical practice guidelines on sclerosing cholangitis. J Hepatol. 2022;77(3):761–806.
4. Bonomi A, Overdevest AG, Busch OR, Kazemier G, Zonderhuis BM, Erdmann JI, et al. Towards a 'step-up approach' for the treatment of recurrent non-stenotic cholangitis after hepaticojejunostomy: systematic review. HPB (Oxford). 2024;26(9):1114–22.
5. Kimura Y, Takada T, Kawarada Y, Nimura Y, Hirata K, Sekimoto M, et al. Definitions, pathophysiology, and epidemiology of acute cholangitis and cholecystitis: Tokyo guidelines. J Hepato-Biliary-Pancreat Surg. 2007;14(1):15–26.
6. Lindor KD, Bowlus CL, Boyer J, Levy C, Mayo M. Primary biliary cholangitis: 2018 practice guidance from the American Association for the study of liver diseases. Hepatology. 2019;69(1):394–419.
7. Buxbaum JL, Buitrago C, Lee A, Elmunzer BJ, Riaz A, Ceppa EP, et al. ASGE guideline on the management of cholangitis. Gastrointest Endosc. 2021;94(2):207–21.

Chapter 36
Approach to Mesenteric Ischemia in the ICU

36.1 Introduction

Acute mesenteric ischemia (AMI), characterized by reduced blood flow to the intestines, can lead to intestinal necrosis and sepsis if untreated. AMI is a high-mortality emergency, particularly when diagnosis and intervention are delayed. This chapter provides a step-by-step approach to managing AMI in the ICU, addressing the early identification of symptoms, diagnostic steps, and specific management pathways based on patient presentation [1] [Ref: Algorithm 36.1].

36.2 Initial Assessment

- Presenting Symptoms: Key symptoms include severe, disproportionate abdominal pain, nausea, vomiting, and sometimes bloody stools. Recognizing this classic pain-to-findings discrepancy is critical for early suspicion of AMI.
- Risk Factors: Advanced age, cardiac history (particularly atrial fibrillation), prior embolic events, and hypercoagulability are common risk factors in AMI patients. Recent hypotensive episodes and vasopressor use are risk factors for non-occlusive mesenteric ischemia. Identifying these factors early can help stratify patients for immediate investigation and intervention [2].

S. B. Mishra et al., *Mastering ICU Care*,
https://doi.org/10.1007/978-981-95-0179-3_36

36.2.1 Clinical Evaluation

- Physical Examination: Assess for abdominal tenderness and peritoneal signs. Symptoms out of proportion to examination findings should heighten suspicion of acute mesenteric ischemia.

  Vitals and Laboratory Work:

  - Vitals: Monitor for hypotension and tachycardia, which may indicate a compromised cardiovascular state.
  - Laboratory Markers: Include lactate (a marker for tissue hypoxia – serial lactate monitoring), D-dimer, arterial blood gases (to detect metabolic acidosis), and complete blood count. Emerging markers such as neutrophil-to-lymphocyte ratio (NLR), mean platelet volume (MPV), and red cell distribution width (RDW) may support early diagnosis and enhance specificity [3].

36.2.2 Imaging and Diagnosis

- CT Angiography (CTA): As the first-line imaging modality, CTA confirms diagnosis, assesses bowel viability, and identifies specific signs such as mesenteric vessel filling defects, bowel wall thickening, pneumatosis intestinalis, and portal venous gas. This imaging step is essential for diagnosing AMI and differentiating types of acute mesenteric ischemia. CTA has >90% sensitivity and specificity to diagnose AMI – *gold standard.*

  Differential Diagnosis: The CTA findings and clinical context guide differentiation into:

  - Arterial Occlusion: Often from embolic or thrombotic events, requiring immediate attention.
  - Venous Thrombosis: Characterized by mesenteric vein occlusion, commonly managed with anticoagulation.
  - Nonocclusive Mesenteric Ischemia (NOMI): Linked to low-flow states and typically managed with vasodilators [4].

36.3 Predictors of Mortality in AMI

- Significant Predictors: Mortality is higher in patients with advanced age, chronic renal disease, patient dependency, arrhythmias, cardiac failure, hypotension, and delayed surgery. Elevated lactate levels and the need for inotropes correlate with poor prognosis, while timely anticoagulation and revascularization improve survival.

- Risk Stratification: Developing a risk stratification model based on these predictors can help in early identification of high-risk patients and prompt more aggressive monitoring and intervention.

36.4 Management Pathway

No Peritoneal Signs (Early Detection):

- Anticoagulation: Begin systemic anticoagulation, especially in cases with high suspicion of ischemia without bowel necrosis.
- Consider Endovascular Therapy: For embolic or thrombotic obstructions, consider thrombolysis or angioplasty as endovascular options, which are associated with lower short-term mortality compared to open surgery.

Peritoneal Signs Present (Suspected Bowel Infarction):

- Surgical Intervention: Immediate laparotomy is required for suspected bowel necrosis.
- Intraoperative Endovascular Support (Hybrid Technique): In settings with endovascular capabilities, a hybrid approach can offer faster reperfusion and facilitate direct assessment of bowel viability, potentially reducing the need for repeat surgeries [5].

36.4.1 Type-Specific Management

- Arterial Occlusion: Treat with endovascular approaches like angioplasty and thrombolysis for revascularization. Open surgery is necessary when bowel necrosis is suspected.
- Venous Thrombosis: Manage primarily with systemic anticoagulation to dissolve clots and restore blood flow, reducing further ischemic damage. Long-term anticoagulation is typically required to prevent recurrence.
- Nonocclusive Mesenteric Ischemia (NOMI): NOMI requires vasodilators (e.g., intra-arterial papaverine) and management of the underlying low-flow state (e.g., treating hypotension) to restore mesenteric perfusion.

36.4.2 Bowel Viability Assessment

- Resection and Second-Look Surgery: During surgery, remove necrotic bowel segments. If viability remains uncertain, schedule a second-look laparotomy within 24–48 h. This approach helps address evolving ischemia and minimizes risks of severe complications. Fluorescence imaging with indocyanine green (ICG) is emerging for intraoperative assessment.

36.4.3 Postoperative and Follow-Up Care

- Monitor for Reperfusion Injury: Postoperatively, assess for reperfusion injury, indicated by metabolic acidosis, rising lactate levels, and multi-organ dysfunction.
- Long-Term Follow-Up: Chronic mesenteric ischemia cases may require periodic imaging due to recurrence risk. For patients with extensive resections, nutritional support may be essential, especially in cases of short bowel syndrome [6].

36.5 Conclusion

Managing Acute mesenteric ischemia in the ICU requires a structured, evidence-based approach that addresses early symptom identification, diagnostic imaging, and targeted therapeutic strategies based on ischemia type. Clinicians should utilize a combination of risk stratification, laboratory markers, CTA imaging, and tailored endovascular or surgical intervention to improve patient outcomes. Continuous postoperative monitoring, especially for reperfusion injury and recurrence, is essential for ensuring long-term success in managing acute mesenteric ischemia. Early recognition and rapid, coordinated intervention remain the most critical determinants of survival in AMI.

Algorithm 36.1: Approach to acute mesenteric ischemia in the ICU

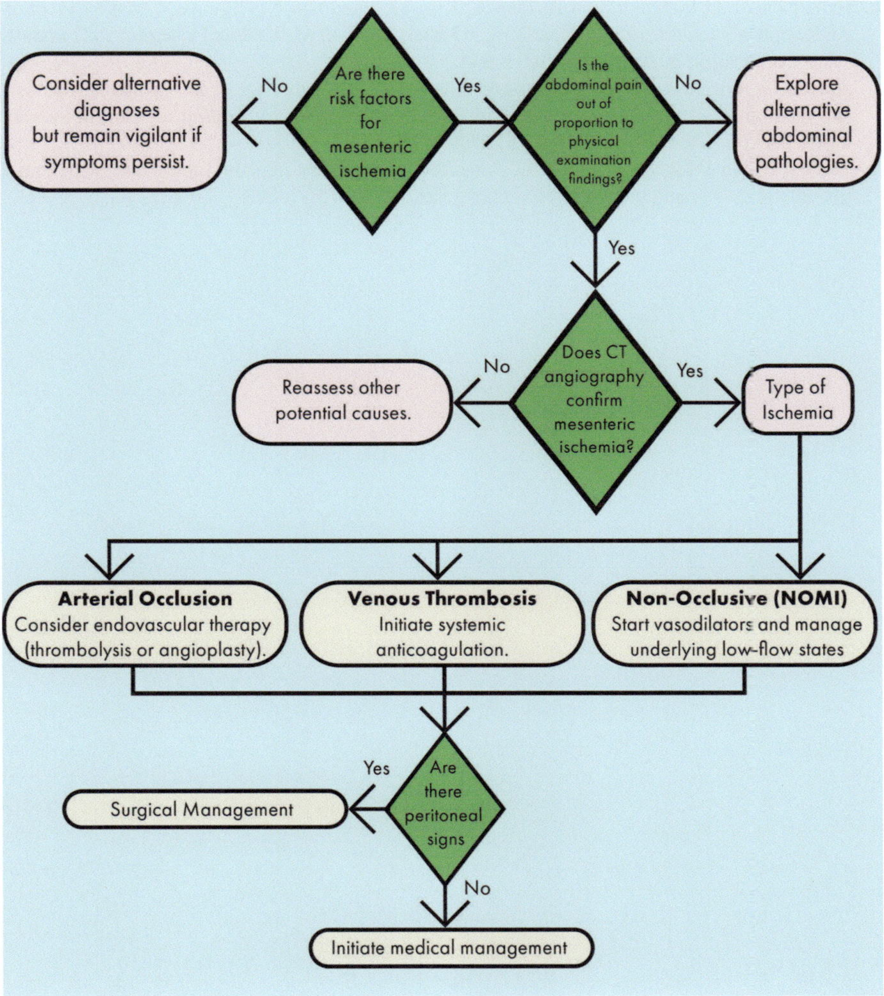

Bibliography

1. Nikoupoor H, Moradi AM, Arasteh P, Shamsaeefar A, Karami MY, Eghlimi H, et al. Guideline for Management of Mesenteric Ischemia: shiraz intestinal failure unit protocol. Arch Iran Med. 2020;23(6):422–5.
2. Zhao Y, Yin H, Yao C, Deng J, Wang M, Li Z, et al. Management of Acute Mesenteric Ischemia: a critical review and treatment algorithm. Vasc Endovasc Surg. 2016;50(3):183–92.

3. Khan SM, Emile SH, Wang Z, Agha MA. Diagnostic accuracy of hematological parameters in acute mesenteric ischemia-a systematic review. Int J Surg. 2019;66:18–27.
4. Expert Panel on Interventional R, Lam A, Kim YJ, Fidelman N, Higgins M, Cash BD, et al. ACR appropriateness criteria(R) radiologic Management of Mesenteric Ischemia: 2022 update. J Am Coll Radiol. 2022;19(11S):S433–S44.
5. Alahdab F, Arwani R, Pasha AK, Razouki ZA, Prokop LJ, Huber TS, et al. A systematic review and meta-analysis of endovascular versus open surgical revascularization for chronic mesenteric ischemia. J Vasc Surg. 2018;67(5):1598–605.
6. Sumbal R, Ali Baig MM, Sumbal A. Predictors of mortality in acute mesenteric ischemia: a systematic review and meta-analysis. J Surg Res. 2022;275:72–86.

Chapter 37
Approach to Intestinal Perforation or Obstruction in the ICU

37.1 Introduction

Intestinal perforation and obstruction are critical conditions encountered in the ICU setting, requiring immediate and structured management due to the risks of sepsis, peritonitis, and rapid deterioration. These conditions commonly arise from underlying diseases such as adhesions following previous surgeries, colorectal cancer, and inflammatory conditions. This chapter provides an evidence-based approach to managing intestinal perforation and obstruction, emphasizing the importance of prompt diagnostic evaluation, appropriate patient stratification, and interprofessional collaboration [1] [Ref: Algorithm 37.1].

37.2 Epidemiology and Risk Factors

- Adhesive Small Bowel Obstruction (ASBO): ASBO is one of the most frequent causes of small bowel obstruction, especially in patients with a history of prior abdominal surgeries, as postoperative adhesions can kink the bowel and obstruct passage. ASBO accounts for a significant number of surgical emergencies in ICU patients.
- Large Bowel Obstruction (LBO): Colorectal cancer, particularly in the sigmoid colon, is the leading cause of LBO. The incidence of LBO varies based on geographic region, dietary habits, and age. LBO is particularly common in older adults, with increasing incidence as the global population ages.
- Perforation Risks: Bowel perforation is often caused by conditions such as duodenal ulcers, diverticulitis, and obstructive tumors, especially in elderly populations. Other causes include inflammatory bowel diseases and trauma, which

S. B. Mishra et al., *Mastering ICU Care*,
https://doi.org/10.1007/978-981-95-0179-3_37

compromise the integrity of the bowel wall, leading to perforation and subsequent peritonitis [1].

37.3 Pathophysiology and Types of Obstructions

Classification of Obstructions

- Partial Obstruction: Allows some passage of intestinal contents but may still cause significant discomfort and distension.
- Complete Obstruction: Prevents all movement of contents, leading to severe distension and rapid progression of symptoms.
- Closed-Loop Obstruction: Occurs when a segment of the bowel is occluded at two points, resulting in ischemia due to trapped contents and compromised blood supply. This type of obstruction carries a high risk of perforation and requires urgent intervention [2].

Mechanism of Perforation

- Perforation can result from ischemia (as in bowel obstruction where decreased blood flow leads to necrosis), inflammation (as in conditions like diverticulitis), erosion (caused by malignancies or ulcers that degrade the bowel wall), and physical disruption (due to trauma or iatrogenic causes during endoscopy). Understanding the underlying cause is essential for timely and effective treatment.

37.4 Detailed Diagnostic Approach

Imaging

Imaging plays a central role in diagnosing and assessing the severity of both bowel obstruction and perforation. Choosing the appropriate imaging modality is crucial, as it directly impacts the quality and speed of diagnosis and, consequently, patient outcomes [3].

CT Scans

- CT (computed tomography) scans are the gold standard for evaluating suspected bowel obstruction and perforation due to their high sensitivity and specificity. A CT scan provides a detailed view of the abdominal structures, enabling precise identification of the location, cause, and severity of the obstruction or perforation.
- CT imaging is invaluable in detecting complications that may arise from obstruction or perforation, such as abscesses, strangulation, or ischemia. In cases of perforation, CT scan can reveal the presence of free air or fluid in the abdominal cavity, along with any local inflammatory response or abscess formation.

- When bowel obstruction is suspected, the CT scan can determine whether it is a partial or complete blockage and identify any closed-loop or strangulated obstructions, which require urgent intervention due to the risk of ischemia and necrosis.
- Contrast-enhanced CT scans are often preferred as they provide better visualization of blood flow and tissue integrity, helping to assess bowel viability and identify signs of ischemia or necrosis.

Bedside Ultrasound and Plain Abdominal X-rays

- For critically ill patients who cannot be easily transported to radiology for a CT scan, bedside ultrasound or plain abdominal X-rays can be valuable initial imaging tools.
- Ultrasound is particularly useful for evaluating abdominal distension and detecting free fluid. Though it is operator-dependent and less comprehensive than CT, ultrasound can quickly identify signs of bowel dilation and guide further management.
- Plain abdominal X-rays are useful for identifying free air under the diaphragm in cases of suspected perforation and can also demonstrate signs of bowel obstruction, such as air-fluid levels and dilated bowel loops. X-rays are less sensitive than CT but may be used in emergencies or as an adjunct when CT is not immediately available.

Laboratory Tests

In addition to imaging, a comprehensive panel of laboratory tests is essential to assess the patient's overall condition and to help identify underlying causes or complications associated with bowel obstruction and perforation.

Basic Laboratory Tests

- A complete blood count (CBC) is critical for identifying leukocytosis, which may suggest infection or inflammation, and anemia, which can indicate chronic blood loss or underlying malignancy.
- Electrolyte levels are assessed to detect imbalances common in bowel obstruction due to vomiting, dehydration, and sequestration of fluids within the bowel lumen. Close monitoring of sodium, potassium, and chloride levels is necessary, as these imbalances can impact patient stability and complicate management.
- C-reactive protein (CRP) and lactate levels are useful inflammatory and metabolic markers. Elevated CRP indicates an inflammatory response, while lactate levels help detect tissue hypoperfusion or ischemia, particularly relevant in strangulated bowel obstruction or perforation cases.

Additional Laboratory Tests

- Liver Function Tests (LFTs): These tests are valuable for identifying liver dysfunction, which may complicate the clinical picture, particularly in cases where the obstruction or perforation has affected the hepatobiliary system or led to secondary sepsis. Elevated liver enzymes could also suggest involvement of the liver or biliary tree, necessitating targeted management.

- Lipase: Pancreatic involvement or secondary pancreatitis may occur in cases of upper gastrointestinal perforation or severe abdominal inflammation, making lipase an important marker to assess. Elevated lipase levels indicate pancreatic involvement, which requires additional supportive management.
- Blood Cultures: In cases with suspected sepsis, blood cultures should be drawn to identify the causative organism and guide antibiotic therapy. Positive blood cultures confirm systemic infection and help tailor antimicrobial therapy for improved outcomes.

37.5 Criteria for Conservative Versus Surgical Management

Non-surgical/Conservative Candidates

Conservative management is an effective approach for certain patients with intestinal obstruction, particularly those with partial obstructions who exhibit no clinical signs of peritonitis or systemic instability. Partial obstruction allows some passage of intestinal contents, making it possible for symptoms to resolve with supportive measures without the need for surgery. The goal of conservative treatment is to relieve symptoms, prevent progression to complete obstruction, and provide support while monitoring for any signs of deterioration [1].

Key Components of Conservative Management

- NPO (Nothing by Mouth/Nil per oral): Patients are kept strictly off oral intake to reduce gastrointestinal motility and minimize the risk of exacerbating the obstruction. This approach helps prevent further distension, reduces vomiting, and lowers the risk of aspiration.
- IV Fluid and Electrolyte Administration: Maintaining adequate hydration and electrolyte balance is critical, as patients with bowel obstruction are at high risk for dehydration and electrolyte disturbances due to vomiting, decreased oral intake, and fluid shifts into the bowel lumen. Isotonic saline or balanced crystalloid solutions are typically used to restore intravascular volume and correct electrolyte imbalances.
- Nasogastric (NG) Tube Decompression: An NG tube is inserted to decompress the stomach and relieve distension by draining fluid and gas that accumulate proximal to the obstruction. This intervention helps alleviate nausea, vomiting, and abdominal discomfort and can reduce the risk of aspiration in patients with significant distension [4].

Indications for Monitoring and Gradual Advancement

- Regular assessments are performed to evaluate symptom improvement, abdominal examination findings, and radiographic changes. If the patient shows clinical improvement, gradual advancement of diet may be considered under careful supervision.

Contraindications for Conservative Management:

- Signs of Peritonitis: The presence of peritonitis, indicated by abdominal tenderness, guarding, and rebound tenderness, signals a more serious intra-abdominal pathology, such as bowel ischemia or perforation, necessitating surgical intervention.
- Ischemia: Symptoms such as increasing abdominal pain, leukocytosis, and elevated lactate suggest ischemia, particularly in a setting of closed-loop obstruction. Surgical exploration is crucial to prevent progression to necrosis.
- Strangulation: If there is evidence of bowel strangulation (compromised blood supply due to twisting or pressure on the bowel), conservative management is contraindicated, as this condition can rapidly lead to ischemia and perforation. Immediate surgery is required to relieve the obstruction and restore blood flow.

Close monitoring is essential in all patients managed conservatively to detect any signs of clinical deterioration that would necessitate surgical assessment. If symptoms do not improve within 24–48 h, or if there are any signs of worsening, surgical evaluation is typically recommended [5].

Surgical Candidates

Surgical intervention is the preferred approach in patients with complete obstruction, intestinal perforation, or peritonitis. These conditions often require immediate surgical resolution to avoid the complications associated with prolonged obstruction or bowel compromise, such as necrosis, sepsis, and multi-organ dysfunction.

Indications for Surgery

- Complete Obstruction: A complete blockage of the bowel prevents any passage of contents, leading to rapid progression of symptoms and potential bowel ischemia. Surgery aims to remove the cause of obstruction and prevent the complications associated with closed-loop or strangulated obstruction.
- Perforation: Bowel perforation results in the leakage of intestinal contents into the peritoneal cavity, leading to peritonitis and systemic infection. Prompt surgical intervention is necessary to repair the perforation, control contamination, and reduce the risk of sepsis.
- Peritonitis: Generalized peritonitis, characterized by widespread abdominal tenderness, fever, and signs of sepsis, indicates an acute abdomen requiring surgical exploration. The goal is to identify and treat the source of peritoneal inflammation, whether due to ischemia, perforation, or abscess formation.

Approach to Surgical Management

- Laparoscopic Surgery: In cases of ASBO, laparoscopic surgery may be a suitable option, particularly for selected patients without significant abdominal distension or dense adhesions. Laparoscopy offers a minimally invasive option that reduces postoperative pain, shortens recovery time, and lowers the risk of postoperative adhesion formation compared to open surgery.
- Open Surgery: In cases where there is a high risk of bowel ischemia, extensive adhesions, or suspected perforation, open surgery may be necessary to provide

better access and control. Open approaches are also preferred in critically ill patients where rapid access to the abdominal cavity is needed.

Considerations in the Surgical Approach

- Sepsis and Severe Ischemia: For patients showing signs of sepsis or bowel ischemia, time is of the essence. Prompt surgery can prevent further deterioration by addressing the underlying obstruction, restoring bowel perfusion, and preventing necrosis. Delayed intervention in these patients risks progression to bowel infarction, septic shock, and multi-organ failure.
- Damage Control Surgery: In severely unstable patients, especially those with peritonitis and sepsis, a damage control approach may be employed. This involves controlling the immediate source of infection or obstruction and then allowing the patient to stabilize before definitive repair. Temporary abdominal closure may be considered, with reexploration after resuscitation and hemodynamic improvement.

37.6 Perioperative and Postoperative Care

Antibiotics and Fluid Resuscitation

Effective perioperative management begins with the stabilization of the patient using broad-spectrum antibiotics and aggressive fluid resuscitation. These interventions are particularly important for patients presenting with suspected bowel perforation or obstruction, as they are at risk for sepsis and multi-organ failure.

Broad-Spectrum Antibiotics

- In cases of suspected bowel perforation or obstruction, empiric broad-spectrum antibiotics are administered immediately to combat potential infections from bowel flora, which includes a high load of Gram-negative and anaerobic bacteria. The choice of antibiotics should cover common enteric pathogens (e.g., *Escherichia coli*, *Bacteroides fragilis*) and be adjusted as necessary based on local antibiograms, infection severity, and the patient's previous antibiotic history.
- For distal perforations, especially involving the large intestine where the bacterial load is higher, antibiotic coverage is critical to prevent peritoneal contamination from progressing to sepsis. Initial antibiotic therapy is often guided by broad-spectrum agents like piperacillin-tazobactam or a combination of cephalosporins and metronidazole until cultures can confirm the exact pathogens involved.
- Antibiotics are typically administered preoperatively and continued postoperatively, with adjustments based on intraoperative findings and the patient's clinical course. The duration of therapy may be prolonged in cases of abscess formation or peritoneal contamination, extending beyond the usual perioperative period to ensure infection control [6].

Fluid Resuscitation

- Fluid resuscitation is a cornerstone of care in bowel obstruction and perforation cases, as these patients often present with significant dehydration, electrolyte imbalances, and hypotension. Vomiting, reduced oral intake, and third-spacing (fluid shifting into the bowel lumen and peritoneal cavity) exacerbate volume loss.
- Isotonic crystalloid solutions, such as normal saline or lactated Ringer's, are typically used to restore intravascular volume and maintain blood pressure, thus preventing hypoperfusion and organ dysfunction. Resuscitation should be guided by hemodynamic parameters, urine output (with a goal of maintaining at least 0.5 mL/kg/hr), and lactate levels to ensure adequate tissue perfusion.
- In patients with signs of sepsis or septic shock, early aggressive fluid resuscitation is critical, with adjustments based on the patient's response to fluids, ensuring that the resuscitation is sufficient to maintain organ perfusion but does not lead to fluid overload.

Nutrition

Nutritional support is a key component of postoperative care, especially in patients with prolonged recovery or delayed return of bowel function.

- Parenteral Nutrition (PN)
  - In patients unable to tolerate enteral nutrition due to ongoing bowel dysfunction, prolonged ileus, or extensive bowel resection, parenteral nutrition becomes necessary. PN provides essential macronutrients (proteins, fats, carbohydrates) and micronutrients (electrolytes, vitamins, trace elements) via the intravenous route, bypassing the gastrointestinal tract and preventing malnutrition.
  - Early initiation of parenteral nutrition within 3–7 days is considered in cases where enteral feeding is expected to be delayed for over a week, as prolonged malnutrition can impair immune function, delay wound healing, and increase the risk of postoperative complications.
  - Transition to enteral nutrition is preferred as soon as feasible, as enteral feeding helps preserve gut integrity and reduces the risk of infection associated with PN. Gradual reintroduction of enteral feeding can be initiated based on the patient's tolerance, with careful monitoring for signs of intolerance, such as abdominal distension, vomiting, or increased nasogastric tube output.

Complication Monitoring

Postoperative monitoring is essential for early detection and management of complications, which can range from minor wound infections to more severe issues such as sepsis, abscess formation, or fistula development.

Infection Surveillance

- Patients are at high risk for surgical site infections, intra-abdominal abscesses, and, in cases of bowel perforation, peritonitis. Postoperative monitoring includes daily assessment of the wound for signs of infection (redness, warmth, discharge), and regular monitoring of inflammatory markers (e.g., white blood cell count, CRP levels) and temperature.

- Blood cultures and imaging (e.g., ultrasound or CT scan) should be considered if there are signs of systemic infection or localized abscesses, especially in patients with persistent fever or unexplained leukocytosis. Prompt detection and drainage of abscesses can prevent sepsis and improve outcomes.

Fistula Monitoring and Management

- Fistulas, abnormal connections between the bowel and other organs or skin, can develop due to incomplete healing of the bowel wall, particularly in patients with significant inflammation or ischemia. Signs of a fistula may include persistent drainage, fever, or abdominal pain. Nutritional support and infection control are crucial in managing fistulas, and in some cases, additional surgical interventions may be required.
- Monitoring for Signs of Ileus and Bowel Function Recovery:
  - Postoperative ileus is common in bowel obstruction or perforation cases, especially after extensive bowel manipulation or resection. Monitoring includes assessing bowel sounds, nasogastric tube output, and signs of abdominal distension or discomfort.
  - Gradual reintroduction of oral intake should be considered only once bowel sounds return and the patient demonstrates the ability to tolerate minimal oral intake without nausea or vomiting. Persistent ileus may require prolonged decompression and supportive care, with careful monitoring to ensure nutritional and electrolyte needs are met.

Vital Sign Monitoring and Sepsis Screening

- Regular assessment of vital signs (temperature, heart rate, respiratory rate, and blood pressure) is essential for early detection of complications such as sepsis. Close attention is given to subtle changes in clinical status, as sepsis can rapidly progress, particularly in patients with ongoing contamination from bowel contents.
- In cases of suspected sepsis, immediate escalation of care, including blood cultures, fluid resuscitation, and appropriate antibiotic adjustments, is essential to reduce morbidity and improve survival.

37.7 Special Considerations and Patient Stratification

Colorectal Cancer Emergencies

- For obstructions or perforations related to colorectal cancer, emergency resection may be necessary. However, stenting may be considered as a bridge to surgery in certain patients. This approach allows temporary relief of obstruction while enabling oncologic planning. The potential oncologic risks associated with emergency surgery should be weighed against the immediate need for intervention.

Risk Factors and Recurrence

- Younger patients with ASBO have a higher risk of recurrence due to adhesion formation. The use of adhesion prevention techniques during surgery, such as the application of adhesion barriers and minimally invasive techniques, can help reduce the risk of future obstructions.

37.8 Role of Interprofessional Care

Team Coordination

- Effective management of intestinal perforation and obstruction requires an interprofessional team approach. Early involvement of surgeons, radiologists, critical care specialists, and pharmacists is essential for timely imaging, surgical intervention, and optimized antibiotic regimens. Collaborative care improves outcomes, particularly for ICU patients with multiple comorbidities and complex presentations.

37.9 Conclusion

Managing intestinal perforation and obstruction in the ICU is a structured process that requires thorough diagnostic evaluation, timely decision-making, and interprofessional coordination. Conservative management may be appropriate in selected cases of partial obstruction, but surgical intervention is often necessary, especially in complete obstruction or perforation cases. Postoperative monitoring and care are crucial to prevent complications and improve patient outcomes. This approach underscores the importance of early intervention, adherence to evidence-based protocols, and teamwork in the ICU.

Algorithm 37.1: Approach to intestinal perforation or obstruction in the ICU

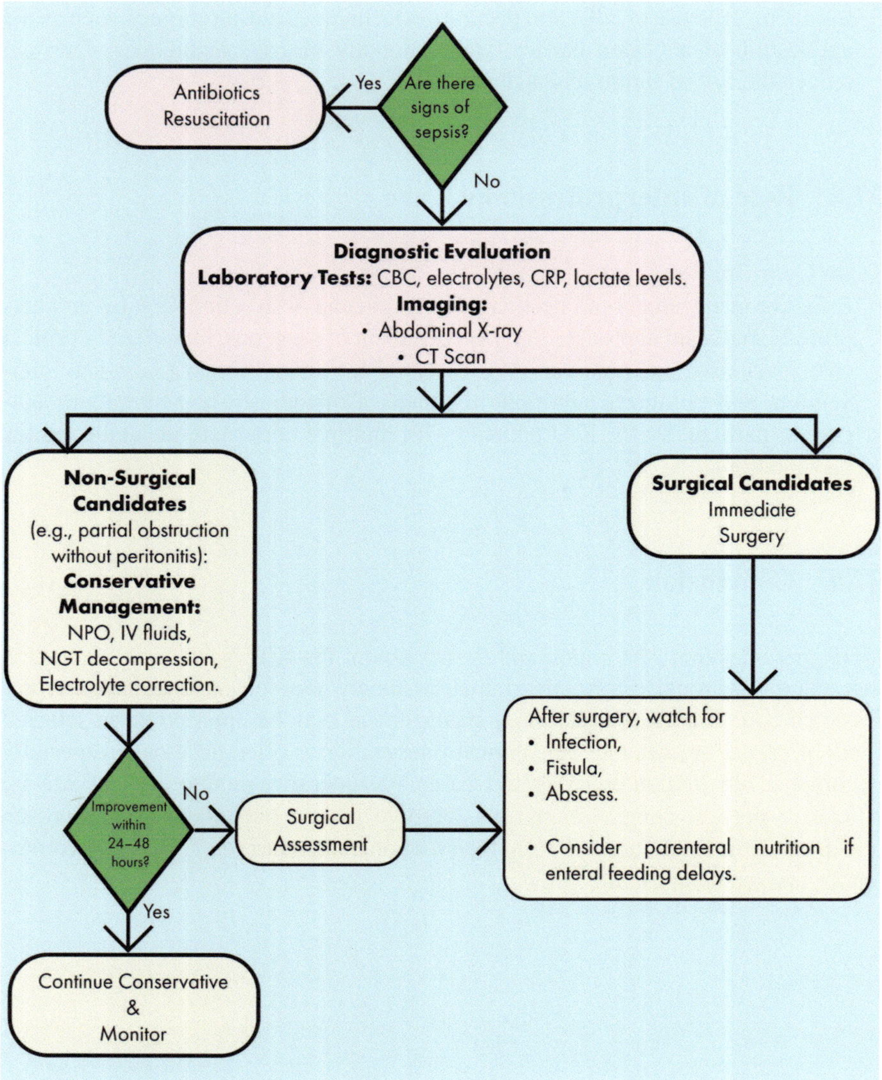

Bibliography

1. Pisano M, Zorcolo L, Merli C, Cimbanassi S, Poiasina E, Ceresoli M, et al. 2017 WSES guidelines on colon and rectal cancer emergencies: obstruction and perforation. World J Emerg Surg. 2018;13:36.
2. Long B, Robertson J, Koyfman A. Emergency medicine evaluation and management of small bowel obstruction: evidence-based recommendations. J Emerg Med. 2019;56(2):166–76.

3. Song WC, Lv WW, Gao XZ. Iatrogenic gastrointestinal perforation following therapeutic endoscopic procedures: management and outcome. J Coll Physicians Surg Pak. 2017;27(9):563–5.
4. Biffl WL, Leppaniemi A. Management guidelines for penetrating abdominal trauma. World J Surg. 2015;39(6):1373–80.
5. Ten Broek RPG, Krielen P, Di Saverio S, Coccolini F, Biffl WL, Ansaloni L, et al. Bologna guidelines for diagnosis and management of adhesive small bowel obstruction (ASBO): 2017 update of the evidence-based guidelines from the world society of emergency surgery ASBO working group. World J Emerg Surg. 2018;13:24.
6. Li PH, Tee YS, Fu CY, Liao CH, Wang SY, Hsu YP, et al. The role of noncontrast CT in the evaluation of surgical abdomen patients. Am Surg. 2018;84(6):1015–21.

Chapter 38
Approach to Upper Gastrointestinal Bleeding (UGIB) in the ICU

38.1 Introduction and Epidemiology

Upper gastrointestinal bleeding (UGIB) is a potentially life-threatening condition that originates from the esophagus, stomach, or duodenum. It can manifest as hematemesis (vomiting blood), melena (black tarry stools), or, in cases of massive bleeding, hematochezia (fresh blood per rectum). Prompt diagnosis and intervention are essential, as UGIB is associated with significant morbidity and mortality, especially in ICU settings. The overall mortality rate for UGIB ranges from 2% to 10%, and outcomes are often worse in patients with comorbid conditions like chronic kidney disease and cardiovascular disease.

In recent years, the epidemiology of UGIB has shifted. While peptic ulcer disease remains a major cause, its incidence has decreased due to widespread *Helicobacter pylori* eradication and the increased use of acid-suppressing medications. Conversely, other causes, including vascular lesions and malignancy, have become more prevalent. This evolving landscape emphasizes the need for careful diagnostic evaluation to identify the underlying etiology and tailor management appropriately [1] [Ref: Algorithm 38.1].

38.2 Initial Assessment and Resuscitation

38.2.1 Airway, Breathing, and Circulation (ABCs)

The initial step in UGIB management involves assessing and stabilizing the patient's airway, breathing, and circulation. In patients with severe hematemesis or altered mental status, intubation may be necessary to protect the airway, especially if the

S. B. Mishra et al., *Mastering ICU Care*,
https://doi.org/10.1007/978-981-95-0179-3_38

gag reflex is compromised. Hemodynamic stability is equally critical, with target goals to maintain mean arterial pressure (MAP) > 65 mm Hg. Secure two large-bore intravenous lines for rapid fluid and blood product administration if necessary.

38.2.2 *Fluid Resuscitation and Transfusion Strategy*

For patients presenting with severe bleeding, judicious fluid resuscitation is critical to prevent hemodilution and fluid overload. In hemodynamically stable patients, restrictive transfusion strategies are recommended, with a hemoglobin threshold of 7 g/dL. However, patients with ongoing hemorrhage and signs of hypoperfusion may require a higher threshold to stabilize their condition. Blood product selection and administration should be guided by coagulation parameters, platelet count, and the extent of blood loss.

38.2.3 *Timing of Endoscopy*

Endoscopy should be performed within 24 hours for most patients with UGIB to identify the bleeding source and facilitate endoscopic therapy. For hemodynamically unstable patients, endoscopy is prioritized as soon as the patient is stabilized, as early intervention in these cases has been shown to reduce mortality and improve outcomes.

38.3 Risk Stratification Tools

Risk assessment tools are crucial in managing patients with upper gastrointestinal bleeding (UGIB). These tools help clinicians identify patients at higher risk for complications, determine the need for urgent interventions, and establish whether a patient can be safely managed as an outpatient or requires inpatient care. Below are descriptions of the most widely used risk stratification tools in UGIB: the Glasgow-Blatchford Score (GBS), the Rockall Score, and the Forrest Classification [2].

38.3.1 *Glasgow-Blatchford Score (GBS)*

The Glasgow-Blatchford Score (GBS) is a pre-endoscopic scoring system used primarily upon a patient's initial presentation to assess the need for medical intervention, such as blood transfusions or endoscopic therapy. GBS evaluates clinical and laboratory parameters without requiring endoscopic findings, making it especially useful in emergency departments to triage patients before endoscopy.

Components of the GBS
The GBS score is calculated based on several variables:

1. Hemoglobin Level: Lower hemoglobin levels contribute to a higher score, as anemia often indicates more significant blood loss.
2. Blood Urea Nitrogen (BUN): Elevated BUN levels suggest upper GI bleeding since blood proteins are broken down in the gastrointestinal tract and absorbed, raising BUN.
3. Systolic Blood Pressure: Lower systolic blood pressure scores higher, indicating possible hypovolemic shock or hemodynamic instability.
4. Pulse Rate: A higher pulse rate reflects compensatory tachycardia due to blood loss.
5. Presence of Melena: Melena (black tarry stools) suggests ongoing or recent upper GI bleeding.
6. History of Syncope: Syncope indicates significant blood loss, leading to hypoperfusion and potential fainting episodes.
7. History of Liver Disease or Heart Failure: Comorbidities such as liver disease or heart failure place patients at increased risk of severe bleeding.

Scoring and Interpretation

- A GBS score of 0 indicates very low risk, where patients are unlikely to require urgent intervention. These low-risk patients may be managed as outpatients.
- Scores above 1 suggest a need for more intensive evaluation, and scores of 2 or higher indicate a higher risk of requiring interventions like transfusion or endoscopy.
- High GBS scores (>3) often warrant admission and rapid endoscopic assessment, as they correlate with increased risk for adverse outcomes and the need for more aggressive management.

GBS is particularly helpful in distinguishing patients who may be safely discharged from those who require immediate intervention.

38.3.2 Rockall Score

The Rockall Score is used both pre- and post-endoscopy to evaluate a patient's risk of mortality and rebleeding. It is designed to be applied initially based on clinical presentation (pre-endoscopy) and then recalculated after endoscopic findings are obtained (post-endoscopy). The Rockall Score is effective for stratifying patients based on their long-term outcomes, especially their risk of death.

Components of the Rockall Score

1. Age: Older age is a strong independent predictor of mortality in UGIB.
2. Shock: Determined based on blood pressure and heart rate, the presence of shock (systolic BP <100 mmHg) indicates severe bleeding and a higher risk of poor outcomes.
3. Comorbidities: Comorbid conditions, such as renal failure, liver failure, heart disease, or malignancy, increase the risk of mortality and are heavily weighted.
4. Endoscopic Diagnosis: This includes findings like ulcers, Mallory-Weiss tears, or tumors. Higher-risk lesions (e.g., actively bleeding ulcers) score higher.
5. Stigmata of Recent Hemorrhage: Endoscopic signs of active or recent bleeding, such as spurting vessels, visible vessels, or adherent clots, indicate an increased risk of rebleeding and mortality.

Scoring and Interpretation

- Pre-endoscopy Rockall Score: This initial score, which excludes endoscopic findings, helps assess mortality risk based on age, shock status, and comorbidities.

- Post-endoscopy Rockall Score: After endoscopic evaluation, findings are incorporated to refine the risk assessment. Scores range from 0 to 11, with higher scores indicating greater mortality risk.
- A score of 0–2 suggests low risk, where patients generally have low mortality risk and may require less intensive monitoring.
- A score above 5 correlates with a high risk of mortality, indicating the need for aggressive monitoring and intervention.
- A score above 7 is associated with an 80% risk of rebleeding, emphasizing the need for close follow-up and possibly repeated intervention.

The Rockall Score is particularly valuable post-endoscopy, where it incorporates endoscopic findings, allowing clinicians to stratify patients by their risk for rebleeding and death and tailor post-endoscopic management accordingly.

38.3.3 Forrest Classification

The Forrest Classification is an endoscopic classification system specifically designed to stratify the risk of rebleeding in patients with peptic ulcer disease, based on the visual appearance of the ulcer during endoscopy. It categorizes ulcers into high- and low-risk groups and helps guide the urgency and type of intervention required.

Forrest Classification Categories

1. Forrest Ia (Active Spurting Hemorrhage): Represents active arterial bleeding with visible spurting. This is an emergency situation with the highest risk of rebleeding, requiring immediate hemostatic intervention.

2. Forrest Ib (Active Oozing Hemorrhage): Continuous oozing of blood indicates ongoing, albeit slower, bleeding. Urgent endoscopic intervention is still necessary, though the immediate risk may be slightly lower than with spurting.
3. Forrest IIa (Non-bleeding Visible Vessel): A visible vessel in the ulcer bed suggests recent hemorrhage and a high risk of rebleeding. Endoscopic therapy is indicated to prevent further bleeding.
4. Forrest IIb (Adherent Clot): The presence of an adherent clot over the ulcer base indicates prior bleeding with a moderate risk of rebleeding. Vigorous irrigation may be attempted to dislodge the clot, followed by endoscopic treatment if high-risk features are revealed.
5. Forrest IIc (Flat Pigmented Spot): Flat, pigmented lesions indicate that bleeding has ceased and that the risk of rebleeding is low. Generally, no endoscopic intervention is needed, though acid suppression therapy may be initiated.
6. Forrest III (Clean Ulcer Base): An ulcer with a clean base has the lowest risk of rebleeding, and these patients may be managed conservatively with supportive care.

Scoring and Interpretation

- High-Risk Lesions (Forrest Ia, Ib, IIa): These are actively bleeding or recently bleeding lesions with a high likelihood of rebleeding and require urgent endoscopic therapy.

- Moderate-Risk Lesions (Forrest IIb): These are generally managed with endoscopic intervention after clot removal to determine the lesion's status.
- Low-Risk Lesions (Forrest IIc, III): These patients typically do not require endoscopic therapy and can often be managed with conservative treatment, such as acid suppression.

Forrest classification is instrumental in determining the type and urgency of endoscopic intervention, helping guide therapy and predict rebleeding risk.

38.3.4 Comparison of GBS, Rockall, and Forrest Classification

Each of these tools serves a unique function in the assessment of UGIB:

- GBS: Primarily used pre-endoscopy to assess the need for urgent intervention and identify patients suitable for outpatient management.
- Rockall Score: Used both pre- and post-endoscopy to evaluate mortality risk, with higher scores indicating a need for closer monitoring and possible interventions.
- Forrest Classification: Applied during endoscopy to assess the visual appearance of ulcers and stratify them based on rebleeding risk, guiding the urgency and approach of therapeutic interventions.

The combined use of GBS, Rockall, and Forrest Classification allows a comprehensive risk assessment in UGIB patients, from initial triage through post-endoscopic management. Each tool supports clinical decision-making, enabling targeted and effective patient care based on specific risk profiles and treatment needs.

38.4 Pre-endoscopic Management

38.4.1 Proton Pump Inhibitors (PPIs)

The use of PPIs before endoscopy in patients with UGIB remains a point of debate. Although routine pre-endoscopic PPI administration has not shown a significant reduction in mortality or urgent intervention need, it may have potential benefits. PPIs work by inhibiting gastric acid secretion, which in turn helps stabilize blood clots formed at the site of bleeding lesions. Lower gastric acidity reduces clot dissolution, enhancing clot stability and minimizing the risk of rebleeding in high-risk lesions, such as peptic ulcers [3].

After endoscopy, high-dose PPI therapy is strongly recommended, especially in patients with confirmed high-risk lesions (e.g., visible vessels or adherent clots). Commonly, this is administered as an 80 mg intravenous bolus followed by a continuous infusion of 8 mg/hour over 72 hours or via intermittent high dosing (40 mg IV twice daily). Studies have shown that this approach decreases rebleeding rates and promotes better outcomes, particularly within the critical first 3 days post-intervention. For patients with confirmed peptic ulcer bleeding, PPI therapy is continued orally after discharge to support ongoing clot stability and ulcer healing, typically at a twice-daily dose for the initial 2 weeks, then reduced to once daily as maintenance therapy.

38.4.2 Erythromycin as a Prokinetic Agent

Erythromycin, administered intravenously at a dose of 250 mg, acts as a prokinetic agent to promote gastric emptying. It is ideally given 30–90 min before endoscopy to improve gastric visualization, particularly when there is significant blood or clots in the stomach that may obscure endoscopic views. By stimulating gastric motility, erythromycin clears blood and gastric contents, allowing for a clearer assessment of the source and extent of bleeding. Enhanced visualization facilitates effective and targeted endoscopic therapy, which is critical in managing UGIB cases with considerable hemorrhage.

Erythromycin's prokinetic effect has also been associated with reduced procedure time and improved diagnostic yield. While erythromycin administration is generally safe, it should be used cautiously in patients with known QT prolongation or those on medications that can interact with erythromycin.

38.4.3 Anticoagulation Management

For patients on anticoagulant therapy, UGIB management requires balancing the risk of ongoing bleeding with the potential for thromboembolic complications if anticoagulation is withheld. The approach to anticoagulation reversal varies based on the specific agent used:

1. Warfarin: For patients on warfarin, vitamin K administration and prothrombin complex concentrates (PCC) or fresh frozen plasma (FFP) are the primary reversal strategies. PCC is preferred in emergent settings due to its rapid reversal effect and lower volume load compared to FFP. Vitamin K provides a more sustained effect and is typically given alongside PCC for durable reversal.
2. Direct Oral Anticoagulants (DOACs): For patients taking DOACs such as apixaban, rivaroxaban, or dabigatran, options include specific reversal agents where available (e.g., idarucizumab for dabigatran) or nonspecific reversal agents like activated charcoal if the DOAC was taken within the past few hours. Hemodialysis can also be effective in dabigatran cases due to its renal excretion.

Reintroduction of anticoagulants post-hemostasis must be carefully timed and considered based on the patient's bleeding risk and thrombotic profile. In high thrombotic risk patients, early reintroduction may be beneficial, typically after 48–72 hours if hemostasis is confirmed and bleeding has ceased.

38.5 Endoscopic Therapy and Post-endoscopic Management

38.5.1 Endoscopic Hemostasis Techniques

Endoscopy serves both diagnostic and therapeutic roles in UGIB. High-risk lesions—such as those with spurting, oozing, or visible vessels—require immediate intervention. Dual therapy, involving a combination of injection and mechanical or thermal methods, is preferred for high-risk lesions. Commonly used combinations include adrenaline injection followed by mechanical clipping or thermal coagulation.

1. Injection Therapy: Epinephrine injection is often used as the initial hemostatic technique due to its vasoconstrictive properties, which temporarily slows bleeding. However, injection alone is usually insufficient, and it should be combined with another modality.

2. Thermal Coagulation: Methods such as bipolar electrocoagulation or heater probe coagulation provide targeted thermal energy to the bleeding site, facilitating tissue coagulation and hemostasis.
3. Hemostatic Powder: Newer agents like hemostatic powder sprays are effective in refractory cases, forming a physical barrier that promotes clot formation. They are also beneficial in cases where traditional methods are challenging, such as diffuse oozing bleeds.
4. Over-the-Scope Clips (OTSC): These are especially useful in recurrent or challenging bleeds, as they can close larger lesions compared to traditional clips [4].

38.5.2 Managing Recurrent Bleeding

In instances of rebleeding, a repeat endoscopy is typically the first line of management. If hemostasis is not achievable with endoscopic measures, non-endoscopic interventions should be considered:

1. Transcatheter Arterial Embolization (TAE): This radiological technique involves embolizing the bleeding vessel, which is especially useful in cases where endoscopic therapy has failed or for patients unfit for surgery.
2. Transjugular Intrahepatic Portosystemic Shunt (TIPS): TIPS is a viable option in variceal bleeding cases where endoscopic and pharmacologic interventions are ineffective. By reducing portal venous pressure, TIPS minimizes the risk of further variceal hemorrhage, offering a long-term solution for patients with advanced liver disease and portal hypertension.

38.6 Post-discharge and Long-Term Management

38.6.1 Prophylactic Antibiotics

In patients with variceal bleeding, prophylactic antibiotics such as ceftriaxone are strongly recommended. Antibiotic prophylaxis reduces the incidence of spontaneous bacterial peritonitis (SBP) and other infections, which are common complications in patients with cirrhosis and UGIB. Prophylactic antibiotic therapy should ideally be initiated upon presentation and continued for up to 7 days, as this duration has been shown to reduce infection rates and improve survival outcomes in this high-risk group.

38.6.2 Helicobacter pylori *Eradication*

For patients with peptic ulcer disease as the underlying cause of UGIB, testing and treating for *Helicobacter pylori* infection is essential. Eradication of H. pylori significantly lowers the recurrence of peptic ulcers and associated bleeding. Typical treatment regimens include a combination of PPIs with antibiotics such as amoxicillin and clarithromycin for 7–14 days. Confirmatory testing post-treatment ensures eradication, which is essential for long-term ulcer management and prevention of rebleeding.

Long-term management also includes PPI maintenance therapy to support ongoing healing and prevent rebleeding, particularly in high-risk patients. Lifestyle adjustments, such as avoiding NSAIDs, reducing alcohol intake, and quitting smoking, further support ulcer healing and reduce the risk of recurrent UGIB.

38.7 Considerations for Special Populations

38.7.1 Older Adults and Comorbidities

Older adults often have higher risks of UGIB-related complications, exacerbated by comorbidities such as cardiovascular and renal diseases. These patients may require a more conservative approach to fluid resuscitation and transfusion, alongside careful monitoring of end-organ function.

38.7.2 Patients on Antithrombotic Therapy

In patients who require ongoing antithrombotic therapy, careful consideration is required regarding when to resume these medications post-hemostasis. For patients at high thrombotic risk, early reintroduction may be beneficial, but it should be balanced against the potential for rebleeding.

38.8 Conclusion

The management of UGIB in the ICU is a multidisciplinary effort involving gastroenterologists, intensivists, radiologists, and surgeons. Prompt stabilization, risk stratification, timely endoscopy, and appropriate post-endoscopic care are essential in reducing UGIB-associated morbidity and mortality. In complex cases, such as those involving recurrent bleeding or significant comorbid conditions, a collaborative approach among specialties enables optimal care and improves outcomes.

Algorithm 38.1: Approach to upper gastrointestinal bleeding (UGIB) in the ICU

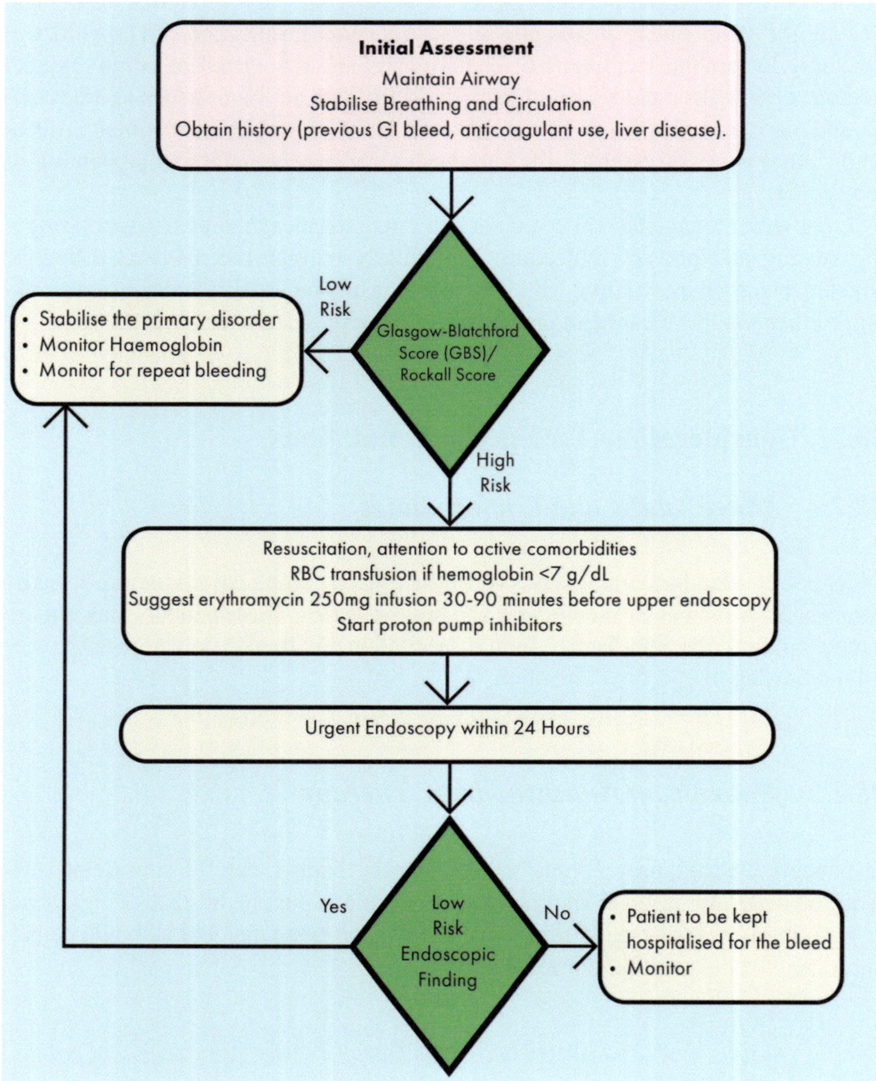

Bibliography

1. Laine L, Barkun AN, Saltzman JR, Martel M, Leontiadis GI. ACG clinical guideline: upper gastrointestinal and ulcer bleeding. Am J Gastroenterol. 2021;116(5):899–917.
2. Stanley AJ, Laine L. Management of acute upper gastrointestinal bleeding. BMJ. 2019;364:l536.
3. Monteiro S, Goncalves TC, Magalhaes J, Cotter J. Upper gastrointestinal bleeding risk scores: who, when and why? World J Gastrointest Pathophysiol. 2016;7(1):86–96.
4. Alali AA, Barkun AN. An update on the management of non-variceal upper gastrointestinal bleeding. Gastroenterol Rep (Oxf). 2023;11:goad011.

Chapter 39
Approach to Lower Gastrointestinal Bleeding (LGIB) in the ICU

39.1 Introduction

Lower gastrointestinal bleeding (LGIB) originates distal to the ligament of Treitz, mainly involving the colon, rectum, and anus. Presenting as either acute, overt bleeding (e.g., hematochezia) or chronic, occult bleeding, LGIB is a significant cause of hospitalization, with rising morbidity and mortality rates, particularly among elderly and comorbid patients. Common causes include diverticular disease, angioectasias, hemorrhoids, and ischemic colitis. Effective management aims to stabilize the patient, identify the bleeding source, and provide targeted medical, endoscopic, or surgical interventions [1] [Algorithm 39.1].

39.2 Initial Assessment

The initial assessment focuses on determining the patient's hemodynamic status and bleeding severity, particularly critical in elderly patients and those with comorbidities due to their higher risk for rapid deterioration. Continuous monitoring of vital signs, especially blood pressure, heart rate, and oxygenation, is recommended.

Key Considerations

- Vital Signs: Observe for hypotension, tachycardia, or signs of shock.
- Comorbid Impact: Conditions such as cardiovascular disease complicate outcomes, stressing the need for immediate and targeted interventions.
- Routine Assessment: Physical examination, including a digital rectal exam (DRE), helps identify signs of active bleeding or hematochezia, as advised by ESGE guidelines.

S. B. Mishra et al., *Mastering ICU Care*,
https://doi.org/10.1007/978-981-95-0179-3_39

39.2.1 Shock Index Assessment

The shock index (SI), calculated by dividing the heart rate by systolic blood pressure, is a practical tool to gauge hemodynamic compromise, especially for patients with suspected significant blood loss. Beyond its threshold of 1, the SI is enhanced by integrating clinical features such as ongoing bleeding.

- Shock Index >1: Indicates hemodynamic instability and suggests significant blood loss, typically warranting urgent resuscitation and invasive diagnostic steps like CT angiography.
- Limitations: In cases with baseline tachycardia or hypotension due to chronic conditions or medications, the shock index should be complemented by clinical judgment, aligning with ACG recommendations.

39.3 Resuscitation

Fluid Resuscitation Strategy
The ACG and ESGE guidelines recommend using blood products preferentially over IV fluids to manage hemodynamic stability in LGIB, particularly in elderly or cardiac-compromised patients who are at a higher risk of complications from fluid overload. Excessive IV fluids can dilute blood components, reducing hemoglobin concentration and impeding adequate oxygen delivery to tissues. This hemodilution effect, especially in patients with significant blood loss, may exacerbate hypotension and tissue hypoxia [2].

Blood transfusions are therefore prioritized when hemoglobin levels fall below critical thresholds (typically 7–9 g/dL for most patients or 8–10 g/dL for those with cardiac conditions). This strategy helps maintain a stable hemoglobin concentration, which supports oxygen-carrying capacity and optimizes tissue perfusion without risking fluid overload, a particularly crucial consideration for patients with congestive heart failure or renal impairment. Monitoring of vital signs and hemodynamic parameters during resuscitation is essential, as is adjusting the approach based on real-time responses to intervention.

Anticoagulation Reversal
For patients on anticoagulation therapy, especially those presenting with life-threatening bleeds, immediate anticoagulation reversal is critical to reduce bleeding severity and allow other hemostatic interventions. The ESGE guidelines recommend a stratified approach to anticoagulation reversal based on the thrombotic risk profile and International Normalized Ratio (INR) levels. For patients on vitamin K antagonists, INR levels can guide the urgency and extent of reversal, with agents like prothrombin complex concentrate (PCC) and vitamin K recommended for rapid INR normalization.

For patients on direct oral anticoagulants (DOACs) like dabigatran, specific reversal agents such as idarucizumab are indicated, while andexanet alfa can be used to reverse factor Xa inhibitors, including apixaban and rivaroxaban. In scenarios where these agents are not available, activated charcoal (if ingestion was within the previous hours) or prothrombin complex concentrates may be considered for partial reversal. Prompt reversal is especially warranted when active bleeding compromises hemodynamic stability, underscoring the need for quick identification of anticoagulant use in patient history during initial assessment.

39.4 CT Angiography (CTA)

Utility
CT angiography is a noninvasive diagnostic imaging technique that can identify the active site of bleeding with high precision, particularly in hemodynamically unstable patients or those with rapid blood loss. CTA allows for detailed vascular imaging, providing clinicians with a roadmap for potential therapeutic interventions, such as embolization, should endoscopic approaches prove insufficient. ACG and ESGE guidelines highlight CTA as the preferred imaging modality due to its rapid acquisition and ability to visualize active extravasation, which helps in planning subsequent endoscopic or interventional radiology procedures.

A positive CTA—showing active extravasation—generally necessitates referral to interventional radiology for possible transcatheter embolization. However, a negative CTA might indicate either a cessation of active bleeding or an undetectable slow bleed. This negative result could prompt further workup, including upper GI endoscopy, especially if clinical suspicion of a non-colonic source persists. In certain cases, conservative management might be sufficient if the patient's hemodynamics stabilize without further evidence of bleeding.

Criteria for CTA Referral
CTA is particularly recommended in cases of:

- Persistent hypotension despite adequate initial fluid resuscitation, as this suggests continued blood loss and risk of shock.
- High clinical suspicion of massive hemorrhage, particularly if initial endoscopy is inconclusive or not immediately available.
- Uncertain localization of the bleeding source where endoscopic visualization is limited or delayed.

Aligning with ESGE guidelines, CTA should ideally be performed within 60 min of patient stabilization for prompt and effective management.

39.4.1 *Negative CTA Results*

Follow-Up
In instances where CTA does not identify an active bleeding site, additional diagnostic steps are necessary to rule out other potential sources, particularly from the upper GI tract. This approach is endorsed by the British Society of Gastroenterology (BSG), which emphasizes the importance of ruling out upper GI causes when a clear source is not visualized in CTA. An upper GI endoscopy may be indicated in cases where aortic aneurysms, peptic ulcers, or aortoenteric fistulas are suspected but not initially visible on CTA.

The algorithm in this case would proceed as follows:

1. Reassess the patient's hemodynamic stability post-CTA.
2. Upper GI endoscopy should be performed if symptoms or clinical history suggest possible upper GI sources, including scenarios where hematemesis or melena are present.
3. If upper GI endoscopy is negative, a conservative observation approach with close monitoring may be considered, especially if the patient stabilizes without recurrent bleeding.

This systematic approach ensures that other potentially serious bleeding sources are not overlooked, preventing premature cessation of the diagnostic workup.

39.5 Oakland Score Assessment

The Oakland Score is a risk stratification tool used in patients with LGIB to estimate the likelihood of adverse outcomes, such as rebleeding or the need for urgent intervention. By incorporating easily measurable clinical parameters, it assists clinicians in determining whether a patient is suitable for outpatient management or requires inpatient care. A score of 8 or below generally indicates a low risk of complications, allowing for conservative management with outpatient follow-up. Conversely, patients scoring above 8 may be at higher risk, warranting closer monitoring and inpatient intervention [3].

Components of the Oakland Score
The Oakland Score is calculated based on the following factors:

1. Age: Age is a significant factor due to the increased risk of adverse outcomes with advancing age.
   - <40 years: 0 points
   - 40–69 years: 1 point
   - ≥70 years: 2 points.

2. Gender: Males tend to have a higher risk for complications from LGIB.
   - Female: 0 points.
   - Male: 1 point.
3. Previous Admission with LGIB: A history of LGIB suggests a greater likelihood of rebleeding and complications.
   - No prior admission for LGIB: 0 points.
   - Prior admission for LGIB: 1 point.
4. Digital Rectal Examination (DRE) Findings: DRE results help determine the likelihood of active or recent bleeding.
   - No blood detected: 0 points.
   - Blood present on DRE: 1 point.
5. Heart Rate: Elevated heart rate may indicate ongoing bleeding or hypovolemia.
   - <70 beats per minute (bpm): 0 points
   - 70–89 bpm: 1 point
   - 90–109 bpm: 2 points
   - ≥110 bpm: 3 points.
6. Systolic Blood Pressure: Lower blood pressure is associated with hypoperfusion and significant blood loss.
   - ≥160 mmHg: 0 points
   - 130–159 mmHg: 2 points
   - 120–129 mmHg: 3 points
   - 90–119 mmHg: 4 points
   - <90 mmHg: 5 points.
7. Hemoglobin Level: Low hemoglobin levels indicate significant blood loss and are predictive of severe bleeding.
   - ≥160 g/L: 0 points
   - 130–159 g/L: 4 points
   - 110–129 g/L: 8 points
   - 90–109 g/L: 13 points
   - 70–89 g/L: 17 points
   - <70 g/L: 22 points.

Interpretation and Clinical Use

- Score ≤ 8: A score of 8 or below is considered low risk, indicating a 95% probability of safe discharge without needing urgent inpatient intervention. These patients can often be managed conservatively with outpatient follow-up.
- Score > 8: A score above 8 suggests a higher risk of serious complications, such as rebleeding or the need for transfusion. For these patients, inpatient care is recommended, along with close monitoring and timely diagnostic procedures, potentially including an urgent colonoscopy.

Stratification and Conservative Management

For patients scoring 8 or below, outpatient management may include the following steps:

1. Clear Discharge Instructions: Educate patients on recognizing rebleeding symptoms and advise them on when to seek emergency care.
2. Elective Colonoscopy or Imaging: Schedule these diagnostic tests within a reasonable timeframe, depending on clinical judgment, to further investigate the source of bleeding.
3. Regular Follow-Up: Arrange follow-up visits to monitor for any delayed complications or recurrence, ensuring the patient remains stable.

This scoring system allows healthcare providers to optimize resource use and patient safety, targeting high-risk patients for more intensive care while minimizing unnecessary admissions for low-risk individuals.

39.6 Colonoscopy

Colonoscopy is essential in both diagnosing and treating lower gastrointestinal bleeding (LGIB), as it provides direct visualization and allows therapeutic intervention at the bleeding site. Current guidelines from ESGE and ACG recommend that the timing of colonoscopy should be based on the patient's stability and bleeding activity rather than routinely performed within 24 hours. For patients with resolved bleeding or those who are hemodynamically stable, elective colonoscopy within 24–72 hours is often appropriate and can improve diagnostic yield by allowing for adequate bowel preparation.

39.6.1 Diagnostic and Therapeutic Interventions

Endoscopic Techniques for Hemostasis

- Through-the-Scope (TTS) Clips: TTS clips are commonly used to mechanically compress the bleeding vessel, especially effective in cases of diverticular bleeding. They are applied directly to the source of bleeding and can rapidly achieve hemostasis.
- Band Ligation: Primarily used in cases of hemorrhoidal or diverticular bleeding, band ligation can occlude blood flow to the bleeding vessel by placing a small rubber band at its base. This technique is particularly beneficial in patients where the bleeding site is clearly identifiable.
- Argon Plasma Coagulation (APC): APC is a noncontact thermal method used to coagulate small bleeding vessels, which is effective for angioectasias and other vascular lesions. By controlling the depth of tissue coagulation, APC can reduce the risk of tissue perforation and is especially useful in diffuse bleeding.

Considerations for Timing

- In actively bleeding patients who are hemodynamically unstable, urgent colonoscopy is advised as it enables real-time diagnosis and immediate therapeutic intervention. For patients with hemodynamic stability but active or recent bleeding, urgent colonoscopy remains beneficial, as it can help identify and treat bleeding sources before rebleeding occurs.
- For stable patients or those with self-limited bleeding, a nonurgent colonoscopy may be scheduled within 24–72 hours. This delayed timing ensures proper bowel preparation, which increases visualization quality and diagnostic accuracy, and reduces the need for emergency procedures. This also aligns with ACG and ESGE recommendations, as evidence suggests that nonurgent colonoscopy does not adversely impact outcomes in stable patients.

39.7 Management of Persistent Active Bleeding

For patients whose bleeding persists despite initial endoscopic interventions, a stepwise approach incorporating interventional radiology and, if necessary, surgical options is recommended.

Angiographic Embolization

- Following a positive CTA that identifies the bleeding site, angiographic embolization can be performed to selectively occlude the bleeding vessel. Embolization is highly effective for localized bleeding sources that are inaccessible or unsuitable for endoscopic treatment.
- ESGE guidelines recommend that embolization should ideally occur within 60 min in centers with 24/7 interventional radiology capabilities. This approach ensures rapid intervention, minimizing the risk of ongoing hemorrhage and hemodynamic compromise. Additionally, centers without immediate access to interventional radiology should establish referral pathways to ensure timely patient transfer.

Surgical Intervention

- Surgery is considered a last-resort option for patients with refractory bleeding who have not responded to endoscopic or radiologic interventions. The ESGE and ACG guidelines both advise against emergency laparotomy unless all other measures have been exhausted. Laparotomy, a highly invasive procedure, carries significant risks, especially in elderly or critically ill patients, and is generally reserved for life-threatening bleeds or cases where other methods are technically unfeasible.
- For patients requiring surgery, preoperative localization of the bleeding site via imaging or endoscopy is critical to guide the surgical approach and improve the likelihood of successful bleeding control.

39.8 Special Considerations

Anticoagulation and Antiplatelet Management

Anticoagulant Reversal:

- For patients actively bleeding while on anticoagulants, stopping and reversing anticoagulation based on bleeding severity and thrombotic risk is necessary. Warfarin, a vitamin K antagonist, can be reversed using vitamin K and prothrombin complex concentrate (PCC) to quickly correct INR and reduce bleeding. For patients on direct oral anticoagulants (DOACs), specific reversal agents such as idarucizumab for dabigatran or andexanet alfa for factor Xa inhibitors should be administered if available.
- It is essential to consider the patient's thrombotic risk before and during anticoagulation reversal. For patients with high thrombotic risk (e.g., those with prosthetic heart valves), resumption of anticoagulation should be discussed with a multidisciplinary team once bleeding is controlled.

Antiplatelet Therapy:

- For patients on antiplatelet therapy, especially those taking aspirin for secondary cardiovascular prevention, a more nuanced approach is required. Continuation of aspirin may be appropriate in certain patients (e.g., those with coronary artery stents) due to the elevated thrombotic risk associated with stopping therapy. Decisions to continue or hold antiplatelet therapy should be individualized, involving input from a cardiologist for patients on dual antiplatelet therapy to balance bleeding risk with thrombotic risk.

Blood Transfusion Strategy
Restrictive Transfusion Thresholds:

- A restrictive approach to blood transfusion is recommended, aiming to maintain hemoglobin levels within 7–9 g/dL, except in patients with cardiovascular disease, where the threshold is slightly higher at 8–10 g/dL. This approach minimizes the risks associated with over-transfusion, including fluid overload, potential cardiac stress, and immunomodulation.
- Evidence suggests that a restrictive transfusion strategy is safe and effective in most patients with LGIB, as it prevents excessive transfusions and associated complications while supporting adequate tissue oxygenation. Hemoglobin levels should be monitored regularly, and transfusion decisions adjusted based on the patient's clinical status and response to treatment.

39.9 Conclusion

The management of LGIB requires a structured, evidence-based approach, starting with patient stabilization and risk stratification using tools like the shock index and Oakland score. These tools help guide the urgency of interventions such as CTA, colonoscopy, and embolization. Evidence-based thresholds for transfusion, selective use of CTA, and outpatient management of low-risk patients can optimize outcomes while reducing unnecessary healthcare utilization. Early, guided intervention and individualized management based on risk profiles improve the efficacy of LGIB management and patient prognosis.

Algorithm 39.1: Approach to lower gastrointestinal bleeding (LGIB) in the ICU

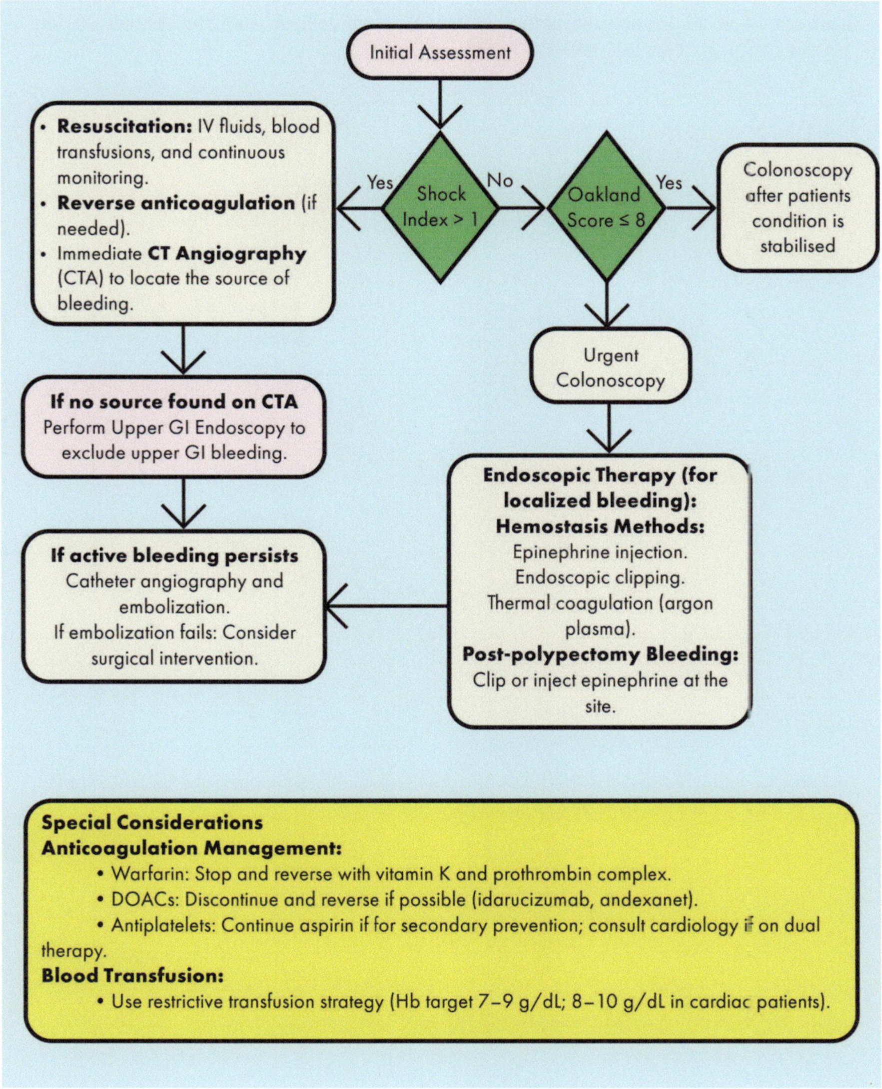

Bibliography

1. Sengupta N, Feuerstein JD, Jairath V, Shergill AK, Strate LL, Wong RJ, et al. Management of patients with acute lower gastrointestinal bleeding: an updated ACG guideline. Am J Gastroenterol. 2023;118(2):208–31.
2. Triantafyllou K, Gkolfakis P, Gralnek IM, Oakland K, Manes G, Radaelli F, et al. Diagnosis and management of acute lower gastrointestinal bleeding: European Society of Gastrointestinal Endoscopy (ESGE) guideline. Endoscopy. 2021;53(8):850–68.
3. Oakland K, Chadwick G, East JE, Guy R, Humphries A, Jairath V, et al. Diagnosis and management of acute lower gastrointestinal bleeding: guidelines from the British Society of Gastroenterology. Gut. 2019;68(5):776–89.

Chapter 40
Approach to Ileus in the ICU

40.1 Introduction

Ileus refers to a functional disruption of the normal propulsive activity of the gastrointestinal (GI) tract, resulting in delayed passage of contents. This condition can affect any part of the GI system but most commonly impacts the small and large intestines. The condition manifests as abdominal discomfort, distension, nausea, vomiting, and the inability to pass flatus or stool, leading to complications such as bacterial overgrowth, sepsis, and multi-organ failure. Ileus often develops postoperatively or due to electrolyte imbalances, infections, or medications, especially opioids. Prompt recognition and effective management are critical to preventing severe complications like bowel perforation or ischemia [1, 2] [Ref: Algorithm 40.1].

40.2 Pathophysiology and Mechanisms

The pathophysiology of ileus, especially in critically ill patients, is multifactorial, involving both neuronal and inflammatory mechanisms:

- Neuronal Mechanisms: Ileus is influenced by the autonomic nervous system, where an imbalance between sympathetic and parasympathetic activity results in reduced GI motility. Postoperative ileus is particularly linked to increased sympathetic activity, leading to decreased peristalsis. Additionally, enhanced release of inhibitory neuromodulators like nitric oxide from inhibitory motor neurons contributes to motility reduction.

S. B. Mishra et al., *Mastering ICU Care*,
https://doi.org/10.1007/978-981-95-0179-3_40

- Inflammatory Mechanisms: Surgery or systemic inflammation can activate local inflammatory responses within the intestinal muscularis, releasing cytokines, nitric oxide, and prostaglandins. These substances, produced by activated macrophages and other immune cells, suppress coordinated intestinal contractions. This mechanism is particularly relevant in critically ill patients, where inflammation, often compounded by sepsis or trauma, leads to prolonged ileus.

Understanding these mechanisms helps explain the therapeutic efficacy of agents like neostigmine, which enhances parasympathetic tone, and peripherally acting opioid antagonists, which counteract opioid-induced motility suppression [3].

40.3 Risk Factors and Etiology

Ileus in critically ill patients often arises from complex, interrelated factors:

- Primary vs. Secondary Ileus: Primary ileus usually results from direct GI trauma or abdominal surgery. In contrast, secondary ileus is a consequence of systemic conditions like sepsis, multi-organ failure, or metabolic disturbances (inadequate fluid resuscitation, excess fluid administration, hyperglycemia, hypothyroidism, uremia, acidosis) that impact GI motility without direct GI injury.
- Critical Illness Factors: The pathogenesis of ileus in the ICU setting involves multiple contributors, including:
  - Mechanical Ventilation: Prolonged ventilation is associated with increased intra-abdominal pressure and decreased diaphragm movement, both of which impair GI motility.
  - Medications: Sedatives and opioids, commonly used in the ICU, decrease bowel motility by reducing neural signaling to the GI tract. Anticholinergics, calcium channel blockers.
  - Immobility.
  - Electrolyte Imbalances: Hypokalemia, hypomagnesemia, and hypercalcemia are frequent in critically ill patients and can significantly impair smooth muscle function, contributing to ileus [4].

Understanding these risk factors allows for targeted interventions to reduce the incidence and severity of ileus in the ICU.

40.4 Monitoring and Diagnosis

Accurate diagnosis of ileus involves both clinical assessment and judicious use of diagnostic tools:

- Limitations of Gastric Residual Volume (GRV): Although GRV measurement is commonly used to assess gastric emptying, its clinical utility in managing ileus is debated. Recent evidence suggests that relying solely on GRV may not accurately predict the risk of aspiration or the severity of ileus, as endogenous secretions can confound the readings. Instead, a focus on clinical symptoms like vomiting, distension, and feeding intolerance is recommended for more effective monitoring.
- Advanced Diagnostic Tools: Newer methods, such as the 13C-octanoate breath test, offer a less invasive approach to assessing gastric emptying and could serve as an alternative to traditional methods like scintigraphy. However, the availability and practicality of such tests in the ICU remain limited.

40.5 Pharmacological Management

Managing ileus pharmacologically requires a tailored approach based on the underlying causes and severity:

- Laxatives/Stool softeners:
  - Lactulose: 13 g three times daily should be given until stool passage and then as needed (on SOS basis).
  - PEG (polyethylene glycol): 13.125 g three times daily in 100 ml water.
  - Psyllium.
  - Coloxyl.
- Prokinetics: Metoclopramide (10 mg four times a day for a maximum of 7 days) and erythromycin are common choices for stimulating gastric motility. However, their long-term use is limited by potential side effects like tardive dyskinesia and tachyphylaxis, respectively. Erythromycin, at doses of 250 mg IV every 8 hours, can be effective for short-term use. 5-HT4 agonists—Cisapride, Levosulpiride (25 mg three times a day)—can also be used.
- Neostigmine: As an acetylcholinesterase inhibitor, neostigmine is particularly effective for treating colonic pseudo-obstruction by increasing parasympathetic activity, thus enhancing motility. Continuous infusion is often preferred over bolus doses to minimize the risk of bradycardia (dose: intravenous infusion 0.4–0.8 mg/h for 24 hours (watch for bradycardia).
- Peripherally Acting Mu-Opioid Receptor Antagonists: Agents like methylnaltrexone and alvimopan specifically target opioid-induced constipation without affecting central analgesia. Their use is critical in reversing opioid-induced ileus, especially in postoperative patients [5].

40.6 Prevention and Early Intervention

Prevention plays a pivotal role in reducing the incidence of ileus in critically ill patients:

- Early Mobility: Mobilizing patients early and reducing the duration of immobility can significantly stimulate bowel motility. Early ambulation has been shown to reduce the duration of ileus postoperatively.
- Minimizing Opioid Use: Judicious use of opioids, alongside non-opioid analgesics, helps prevent opioid-induced suppression of GI motility. The use of multimodal analgesia is often preferred.
- Optimal Nutritional Strategies: Early initiation of enteral nutrition, using small volumes and advancing slowly, supports gut function and reduces the risk of ileus. When enteral feeding is not possible, intravenous fluids should be carefully managed to maintain hydration.

40.7 Detailed Treatment Pathways

A stepwise approach to managing ileus ensures timely intervention and minimizes complications:

1. Initial Assessment and Stabilization:
    - Ensure airway protection and stabilize circulation. Consider fluid resuscitation or vasopressors for hypotensive patients while avoiding fluid overload.
    - Hold enteral feeding temporarily if signs of intolerance are present and initiate nasogastric decompression for symptomatic relief.
2. Medical Management:
    - Correct electrolyte imbalances and discontinue medications that impair motility.
    - Start prokinetic agents if there is no evidence of mechanical obstruction and escalate to neostigmine or other specific therapies in refractory cases.
3. Escalating Care and Surgical Consultation:
    - If symptoms persist despite medical management, consider abdominal CT to rule out complications like ischemia or perforation.
    - Surgical consultation is necessary for cases with suspected bowel ischemia, perforation, or mechanical obstruction.

Surgical Decompression:

(a) Sigmoidoscopy.
(b) Colonoscopy.
(c) Surgical decompression.
(d) Cecostomy, colectomy, ileostomy, and Hartmann procedure.

40.8 Impact on Patient Outcomes

Effective management of ileus significantly improves outcomes in critically ill patients:

- Reduced ICU Stay and Morbidity: Timely intervention can shorten the duration of mechanical ventilation and ICU length of stay by enabling early resumption of enteral nutrition.
- Prevention of Complications: Proper management reduces the risk of aspiration pneumonia and other complications like bacterial translocation, which can lead to sepsis.
- Improved Survival Rates: Addressing ileus and its underlying causes helps prevent multi-organ failure, ultimately improving patient survival.

40.9 Conclusion

The management of ileus in critically ill patients requires a comprehensive and systematic approach that addresses the underlying pathophysiology, closely monitors clinical symptoms, and applies targeted pharmacological and supportive therapies. Early intervention and a multidisciplinary approach can significantly improve patient outcomes, reducing morbidity and mortality associated with this condition.

Algorithm 40.1: Approach to ileus in the ICU

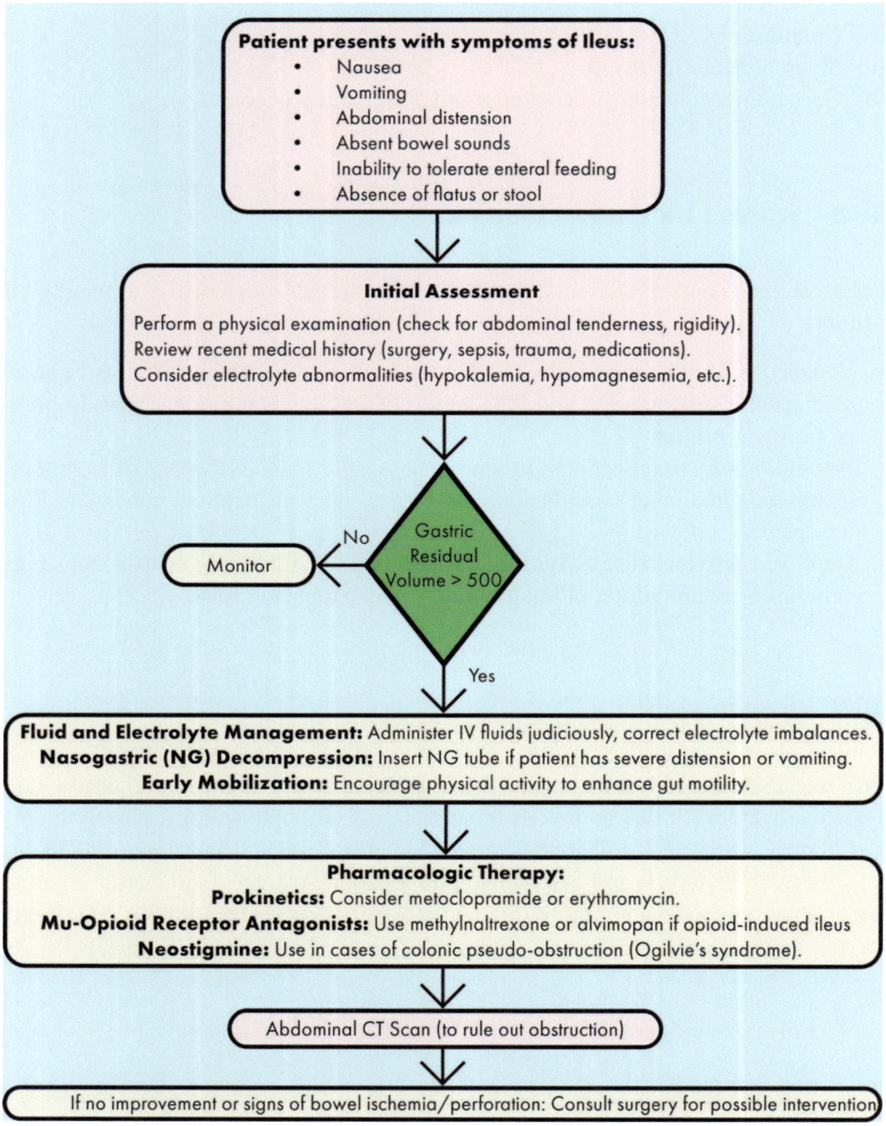

Bibliography

1. Bauer AJ, Schwarz NT, Moore BA, Türler A, Kalff JC. Ileus in critical illness: mechanisms and management. Curr Opin Crit Care. 2002;8(2):152–7.
2. Govil D, Pal D. Gastrointestinal motility disorders in critically ill. Indian J Crit Care Med. 2020;24(Suppl 4):S179–s82.
3. Aries P, Huet O. Ileus in the critically ill: causes, treatment and prevention. Minerva Anestesiol. 2020;86(9):974–83.
4. Ladopoulos T, Giannaki M, Alexopoulou C, Proklou A, Pediaditis E, Kondili E. Gastrointestinal dysmotility in critically ill patients. Ann Gastroenterol. 2018;31(3):273–81.
5. Vazquez-Sandoval A, Ghamande S, Surani S. Critically ill patients and gut motility: are we addressing it? World J Gastrointest Pharmacol Ther. 2017;8(3):174–9.

Chapter 41
Approach to Diarrhea in the ICU

41.1 Introduction

Diarrhea in critically ill patients can significantly affect their recovery, contributing to dehydration, electrolyte imbalances, skin breakdown, and even sepsis. Studies indicate that diarrhea affects 15–38% of ICU patients, highlighting the importance of effective management. The challenge lies in distinguishing true diarrhea from other changes in bowel habits, such as those caused by altered gut motility or enteral feeding. Accurate diagnosis and timely intervention are essential to prevent further complications and improve outcomes. This write-up provides a stepwise explanation of the management process, focusing on clinical decision points, diagnostic tools, and therapeutic interventions [1, 2] [Ref: Algorithm 41.1].

41.2 Criteria for Diarrhea

The initial step in managing diarrhea involves confirming its presence based on established criteria:

- Stool frequency: More than three stools per day.
- Stool weight: Greater than 200 grams per day.
- Consistency: Classified according to the Bristol Stool Chart (Type 5–7 indicates diarrhea).

Additionally, the World Health Organization (WHO) defines diarrhea as the passage of three or more liquid stools per day. Incorporating tools like the Bristol Stool Chart and Bliss Stool Classification System provides a robust framework for assessing stool consistency, ensuring accurate diagnosis and guiding treatment.

S. B. Mishra et al., *Mastering ICU Care*,
https://doi.org/10.1007/978-981-95-0179-3_41

41.3 Etiology

- Infective: Bacteria—*Vibrio cholerae*, *Salmonella*, *Shigella*, *Campylobacter*, *Escherichia coli*, *Clostridioides difficile*.
  - Virus—Rotavirus, Adenovirus, Norovirus.
  - Parasite—*Giardia*, *Amoeba (Entamoeba histolytica)*, *Strongyloides*, *Microsporidium*, *Cryptosporidium*, *Cyclospora*.
- Inflammatory: Inflammatory bowel disease, Ischemic colitis, Diverticulitis, Appendicitis.
- Food poisoning/Toxins/Poisoning (Organophosphorus).
- Immunosuppressants: Transplant patients, HIV patients.
- Irritable bowel syndrome.
- Endocrine: Adrenal dysfunction, bile acid malabsorption, pancreatic exocrine insufficiency, thyroid disorder.
- Drugs: Histamine receptor antagonists, Proton pump inhibitors, Potassium chloride, Antibiotics, NSAIDs, Cardiac (Quinidine, Digitalis, Theophylline), Prokinetics (Metoclopramide, 5HT4 agonists, Erythromycin), Anti-cancer drugs, Laxatives, Cholinergics.
- Enteral feeds, Hyperosmolar feeds.

41.4 Investigations

- Identify the cause of diarrhea. Send complete blood culture (hemoglobin, hematocrit, total leukocyte count), serum electrolytes, renal function tests, blood glucose levels.
- Stool tests: Stool routine microscopy for ova and parasites (if persists >7 days), hanging drop, culture. Look for fecal WBCs (mucosal invasion in Shigella, Campylobacter, Enterohemorrhagic and Enteroinvasive *E. coli*). Send for C. difficile toxins, Glutamate dehydrogenase. PCR for viral and bacterial toxins).
- Imaging: Abdominal X-ray may show signs of ischemia, partial obstruction, perforation, or a toxic megacolon associated with colitis. CECT abdomen may also be done if X-ray does not help or to assess the extent of the disease.
- Flexible or rigid proctosigmoidoscopy is useful in diagnosing antibiotic-associated colitis, distal ischemic colitis, GVHD, and vasculitis, to name a few.
- Other/Specific—*Giardia*, Rotavirus antigen, ELISA and PCR for viruses, Dark field/phase contrast microscopy for Campylobacter. Stool osmolal gap to rule out osmotic diarrhea (Stool osmolality—2*(Na + K)).

41.5 Evaluate Fluid and Electrolyte Status

Diarrhea in critically ill patients can cause rapid and significant fluid and electrolyte losses, leading to risks such as hemodynamic instability, cardiac arrhythmias, or acute renal failure. Early and accurate assessment of fluid and electrolyte status is vital to prevent severe complications and stabilize the patient.

41.5.1 Stable Fluid and Electrolyte Status

- Conservative Management: If the patient's fluid balance and electrolytes are within normal ranges, conservative management is recommended.
- Monitoring: Continuous monitoring of vital signs (blood pressure, heart rate), urine output, and serum electrolyte levels (sodium, potassium, magnesium) is crucial to detect early changes.
- Adjustments in Medication: Discontinue any nonessential medications, especially laxatives or diuretics, that could worsen fluid loss or electrolyte imbalances.

41.5.2 Deranged Fluid and Electrolyte Status

- Recognition and Signs of Hypovolemia: Tachycardia, hypotension, decreased urine output (<0.5 mL/kg/hour), and dry mucous membranes should prompt immediate intervention.
- Isotonic Fluid Administration: Start with isotonic fluids like normal saline or Ringer's lactate to rapidly restore intravascular volume. Adjust the volume based on severity, aiming for hemodynamic stability [3].

41.5.3 Electrolyte Replacement

- Potassium: Aim to keep serum potassium levels above 4.0 mEq/L to prevent cardiac arrhythmias. Intravenous potassium chloride can be administered, typically starting with 20–40 mEq over several hours, adjusting based on severity and monitoring serum levels.
- Magnesium: Maintain serum magnesium above 2.0 mg/dL to support cardiac and neuromuscular function. Magnesium sulfate can be given intravenously, typically 1–2 grams over 1–2 hours, depending on the deficit.
- Sodium and Hyponatremia: In cases of hyponatremia, careful correction is necessary to avoid rapid shifts that can lead to osmotic demyelination. Hypertonic saline (3%) may be used in severe cases, but isotonic saline is typically preferred for gradual correction.

41.5.4 Addressing Metabolic Acidosis

- Severe Acidosis: If metabolic acidosis is significant (e.g., bicarbonate <15 mEq/L), administer sodium bicarbonate cautiously. The typical dose is calculated based on the patient's base deficit, but a standard approach starts with 1–2 amps (50–100 mEq) diluted in intravenous fluids.
- Frequent Monitoring: Monitor arterial blood gases (ABGs) and serum bicarbonate levels to assess the effectiveness of treatment and adjust dosages accordingly.

41.5.5 Re-evaluation and Adjustments

- Continuous Assessment: Reevaluate fluid and electrolyte status every 4–6 hours in the acute phase to ensure the patient remains stable and to adjust treatment plans.
- Urine Output as a Marker: Aim for a urine output of 0.5–1 mL/kg/hour, as it serves as an important marker of adequate fluid resuscitation and renal function [4].

41.6 Assess for Infection

Infectious diarrhea is a critical concern in ICU patients, particularly in those with recent antibiotic use, immunosuppression, or enteral feeding. Testing for *Clostridioides difficile* (*C. difficile*) and other pathogens based on clinical suspicion is essential.

- Yes (Infected): If an infection is suspected or confirmed, targeted antibiotic therapy should be initiated:

  C. difficile infection:

  - Oral Fidaxomicin: 200 mg twice daily.
  - Oral Vancomycin: 125 mg four times daily, or 500 mg four times daily in severe cases. For ileus, rectal vancomycin (250 mg every 6 hours) may be used.
  - Oral Metronidazole: 500 mg every 8 hours.
  - Monitor for complications like abdominal distension and toxic megacolon. Discontinue broad-spectrum antibiotics when possible and consider fecal microbiota transplantation (FMT) for recurrent CDI.

Other infections:

- *Salmonella*: Ciprofloxacin 400 mg IV twice daily for 14 days or Ceftriaxone 2 g IV twice daily for 14 days. Transition to oral therapy when tolerated. Alternative options include Azithromycin 500 mg twice daily or Co-trimoxazole.
- Giardiasis/Amebiasis: Treated with Metronidazole.
- Strongyloidiasis: Managed with Ivermectin and Albendazole.

- No (Noninfectious Causes): If infection is ruled out, the focus shifts to other factors like enteral feeding formulas and medications [5].

41.7 Review Risk Factors and Noninfectious Causes

Diarrhea in ICU patients is often multifactorial, meaning that multiple contributing factors may be involved. Identifying and managing these factors is crucial for effective treatment. Noninfectious causes are common in this setting and may stem from medications, nutrition, and underlying systemic conditions like hypoalbuminemia. A comprehensive approach to managing these factors can help prevent the worsening of symptoms and promote recovery.

Adjustments to Enteral Feeding: Enteral feeding is a vital part of nutrition management in ICU patients, but it can contribute to diarrhea, particularly if high-osmolality formulas are used. High-osmolality feeds draw water into the intestine, which can increase stool frequency and volume. To mitigate this, switching to low-osmolality formulas can reduce the osmotic load on the gut, decreasing the likelihood of diarrhea. Additionally, fiber-enriched formulas can help improve stool consistency by absorbing excess water and promoting a more formed stool. Fiber can also provide a substrate for beneficial gut bacteria, potentially improving gut health. In cases where digestion is impaired, predigested or peptide-based formulas may be used, as these contain partially hydrolyzed proteins and fats, making them easier to absorb and reducing the gastrointestinal burden.

Medication Review: A detailed review of the patient's medication regimen is essential, as many commonly used drugs in the ICU can contribute to diarrhea. Antibiotics, especially broad-spectrum types, can disrupt the normal gut flora, leading to conditions like *Clostridioides difficile* infections or generalized antibiotic-associated diarrhea. Proton pump inhibitors (PPIs), used to reduce gastric acidity, can alter gut pH, promoting an environment that favors pathogenic bacteria. Laxatives, whether prescribed or given inadvertently through enteral formulas, can exacerbate diarrhea. Adjusting or discontinuing such medications when possible, while balancing the need for their therapeutic effects, can significantly reduce diarrhea risk. Deprescribing or substituting medications with less gastrointestinal side effects may be considered as part of a tailored approach to each patient.

Address Systemic Factors: Underlying systemic conditions can significantly impact gastrointestinal function. Hypoalbuminemia, a common condition in critically ill patients, can lead to gut edema and impaired barrier function, which may contribute to diarrhea. This condition reduces the oncotic pressure in the blood vessels, leading to fluid leakage into the intestinal lumen and resulting in loose stools. Correcting hypoalbuminemia through appropriate albumin supplementation or optimizing overall protein intake can improve bowel function. Other systemic factors, such as diabetes or thyroid disorders, should also be addressed as part of comprehensive care to ensure that they do not complicate the clinical picture further [6].

41.8 Prevent Complications

Diarrhea in critically ill patients can lead to a range of complications, requiring a proactive and comprehensive approach to minimize adverse outcomes:

- Skin Protection: Frequent, watery stools can lead to skin breakdown, which increases the risk of pressure ulcers and infection. Using barrier creams or zinc oxide ointments can protect the skin from moisture damage. Additionally, implementing a repositioning schedule helps reduce the risk of pressure sores, particularly in patients who are immobile. Maintaining meticulous skin care is vital to prevent secondary infections and promote comfort.
- Infection Control: In cases of infectious diarrhea, especially with pathogens like C. difficile, stringent contact precautions are essential to prevent the spread of infection to other patients and staff. Isolation protocols should be followed, and proper hand hygiene practices enforced. Healthcare workers should use personal protective equipment (PPE) appropriately to minimize cross-contamination. Implementing these measures is crucial for containing outbreaks within the ICU.
- Nutritional Optimization: Continuous diarrhea can hinder the absorption of nutrients, leading to malnutrition and weakening the patient's overall condition. Adjusting enteral feeding rates to match the patient's tolerance, using predigested formulas, or selecting formulas with medium-chain triglycerides can help improve nutrient absorption. It is important to ensure that the caloric and protein needs are met, either through enteral or parenteral nutrition, to support tissue repair and immune function. Regular assessments of nutritional status help to adapt feeding strategies according to the patient's evolving needs.

41.9 Symptom Relief

Managing symptoms of diarrhea can improve comfort and quality of life for patients, particularly when the underlying cause is noninfectious:

- Loperamide: An antidiarrheal that reduces bowel motility, loperamide (2–4 mg up to four times daily) can be effective in managing diarrhea caused by chemotherapy or other noninfective conditions. It should be used cautiously in infectious cases, as reducing motility can worsen infections.
- Racecadotril: As an antisecretory agent, racecadotril (100 mg three times daily) works by reducing intestinal water and electrolyte secretion, making it effective in reducing the volume of diarrhea.
- Somatostatin Analogues (Octreotide): Octreotide (50–250 mcg subcutaneously three times daily) is particularly useful in conditions like graft-versus-host disease (GVHD) or immunodeficiency, where it helps reduce gastrointestinal secretions and motility.
- Probiotics/Prebiotics: These can aid in restoring a healthy gut microbiome, potentially reducing diarrhea symptoms. However, they should be used with caution in immunocompromised patients due to the risk of systemic infection.
- Fiber-Enriched Formulas: These are especially beneficial in reducing stool frequency and improving the consistency of stools. They provide a substrate for beneficial bacteria and help bulk up stool, making them a valuable part of enteral feeding regimens for patients with diarrhea.

These measures ensure a comprehensive approach to managing diarrhea, addressing not only the symptoms but also the underlying causes and preventing complications in critically ill patients.

41.10 Conclusion

The management of diarrhea in critically ill patients requires a structured, evidence-based approach, focusing on the evaluation of fluid and electrolyte balance, assessment of infectious and noninfectious causes, and correction of contributing factors. Evidence-based protocols have been shown to reduce the incidence of diarrhea and improve patient outcomes, with a reported 13% reduction in diarrhea rates after protocol implementation. Preventing complications such as skin breakdown, malnutrition, and infection spread is essential for comprehensive care. Early recognition and intervention are crucial in preventing severe outcomes, ensuring better recovery and shorter ICU stays for patients.

Algorithm 41.1: Approach to diarrhoea in the ICU

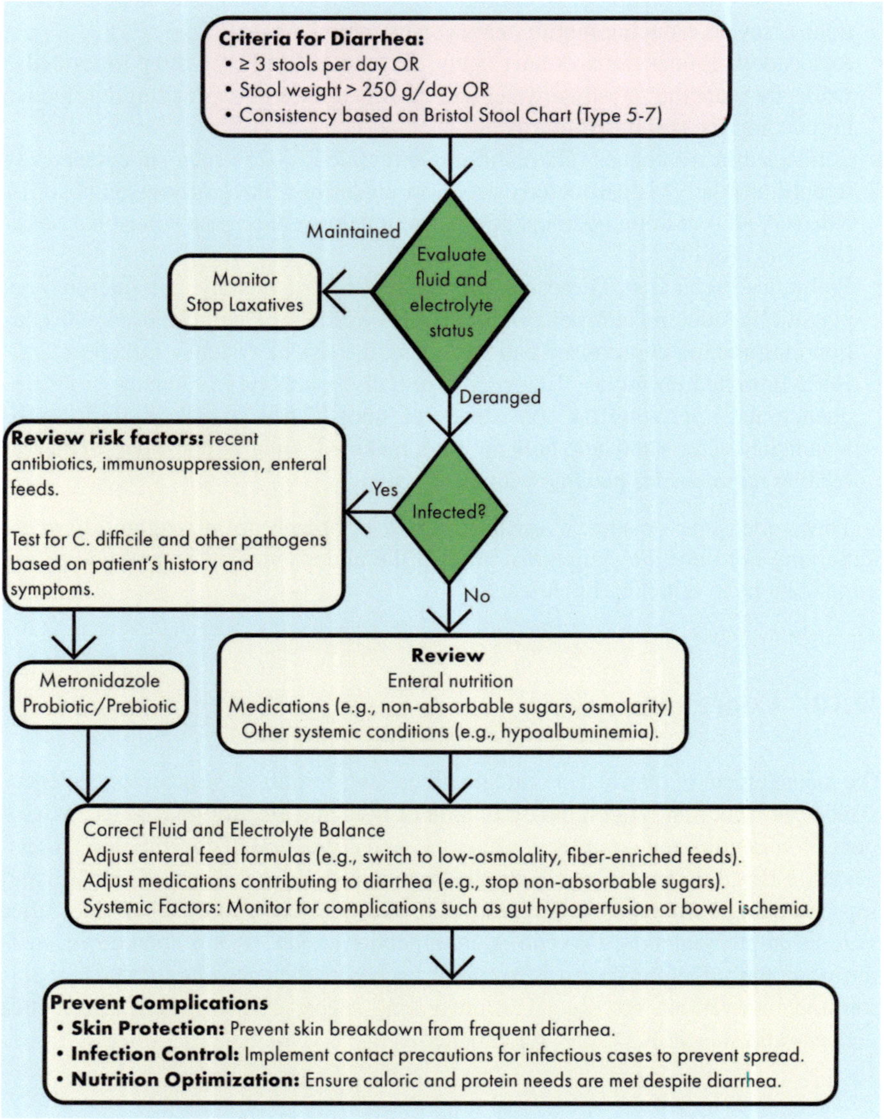

Bibliography

1. Dionne JC, Sullivan K, Mbuagbaw L, Takaoka A, Duan EH, Alhazzani W, et al. Diarrhoea: interventions, consequences and epidemiology in the intensive care unit (DICE-ICU): a protocol for a prospective multicentre cohort study. BMJ Open. 2019;9(6):e028237.
2. Adelman MW, Woodworth MH, Shaffer VO, Martin GS, Kraft CS. Critical Care Management of the Patient with Clostridioides difficile. Crit Care Med. 2021;49(1):127–39.
3. Tirlapur N, Puthucheary ZA, Cooper JA, Sanders J, Coen PG, Moonesinghe SR, et al. Diarrhoea in the critically ill is common, associated with poor outcome, and rarely due to Clostridium difficile. Sci Rep. 2016;6:24691.
4. Johnson S, Lavergne V, Skinner AM, Gonzales-Luna AJ, Garey KW, Kelly CP, et al. Clinical practice guideline by the Infectious Diseases Society of America (IDSA) and Society for Healthcare Epidemiology of America (SHEA): 2021 focused update guidelines on management of clostridioides difficile infection in adults. Clin Infect Dis. 2021;73(5):e1029–e44.
5. Ferrie S, East V. Managing diarrhoea in intensive care. Aust Crit Care. 2007;20(1):7–13.
6. Reintam Blaser A, Deane AM, Fruhwald S. Diarrhoea in the critically ill. Curr Opin Crit Care. 2015;21(2):142–53.

Chapter 42
Approach to *Clostridioides Difficile* (*C. Difficile*) Infection in the ICU

42.1 Introduction

Clostridioides difficile infection (CDI) is a significant cause of healthcare-associated infections, ranging from mild diarrhea to life-threatening colitis. CDI typically occurs after antibiotic use, which disrupts the normal gut microbiota, allowing *C. difficile* to proliferate. Early and accurate identification of CDI severity is critical for effective management and to prevent complications. Management of CDI is guided by clinical severity, with treatments tailored for non-severe, severe, or fulminant presentations. Recurrent infections are common, requiring specific protocols for effective treatment. Recent updates in the management of CDI emphasize newer agents like fidaxomicin and adjunctive therapies such as bezlotoxumab, offering better outcomes in preventing recurrences [1–3] [Ref: Algorithm 42.1].

42.2 Initial Evaluation

The initial step in managing CDI involves assessing the severity of the infection to guide treatment:

- Non-severe CDI: Defined by a white blood cell count (WBC) ≤15,000 cells/μL and serum creatinine (Cr) <1.5 mg/dL. Patients typically present with diarrhea but without systemic toxicity.
- Severe CDI: Characterized by WBC >15,000 cells/μL or serum creatinine ≥1.5 mg/dL. These patients have a higher risk of complications, warranting more intensive treatment.
- Fulminant CDI: The most critical form, marked by hypotension, shock, ileus, or megacolon. Patients often require a combination of oral and intravenous (IV) treatments and may need ICU care.

S. B. Mishra et al., *Mastering ICU Care*,
https://doi.org/10.1007/978-981-95-0179-3_42

42.3 Non-severe CDI: First-Line Treatment

The primary goal in treating non-severe CDI is to eradicate the infection while minimizing the risk of recurrence. Updated guidelines highlight:

- Fidaxomicin (200 mg orally twice daily for 10 days) is preferred over vancomycin due to a lower risk of recurrence.
- Vancomycin (125 mg orally four times daily for 10 days) remains a suitable alternative, particularly when fidaxomicin is unavailable.
- Metronidazole (500 mg orally three times daily for 10 days) is reserved as an alternative when neither fidaxomicin nor vancomycin is available, though it is less effective, especially in recurrent cases.

42.4 Severe CDI: First-Line Treatment

For severe CDI, therapy aims to control bacterial overgrowth while closely monitoring for systemic complications:

- Fidaxomicin (200 mg orally twice daily for 10 days) is preferred due to better outcomes in preventing recurrences.
- Vancomycin (125 mg orally four times daily for 10 days) is a viable alternative when fidaxomicin is not feasible.
- Adjunctive bezlotoxumab should be added for primary CDI if other risk factors for recurrence (age $\geq$ 65 years, immunocompromised host) or if an episode of CDI in the last 6 months is present.
- Treatment should be accompanied by close monitoring of hydration status, potential complications, and prompt adjustments in therapy based on the patient's clinical response.

42.5 Fulminant CDI: First-Line Treatment

Managing fulminant CDI requires aggressive intervention to reduce morbidity and mortality:

- Vancomycin (500 mg orally or via nasogastric tube four times daily) is recommended, with consideration for rectal vancomycin (500 mg in 100 mL of normal saline every 6 hours) if the patient has ileus.

And

Intravenous metronidazole (500 mg every 8 hours) is added to ensure systemic coverage, particularly when oral delivery is compromised.

- As per ESCIMD guidelines, IV tigecycline 100 mg loading then 50 mg 12 hourly can also be used as an alternative regimen.
- This regimen is essential to ensure the medication reaches the colon effectively, even in the presence of intestinal paralysis.

42.6 Recurrent CDI

Recurrence is a common challenge in CDI, affecting about 20–30% of cases. Management strategies are adjusted based on previous treatments:

First Recurrence:

- If previously treated with metronidazole, transition to vancomycin (125 mg orally four times daily for 10 days).
- If vancomycin was used initially, switch to fidaxomicin (200 mg orally twice daily for 10 days).
- A vancomycin taper and pulse regimen can also be used, gradually reducing the dose over weeks to enhance the suppression of *C. difficile*, and adjunctive bezlotoxumab should be given if prior episode is present in the last 6 months.

Second or Subsequent Recurrences:

- Use vancomycin in a tapered and pulsed regimen, such as 125 mg four times daily for 10–14 days, then gradually tapering over 2–8 weeks. Adjunctive bezlotoxumab should be added if prior episode is present in the last 6 months.
- Fidaxomicin remains a viable option if not previously utilized.
- For patients with multiple recurrences, fecal microbiota transplantation (FMT) is recommended, restoring normal gut flora and reducing recurrence risk.

42.7 Adjunctive Therapies

Several adjunctive measures can support recovery and reduce recurrence risk:

- Bezlotoxumab: A monoclonal antibody targeting *C. difficile* toxin B, it is considered for patients at high risk of recurrence (e.g., those aged ≥65, immunocompromised). It is administered as a single IV dose of 10 mg/kg during antibiotic therapy. However, caution is advised for patients with congestive heart failure due to potential risks.

- Stopping the inciting antibiotic: Discontinuing unnecessary antibiotics helps restore gut microbiota, reducing the risk of recurrence.
- Avoiding anti-motility agents (e.g., loperamide): These can slow the clearance of the bacteria and increase the risk of toxic megacolon.
- Maintaining adequate hydration and electrolyte balance: Addressing dehydration and electrolyte disturbances from diarrhea is critical.
- Infection control: Contact precautions, hand hygiene, and isolation are vital to prevent the spread of CDI in healthcare settings.

42.8 Early Diagnosis

Accurate and timely diagnosis is fundamental in CDI management. Implementing a multistep testing algorithm—such as using glutamate dehydrogenase (GDH) and toxin assays or a combination of nucleic acid amplification tests (NAATs)—ensures that patients with clinically significant CDI are appropriately identified and treated. This approach helps reduce the risk of overtreatment and improves patient outcomes.

42.9 Conclusion

Management of *Clostridioides difficile* infection (CDI) is tailored to clinical severity, with a focus on preventing complications like recurrence, fulminant colitis, or toxic megacolon. Updated guidelines favor fidaxomicin over vancomycin for its lower recurrence rates, with metronidazole as an alternative in resource-limited settings. In cases of recurrence, strategies such as vancomycin taper regimens or fecal microbiota transplantation provide effective options. Early recognition and appropriate treatment are key to reducing CDI-related morbidity and mortality. Adherence to current guidelines, particularly in using newer therapeutic options and adjunctive measures, ensures improved outcomes in managing this challenging condition.

Algorithm 42.1: Approach to *Clostridioides difficile* (*C. Difficile*) infection in the ICU

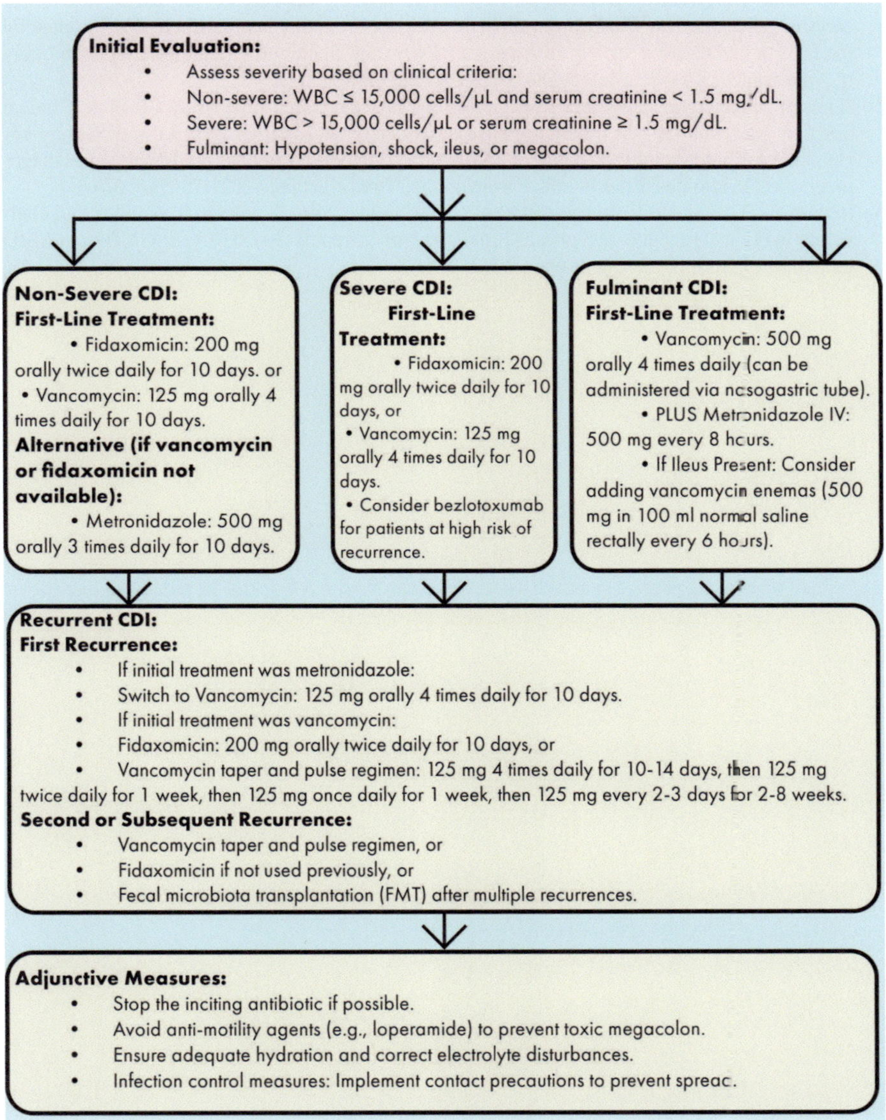

Bibliography

1. McDonald LC, Gerding DN, Johnson S, Bakken JS, Carroll KC, Coffin SE, et al. Clinical practice guidelines for Clostridium difficile infection in adults and children: 2017 update by the Infectious Diseases Society of America (IDSA) and Society for Healthcare Epidemiology of America (SHEA). Clin Infect Dis. 2018;66(7):e1–e48.
2. Johnson S, Lavergne V, Skinner AM, Gonzales-Luna AJ, Garey KW, Kelly CP, et al. Clinical practice guideline by the Infectious Diseases Society of America (IDSA) and Society for Healthcare Epidemiology of America (SHEA): 2021 focused update guidelines on management of clostridioides difficile infection in adults. Clin Infect Dis. 2021;73(5):e1029–e44.
3. Bishop EJ, Tiruvoipati R. Management of Clostridioides difficile infection in adults and challenges in clinical practice: review and comparison of current IDSA/SHEA, ESCMID and ASID guidelines. J Antimicrob Chemother. 2022;78(1):21–30.

Chapter 43
Approach to Hepatic Encephalopathy in the ICU

43.1 Introduction

Hepatic encephalopathy (HE) is a neuropsychiatric syndrome that arises from liver dysfunction, typically associated with cirrhosis. It can present with a range of symptoms, from subtle cognitive changes to deep coma. Up to 30–50% of patients with cirrhosis will develop some form of HE during their lifetime, significantly affecting one-year mortality rates. Early recognition and targeted management are essential to prevent complications and improve patient outcomes.

The pathophysiology of HE involves the buildup of neurotoxins like ammonia and manganese due to impaired liver detoxification and portosystemic shunting. These toxins cross the blood-brain barrier, leading to astrocyte swelling, changes in neurotransmitter levels, and brain edema. Understanding these mechanisms helps guide treatment strategies, focusing on reducing neurotoxic burden and stabilizing neurological function [1, 2] [Ref: Algorithm 43.1].

43.2 Assess if the Patient's Airway Is Compromised

- Severe cases of HE, especially those resulting from acute liver failure, can lead to cerebral edema, increasing intracranial pressure and potentially causing brainstem compression. Early airway protection is critical, particularly in patients with fulminant liver failure, to prevent hypoxia and secondary brain injury. Intubation should be considered for patients with significantly impaired consciousness (e.g., low Glasgow Coma Scale score).
- The use of sedatives should be minimized, as they can exacerbate encephalopathy. If sedation is necessary, it is advisable to use agents with minimal hepatic metabolism, such as propofol [3].

S. B. Mishra et al., *Mastering ICU Care*,
https://doi.org/10.1007/978-981-95-0179-3_43

43.3 Staging

43.3.1 West Haven Criteria [4]

- **Grade 1:** Characterized by a lack of awareness, euphoria or anxiety, reduced attention span, and difficulty with simple tasks such as addition or subtraction.
- **Grade 2:** Marked by lethargy or apathy, slight disorientation to time, place, or person, personality changes, inappropriate behavior, and the presence of a flapping tremor (asterixis).
- **Grade 3:** The patient is somnolent to semi-stuporous but still responsive to verbal stimuli, with significant confusion and marked disorientation.
- **Grade 4:** Represents coma, with no response to verbal commands and complete unresponsiveness.

This classification helps guide clinical management and monitor disease progression.

43.3.2 Classification Based on the Underlying Cause [4]

Type A (Acute): Associated with acute liver failure, this form of HE often presents rapidly and is commonly linked with cerebral edema and increased intracranial pressure.

Type B (Bypass): Occurs due to portal-systemic shunting in the absence of intrinsic liver disease. The shunt allows toxins to bypass the liver, leading to neuropsychiatric symptoms.

Type C (Cirrhosis): Seen in patients with chronic liver disease or cirrhosis. It is further categorized into:

- **Episodic:** Intermittent episodes triggered by precipitating factors.
- **Persistent:** Chronic, ongoing symptoms of encephalopathy.
- **Minimal (or Covert):** Subtle cognitive and psychomotor deficits without overt clinical signs, often requiring specialized testing for diagnosis.

This classification aids in identifying the etiology and tailoring appropriate treatment strategies.

43.3.3 Overt HE

This refers to clinically apparent episodes of neuropsychiatric dysfunction. It can be **episodic**, occurring as isolated events, or **recurrent**, defined as more than one episode within a six-month period.

43.3.4 Persistent HE

In this form, patients do not return to their baseline neuropsychiatric status between episodes. Symptoms are continuous or fluctuate without complete resolution, indicating a chronic impairment in cognitive and neurological function.

43.4 Presence of Precipitating Factors

- Identifying and managing precipitating factors is crucial, as they can often trigger or worsen HE. Common precipitating factors include infections (e.g., spontaneous bacterial peritonitis), electrolyte imbalances such as hyponatremia, renal failure, and the excessive use of diuretics, gastrointestinal bleeding, medicine noncompliance, dehydration (due to diarrhea, vomiting, fluid restriction), alcohol consumption, and use of sedatives or specific analgesics. Targeted management of these factors can significantly improve patient outcomes.
- Diagnostic workup should include cultures, serum electrolytes, blood urea nitrogen (BUN) levels, and ammonia levels, although ammonia levels may not always directly correlate with the severity of HE [5, 6].

43.5 Focus on General Supportive Care and Continue Evaluation

- Supportive care is essential for stabilizing patients with HE. This includes maintaining adequate caloric intake (35–40 kcal/kg/day) and protein intake (1.2–1.5 g/kg/day) to prevent catabolism. Contrary to earlier beliefs, protein restriction is not recommended due to the risk of malnutrition; instead, a balanced diet with a higher vegetable protein content is preferable. Small meals or liquid nutritional supplements evenly distributed throughout the day and a late-night snack should be offered.
- Ongoing evaluation should include monitoring neurological status and conducting further tests, such as cultures or imaging, to identify other contributing factors to encephalopathy.

43.6 If the Patient Is Not Responding to Lactulose, Consider Rifaximin or Alternative Therapies

- Lactulose is a cornerstone of HE therapy due to its ability to lower systemic ammonia. It promotes conversion of ammonia (NH_3) into ammonium (NH_3^+) in the gut by acidifying the colon, which also inhibits ammonia-producing bacterial strains. Additionally, lactulose increases colonic motility, reducing the duration available for ammonia reabsorption, and supports nitrogen excretion by acting osmotically. Dose: 30 ml 3–4 times /day. Enema can also be given if there is inadequate response or there is intolerance to oral/enteral feed. Target 2–4 soft/loose stools per day.

Rifaximin enhances treatment by decreasing the population of gut flora that produce ammonia. It acts locally in the gut without systemic absorption and inhibits bacterial RNA synthesis, thus further lowering neurotoxin production. Dose: 550 mg twice daily or 400 mg thrice daily.

- Alternatives like L-ornithine L-aspartate (LOLA) may be considered to further reduce ammonia levels in patients not responding to lactulose and rifaximin. Emerging therapies, such as fecal microbiota transplants, are also being explored for managing refractory cases of HE.

43.7 If the Patient Still Does Not Respond, Reevaluate for Other Complications

- When standard therapy fails, it is essential to reassess for other potential complications or underlying conditions. Persistent HE may indicate the presence of intracranial pathologies, such as subdural hematoma or stroke, which can mimic or worsen encephalopathy.
- In such cases, advanced imaging like MRI or CT scans, along with EEG, can help identify conditions such as non-convulsive status epilepticus. Additionally, evaluate the need for adjusting or closing a transjugular intrahepatic portosystemic shunt (TIPS) if it is contributing to persistent HE [7]

43.8 Is the Patient a Candidate for Liver Transplant?

- In individuals experiencing frequent or treatment-resistant episodes of hepatic encephalopathy, liver transplantation offers a curative approach by correcting the primary hepatic insufficiency. The MELD score plays a pivotal role in determining transplant candidacy by evaluating disease severity.
- Timely consultation with a transplant center is crucial when medical therapy fails to yield adequate results, as delayed referrals may adversely affect prognosis. Alongside clinical eligibility, factors such as daily functioning and overall quality of life should be weighed, considering the profound burden HE imposes on patients.

43.9 Conclusion

Managing hepatic encephalopathy requires a structured approach that includes stabilizing the patient, identifying and treating precipitating factors, and considering advanced treatments such as liver transplantation. Preventing recurrence is a key focus, with secondary prophylaxis using lactulose and rifaximin playing an important role in reducing future episodes. A multidisciplinary approach, involving hepatologists, dietitians, and neurologists, ensures comprehensive care for patients with HE. Individualized care plans and timely interventions are essential to improving outcomes for this complex condition.

Algorithm 43.1: Approach to hepatic encephalopathy in the ICU

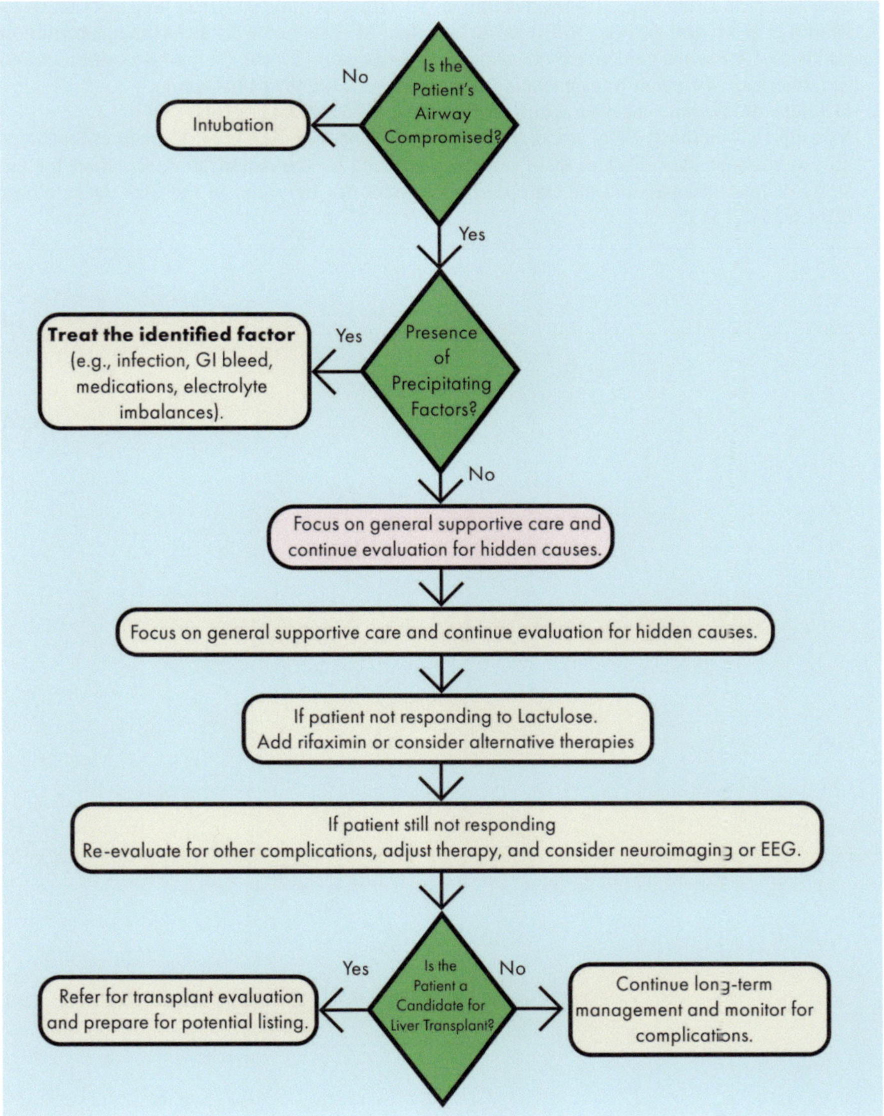

Bibliography

1. European Association for the Study of the Liver. Electronic address EEE, European Association for the Study of the L. EASL clinical practice guidelines on the management of hepatic encephalopathy. J Hepatol. 2022;77(3):807–24.
2. Hoilat GJ, Suhail FK, Adhami T, John S. Evidence-based approach to management of hepatic encephalopathy in adults. World J Hepatol. 2022;14(4):670–81.
3. Korean Association for the Study of the L. KASL clinical practice guidelines for liver cirrhosis: varices, hepatic encephalopathy, and related complications. Clin Mol Hepatol. 2020;26(2):83–127.
4. American Association for the Study of Liver Diseases; European Association for the Study of the Liver. Hepatic encephalopathy in chronic liver disease: 2014 practice guideline by the European Association for the Study of the liver and the American Association for the study of liver diseases. J Hepatol. 2014 Sep;61(3):642–59. https://doi.org/10.1016/j.jhep.2014.05.042.
5. Martin P, DiMartini A, Feng S, Brown R Jr, Fallon M. Evaluation for liver transplantation in adults: 2013 practice guideline by the American Association for the study of liver diseases and the American Society of transplantation. Hepatology. 2014;59(3):1144–65.
6. Wijdicks EF. Hepatic encephalopathy. N Engl J Med. 2016;375(17):1660–70.
7. Vilstrup H, Amodio P, Bajaj J, Cordoba J, Ferenci P, Mullen KD, et al. Hepatic encephalopathy in chronic liver disease: 2014 practice guideline by the American Association for the study of liver diseases and the European Association for the study of the liver. Hepatology. 2014;60(2):715–35.

Chapter 44
Approach to Raised Intra-abdominal Pressure in the ICU

44.1 Introduction

Abdominal compartment syndrome (ACS) is a critical condition characterized by increased intra-abdominal pressure (IAP), leading to potential organ dysfunction and high mortality if not managed appropriately. It is essential to distinguish between intra-abdominal hypertension (IAH) and ACS: IAH refers to a sustained or repeated pathological elevation of IAP $\geq$ 12 mm Hg, while ACS involves a sustained IAP > 20 mm Hg with associated new organ dysfunction or failure. The concept of abdominal perfusion pressure (APP), defined as mean arterial pressure (MAP) minus IAP, serves as a crucial marker of abdominal organ perfusion. Maintaining adequate APP is vital to ensure sufficient blood flow to the abdominal organs [1, 2] [Ref: Algorithm 44.1].

44.2 Epidemiology

IAH is a relatively common condition in the intensive care unit (ICU), affecting up to 25% of ICU patients, with a smaller subset progressing to ACS. This condition often goes underdiagnosed, which underscores the importance of regular monitoring and maintaining a high index of suspicion, especially in at-risk patients. Without timely intervention, the mortality rate for untreated ACS can reach up to 40% due to the progression to multiorgan failure.

S. B. Mishra et al., *Mastering ICU Care*,
https://doi.org/10.1007/978-981-95-0179-3_44

44.3 Pathophysiology

The pathophysiological mechanisms of ACS include increased IAP, which impairs venous return, elevates intrathoracic pressure, and compromises diaphragmatic movement. This results in decreased cardiac output, reduced renal perfusion, and impaired respiratory mechanics, leading to potential organ dysfunction. Understanding these mechanisms helps ICU staff appreciate the systemic impact of elevated IAP and underscores the urgency of timely management to prevent irreversible organ damage [3].

44.4 Measurement of IAP

Measurement of IAP is crucial for early diagnosis and management of IAH and ACS. The bladder-based method remains the gold standard for IAP measurement, involving measurement of pressure via the bladder with a Foley catheter. Measurements should be taken at end-expiration and with a standardized technique to avoid erroneous readings. The transducer must be zeroed at the mid-axillary line, ensuring that abdominal muscle contractions are minimized during the measurement. Alternative measurement techniques, such as gastric or rectal pressure monitoring, can be considered for specific clinical scenarios. IAP should be monitored regularly in patients with risk factors like sepsis, trauma, or recent abdominal surgeries.

44.5 IAH and Its Grading

IAH is classified into four grades based on IAP measurements:

- Grade I: IAP 12–15 mm Hg.
- Grade II: IAP 16–20 mm Hg.
- Grade III: IAP 21–25 mm Hg.
- Grade IV: IAP > 25 mm Hg.

This grading helps tailor management strategies according to the severity of IAP. For instance, Grade I may only require close monitoring, while higher grades might necessitate more aggressive interventions.

44.6 Management of Elevated IAP (> 12 mm Hg)

44.6.1 Conservative Measures

- Fluid Management: Optimizing fluid balance is critical, as excessive fluid can exacerbate IAH by increasing intra-abdominal volume. Strategies to achieve a negative fluid balance can help prevent further IAP elevation.

- Patient Positioning: Adjusting the patient's position to a semi-recumbent position can reduce IAP by improving venous return.
- Sedation and Neuromuscular Blockade: These can be employed to decrease abdominal wall muscle tone, which can help lower IAP when conservative measures alone are insufficient.
- Minimally Invasive Techniques: Consider percutaneous catheter drainage in cases where intraluminal or extraluminal fluid needs to be reduced without resorting to surgery.

44.6.2 Decision-Making for Surgical Intervention (Decompressive Laparotomy)

44.6.2.1 Indications

A decompressive laparotomy is indicated for patients with IAP > 20 mm Hg who exhibit signs of ongoing organ dysfunction that are unresponsive to conservative measures, such as optimizing fluid balance, adjusting patient positioning, and using pharmacological interventions like neuromuscular blockade. Indications include persistent hypotension despite adequate fluid resuscitation, oliguria or anuria indicating renal compromise, worsening respiratory parameters due to decreased lung compliance, and increasing lactate levels suggesting tissue hypoperfusion. The goal of decompressive laparotomy is to rapidly relieve intra-abdominal pressure, allowing improved perfusion to vital organs such as the kidneys, liver, and intestines, and to prevent further progression to multiorgan failure [4].

44.6.2.2 Risks

While decompressive laparotomy can be lifesaving, it carries several potential risks that must be carefully weighed before proceeding:

- Wound Complications: The open abdomen can lead to difficulties in wound healing, including delayed closure and a higher risk of wound infections. Wound management is critical to prevent infection and sepsis, which can further complicate patient outcomes.
- Entero-atmospheric Fistulas: These abnormal connections between the intestines and the open wound can develop when bowel loops are exposed and become adherent to the wound edges. They are difficult to manage and can lead to significant fluid and electrolyte imbalances, increasing patient morbidity.
- Need for Abdominal Wall Reconstruction: Patients who undergo decompressive laparotomy may eventually require reconstructive surgery to close the abdominal wall, especially if delayed primary closure is not possible. This can include complex procedures such as skin grafting or the use of biological or synthetic mesh. These secondary procedures add to the overall burden of care and can extend the patient's ICU and hospital stay.

The decision to proceed with decompressive laparotomy should involve multidisciplinary input, including critical care specialists, surgeons, and possibly a wound care team, to ensure that the benefits of intervention outweigh the risks.

44.7 Open Abdomen Management

Open abdomen management is a crucial aspect of care following a decompressive laparotomy. This technique involves intentionally leaving the abdominal cavity open using temporary abdominal closure (TAC) techniques. The open abdomen approach allows for:

- Relief of Continued Swelling: After decompressive laparotomy, ongoing edema and inflammation can maintain elevated intra-abdominal pressures. TAC allows for continued decompression and access for subsequent surgical interventions if needed.
- Planned Reexplorations: It facilitates planned re-exploratory surgeries, where the surgical team can reenter the abdomen to address bleeding, infection, or other complications without having to reopen a fully closed abdomen.
- Techniques for Temporary Closure: Common methods include negative pressure wound therapy (NPWT) with vacuum-assisted closure devices, which help remove excess fluid, reduce edema, and promote granulation tissue formation. Other options include using absorbable meshes or silastic sheets to protect the exposed organs while maintaining some degree of coverage.

Early fascial closure is a key objective once the patient's condition stabilizes and IAP is under control. This involves closing the abdominal wall within 7–10 days to minimize complications associated with a prolonged open abdomen, such as the development of a frozen abdomen, where adhesions make future closure difficult. Achieving early closure can reduce the risk of further infections and improve long-term outcomes, including the likelihood of successful abdominal wall reconstruction [5].

44.8 Post-decompression Care

44.8.1 Fluid Resuscitation

Following decompressive laparotomy, careful management of fluid therapy is essential to prevent reperfusion injury. Reperfusion injury can occur when blood flow is suddenly restored to previously ischemic tissues, leading to oxidative stress and inflammation. Therefore, fluid resuscitation should be gradual and carefully titrated, focusing on maintaining adequate perfusion without causing a sudden rise in fluid volume that could increase IAP again. The use of balanced crystalloids and close monitoring of fluid status, such as through daily weight measurements and central venous pressure (CVP) monitoring, can help guide appropriate resuscitation.

44.8.2 Complication Management

The postoperative phase also requires vigilant monitoring for complications to ensure optimal patient recovery:

- Bleeding and Coagulopathy: Patients who have undergone decompressive laparotomy may be at risk for bleeding due to surgical trauma and possible coagulopathy. Coagulopathy should be addressed promptly with blood products like platelets or fresh frozen plasma, guided by regular coagulation profiles.
- Infections: The open abdomen presents a significant risk for abdominal and wound infections, which can progress to sepsis if not controlled. Prophylactic antibiotics and strict aseptic techniques during dressing changes are critical components of infection prevention. Early signs of infection, such as fever or purulent wound drainage, should prompt immediate intervention.
- Nutritional Support: Due to high catabolic demands and protein losses from the open abdomen, early enteral nutrition is recommended as soon as it is feasible to support healing and immune function.

44.8.3 Ongoing Monitoring

Regular IAP monitoring remains crucial even after surgical decompression to detect early signs of recurrent intra-abdominal hypertension. IAP should be measured every 4–6 hours during the initial postoperative period or whenever there are signs of hemodynamic instability. This allows for timely interventions such as adjusting fluid therapy or considering further decompressive measures if pressures rise again. Continuous assessment of organ function, including renal output, liver enzymes, and arterial blood gases, helps gauge the patient's response to decompression and guide ongoing treatment strategies.

Together, these steps aim to stabilize the patient post-laparotomy and improve the chances of recovery while mitigating the complications associated with ACS and its surgical treatment.

44.9 Conclusion

Effective management of IAH and ACS requires a systematic and patient-specific approach. Regular monitoring, timely conservative interventions, and judicious decision-making regarding surgical decompression are essential for optimizing patient outcomes. It is crucial to adapt the management strategy to the dynamic evolution of each patient's condition, integrating insights from a multidisciplinary team of critical care physicians, surgeons, and nurses. Recognizing the interplay between IAP and systemic physiology allows for a more tailored approach, improving survival rates and reducing long-term morbidity for patients with IAH and ACS.

Algorithm 44.1: Approach to raise intra-abdominal pressure in the ICU

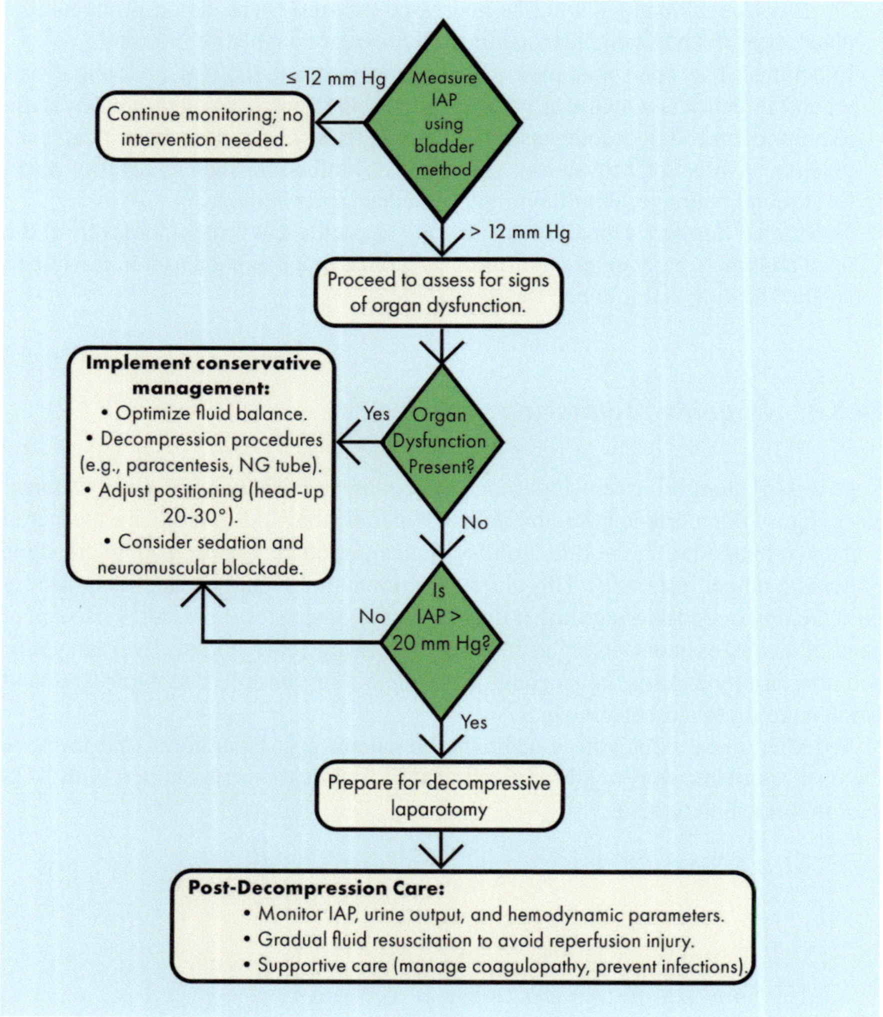

Bibliography

1. Kirkpatrick AW, Roberts DJ, De Waele J, Jaeschke R, Malbrain ML, De Keulenaer B, et al. Intra-abdominal hypertension and the abdominal compartment syndrome: updated consensus definitions and clinical practice guidelines from the world society of the abdominal compartment syndrome. Intensive Care Med. 2013;39(7):1190–206.
2. Coccolini F, Roberts D, Ansaloni L, Ivatury R, Gamberini E, Kluger Y, et al. The open abdomen in trauma and non-trauma patients: WSES guidelines. World J Emerg Surg. 2018;13:7.
3. Jang H, Lee N, Jeong E, Park Y, Jo Y, Kim J, et al. Abdominal compartment syndrome in critically ill patients. Acute Crit Care. 2023;38(4):399–408.
4. De Laet IE, Malbrain M, De Waele JJ. A clinician's guide to management of intra-abdominal hypertension and abdominal compartment syndrome in critically ill patients. Crit Care. 2020;24(1):97.
5. Montalvo-Jave EE, Espejel-Deloiza M, Chernitzky-Camaño J, Peña-Pérez CA, Rivero-Sigarroa E, Ortega-León LH. Abdominal compartment syndrome: current concepts and management. Revista de Gastroenterología de México (English Edition). 2020;85(4):443–51.

Chapter 45
Approach to Acute Liver Failure in the ICU

45.1 Introduction

Acute liver failure (ALF) is a critical condition characterized by the rapid deterioration of liver function in patients without preexisting liver disease. This condition can progress rapidly and lead to life-threatening complications, including cerebral edema, coagulopathy, and multi-organ failure. The management of ALF in the intensive care unit (ICU) requires a systematic approach to stabilize the patient, prevent complications, and evaluate for potential liver transplantation. This chapter outlines a comprehensive approach to managing ALF, integrating the latest clinical guidelines and considerations [1, 2] [Ref: Algorithm 45.1].

Definition ALF is defined as the development of severe acute liver injury with encephalopathy and impaired synthetic function (INR of 1.5 or higher) in a patient without cirrhosis or preexisting liver disease and with an illness of fewer than 26 weeks duration.

45.2 Etiological Assessment

- Viral Causes: ALF can be triggered by viral infections like hepatitis B, A, E, herpes simplex virus, and cytomegalovirus (CMV). These infections are particularly relevant in certain geographic regions, and immunosuppressed patients (e.g., those undergoing chemotherapy) are at higher risk for viral reactivation leading to ALF.
- Drug-Induced Liver Injury (DILI): Acetaminophen remains the most common cause of ALF in developed countries; however, idiosyncratic reactions to other drugs, such as antibiotics, also contribute significantly to cases. A thorough

S. B. Mishra et al., *Mastering ICU Care*,
https://doi.org/10.1007/978-981-95-0179-3_45

review of the patient's medication history is critical to identify potential drug-related causes.
- Wilson's Disease and Other Specific Causes: Rare etiologies like Wilson's disease and acute Budd-Chiari syndrome should be considered, as these require specific diagnostic approaches. Early recognition of these conditions is essential, as they often necessitate urgent liver transplantation for improved outcomes.

45.3 Management

1. **Airway Management**
   - Decision Point: Is the patient able to maintain airway?
   - If no, intubate the patient to protect the airway. Intubation is crucial in patients with encephalopathy or altered mental status to prevent aspiration and ensure proper oxygenation and ventilation.
   - If yes, proceed with the management of hemodynamic stability and cerebral edema prevention.
2. **Prevention and Management of Cerebral Edema**
   - Head Elevation: Keep the head of the bed elevated at 30 degrees to reduce intracranial pressure (ICP) and minimize the risk of cerebral edema.
   - Serum Sodium Management: Maintain serum sodium levels between 145 and 155 mmol/L using hypertonic saline as needed. This approach helps to minimize cerebral edema, especially in patients with elevated ICP.
   - Intracranial Pressure Monitoring: Consider ICP monitoring in patients with advanced hepatic encephalopathy who are awaiting liver transplantation. This helps guide the use of osmotic therapies like mannitol or hypertonic saline.
   - Role of Hypothermia: Mild hypothermia may serve as a bridge therapy for patients with refractory intracranial hypertension, particularly in centers experienced with this technique.
   - Sedation: Sedating with Propofol can aid in controlling agitation and reducing cerebral metabolic demands, but careful monitoring is essential to avoid excessive sedation [3].
3. **Hemodynamic Support**
   - Maintain Mean Arterial Pressure (MAP) > 65 mm Hg: Adequate MAP ensures sufficient organ perfusion, especially in the setting of compromised liver function. Vasopressors may be used if required to maintain target pressures.
4. **Management of Hyperammonemia**
   Hyperammonemia is a hallmark of ALF and contributes significantly to the development of hepatic encephalopathy and cerebral edema. Elevated ammonia levels result from impaired liver function, which reduces the organ's ability to

detoxify ammonia produced by gut bacteria. In ALF, managing hyperammonemia is crucial to prevent worsening neurological status and other complications.

5. **Ammonia Management**

- Lactulose Caution: While lactulose is frequently used in chronic liver disease to reduce ammonia levels, its role in ALF is less clear. Lactulose works by acidifying the gut and promoting the conversion of ammonia into ammonium, which is then excreted in the stool. However, in ALF, lactulose should be used with caution due to the potential for bowel distension and the risk of aspiration, especially in patients with altered mental status who are not intubated. Lactulose can increase the risk of abdominal bloating and discomfort, which can complicate care in the ICU setting.
- CRRT as Preferred Therapy: Continuous Renal Replacement Therapy (CRRT) is the preferred method for managing severe hyperammonemia in ALF patients. CRRT offers several advantages, including the ability to provide consistent removal of ammonia from the blood, management of fluid balance, and correction of acid-base imbalances. This is especially beneficial in ALF, where rapid changes in fluid status and electrolytes can exacerbate cerebral edema. CRRT is often initiated when ammonia levels are significantly elevated and not responding to conservative measures, making it a critical tool for ammonia control in the ICU.

Are Ammonia Levels Elevated (>100 µmol/L)?
If Yes:

- Initiate CRRT: When ammonia levels exceed 100 µmol/L, this is considered a threshold where the risk of cerebral edema increases significantly. Initiating CRRT at this point helps to actively reduce circulating ammonia, thus lowering the risk of further neurological deterioration. CRRT is especially indicated in cases where other methods like lactulose are ineffective or contraindicated.
- Adjust Serum Sodium Levels: Concurrently, maintaining serum sodium levels in the high-normal range (145–155 mmol/L) using hypertonic saline can help to reduce the risk of cerebral edema. This osmotic strategy helps to shift water out of the brain, countering the effects of ammonia-induced astrocyte swelling. Adjusting serum sodium is crucial in managing elevated intracranial pressure in patients with severe hyperammonemia.
- **If No:**
- Continue Monitoring: In cases where ammonia levels are below the threshold, it is essential to continue regular monitoring of ammonia levels and the patient's neurological status. Even moderate elevations in ammonia can lead to a gradual decline in mental status, and timely adjustments in management are critical. Frequent assessments help in detecting early signs of worsening encephalopathy, guiding the need for more aggressive interventions like CRRT or adjustment of sodium levels.

- Neurological Monitoring: Close monitoring of the patient's neurological status is crucial, as changes can indicate an increase in cerebral edema. Tools such as serial neurological exams, Glasgow Coma Scale (GCS) scoring, and consideration of intracranial pressure monitoring can help in detecting early signs of intracranial hypertension. This allows for prompt escalation in therapy if needed.

6. **N-Acetylcysteine (NAC):** Administering N-acetylcysteine (NAC) is often used in clinical settings to manage acetaminophen toxicity and in other off-label uses, such as treating non-acetaminophen-induced acute liver failure and certain oxidative stress conditions [4]. Below is a detailed approach to dosing NAC for different indications:

   Acetaminophen Overdose

- Oral Route:
  - Loading Dose: 140 mg/kg of NAC given as a single dose.
  - Maintenance Dose: 70 mg/kg every 4 hours for 17 doses (total duration: 72 hours).
  - The solution is typically diluted to 5% (diluted with a suitable liquid like water, juice, or cola) to improve palatability and reduce the risk of gastrointestinal side effects.
- Intravenous Route:
  - Loading Dose: 150 mg/kg over 60 minutes.
  - Second Dose: 50 mg/kg over 4 hours.
  - Third Dose: 100 mg/kg over the next 16 hours (total duration: 21 hours).
  - Some protocols may continue the infusion beyond 21 hours based on the patient's clinical status and acetaminophen levels.

Key Considerations

- Adverse Reactions: Oral NAC is generally well-tolerated, though it may cause gastrointestinal discomfort, nausea, or vomiting. IV administration can cause anaphylactoid reactions in some patients, including rash, bronchospasm, and hypotension, particularly with rapid infusion rates.
- Monitoring: During IV administration, monitor liver function tests, serum electrolytes, and clinical signs of improvement or adverse reactions. For acetaminophen overdose, continue monitoring serum acetaminophen levels until they reach nontoxic levels and liver function normalizes.
- Dilution: When given intravenously, NAC should be diluted in dextrose 5% or sodium chloride solution to avoid vein irritation.

NAC is a versatile agent with multiple therapeutic applications in the ICU and emergency settings, and careful dosing and monitoring are crucial to ensure its safety and efficacy.

45.4 Management of Complications

Coagulopathy:

- Treat active bleeding or if any procedures are planned. Coagulopathy in ALF is common due to impaired production of clotting factors by the liver.
- Consider transfusion of blood products such as fresh frozen plasma (FFP) or platelets if clinically indicated.

Infection Management:

- Empirical Antibiotics: Initiate broad-spectrum antibiotics empirically due to the high risk of infections in ALF patients. Infection remains a major cause of morbidity and mortality in this population.
- Fungal Infection Considerations: Given the risk of fungal infections in ALF, especially in cases of prolonged ICU stay, antifungal agents should be considered for high-risk patients.

45.5 Transplant Criteria and Timing

Liver transplantation is often the definitive treatment for patients with ALF who do not show signs of spontaneous recovery. Determining which patients may benefit from transplantation is crucial, as timing can significantly impact outcomes. Using structured criteria and ensuring early coordination with liver transplant centers helps optimize the chances of survival and recovery.

Prognostic Scoring Systems:

- MELD Score (Model for End-Stage Liver Disease): The MELD score is widely used to assess the severity of liver disease and prioritize patients for transplantation based on their risk of mortality without a transplant. It considers laboratory values such as serum bilirubin, serum creatinine, and INR (International Normalized Ratio). In ALF, the MELD score can help identify patients at high risk of deterioration. While MELD is traditionally used for chronic liver diseases, recent evidence suggests it can also be valuable in ALF, especially when combined with clinical judgment to assess overall prognosis.
- King's College Criteria (KCC): KCC is a well-established set of criteria specifically designed for predicting outcomes in ALF. It helps clinicians identify patients who are unlikely to recover without transplantation. The criteria include parameters such as arterial pH, serum lactate, prothrombin time, and the presence of encephalopathy. For example:
  - In acetaminophen-induced ALF, KCC criteria include factors like arterial $pH < 7.3$ or the presence of severe coagulopathy ($INR > 6.5$) alongside renal failure and grade 3 or 4 encephalopathy.

- In non-acetaminophen ALF, KCC looks at prolonged prothrombin time (INR > 6.5) or the presence of grade 3 or 4 encephalopathy, often combined with other markers such as bilirubin levels.

- Use of Scoring Systems in Practice: Both MELD and KCC provide valuable guidance but should not be the sole determinants of transplantation decisions. A holistic evaluation of the patient's condition, including the speed of clinical decline, comorbidities, and response to supportive care, should complement these scores. This integrated approach allows for better prediction of outcomes and decision-making regarding the timing of liver transplantation [5].

45.6 Early Referral to Transplant Centers

- Importance of Timely Communication: Early referral to a liver transplant center is crucial for patients with ALF, as the window for intervention is often narrow. Delayed referral can limit options, especially if complications like cerebral edema or multi-organ failure develop, which can preclude successful transplantation.
- Rapid Assessment and Coordination: Coordination with transplant centers allows for timely evaluation of the patient's eligibility for transplantation, pretransplant optimization, and access to advanced therapies, such as extracorporeal liver support systems. This coordination is particularly important for patients who show signs of rapid clinical deterioration or meet the prognostic criteria for poor outcomes.
- Stabilization and Transfer: In situations where a patient requires transfer to a liver transplant center, stabilizing the patient's condition before transfer is essential. This includes securing the airway if there is altered mental status, maintaining hemodynamic stability with vasopressors if needed, and initiating therapies like CRRT for hyperammonemia. Ensuring a smooth and safe transfer can prevent further complications during transport and enable immediate evaluation upon arrival.
- Consultation for Transplantation Decision-Making: Even if the patient's condition appears to stabilize temporarily, involving a transplant center early allows for a more comprehensive evaluation and helps in determining the ideal timing for listing the patient for transplantation. This proactive approach can provide a critical advantage, especially if the patient's condition worsens unexpectedly.

45.7 Conclusion

The management of acute liver failure in the ICU is a complex and dynamic process that requires vigilance, prompt intervention, and a multidisciplinary approach. This protocol emphasizes securing the airway, preventing cerebral complications, maintaining hemodynamic stability, and addressing complications such as coagulopathy and infection. A key component of the approach is recognizing patients who may benefit from urgent liver transplantation, as it often remains the definitive treatment for those with irreversible liver damage. Incorporating considerations like specific etiologies, tailored infection management, and advanced care measures helps improve outcomes in this critical condition.

Algorithm 45.1: Approach to acute liver failure in the ICU

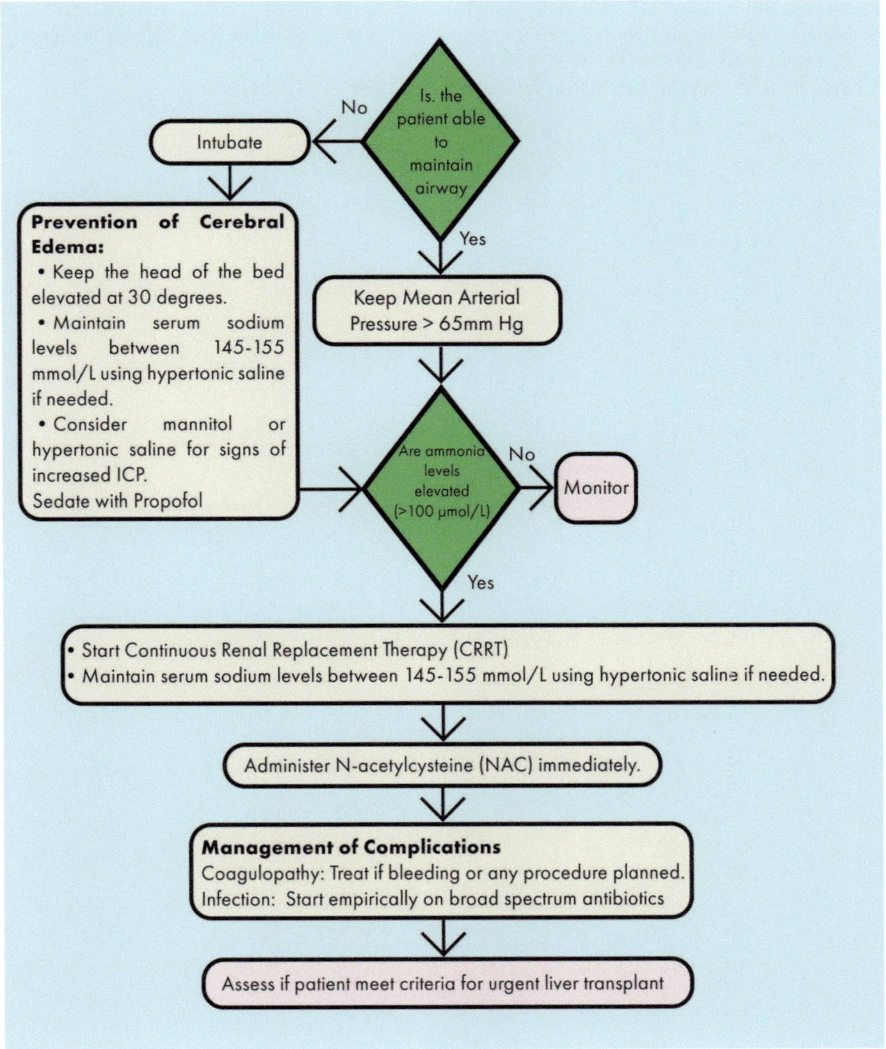

Bibliography

1. Bernal W, Wendon J. Acute liver failure. N Engl J Med. 2013;369(26):2525–34.
2. Flamm SL, Yang YX, Singh S, Falck-Ytter YT, Committee AGAICG. American Gastroenterological Association Institute guidelines for the diagnosis and management of acute liver failure. Gastroenterology. 2017;152(3):644–7.
3. Escorsell À, Castellote J, Sánchez-Delgado J, Charco R, Crespo G, Fernández J. Management of acute liver failure. Clinical guideline from the Catalan Society of Digestology. Gastroenterología y Hepatología (English Edition). 2019;42(1):51–64.
4. Stravitz RT, Kramer AH, Davern T, Shaikh AO, Caldwell SH, Mehta RL, et al. Intensive care of patients with acute liver failure: recommendations of the U.S. acute liver failure study group. Crit Care Med. 2007;35(11):2498–508.
5. Stravitz RT, Lee WM. Acute liver failure. Lancet. 2019;394(10201):869–81.

Chapter 46
Approach to Jaundice in the ICU

46.1 Introduction

Jaundice in the ICU is a frequent yet complex clinical issue, reflecting a spectrum of underlying hepatic and systemic disorders. It is defined by the yellowish discoloration of the skin and sclera due to elevated bilirubin levels, typically noticeable when serum bilirubin exceeds 2.5–3 mg/dL. Jaundice can be a marker of liver dysfunction, systemic infections like sepsis, or other critical illnesses, requiring a systematic approach to diagnosis and management. This chapter provides an in-depth analysis of the pathophysiology, diagnostic strategies, and management of jaundice in critically ill patients [1, 2]. [Ref: Algorithm 46.1].

46.2 Pathophysiology and Classification of Hyperbilirubinemia

Mechanisms of Hyperbilirubinemia:

- Bilirubin metabolism involves the breakdown of heme from red blood cells into unconjugated bilirubin, which is transported to the liver. Hepatocytes convert this into conjugated bilirubin through the action of the enzyme UDP-glucuronosyltransferase (UGT). Conjugated bilirubin is then excreted into bile ducts. Disruptions at any stage—ranging from hemolysis to impaired hepatic conjugation or biliary obstruction—can lead to different forms of jaundice.
- Unconjugated hyperbilirubinemia occurs when there is increased bilirubin production (e.g., hemolysis, resorption from hematomas) or impaired hepatic uptake/conjugation (e.g., Gilbert syndrome). It is characterized by elevated indirect bilirubin.

S. B. Mishra et al., *Mastering ICU Care*,
https://doi.org/10.1007/978-981-95-0179-3_46

- Conjugated hyperbilirubinemia suggests hepatocellular dysfunction or cholestasis, where conjugated bilirubin cannot be effectively secreted into the bile ducts, leading to elevated direct bilirubin levels.

Comprehensive Classification:
Jaundice can be classified into:

- Intrahepatic Causes: Hepatocellular injury due to viral hepatitis, sepsis-induced cholestasis, total parenteral nutrition (TPN) related cholestasis, or drug-induced liver injury.
- Extrahepatic Causes: Mechanical obstruction from choledocholithiasis, strictures, or tumors compressing the biliary tree. Differentiating between these is crucial for guiding further imaging and interventions.

46.3 Diagnostic Approach: Tests and Imaging

Laboratory Evaluation:

- Liver Function Tests (LFTs): Evaluate levels of alanine aminotransferase (ALT), aspartate aminotransferase (AST), alkaline phosphatase (ALP), gamma glutamyl transferase (GGT), and bilirubin (direct and total). Elevated ALP with GGT suggests a hepatobiliary origin, while a marked rise in AST/ALT indicates hepatocellular injury.
- Markers of Liver Function and Synthetic Capacity: PT/INR and albumin levels assess the liver's ability to synthesize proteins and clotting factors. Elevated INR with low albumin may indicate chronic liver disease.
- Hemoglobin Levels, Haptoglobin Levels, Peripheral Smear Comment, Reticulocyte Count, Lactate Dehydrogenase Levels, Coombs Test: To diagnose and identify hemolysis.

Imaging Modalities:

- Ultrasound: The initial imaging choice due to its high specificity for identifying gallstones and bile duct dilation. It is noninvasive and suitable for unstable ICU patients.
- Magnetic Resonance Cholangiopancreaticography (MRCP) and Computed Tomography (CT): Recommended if ultrasound is inconclusive or for better visualization of the biliary tree and pancreatic structures. MRCP is noninvasive and avoids radiation, making it a good alternative to Endoscopic retrograde cholangiopancreaticography (ERCP) in certain cases.
- ERCP/Percutaneous Transhepatic Catheter (PTC): Used for both diagnosis and therapeutic intervention in cases of confirmed biliary obstruction. ERCP is preferred for stone removal and stent placement, while PTC may be required if ERCP is unsuccessful.

46.4 Management Strategies for ICU-Associated Jaundice

Obstructive Jaundice:

- Choledocholithiasis and Cholangitis: ERCP for stone removal and biliary drainage is essential. Early intervention can prevent sepsis and reduce the risk of complications like biliary peritonitis.
- Malignancies: Surgical intervention or stenting may be needed for tumors causing biliary obstruction. Biopsy during ERCP can help confirm the diagnosis.

Nonobstructive Jaundice:

- Sepsis-Induced Cholestasis: Treat underlying infections with appropriate antibiotics and manage septic shock with fluid resuscitation and vasopressors. Early source control is critical.
- TPN-Related Cholestasis: Transitioning from continuous to cyclic TPN can mitigate liver damage. Emphasize early enteral feeding where possible to reduce reliance on TPN.
- Shock Liver (Ischemic Hepatitis): Focus on restoring hemodynamic stability through aggressive fluid resuscitation and the use of inotropes to improve liver perfusion.

ICU-Specific Challenges:

- Hemodynamic Management: Avoid excessive use of positive end-expiratory pressure (PEEP) in mechanically ventilated patients, as this can reduce liver perfusion and exacerbate hepatic congestion. Adjust vasoactive medications carefully to balance cardiac output and liver blood flow.

46.5 Prognostic Implications and Complications

Prognosis of Persistent Jaundice:

- Persistent jaundice in critically ill patients is associated with increased morbidity and mortality, often indicating underlying sepsis or multi-organ dysfunction. Monitoring trends in bilirubin levels and liver enzymes can help assess the progression of underlying disease.
- Multi-organ Failure: Jaundice that worsens despite intervention may indicate impending or ongoing multi-organ failure, necessitating prompt escalation of care and consideration for liver support therapies or referral for transplantation.

Managing Complications:

- Biliary Sepsis: Requires urgent biliary decompression via ERCP or PTC and broad-spectrum antibiotics targeting common gram-negative organisms.

- Hepatic Encephalopathy: In severe cases of hyperbilirubinemia, particularly with synthetic dysfunction, hepatic encephalopathy may develop. Management includes lactulose to reduce ammonia levels and close monitoring for neurological changes.

46.6 Conclusion

Managing jaundice in the ICU requires a thorough understanding of its pathophysiology, a structured diagnostic approach, and tailored therapeutic strategies. Clinicians should be equipped to differentiate between obstructive and nonobstructive causes and to address the specific needs of critically ill patients, using updated clinical guidelines. Recognizing the potential complications of persistent jaundice and intervening appropriately can significantly impact patient outcomes, emphasizing the importance of a systematic and informed approach.

Algorithm 46.1: Approach to jaundice in the ICU

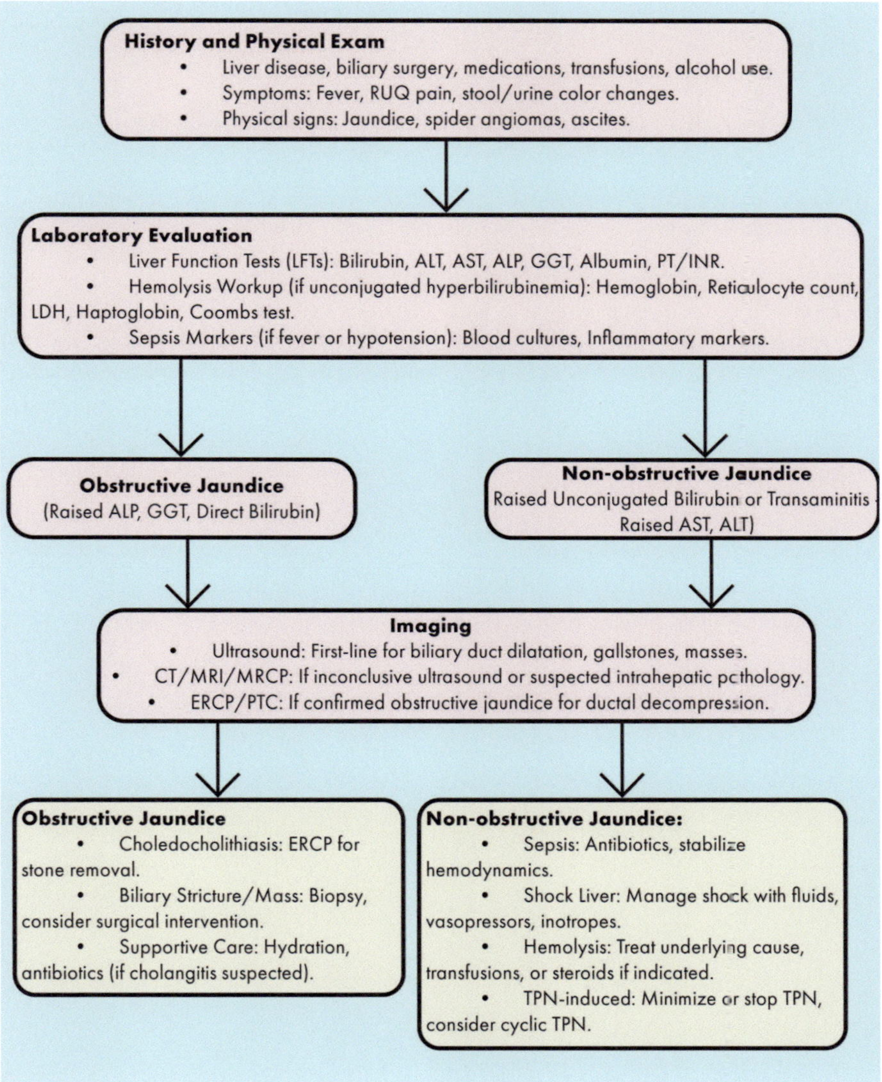

Bibliography

1. Bansal V, Schuchert VD. Jaundice in the intensive care unit. Surg Clin North Am. 2006;86(6):1495–502.
2. Gondal B, Aronsohn A. A systematic approach to patients with jaundice. Semin Intervent Radiol. 2016;33(4):253–8.

Chapter 47
Approach to Nutrition in the ICU

47.1 Introduction

Proper nutritional support is a crucial aspect of managing critically ill patients in the ICU. Adequate nutrition can significantly influence recovery, immune function, and overall outcomes. In the ICU, a structured approach is essential to assess nutritional risk, determine the appropriate method of feeding, and adjust caloric and protein intake [1, 2] [Ref: Algorithm 47.1].

47.2 Assess Nutritional Risk

- Tools: Use validated scoring systems such as the NUTRIC or NRS 2002 score to evaluate a patient's risk for malnutrition.
- Purpose: Identifying high-risk patients allows early intervention, which is critical to prevent further nutritional decline.
- Considerations: It's also important to check for contraindications to enteral nutrition (EN), such as bowel ischemia, which could necessitate alternative feeding strategies.

47.3 Determine Feeding Ability

Can the Patient Feed Orally?

- Yes: If the patient can feed orally, initiate oral intake but ensure it meets their caloric needs. This is often limited to patients with intact swallowing reflexes and a stable mental status.

S. B. Mishra et al., *Mastering ICU Care*,
https://doi.org/10.1007/978-981-95-0179-3_47

- No: If the patient cannot feed orally due to critical illness or other factors, consider other methods like enteral feeding.

47.4 Enteral Feeding Pathway

- High-Risk Patients.
  - For patients identified as high-risk, proceed directly to enteral feeding (EN) unless contraindicated. EN should be initiated early, ideally within 24–48 hours, to help maintain gut integrity and reduce infection risks.
- Not High-Risk Patients.
- Assess whether the patient can tolerate oral feeding. If not, transition to enteral feeding as a primary method, with the same emphasis on early initiation.

47.5 Start Enteral Feeding

- Begin EN with a Hypocaloric Approach: Start feeding within the range of 12–25 kcal/kg/day during the initial 7–10 days. Prefer hypocaloric feeding (up to 70% of energy needs), especially in the first 48–72 hours to prevent overfeeding.
- Rationale: This gradual increase helps avoid complications like hyperglycemia and refeeding syndrome, allowing metabolic adaptation during the critical illness phase.
- Special Conditions: EN is recommended even in certain complex clinical scenarios such as traumatic brain injury, therapeutic hypothermia, and severe acute pancreatitis. Tailoring EN in these cases supports gut function while considering specific clinical needs.
- EN may be withheld in a setting of hemodynamic compromise or instability. EN should be started as soon as possible when the patient gets stable or with caution when there is initiation of withdrawal of vasopressor support.

47.6 Caloric Delivery Monitoring

- Ensure 70% of caloric intake by day 3/7.
- Goal: Achieve 70% of the calculated caloric target by day 3 for high-risk patients or by day 7 for lower-risk patients to prevent caloric deficits.
- If Not Achieved: Supplemental parenteral nutrition (PN) should be considered to meet the deficit.
- Rationale: A hypocaloric approach initially followed by progressive increases ensures caloric needs are met without overfeeding, helping to balance energy requirements with the body's metabolic state.

47.7 Timing of Parenteral Nutrition (PN)

- ASPEN guidance: there was no clinically significant difference in outcomes between exclusive PN and EN during first week of critical illness. It must be noted that PN was not found to be superior to EN, and both had similar risk profiles with improved catheter care, glycemic control, and avoidance of overfeeding energy in PN. It must be kept in mind that PN must be started early (within first 3 days of ICU admission) and must be continued for a shorter duration (5–7 days) and not for longer periods (weeks). This is for the cohort that may be candidates for EN and is to be followed in first week of ICU therapy. However, there is no role for supplemental parenteral nutrition to EN during the first week of ICU stay.
- ESPEN guidance: Start PN if needed: PN should be initiated cautiously, preferably after all strategies to improve EN tolerance have been exhausted. For most patients, initiating supplemental PN before day 7 is not recommended unless they are severely malnourished. PN should be initiated within 3–7 days if there is contra-indication to oral and EN. In patients who do not tolerate full-dose EN during the first week in the ICU, the safety and benefits of initiating PN should be weighed on a case-by-case basis.
- Rationale: Delaying PN helps minimize the risks of infections and hyperglycemia associated with early PN, allowing time for EN tolerance to develop.

47.8 Provision of Dextrose and Amino Acids

- Indication: For patients who cannot receive EN or oral feeds, dextrose and amino acids can be used as temporary measures to provide basal energy and protein requirements.
- Rationale: This ensures that even in the absence of full caloric support, the patient receives some macronutrients to support metabolic functions.

47.9 Provision of Fats/Lipids

ASPEN Guidance

- There is a weak recommendation against a backdrop of low evidence to provide either mixed-oil lipid injectable emulsion (ILE) or 100% soybean oil (SO) ILE to critically ill patients who are appropriate candidates for initiation of PN, including within the first week of ICU admission. It should be limited to a maximum of 100 g/week if there is suspicion of deficiency of essential fatty acids.

47.10 Miscellaneous

ESPEN Guidance

- Postpyloric or jejunal feeds must be initiated in patients with high risk of aspiration (ASPEN definition of high risk of aspiration: inability to protect the airways, support with mechanical ventilation, age > 70 years, reduced level of consciousness, poor oral care, inadequate nurse: patient ratio, supine positioning, neurologic deficits, gastroesophageal reflux, transport out of the ICU, and use of bolus intermittent EN).
- Continuous EN is preferred to intermittent bolus EN.
- First preference is always oral feeding, followed by gastric feeding (EN).
- Prokinetic agents may be used if there is initial intolerance to gastric feeds. Intravenous erythromycin should be used as first-line prokinetic therapy. Intravenous metoclopramide can be used as a second-line agent or can be given along with Erythromycin.
- Enteral feeding should be delayed only if there is a gastric residual volume (GRV) of >500 mL over 6 hours.
- Post pyloric feeding should be initiated if there is no response to prokinetic agents.

ASPEN Guidance

- Inappropriate cessation of EN should be avoided for diagnostic procedures or tests.
- GRV should not be used routinely to assess tolerance to EN. Even if it is routinely used at some centers, then holding feeds with GRV < 500 mL should be avoided.
- High GRV should only lead to implementation of measures to reduce risk of aspiration.
- In all intubated ICU patients receiving EN, the head of the bed should be elevated 30°–45°, and the use of chlorhexidine mouthwash twice a day should be considered. 10–20 g of a fermentable soluble fiber supplement should be given in divided doses over 24 hours as adjunctive therapy if there is evidence of diarrhea.
- EN should not be interrupted in diarrhea till evaluation of the cause.
- Standard polymeric formula should be used in EN initiation.
- Supplemental PN should be considered only after 10 days of unmet targets of energy and protein requirements (60%).
- PN should be discontinued when 60% of the requirement is achieved through EN.
- Fluid-restrictive, energy-dense formula should be used in patients with acute respiratory distress syndrome to limit total intake.
- Similar caloric and protein targets should be aimed even in acute kidney injury (AKI).
- Trophic feeds should be given in moderate to severe acute pancreatitis (after 24–48 hours) and gradually increased to achieve target energy and protein intake.
- Use of PN should be considered in severe acute pancreatitis only after 1 week.

47.11 Caloric, Protein, and Micronutrient Requirements

1. **Gradual Approach to Caloric Intake.**
    - ASPEN Guidance: Feed within a range of 12–25 kcal/kg/day during the first 7–10 days to avoid overfeeding.
    - ESPEN Guidance: Focus on hypocaloric feeding up to 70% of energy needs, especially in the initial 48–72 hours.
    - Incorporation: Starting with a hypocaloric approach and gradually increasing to 70–100% of energy expenditure helps to reduce the risks of refeeding syndrome and metabolic complications during the early phase of critical illness.
2. **Protein Provision Strategy.**
    - ASPEN Guidance: Recommends 1.2–2.0 g/kg/day of protein.
    - ESPEN Guidance: Suggests starting with 1.3 g/kg/day and progressively increasing as the patient stabilizes. Protein requirement should be increased to 2.5 g/kg/day in patients needing frequent dialysis or continuous renal replacement therapy.
    - Incorporation: Clarify that protein requirements should be adjusted progressively during the first week, aligning with the patient's metabolic state and organ function. Higher targets may be needed for patients on dialysis or with significant protein loss.
3. **Micronutrient Supplementation.**
    - Include daily multivitamins to ensure micronutrient needs are met.
    - Supplement with trace elements like zinc, copper, selenium, and others as part of the regimen.
    - Rationale: Critical illness can lead to increased micronutrient losses, and supplementation supports overall metabolic processes.
    - Glutamine should be administered to only burn and critically ill trauma patients and should be avoided in liver and renal failure patients.
    - Daily dose of glutamine (0.2–0.3 g/kg/day) can be administered to critically ill trauma patients for the first 5 days and may be extended to 10–15 days in case of delayed wound healing.
4. **Monitoring and Adjustments.**
    - ASPEN Guidance: Recommends regular monitoring of glycemic control and lipid levels during PN administration.
    - ESPEN Guidance: Stresses the use of indirect calorimetry to guide energy targets and prevent overfeeding. Glucose levels must be kept below 180 mg/dL, necessitating the use of insulin otherwise. Electrolytes must be monitored daily and the blood glucose levels must be monitored every 4 hourly for the first 2 days in general.

- Incorporation: Emphasize the importance of using indirect calorimetry where available or other markers like CO_2 production to tailor energy needs. Adjustments should be made based on metabolic responses to prevent both under- and overfeeding, thereby ensuring optimal nutritional support.

47.12 Conclusion

The structured approach to nutrition in the ICU aims at minimizing the risk of malnutrition, optimizing immune function, and supporting recovery. By prioritizing early enteral nutrition and delaying parenteral nutrition until necessary, it helps to ensure that the unique needs of each patient are met. Adopting a hypocaloric approach initially and gradually increasing to full caloric targets helps prevent metabolic complications. Regular monitoring and adjusting nutritional support based on clinical responses ensure the best outcomes for critically ill patients.

Algorithm 47.1: Approach to nutrition in the ICU

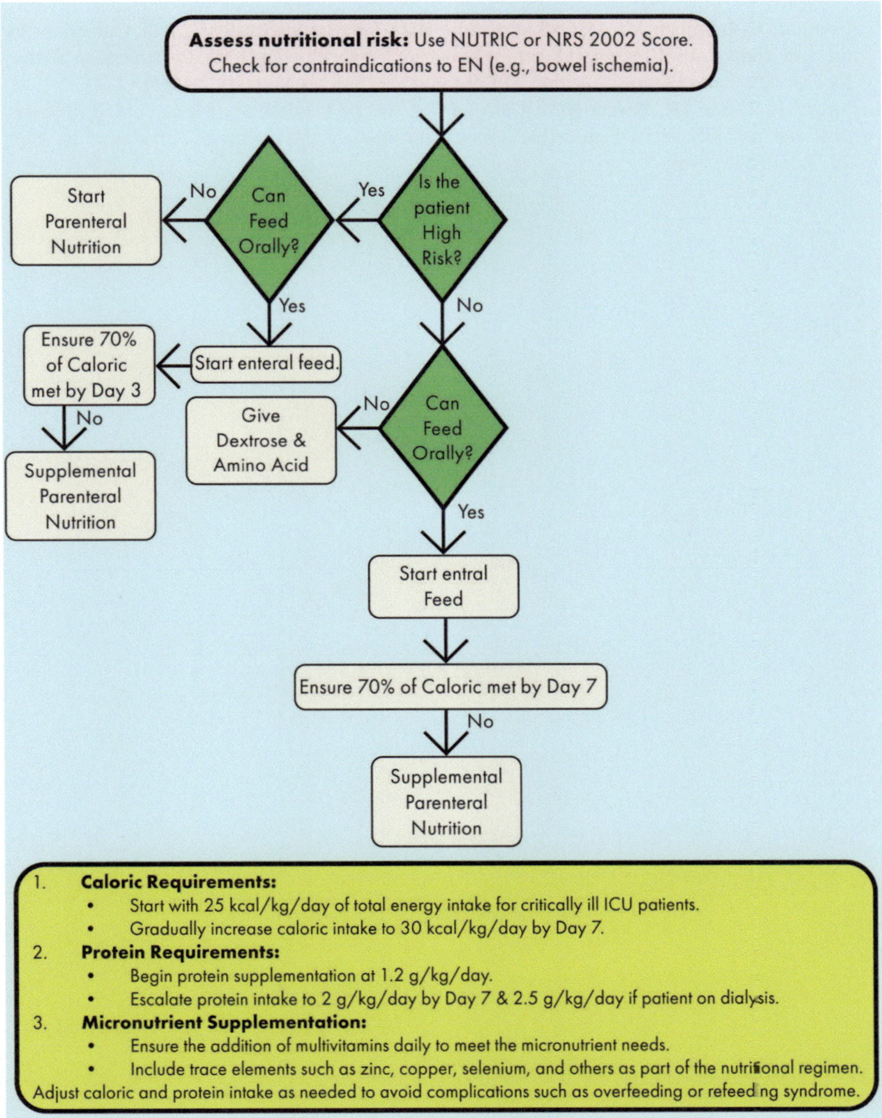

Bibliography

1. Compher C, Bingham AL, McCall M, Patel J, Rice TW, Braunschweig C, et al. Guidelines for the provision of nutrition support therapy in the adult critically ill patient: the American Society for Parenteral and Enteral Nutrition. JPEN J Parenter Enteral Nutr. 2022;46(1):12–41.
2. Singer P, Blaser AR, Berger MM, Calder PC, Casaer M, Hiesmayr M, et al. ESPEN practical and partially revised guideline: clinical nutrition in the intensive care unit. Clin Nutr. 2023;42(9):1671–89.

Part IV
Endocrinology

Chapter 48
Approach to Hyperglycemia in the ICU

48.1 Introduction

Hyperglycemic crises, particularly diabetic ketoacidosis (DKA) and hyperosmolar hyperglycemic syndrome (HHS), are life-threatening emergencies common in ICU settings. Their occurrence can be associated with both type 1 and type 2 diabetes and, without timely intervention, can lead to severe complications and high healthcare costs. The structured approach outlined here offers a comprehensive guide for identifying, assessing, and managing these crises to optimize outcomes and reduce risks [1–5]. [Ref: Algorithm 48.1].

48.2 Epidemiological and Economic Impact

- Increased Incidence: In recent years, the incidence of both DKA and HHS has surged, often due to delayed diagnosis and the rising prevalence of diabetes globally. This trend has placed a substantial burden on healthcare systems, with DKA and HHS admissions escalating the demand for ICU resources.
- Economic Burden: Management of recurrent hyperglycemic crises is costly. DKA and HHS are responsible for high hospitalization costs, especially with recurrent episodes, which frequently lead to repeat ICU admissions. For effective long-term management, reducing recurrence is paramount to controlling these costs [6].

S. B. Mishra et al., *Mastering ICU Care*,
https://doi.org/10.1007/978-981-95-0179-3_48

48.2.1 *Risk Factors and Preventative Measures*

- Risk Factors: Key risk factors include infections, intercurrent illnesses, psychological stress, and omission or insufficient use of insulin therapy. Of these, infection is the most common trigger worldwide. Urinary tract infection and pneumonia are the most common infectious causes leading to DKA and HHS. Stroke, alcohol and substance use, pancreatitis, pulmonary embolism, myocardial infarction, and trauma are the other acute factors that can precipitate DKA. Among the type 1 diabetes patients, omission of insulin therapy, often in the setting of psychological and socioeconomic factors, is a major cause of DKA. Younger age, prior history of hyperglycemic and hypoglycemic crises, presence of kidney disease, neuropathy, depression, smoking, alcohol and substance abuse, and high HbA1c are the other factors leading to increased chances of DKA in type 1 diabetes population. For people with type 2 diabetes, presence of comorbidities is another risk factor in addition to the factors mentioned.
- The risk factors for recurrence are insulin omission, psychiatric conditions (such as depression or substance abuse), and poor social support, all of which can increase the likelihood of repeat episodes. Recognizing and addressing these factors can prevent future crises.
- Preventative Education: Educating patients and families on early signs and symptoms, such as excessive thirst, frequent urination, and fatigue, is critical. Awareness of triggers and preventive strategies can empower patients and reduce the severity and frequency of hyperglycemic events [7].

48.3 Pathophysiology and Diagnostic Nuances

- Differentiation of DKA and HHS:

- Diabetic ketoacidosis (DKA) and hyperosmolar hyperglycemic syndrome (HHS) represent two distinct clinical syndromes along the spectrum of hyperglycemic crises, each with unique pathophysiology and management implications.
- DKA occurs predominantly in patients with type 1 diabetes but can also affect those with type 2 diabetes under extreme stress or during critical illness. It is characterized by an absolute insulin deficiency, which leads to an unregulated breakdown of fatty acids, resulting in ketonemia (elevated ketones) and anion gap metabolic acidosis. In DKA, hyperglycemia is typically present but is less pronounced than in HHS.
- HHS often occurs in patients with type 2 diabetes, particularly elderly individuals with concomitant infections or other stressors. Here, relative insulin deficiency allows for severe hyperglycemia, which causes an osmotic diuresis and leads to extreme dehydration and hyperosmolality (often exceeding 320 mOsm/

kg). However, because there is usually a minimal increase in lipolysis, ketosis and acidosis are absent or mild.

- Differentiating DKA from HHS is essential as they involve different risks and treatment approaches. DKA requires prompt correction of acidosis and careful electrolyte management, while HHS management emphasizes gradual correction of hyperosmolality and rehydration to avoid complications like cerebral edema. This distinction guides treatment priorities, especially regarding fluid management and insulin therapy initiation.
- Euglycemic DKA:
- Euglycemic DKA (eDKA) is a variant of DKA where patients present with the classical metabolic acidosis and ketonemia of DKA but with normal to only moderately elevated blood glucose levels (often <250 mg/dL). This condition is increasingly recognized, especially in patients treated with SGLT2 inhibitors, which promote urinary glucose excretion and can obscure the hyperglycemia typically associated with DKA. Identifying euglycemic DKA can be challenging due to its atypical presentation, as clinicians often rely on elevated glucose levels as a diagnostic marker for hyperglycemic crises. Therefore, in patients taking SGLT2 inhibitors or those with symptoms consistent with DKA (nausea, vomiting, abdominal pain, altered mental status), it is crucial to assess blood ketone levels and blood gas values to detect acidosis.
- Managing eDKA involves similar principles to DKA, focusing on correcting acidosis, managing ketonemia, and stabilizing electrolytes, with the added emphasis on monitoring for hypoglycemia since blood glucose levels may not be significantly elevated. Regular ketone monitoring and close observation for acidosis resolution are necessary throughout treatment [8].
- Diagnostic criteria DKA:
  - Glucose $\geq$200 mg/dL (11.1 mmol/L) OR prior history of diabetes.
  - β-Hydroxybutyrate concentration $\geq$ 3.0 mmol/L (3.8 mg/dL) OR urine ketone strip 2+ or greater,
  - pH < 7.3 and/or bicarbonate levels <18 mmol/L.

Presence of all 3 is necessary to make a diagnosis of DKA.

Serum ketone (β-hydroxybutyrate) levels are more specific than urine ketone (acetoacetate). Urine ketone testing can underestimate the severity of ketonemia early in the course of DKA because of a lag in the formation of acetoacetate, and conversely, overestimate its severity later in the course of DKA when β-hydroxybutyrate is being cleared and converted into acetoacetate. DKA patients usually present with a high anion gap metabolic acidosis.

DKA can be graded into mild, moderate, and severe based on metabolic acidosis, ketonemia, and mental status.

	Mild DKA	Moderate DKA	Severe DKA
Blood glucose levels/history of DM	Glucose ≥200 mg/dL	Glucose ≥200 mg/dL	Glucose≥200 mg/dL
Ketonemia	β-Hydroxybutyrate 3.8–7.6 mg/dL	β-Hydroxybutyrate 3.8–7.6 mg/dL	β-Hydroxybutyrate>7.6 mg/dL
Acidosis	pH >7.25 to<7.30 and Bicarbonate 15–18 mmol/L	pH 7.00–7.25 and Bicarbonate 10–15 mmol/L	pH <7.00 and Bicarbonate <10 mmol/L
Mental status	Alert	Alert/drowsy	Stupor/coma

- Diagnostic criteria HHS: hyperglycemia and hyperosmolality in the absence of severe ketonemia and metabolic acidosis.
  - Plasma glucose ≥600 mg/dL (33.3 mmol/L).
  - Calculated effective serum osmolality >300 mOsm/kg (calculated as [2xNa + (mmol/L) + glucose (mmol/L)]), OR total serum osmolality >320 mOsm/kg [(2xNa + (mmol/L) + glucose (mmol/L) + urea (mmol/L)].
  - β-Hydroxybutyrate concentration <; 3.8 mg/dL or urine ketone showing <;2+ on strip.
  - pH ≥7.3 and bicarbonate concentration ≥ 15 mmol/L (absence of acidosis).

Clinical presentation:
DKA:

- Develops over hours to days.
- Usually alert.
- Polyuria, polydipsia, weight loss, and dehydration.
- Nausea, vomiting, and abdominal pain.
- Kussmaul respiration.

HHS:

- Develops over days to a week.
- Change in cognitive state common.
- Polyuria, polydipsia, weight loss, and dehydration.
- Often co-presenting with other acute illness.

48.4 Fluid Management and Electrolyte Considerations

- Guidelines on Fluid Replacement:
- Fluid resuscitation is the cornerstone of initial management for both DKA and HHS, addressing the severe dehydration common in both conditions.

- Initiation: Start with isotonic saline (0.9% NaCl) to quickly expand intravascular volume and prevent hypovolemic shock. In patients with normal cardiac and renal function, give 500–1000 mL/h during the first 2–4 h. The infusion rate is adjusted based on factors like blood pressure, heart rate, and clinical signs of perfusion. In the first few hours, rapid repletion may be necessary to restore hemodynamic stability. In patients with cardiac and renal compromise, small boluses of 250 mL intravenous isotonic crystalloids must be given. and regular hemodynamic assessment must be done.
- Ongoing Management: Estimated fluid deficit should be corrected in 24–48 hours. 5% Dextrose may be used when blood glucose levels are <250 mg/dL, but the ketonemia is not corrected, mandating continuous need of insulin infusion. After initial stabilization, further fluid management is tailored to serum sodium and osmolality levels. For example, in cases of hypernatremia, fluid replacement may shift to hypotonic solutions to avoid worsening hyperosmolarity and minimize the risk of cerebral edema.

In HHS patients, rate of decline in osmolality should be 3–8 mOsm//kg/hr., and sodium correction should be 10 mmol/day.

- Potassium Replacement Protocol:

- Potassium management is a crucial element in treating DKA and HHS due to the shifts in potassium levels induced by insulin therapy and rehydration.
- Initial Assessment: Before initiating insulin therapy, assess serum potassium levels. If potassium levels are low (<3.3 mmol/L), insulin should be delayed until potassium is corrected to avoid life-threatening hypokalemia.
- Replacement Strategy: If serum potassium is within normal range (3.3–5.5 mmol/L), potassium should be supplemented as insulin and fluids are administered, with typical dosing at 20–40 mmol/L in IV fluids. In patients with initial hyperkalemia (>5.5 mmol/L), potassium should be monitored closely, and replacement deferred until levels decrease due to redistribution from insulin and fluid therapy. Regular monitoring every 2–4 hours is essential to adjust potassium replacement based on ongoing levels and avoid hypo- or hyperkalemia [9, 10].

Routine sodium bicarbonate is not recommended. Fluids and insulin usually reverse the deleterious effect of DKA. Bicarbonate may only be given if the pH is <7.0 to reduce several vascular effects like refractory hypotension.

48.5 Monitoring Guidelines and Complication Management

If DKA or HHS is suspected, initial samples should be taken for glucose, serum electrolytes, venous blood gases, complete blood count, and blood or urine ketone levels.

Resolution of DKA is defined as achieving plasma ketone <0.6 mmol/L and venous pH $\geq$7.3 or bicarbonate $\geq$18 mmol/L [2]. Ideally, the blood glucose concentration should also be<200 mg/dL (11.1 mmol/L). The anion gap should not be used as a criterion, as it may be misleading because of the presence of hyperchloremic metabolic acidosis caused by large volumes of 0.9% sodium chloride solution. Because β-hydroxybutyrate is converted into acetoacetate as the acidosis improves, urinary ketone measurement should be avoided as a criterion of DKA resolution.

HHS is resolved when the measured or calculated serum osmolality falls to<300 mOsm/kg, hyperglycemia has been corrected, urine output is >0.5 mL/kg/h, cognitive status has improved, and the blood glucose is<250 mg/dL.

- Bedside Monitoring with Ketone Meters:

- Bedside measurement of blood ketones, specifically 3-β-hydroxybutyrate, provides a direct marker of ketonemia and metabolic derangement, offering a more precise assessment of DKA resolution compared to blood glucose alone.
- Clinical Practice: Ketone levels should be measured frequently, typically every 1–2 hours during the initial phases of treatment. As ketosis resolves and glucose levels approach target ranges, monitoring frequency may be reduced based on clinical stability.
- Managing Cerebral Edema:
- Cerebral edema is a life-threatening complication, particularly in pediatric DKA patients. It is thought to result from rapid osmolar shifts during rehydration, where excessive fluid shifts into the brain, causing swelling.
- Early Warning Signs: Symptoms such as headache, decreased heart rate, altered neurological status (restlessness, drowsiness), and rising blood pressure are early indicators of cerebral edema. Immediate intervention with hypertonic saline or mannitol is critical in suspected cases to reduce intracranial pressure.
- Preparedness: In pediatric and high-risk cases, hyperosmolar therapy supplies should be readily available, and staff trained to respond promptly to early signs of cerebral edema.

Aims of Treatment

- Rate of fall of ketones of at least 0.5 mmol/L/h OR bicarbonate rise 3 mmol/L/h and blood glucose fall 3 mmol/L/h.
- Maintain serum potassium in normal range.
- Avoid hypoglycemia.

48.6 Insulin Therapy Adjustments

Confirmation of hyperglycemia: To confirm that hyperglycemia is persistent and not secondary to another condition or factor that could be causing elevated blood glucose levels, such as medications (e.g., corticosteroids), infections, or underlying medical conditions. Once these other potential causes are ruled out, the focus shifts to treating the hyperglycemia directly with insulin. Short-acting insulin given intravenously is the preferred choice to lower blood glucose levels.

Rationale for Starting IV Insulin Infusion

- Persistent Hyperglycemia Management: When blood glucose levels remain above 200 mg/dL without any identifiable alternative cause, it suggests that the patient may have inadequate insulin activity relative to glucose levels. At this stage, initiating IV insulin infusion is necessary to control glucose levels, as oral agents or subcutaneous insulin may not provide adequate or timely glucose reduction.
- Insulin Infusion Advantages: Intravenous insulin allows for rapid and precise control of blood glucose levels, which is critical in ICU patients where swift adjustments are often required. IV insulin bypasses the absorption variability associated with subcutaneous injections, ensuring immediate availability and better response in acute settings.
- Low-Dose Insulin Protocols:
- Initiating insulin therapy at low doses (0.05–0.1 U/kg/hr) is recommended after adequate fluid resuscitation, especially in HHS, to prevent rapid osmolar shifts. A bolus of 0.1 U/kg is given as a bolus, and then a continuous infusion is started. The target blood glucose levels must be around 200 mg/dL. 5% Dextrose may be started if blood glucose levels fall below the desired levels. Nurse/institute-driven protocol may also be used to titrate the infusion of Insulin. Insulin infusion can be brought down to as low as 0.05 U/kg/hr. However, it must be kept in mind that insulin infusion is to be continued till the correction of acetonemia.
- Benefits of Low-Dose Protocols: Low-dose insulin achieves a gradual reduction in blood glucose without causing a precipitous drop, which can be dangerous in cases of extreme hyperosmolality in HHS. This approach minimizes the risk of hypoglycemia and reduces the potential for electrolyte imbalances.
- Administration Timing: Starting insulin after 1–2 hours of fluid resuscitation allows for initial hemodynamic stabilization and helps assess the patient's potassium status to prevent complications like hypokalemia.
- Continuation of Basal Insulin:
- For patients with a baseline requirement for long-acting (basal) insulin, it is often beneficial to continue their usual dose during crisis management, even while they are receiving insulin infusions. Continuation of basal insulin prevents rebound hyperglycemia once the insulin infusion is tapered and may stabilize glycemic control, facilitating the transition back to subcutaneous insulin therapy. Long-acting basal insulin should be initiated subcutaneously at 0.15–0.3 units/kg.

48.7 Management Algorithm

48.7.1 Initial Glucose Assessment

Begin by measuring blood glucose levels to determine if the patient is experiencing significant hyperglycemia, which in the ICU setting is defined as blood glucose above 200 mg/dL. If glucose is below this threshold, there is no immediate concern for a hyperglycemic crisis, and regular monitoring at standard intervals should continue to ensure stability, especially if the patient has risk factors for metabolic disturbances. However, when blood glucose exceeds 200 mg/dL, this may indicate a potential metabolic crisis such as diabetic ketoacidosis (DKA) or hyperosmolar hyperglycemic syndrome (HHS), both of which require prompt evaluation and intervention due to their potential severity in critically ill patients.

48.7.2 Symptom and Vital Sign Assessment

For patients with glucose levels over 200 mg/dL, assess for signs of severe metabolic imbalance. Key symptoms to look for include dehydration (e.g., dry mucous membranes, poor skin turgor, hypotension, urine output <0.5 mL/kg body weight), altered mental status (such as confusion, lethargy, or coma), and Kussmaul respirations, which are characteristic of acidosis. These symptoms are often indicative of DKA or HHS, and their presence supports the need for immediate diagnostic confirmation and therapeutic intervention. DKA typically presents with rapid breathing and altered mental status due to acidosis, whereas HHS may involve extreme dehydration and profound mental status changes owing to hyperosmolarity. If such symptoms are absent, continue monitoring glucose while exploring other potential causes of hyperglycemia, such as medication effects or stress responses, to avoid unnecessary intervention.

48.7.3 Presence of Ketones and pH Levels

The next step involves determining whether ketones are present in the blood and assessing blood pH levels to differentiate between DKA and HHS, as both conditions can present with high glucose but require different treatment approaches. Elevated ketones combined with a low pH (below 7.3) strongly suggest DKA, whereas HHS is typically indicated by high serum osmolality (often exceeding 320 mOsm/kg) without significant ketonemia and a pH greater than 7.3. Accurate differentiation between DKA and HHS is essential because each condition requires distinct management: DKA focuses on correcting acidosis and reducing ketones, while HHS management prioritizes gradual reduction of hyperosmolality to prevent cerebral edema.

48.7.4 DKA Management

In cases where ketones are positive and pH is below 7.3, DKA is likely, and immediate management is necessary to prevent progression of acidosis and related complications. Begin fluid resuscitation with isotonic saline to restore intravascular volume. After initial stabilization, fluids may be adjusted to 0.45% saline based on serum sodium levels, aiming for gradual volume replacement over 24–48 hours to minimize the risk of cerebral edema. Following fluid resuscitation, initiate an IV insulin infusion at 0.05–0.1 U/kg/h to gradually reduce glucose levels, inhibit ketogenesis, and correct acidosis. Insulin therapy is crucial for stopping ketone production, while slow, controlled fluid replacement reduces the risk of cerebral edema, particularly in younger patients and those prone to rapid osmolar shifts.

48.7.5 HHS Management

If ketones are absent, pH is above 7.3, and serum osmolality exceeds 320 mOsm/kg, HHS is the likely diagnosis, requiring a treatment plan centered on fluid rehydration to safely reduce hyperosmolarity. Aggressive rehydration with isotonic saline is essential to restore hydration and gradually reduce serum osmolality, thereby preventing dehydration-related complications. Careful monitoring of fluid administration is vital to avoid rapid shifts that could elevate the risk of cerebral edema. Insulin therapy, if needed, is initiated at a low dose (0.025–0.05 U/kg/h) only if blood glucose does not decrease adequately with fluid management alone, thereby preventing unnecessary insulin-related complications. The primary focus in HHS is on achieving fluid balance and osmolar correction, with insulin introduced only when fluid therapy alone proves insufficient for glucose control.

48.7.6 Monitoring Potassium Levels

Potassium monitoring is crucial throughout DKA and HHS management, as insulin and fluid therapy can drive potassium into cells, risking hypokalemia, which poses a serious risk for cardiac arrhythmias. If potassium levels are below 5.5 mmol/L, initiate potassium replacement to maintain levels within the safe range of

4–5 mmol/L, typically adding potassium to IV fluids in accordance with the insulin infusion rate and real-time potassium levels. For patients with initial potassium levels above 5.5 mmol/L, immediate replacement may not be necessary, but levels should be monitored closely to detect any rapid declines. Frequent monitoring and appropriate potassium adjustments are essential to prevent cardiac complications, ensuring that electrolyte levels remain stable throughout treatment.

This structured approach to hyperglycemia management in the ICU ensures that each critical step—glucose assessment, symptom evaluation, diagnostic differentiation, and appropriate interventions—is addressed to optimize patient outcomes and reduce the risks associated with DKA and HHS.

48.8 Special Considerations and Populations

- Elderly Patients and Comorbidities: Elderly patients, frequently presenting with HHS, are at higher risk due to comorbid infections or cardiovascular conditions. These patients require gradual osmolar correction and careful monitoring for precipitating conditions that may impact recovery and increase mortality risk.

48.9 Long-Term and Psychosocial Follow-Up

- Psychosocial Interventions for High-Risk Patients: Integrating mental health assessments, social support, and substance use screenings into postcrisis follow-up can prevent recurrent episodes, especially for patients with significant psychosocial barriers. Regular follow-up with diabetes education and social services support can improve adherence and reduce long-term morbidity associated with hyperglycemic crises.

48.10 Conclusion

This structured approach to DKA and HHS management addresses both acute treatment and long-term prevention, emphasizing the importance of individualized care, psychosocial support, and early recognition of complications. Adhering to these guidelines optimizes patient outcomes, decreases healthcare costs, and reduces the frequency of recurrent ICU admissions for hyperglycemic crises.

Algorithm 48.1: Approach to hyperglycemia in the ICU

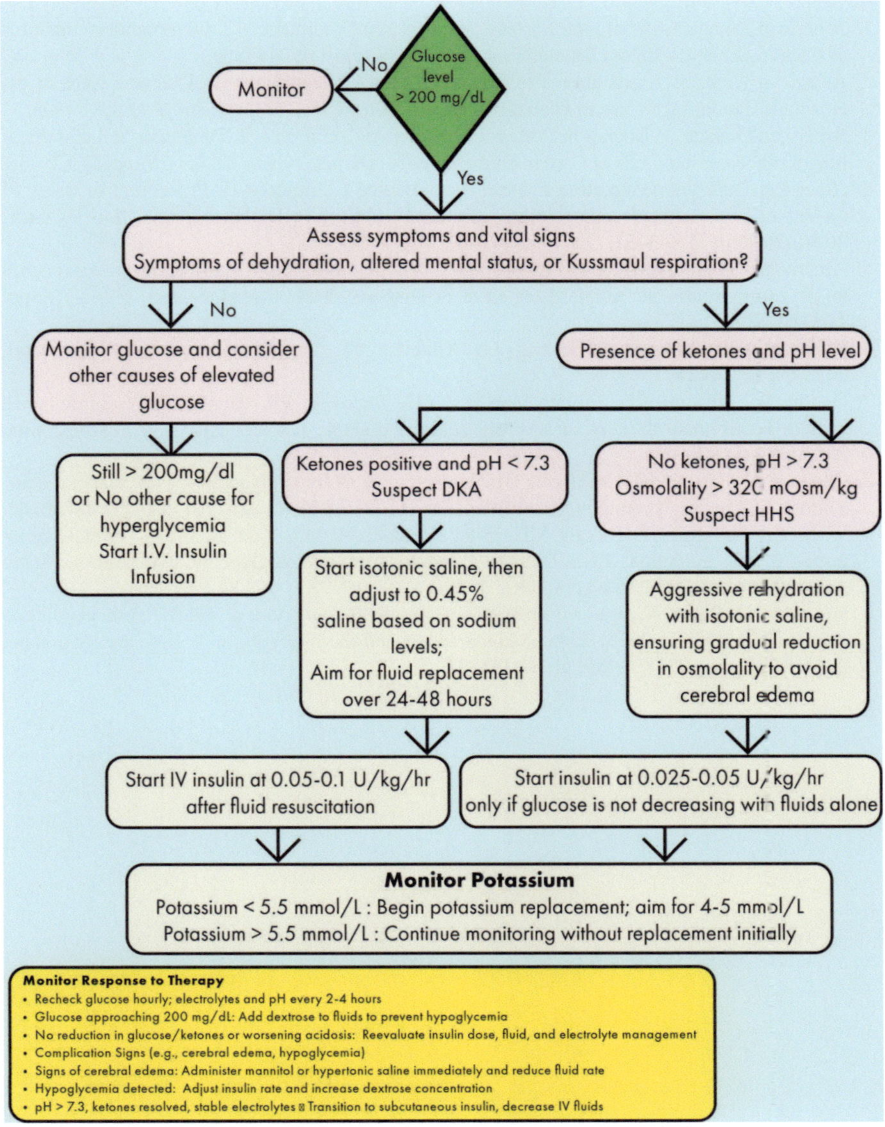

Bibliography

1. American Diabetes Association Professional Practice Committee. 13. Older adults: standards of Care in Diabetes-2024. Diabetes Care. 2024;47(Suppl 1):S244–S57.
2. American Diabetes Association Professional Practice Committee. 16. Diabetes Care in the Hospital: standards of Care in Diabetes-2024. Diabetes Care. 2024;47(Suppl 1):S295–306.
3. American Diabetes Association Professional Practice Committee. 2. Diagnosis and classification of diabetes: standards of Care in Diabetes-2024. Diabetes Care. 2024;47(Suppl 1):S20–42.
4. American Diabetes Association Professional Practice Committee. 3. Prevention or delay of diabetes and associated comorbidities: standards of Care in Diabetes-2024. Diabetes Care. 2024;47(Suppl 1):S43–51.
5. American Diabetes Association Professional Practice Committee. 9. Pharmacologic approaches to Glycemic treatment: standards of Care in Diabetes-2024. Diabetes Care. 2024;47(Suppl 1):S158–S78.
6. Calimag APP, Chlebek S, Lerma EV, Chaiban JT. Diabetic ketoacidosis. Dis Mon. 2023;69(3):101418.
7. Duhon B, Attridge RL, Franco-Martinez AC, Maxwell PR, Hughes DW. Intravenous sodium bicarbonate therapy in severely acidotic diabetic ketoacidosis. Ann Pharmacother. 2013;47(7–8):970–5.
8. Fayfman M, Pasquel FJ, Umpierrez GE. Management of hyperglycemic crises: diabetic ketoacidosis and hyperglycemic hyperosmolar state. Med Clin North Am. 2017;101(3):587–606.
9. Wolfsdorf JI, Allgrove J, Craig ME, Edge J, Glaser N, Jain V, et al. ISPAD clinical practice consensus guidelines 2014. Diabetic ketoacidosis and hyperglycemic hyperosmolar state. Pediatr Diabetes. 2014;15(Suppl 20):154–79.
10. Wolfsdorf JI, Glaser N, Agus M, Fritsch M, Hanas R, Rewers A, et al. ISPAD clinical practice consensus guidelines 2018: diabetic ketoacidosis and the hyperglycemic hyperosmolar state. Pediatr Diabetes. 2018;19(Suppl 27):155–77.

Chapter 49
Approach to Hypoglycemia in the ICU

49.1 Introduction

Hypoglycemia in the intensive care unit (ICU) is a critical condition that can lead to severe neurological impairment and other life-threatening complications if not managed promptly. It is common in patients with diabetes and may also affect nondiabetic patients due to critical illnesses, medication interactions, or metabolic disturbances. A standardized, tiered approach to hypoglycemia management enhances patient safety and helps prevent recurrence, especially in high-risk ICU settings [1, 2]. [Ref: Algorithm 49.1].

49.2 Classification of Hypoglycemia Severity

Hypoglycemia can be classified using the three-tiered approach defined by the International Hypoglycemia Study Group, which provides structured guidelines for the diagnosis and treatment based on severity:

1. Level 1 Hypoglycemia: Blood glucose <70 mg/dL but ≥55 mg/dL. This level typically allows for self-treatment if the patient is conscious and cooperative.
2. Level 2 Hypoglycemia: Blood glucose <55 mg/dL, which requires prompt intervention to raise blood glucose levels due to the increased risk of adverse effects on cognitive function and physical stability.
3. Level 3 Hypoglycemia (Severe): Severe hypoglycemia associated with neuroglycopenic symptoms (e.g., confusion, seizures, unconsciousness) that require external assistance.

S. B. Mishra et al., *Mastering ICU Care*,
https://doi.org/10.1007/978-981-95-0179-3_49

Differentiating between neurogenic (autonomic) symptoms, like sweating, tremors, and palpitations, and neuroglycopenic symptoms, such as confusion, slurred speech, and drowsiness, helps with rapid assessment and informs treatment urgency.

49.3 Addressing Specific Risk Factors for ICU Patients

In the ICU, certain risk factors make patients more susceptible to hypoglycemia. Recognizing and monitoring these can prevent episodes and mitigate risks:

1. Common Risk Factors: These include diabetes treatments (insulin and insulin secretagogues), critical illness, adrenal insufficiency, and sepsis, all of which can disrupt glucose regulation. Highlighting these risks during admission or transfer to the ICU can allow for tailored glucose monitoring protocols in high-risk individuals.
2. Counter-Regulatory Deficits: Patients with autonomic neuropathy, a history of severe hypoglycemia, or hypoglycemia unawareness may have impaired counter-regulatory responses, putting them at higher risk for undetected hypoglycemia. These patients require more frequent blood glucose checks, potentially continuous glucose monitoring, and close observation for any atypical signs of hypoglycemia [3].

49.4 Diagnostic Workup for Nondiabetic Hypoglycemia

In nondiabetic ICU patients experiencing hypoglycemia, a thorough diagnostic workup is essential to determine the underlying cause:

1. Comprehensive Diagnostic Approach: During hypoglycemic episodes, assess plasma glucose, insulin, C-peptide, proinsulin, and β-hydroxybutyrate levels. This aids in identifying causes like endogenous hyperinsulinism (e.g., insulinoma, nesidioblastosis), adrenal insufficiency, or metabolic syndromes.
2. Use of Provocative Testing: When hypoglycemia cannot be observed spontaneously, consider controlled testing, such as supervised fasting or postprandial monitoring, to identify endogenous insulin overproduction or other metabolic abnormalities.

49.5 Interprofessional Management and Patient Education

An effective hypoglycemia management strategy in the ICU relies on collaboration across the healthcare team and proactive patient and caregiver education:

1. Role of Inter-professional Teams: ICU staff, dietitians, pharmacists, and endocrinologists should coordinate to develop individualized care plans for patients at risk. Regular team discussions and medication reviews are essential to adjust therapy and reduce hypoglycemia risk.
2. Education on Hypoglycemia Awareness and Prevention: Educate patients and their families on recognizing hypoglycemia symptoms, understanding its potential triggers, and responding effectively. For patients with recurrent hypoglycemia, involve family or support persons in education about rapid response measures, such as glucose or glucagon administration.

49.6 Prophylactic and Treatment Strategies

Preventing hypoglycemia recurrence in high-risk ICU patients requires both careful monitoring and structured treatment protocols:

1. Enhanced Prophylactic Measures: Continuous glucose monitoring (CGM) can be highly beneficial for ICU patients at high risk of hypoglycemia, as it provides real-time alerts for declining glucose levels. For patients with a history of severe hypoglycemia, glucagon kits should be readily available, and caregivers should be trained on their administration.
2. Treatment Dosage and Timing: For immediate treatment, administer glucose with attention to dosage to avoid rebound hyperglycemia. Once blood glucose stabilizes, provide a 15 g carbohydrate snack plus protein if the next meal is over an hour away. This combination helps maintain glucose levels until the next scheduled meal and prevents rapid glucose fluctuations.

49.7 Management Algorithm

49.7.1 Initial Glucose Monitoring

The first step is to monitor the patient's blood glucose levels. If the glucose level is ≥70 mg/dL, continue routine monitoring without immediate intervention. However, if the glucose level falls below 70 mg/dL, this indicates hypoglycemia and warrants further evaluation and management. Early detection is crucial in preventing complications, especially in the ICU where patients may not display typical symptoms of hypoglycemia due to sedation, intubation, or other conditions that limit their ability to communicate [4].

49.7.2 Assessing Whipple's Triad

If hypoglycemia is detected (glucose <70 mg/dL), the next step is to assess Whipple's Triad, which confirms clinically significant hypoglycemia. Whipple's Triad includes three elements: (1) the presence of hypoglycemic symptoms, (2) a low plasma glucose concentration, and (3) the resolution of symptoms once glucose levels are corrected. If the triad is not present, continue glucose monitoring as part of routine care. However, if Whipple's Triad is confirmed, it validates that the hypoglycemia is indeed symptomatic and clinically relevant, necessitating prompt intervention.

49.7.3 Evaluating Diabetes Status and Medication Use

If Whipple's Triad is confirmed, assess whether the patient has diabetes or is currently using insulin or insulin secretagogues, such as sulfonylureas. If the patient is diabetic or on such medications, it is likely that hypoglycemia is due to their diabetes treatment regimen. This step is critical because it helps differentiate between diabetic and nondiabetic hypoglycemia, directing the clinician toward appropriate management tailored to the patient's underlying condition.

49.7.4 Diabetic Hypoglycemia Management

For diabetic patients, hypoglycemia management involves a detailed assessment of recent insulin administration, timing, dosing adjustments, renal function, and oral intake. These factors can all influence glucose levels. For instance, renal impairment may reduce insulin clearance, leading to prolonged hypoglycemia. Reviewing medication timing and ensuring consistent oral intake are crucial steps in stabilizing glucose levels. Adjusting insulin or medication doses based on this assessment helps prevent further hypoglycemic events.

49.7.5 Nondiabetic Hypoglycemia Investigation

In cases where the patient does not have diabetes and is not on insulin or insulin secretagogues, investigate other possible causes of hypoglycemia. Order specific lab tests, including plasma glucose, insulin, C-peptide, and β-hydroxybutyrate, to identify underlying conditions such as insulinoma, adrenal insufficiency, or sepsis. This comprehensive approach is essential in nondiabetic patients to uncover any metabolic or endocrine disorders that may be contributing to hypoglycemia, ensuring appropriate and targeted treatment.

49.7.6 *Immediate Treatment*

Regardless of the underlying cause, immediate treatment is necessary for all cases of confirmed hypoglycemia. Administer glucose orally if the patient is conscious and able to swallow, or via intravenous (IV) route if the patient is unconscious or at risk of aspiration. In certain cases, glucagon (1 mg glucagon intramuscularly, subcutaneously, or intravenously; repeat in 15 min) may be administered as an alternative or adjunct to glucose, especially when IV access is challenging. Prompt treatment stabilizes glucose levels, alleviates symptoms, and prevents progression to severe hypoglycemia. Nasal spray of 3 mg glucagon in a single nostril can also be tried as an alternative.

49.7.7 *Address Underlying Cause*

Once initial treatment has stabilized the patient, address any underlying conditions contributing to the hypoglycemia. For instance, if sepsis or adrenal insufficiency is identified, initiate appropriate treatment for these conditions to prevent recurrent hypoglycemic episodes. Managing the root cause is essential for long-term glucose stability and reduces the risk of future hypoglycemic events.

49.7.8 *Reassessment and Long-Term Monitoring*

After stabilizing the patient and addressing any underlying causes, reassess the need for continued glucose monitoring and adjust medication regimens as needed. High-risk patients, especially those with recurrent hypoglycemia, may benefit from continuous glucose monitoring (CGM) to detect and prevent further episodes. Additionally, ensure that the patient has a consistent oral intake schedule to maintain stable glucose levels. This ongoing management is vital for preventing hypoglycemia and improving patient outcomes in the ICU setting [5].

49.8 Conclusion

Managing hypoglycemia in the ICU requires a proactive, tiered approach that includes monitoring high-risk patients, educating patients and caregivers, and using structured diagnostic protocols for nondiabetic hypoglycemia. Adopting standardized treatment guidelines, informed by hypoglycemia severity and patient risk factors, can improve outcomes and reduce the likelihood of severe hypoglycemic events in critical care settings.

Algorithm 49.1: Approach to hypoglycemia in the ICU

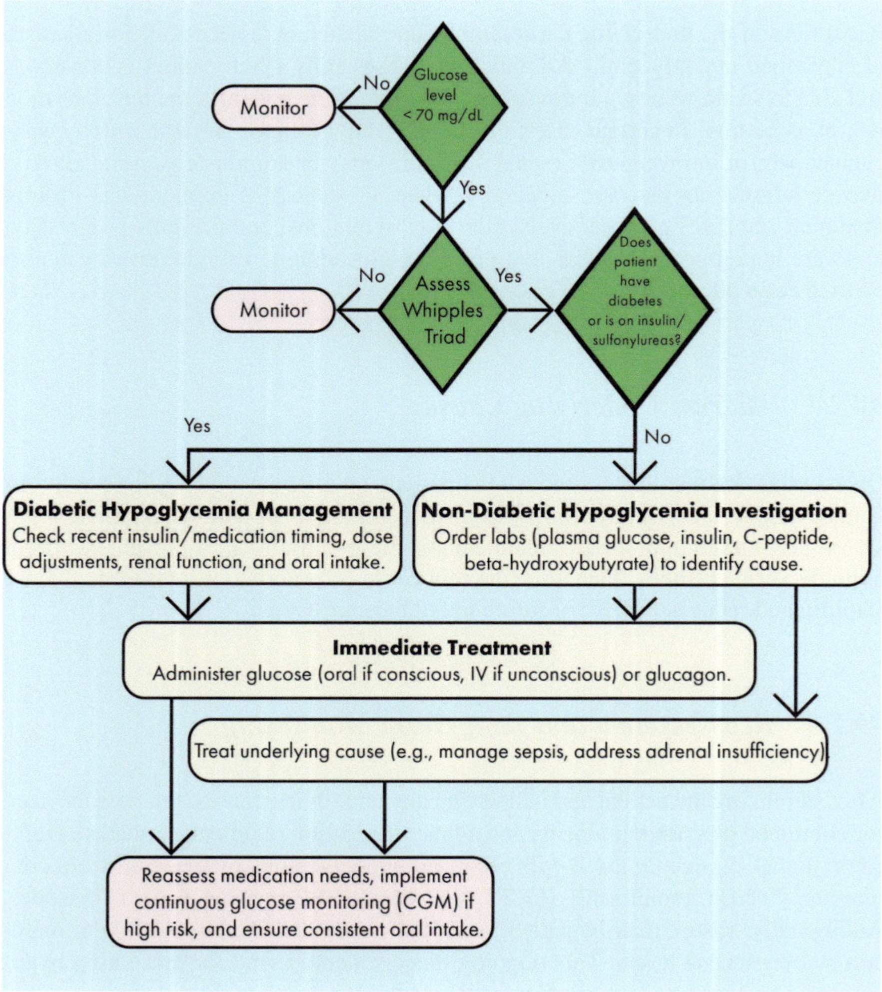

Bibliography

1. Canadian Diabetes Association Clinical Practice Guidelines Expert Committee, et al. Hypoglycemia. Can J Diabetes. 2013;37(Suppl 1):S69–71.
2. Diabetes Canada Clinical Practice Guidelines Expert Working, et al. Hypoglycemia in adults. Can J Diabetes. 2023;47(7):548–59.

3. Cryer PE, Axelrod L, Grossman AB, Heller SR, Montori VM, Seaquist ER, et al. Evaluation and management of adult hypoglycemic disorders: an endocrine society clinical practice guideline. J Clin Endocrinol Metab. 2009;94(3):709–28.
4. Mezquita-Raya P, Reyes-Garcia R, Moreno-Perez O, Munoz-Torres M, Merino-Torres JF, Gorgojo-Martinez JJ, et al. Position statement: hypoglycemia management in patients with diabetes mellitus. Diabetes mellitus working Group of the Spanish Society of endocrinology and nutrition. Endocrinol Nutr. 2013;60(9):517.
5. Reyes-Garcia R, Mezquita-Raya P, Moreno-Perez O, Munoz-Torres M, Merino-Torres JF, Marquez Pardo R, et al. Executive summary: position document: evaluation and management of hypoglycemia in the patient with diabetes mellitus 2020. Diabetes mellitus working Group of the Spanish Society of endocrinology and nutrition. Endocrinol Diabetes Nutr (Engl Ed). 2021;68(4):270–6.

Chapter 50
Approach to Hyperthyroidism in the ICU

50.1 Introduction

Hyperthyroidism in the ICU is a complex and potentially life-threatening condition, particularly in patients experiencing severe thyroid hormone excess, such as in thyroid storm. Early diagnosis and appropriate management are crucial to stabilizing the patient and mitigating risks associated with thyrotoxicosis, including cardiovascular, neurological, and metabolic complications. This chapter provides a detailed approach to managing hyperthyroidism in critically ill patients, emphasizing the assessment of severity, rapid symptom control, and addressing underlying etiologies [1, 2]. [Ref: Algorithm 50.1].

50.2 Order Laboratory Tests (TSH, Free T4, Free T3)

- Rationale: Confirming hyperthyroidism with thyroid function tests is the initial step in evaluation. Suppressed TSH with elevated free T4 and T3 levels typically indicates hyperthyroidism.
- Subclinical Hyperthyroidism: For ICU patients, particularly the elderly, subclinical hyperthyroidism (low TSH with normal T4 and T3) may be relevant. This condition can progress to overt hyperthyroidism or lead to complications like atrial fibrillation and osteoporosis. Treatment may be warranted in patients with TSH <0.1 mIU/L, especially if symptomatic or at risk.

Tests and Interpretation:

- TSH: Low or undetectable in hyperthyroidism.
- Free T4 and T3: Elevated in overt hyperthyroidism; normal in subclinical cases.

S. B. Mishra et al., *Mastering ICU Care*,
https://doi.org/10.1007/978-981-95-0179-3_50

50.3 Assess for Life-Threatening Symptoms

- Rationale: Identifying life-threatening symptoms is critical in the ICU because patients with severe hyperthyroidism or a full-blown thyroid storm can rapidly deteriorate. Thyroid storm is an acute, life-threatening exacerbation of hyperthyroidism marked by a high metabolic state, which places enormous stress on the cardiovascular, neurological, and thermoregulatory systems. Early recognition allows for timely, aggressive intervention to stabilize the patient and prevent multi-organ failure.

Key Symptoms: Classic signs of thyroid storm include:

- Tachycardia: Often severe, with heart rates that may exceed 140 bpm. This reflects high adrenergic activity and increased cardiac output demands, which can lead to arrhythmias, including atrial fibrillation, and high-output heart failure.
- Hyperthermia: Fever is often above 38.5 °C (101.3 °F) and can reach up to 40 °C (104 °F) or higher in severe cases, due to increased metabolic rate and heat production.
- Altered Mental Status: Symptoms range from agitation and delirium to severe confusion, seizures, and even coma. These neurological signs are due to both hyperthermia and the direct effects of excessive thyroid hormone on the brain.
- Arrhythmias: Common in thyroid storm and can include atrial fibrillation, which significantly increases the risk of thromboembolic events, especially stroke.

Other Signs: Diaphoresis, vomiting, diarrhea, and jaundice may also occur, often exacerbating dehydration and electrolyte imbalance, which can further destabilize the patient.

Management Decision:

- Aggressive Intervention: If life-threatening symptoms are present, immediate intensive therapy is needed to control symptoms and prevent progression to multi-organ failure. Treatment should not be delayed for confirmatory testing if clinical signs strongly indicate a thyroid storm.
- Symptomatic Management: For patients with hyperthyroidism but without life-threatening signs, management can focus on controlling symptoms (e.g., with beta-blockers) while confirming the diagnosis and assessing for underlying causes [3].

50.3.1 If Life-Threatening Symptoms Are Present

- **Administer Beta-Blockers (e.g., IV Propranolol or Esmolol)**
  - Purpose: Beta-blockers provide rapid control of tachycardia and reduce cardiac output, essential in managing the adrenergic symptoms of thyroid storm. They block the effects of excess thyroid hormone on the cardiovascular system, improving tachycardia, anxiety, and tremor.

- Choice of Beta-Blocker:
- Propranolol: Preferred for its added benefit of partially inhibits peripheral conversion of T4 to T3, which can help lower the overall hormone activity.
- Esmolol: Often used in patients with contraindications to propranolol or where tighter control is needed due to its ultra-short half-life, allowing for rapid titration.
- Caution: Careful monitoring is necessary, as beta-blockers can lead to hypotension or bradycardia, particularly in elderly or volume-depleted patients. It's crucial to titrate the dose based on heart rate and blood pressure response.

• **Start Antithyroid Drugs (ATDs)**

  - Preferred Drug: Propylthiouracil (PTU) is often the first choice in thyroid storm due to its dual action—blocking both central thyroid hormone synthesis and peripheral T4 to T3 conversion. This additional inhibition of T3 production is particularly valuable in severe cases.
  - Alternative: Methimazole is used if PTU is unavailable. Methimazole is potent and effective in lowering hormone synthesis but lacks PTU's action on peripheral conversion.
  - Considerations: Liver function monitoring is essential because PTU, and to a lesser extent methimazole, can cause hepatotoxicity. Baseline liver function tests are recommended prior to initiation, with careful observation for any signs of hepatic impairment during treatment [4].

• **Administer Iodine Post-ATDs**

  - Example: Potassium iodide is administered after ATDs to inhibit the release of stored thyroid hormones from the thyroid gland, a phenomenon known as the Wolff-Chaikoff effect.
  - Timing: Iodine should only be given after ATDs are initiated to prevent paradoxical stimulation of hormone release. This step helps quickly reduce circulating thyroid hormone levels, providing further stabilization.

• **Add Glucocorticoids (e.g., IV Hydrocortisone or Dexamethasone)**

  - Purpose: Glucocorticoids block peripheral conversion of T4 to T3, reducing the active form of thyroid hormone. They also provide essential support in patients with adrenal insufficiency, which may coexist due to prolonged hyperthyroidism.
  - Dosing and Route: Use intravenous glucocorticoids for immediate effect. Hydrocortisone is commonly chosen due to its dual glucocorticoid and mineralocorticoid effects. Doses are adjusted based on the patient's clinical response, and ongoing assessment is needed to avoid potential adrenal suppression.

50.3.2 Administer Beta-Blockers for Symptomatic Relief (If No Life-Threatening Symptoms)

- Purpose: For patients who do not meet the criteria for thyroid storm but still have symptomatic hyperthyroidism, beta-blockers offer relief from cardiovascular symptoms like tachycardia and reduce the overall adrenergic tone, helping manage tremors and anxiety.
- Choice of Drug and Route:
- IV Propranolol or Esmolol is often used initially to ensure rapid symptom control. Once stabilized, patients can be transitioned to oral beta-blockers, maintaining adequate heart rate control over time.

50.4 Assess for Significant Symptoms or High Burch-Wartofsky Score

The Burch-Wartofsky Point Scale (BWPS) is a clinical scoring system used to assess the likelihood and severity of a thyroid storm. A thyroid storm is an extreme, life-threatening manifestation of thyrotoxicosis, and the BWPS helps clinicians to differentiate between severe hyperthyroidism and true thyroid storm, guiding treatment decisions. Developed by Dr. Henry B. Burch and Dr. Leonard E. Wartofsky, the scale assigns point values based on specific clinical parameters, each reflecting the severity of thyroid hormone excess across various physiological systems.

Components of the BWPS

The BWPS considers six major categories, each with varying points assigned depending on severity:

1. Thermoregulatory Dysfunction (Temperature)
    - Fever is a hallmark of thyroid storm due to increased metabolic activity.
    - Points are assigned based on the degree of hyperthermia, as follows:
    - 37.2–37.7 °C (99–99.9 °F): 5 points
    - 37.8–38.2 °C (100–100.7 °F): 10 points
    - 38.3–38.8 °C (100.8–101.8 °F): 15 points
    - 38.9–39.4 °C (102–102.9 °F): 20 points
    - 39.4–39.9 °C (103–103.9 °F): 25 points
    - ≥40 °C (104 °F or higher): 30 points.
2. Central Nervous System Effects (CNS)
    - Thyroid storm can lead to significant neuropsychiatric symptoms due to heightened adrenergic response and metabolic activity.
    - Points for CNS symptoms:
    - Mild agitation: 10 points.

- Moderate delirium, psychosis, or extreme lethargy: 20 points.
- Seizures or coma: 30 points.

3. Gastrointestinal and Hepatic Dysfunction

- Gastrointestinal and hepatic symptoms occur due to increased metabolic demands, dehydration, and hepatocellular stress.
- Points for symptoms:
- Mild symptoms (nausea, vomiting, diarrhea, or abdominal pain) 10 points.
- Moderate to severe symptoms (jaundice, severe nausea, vomiting, or diarrhea): 20 points.

4. Cardiovascular Dysfunction

- Cardiovascular instability, marked by tachycardia and arrhythmias, is common in thyroid storm.
- Points for heart rate:
- Tachycardia (99–109 bpm): 5 points.
- Moderate tachycardia (110–119 bpm): 10 points.
- Significant tachycardia (120–129 bpm): 15 points.
- Severe tachycardia (≥130 bpm): 20 points.
- Additionally:
- Presence of atrial fibrillation: 10 points.
- Congestive heart failure (CHF): 10 points.

5. Congestive Heart Failure (CHF)

- Often a direct result of high cardiac output, which can exceed cardiac reserves and lead to left ventricular dysfunction.
- Points for CHF:
- Mild CHF (rales only): 10 points.
- Moderate CHF (rales and peripheral edema): 15 points.
- Severe CHF (pulmonary edema): 20 points.

6. Precipitating Event

- Recognizing any underlying or precipitating factor is important, as these can exacerbate hyperthyroidism or trigger thyroid storm.
- Precipitating event (e.g., infection, surgery, trauma, withdrawal of antithyroid drugs): 10 points.

Interpreting the BWPS Score

- Scores >45: Indicative of a high likelihood of thyroid storm. Aggressive intervention is recommended with supportive care, antithyroid drugs, and glucocorticoids.
- Scores 25–44: Suggest impending thyroid storm or severe hyperthyroidism. Close monitoring is advised, with preparations for escalation if symptoms worsen.

- Scores <25: Unlikely to be a thyroid storm. These cases might be managed as severe hyperthyroidism without the full intensive interventions required for thyroid storm.

Utility of BWPS
The BWPS provides a standardized approach to assess thyroid storm, helping guide the urgency and intensity of treatment. By focusing on the most common symptoms of thyroid storm across multiple systems (CNS, cardiovascular, thermoregulatory), the BWPS allows clinicians to identify critical instability early. However, clinical judgment remains crucial, as BWPS is an adjunctive tool rather than a definitive diagnostic criterion.

50.4.1 If Significant Symptoms or High Score Are Absent

- Identify and Confirm Hyperthyroidism Etiology.

Purpose: Differentiating between Graves' disease, toxic multinodular goiter, and thyroiditis aids in selecting appropriate treatment.

- Tests and Markers: Consider TSH receptor antibodies (TRAb) to confirm Graves' disease, especially when etiology is unclear. TRAb testing is also valuable during pregnancy and in assessing relapse risk after ATD therapy.
- Thyroid Imaging Recommendations.

Use Ultrasound: Ultrasound can help evaluate thyroid morphology, identify nodules, and distinguish Graves' disease from nodular goiters. A thyroid scan may also help assess nodules' functional status.

Indications: Nodules or goiters suspected on physical exam, or when malignancy cannot be excluded.

50.5 Track TSH, Free T4, Free T3, and Adjust Therapy as Needed

- Purpose: Regular monitoring is essential to evaluate treatment efficacy and adjust ATDs and beta-blockers as required.
- Considerations: Avoid overtreatment to prevent hypothyroidism. Monitor both lab results and clinical symptoms to fine-tune therapy.

Additional Management Considerations
1. Management of Graves' Orbitopathy

   - Guidelines: For patients with Graves' orbitopathy, avoid radioactive iodine (RAI) in active orbitopathy due to the risk of exacerbation. If RAI is necessary, prophylactic glucocorticoids are recommended for patients with mild-to-moderate orbitopathy to minimize inflammation.

2. Monitoring and Side Effects of Antithyroid Drugs (ATDs)
   - ATD Monitoring: Obtain baseline liver function and complete blood count before starting PTU or methimazole. Monitor for adverse reactions, such as agranulocytosis and hepatotoxicity. Advise patients to report symptoms like fever or sore throat immediately, as these may indicate agranulocytosis.
3. Radioactive Iodine Therapy (RAI)
   - Indications and Preparation: RAI is effective for toxic adenomas and multinodular goiter. Stop ATDs before RAI to enhance uptake, conduct pregnancy testing in women of reproductive age, and carefully select RAI doses based on the patient's clinical status and thyroid uptake studies.
4. Considerations for Thyroidectomy
   - Preoperative Preparation: Beta-blockade, euthyroid status (using ATDs), and iodine (Lugol's solution or potassium iodide) administration reduce thyroid vascularity, aiding surgical outcomes. Thyroidectomy may be preferred in cases of large goiters, obstructive symptoms, or in patients unresponsive to RAI.
5. Management of Hyperthyroid Emergencies (Thyroid Storm)
   - Protocol: In thyroid storm, rapidly administer high-dose beta-blockers, ATDs, and glucocorticoids. Supportive care includes aggressive cooling, electrolyte management, and monitoring for organ dysfunction. Quick, coordinated action is critical to mitigate this life-threatening condition.
6. Follow-Up and Long-Term Management
   - Guidance: For patients post-treatment with RAI or thyroidectomy, regular TSH and free T4 monitoring is crucial to detect hypothyroidism or recurrent hyperthyroidism early. Long-term follow-up ensures timely adjustment of therapy and addresses complications.
7. Special Considerations in Pregnancy
   - Management: PTU is the preferred ATD during the first trimester due to lower teratogenic risk. Switch to methimazole after the first trimester if continued ATD therapy is required. Monitor thyroid function and TRAb levels closely to manage maternal and fetal risks effectively.

50.6 Conclusion

Effective management of hyperthyroidism in the ICU requires a structured approach that prioritizes rapid assessment, appropriate therapy initiation, and continuous monitoring. Identifying the etiology and considering specific patient factors, such as pregnancy or orbitopathy, enables tailored treatment. Regular follow-up with TSH, free T4, and free T3 measurements ensures optimal control, preventing complications and improving outcomes for ICU patients.

Algorithm 50.1: Approach to hyperthyroidism in the ICU

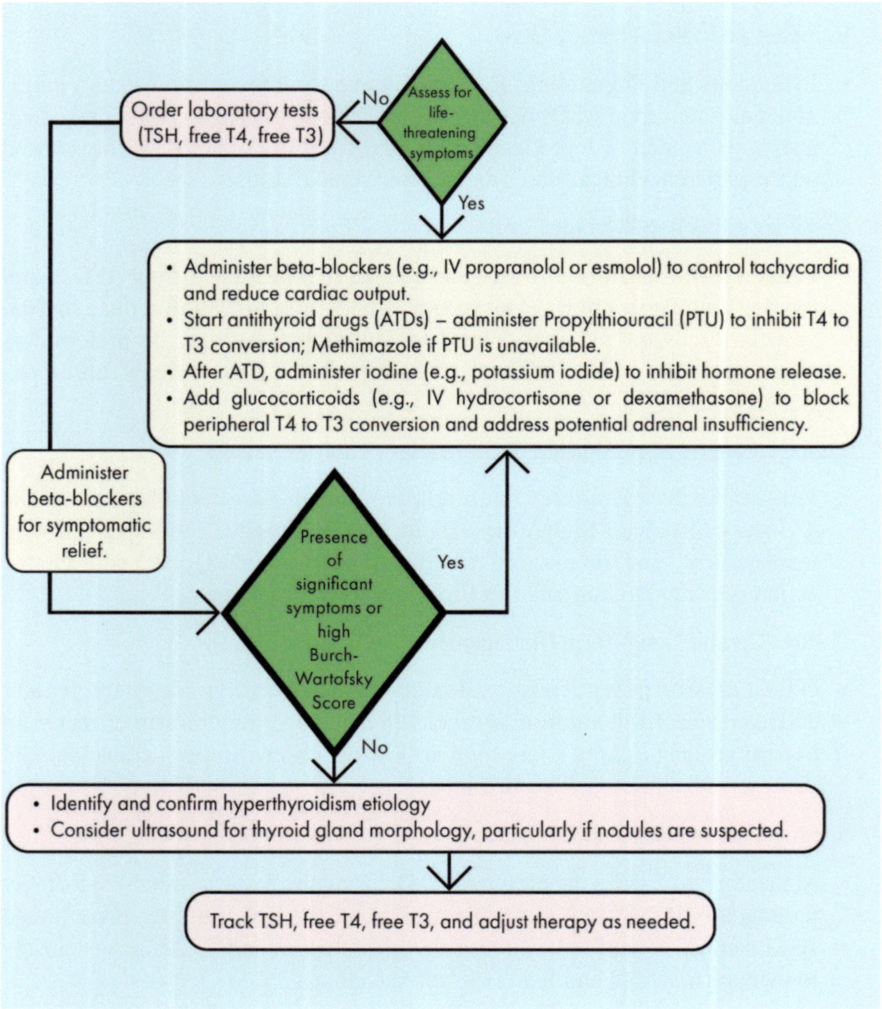

Bibliography

1. Bahn Chair RS, Burch HB, Cooper DS, Garber JR, Greenlee MC, Klein I, et al. Hyperthyroidism and other causes of thyrotoxicosis: management guidelines of the American Thyroid Association and American Association of Clinical Endocrinologists. Thyroid. 2011;21(6):593–646.
2. Kahaly GJ, Bartalena L, Hegedus L, Leenhardt L, Poppe K, Pearce SH. 2018 European thyroid association guideline for the Management of Graves' hyperthyroidism. Eur Thyroid J. 2018;7(4):167–86.
3. Bahn RS, Burch HB, Cooper DS, Garber JR, Greenlee MC, Klein I, et al. Hyperthyroidism and other causes of thyrotoxicosis: management guidelines of the American Thyroid Association and American Association of Clinical Endocrinologists. Endocr Pract. 2011;17(3):456–520.
4. Ross DS, Burch HB, Cooper DS, Greenlee MC, Laurberg P, Maia AL, et al. 2016 American Thyroid Association guidelines for diagnosis and Management of Hyperthyroidism and Other Causes of thyrotoxicosis. Thyroid. 2016;26(10):1343–421.

Chapter 51
Approach to Hypothyroidism in the ICU

51.1 Introduction

Myxedema coma is a rare but life-threatening complication of severe, often long-standing untreated hypothyroidism. It occurs when adaptive mechanisms—such as peripheral vasoconstriction and reduced blood volume—begin to fail. These adaptations can be overwhelmed by precipitating events such as infections or cold exposure, pushing the patient into a critical state requiring immediate intensive care. Early recognition and intervention are crucial, as mortality rates range from 20% to 60% even with advanced ICU support. This chapter provides a detailed, stepwise approach to managing myxedema coma in the ICU, covering initial recognition, diagnostic steps, critical care interventions, hormone replacement therapy, and strategies for addressing precipitating factors [1, 2]. [Ref: Algorithm 51.1].

51.2 Initial Assessment and Recognition

51.2.1 Identification of Symptoms and Signs

Early recognition of myxedema coma is vital due to its subtle presentation and high mortality. Common signs include altered mental status (from confusion to coma), hypothermia, bradycardia, hypotension, and hypoventilation. Importantly, myxedema coma often presents in older adults and during winter months, as cold exposure can exacerbate hypothermia in patients with diminished thermoregulation. A critical red flag is the absence of the mild diastolic hypertension that usually accompanies severe hypothyroidism; its absence may signal impending myxedema coma.

S. B. Mishra et al., *Mastering ICU Care*,
https://doi.org/10.1007/978-981-95-0179-3_51

51.2.2 History Taking

A thorough history is essential, with attention to known hypothyroidism, previous thyroid surgery, or use of medications like lithium and amiodarone, which may contribute to thyroid dysfunction. Recognizing a history of hypothyroidism is critical, as it can direct clinicians to consider this rare but severe diagnosis early.

51.3 Confirming Diagnosis

51.3.1 Laboratory Investigations

Diagnosis relies on serum-free T4 (FT4) and TSH levels. Typically, TSH is elevated in primary hypothyroidism with low FT4. However, TSH can be low or normal in cases of central hypothyroidism or nonthyroidal illness syndrome, complicating diagnosis and highlighting the need for comprehensive testing. Additional laboratory assessments should include tests for anemia, hyponatremia, hypoglycemia, and elevated creatine kinase—common metabolic abnormalities in myxedema coma. Accurate temperature measurement is critical, as automatic thermometers may fail to register the hypothermia typically seen in these patients.

51.4 Immediate Management (Supportive Care)

51.4.1 Respiratory and Cardiovascular Complications

Given the high risk of hypoventilation due to respiratory depression, early intubation and mechanical ventilation are recommended to prevent hypercapnic respiratory failure. Mechanical support stabilizes oxygenation while allowing clinicians to focus on underlying management. In managing hypothermia, active rewarming should be avoided, as peripheral warming may lead to vasodilation and subsequent hypotension. If rewarming is needed, consider central methods like warmed IV fluids, but exercise caution.

51.4.2 Hemodynamic Support

Hypotension, commonly seen in myxedema coma, often results from decreased cardiac output and systemic vascular resistance. Initial management includes cautious fluid resuscitation, but vasopressors may be required if hypotension persists despite adequate fluid support. Careful titration is essential to avoid fluid overload in these patients.

51.5 Hormonal Replacement Therapy

51.5.1 Thyroid Hormone Replacement

The cornerstone of treatment is thyroid hormone replacement, with IV T4 (levothyroxine) preferred for initial administration due to potential gastrointestinal absorption issues. Updated guidelines suggest an initial IV T4 dose of 300–500 μg, followed by daily maintenance at 1.6 μg/kg. If there is no clinical improvement within 24 hours, IV T3 (liothyronine) may be considered, though it should be used cautiously—especially in patients with cardiovascular comorbidities—as high doses may precipitate arrhythmias or myocardial ischemia. A conservative regimen of 10–25 μg IV T3 every 8 hours is recommended, with adjustments based on patient response and cardiovascular risk.

51.5.2 Glucocorticoid Administration

Concurrent adrenal insufficiency is a risk in severe hypothyroidism, as increased metabolic demands from thyroid hormone therapy may precipitate adrenal crisis. IV hydrocortisone (100 mg every 8 hours) is recommended to stabilize the adrenal axis during the acute phase. This prevents adrenal suppression while metabolic rates are restored.

51.6 Monitoring and Addressing Complications

51.6.1 Electrolyte and Glucose Management

Hyponatremia is a frequent complication and can typically be managed with fluid restriction. For severe cases, cautious administration of hypertonic saline may be necessary. In cases resistant to standard management, conivaptan, a vasopressin antagonist, may be considered, although evidence for its use in myxedema coma remains limited. Hypoglycemia, due to impaired gluconeogenesis, should be managed with IV dextrose to maintain stable glucose levels. Continuous monitoring of electrolytes, glucose, and thyroid hormone levels is essential to tailor treatment and monitor response as the patient stabilizes.

51.7 Identification and Treatment of Precipitating Factors

Myxedema coma often results from an acute precipitating event in an already hypothyroid patient. Recognizing and addressing these precipitating factors is crucial:

- Infection: The most common precipitating factor, infection, may not present with fever due to hypothermia. Empiric broad-spectrum antibiotics should be initiated until infection is ruled out.
- Other Triggers: Besides infection, other triggers include cold exposure, trauma, stroke, gastrointestinal bleeding, and certain medications (e.g., sedatives and tranquilizers), which depress respiratory function further. These should be managed or avoided as part of the overall treatment plan.

51.8 Follow-Up and Transition

51.8.1 Transition to Oral Therapy

Once the patient is alert, stable, and able to tolerate oral intake, transitioning from IV to oral thyroid hormone therapy is essential for ongoing management. Oral levothyroxine can be initiated with careful dose titration based on thyroid hormone levels and the patient's clinical response. Gradual increase in oral doses helps to avoid excessive fluctuations in hormone levels during recovery.

51.8.2 Tapering of Glucocorticoids

When the patient stabilizes, glucocorticoid support can be gradually tapered to minimize the risk of adrenal suppression. Monitoring adrenal function as glucocorticoids are withdrawn ensures that the patient's adrenal axis remains intact, supporting a smooth transition out of critical care.

51.9 Conclusion

Managing myxedema coma or severe hypothyroidism in the ICU requires a structured approach, integrating early recognition with targeted thyroid hormone replacement and supportive care. Addressing precipitating factors is equally critical, as these often exacerbate the hypothyroid crisis. Practitioners should balance the need for adequate hormone replacement with caution to avoid excessive cardiovascular stress. Through careful titration of IV T4, selective use of T3, and adrenal support with glucocorticoids, clinicians can optimize care in this life-threatening condition. Early and aggressive intervention, along with a systematic transition to long-term therapy, are central to improving outcomes in myxedema coma management.

Algorithm 51.1: Approach to hypothyroidism in the ICU

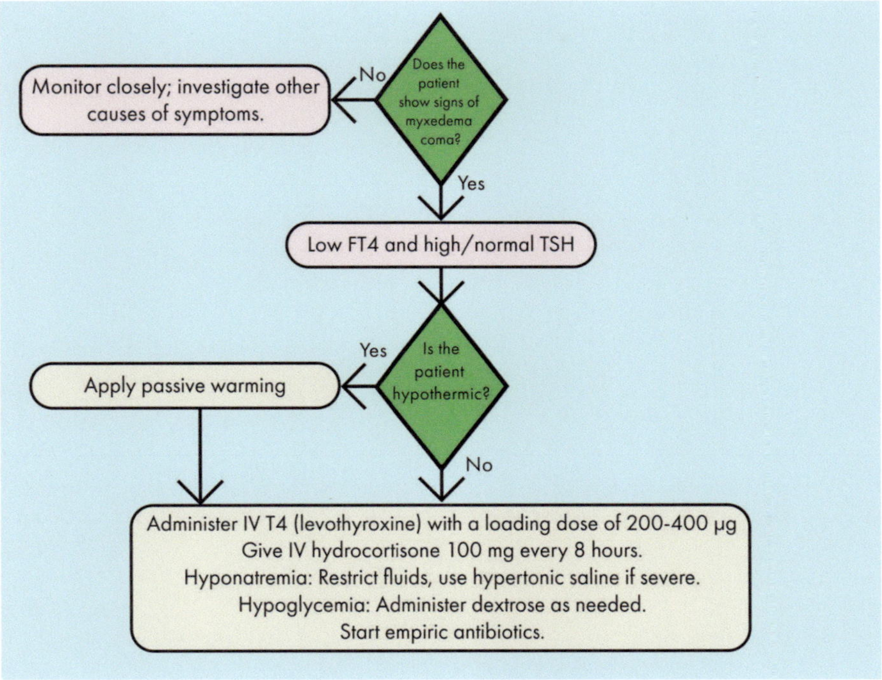

Bibliography

1. Jonklaas J, Bianco AC, Bauer AJ, Burman KD, Cappola AR, Celi FS, et al. Guidelines for the treatment of hypothyroidism: prepared by the american thyroid association task force on thyroid hormone replacement. Thyroid. 2014;24(12):1670–751.
2. Persani L, Brabant G, Dattani M, Bonomi M, Feldt-Rasmussen U, Fliers E, et al. 2018 European thyroid association (ETA) guidelines on the diagnosis and Management of Central Hypothyroidism. Eur Thyroid J. 2018;7(5):225–37.

Part V
Trauma

Chapter 52
Approach to Head Injury in the ICU

52.1 Introduction

Traumatic brain injury (TBI) is a life-threatening condition that demands immediate, structured, and evidence-based management to prevent secondary injuries and optimize neurological outcomes. The primary objectives in the ICU setting include maintaining adequate cerebral perfusion and oxygenation, stabilizing intracranial pressure (ICP), and preventing complications such as hypoxia, hypotension, cerebral edema, and seizures [1, 2]. [Ref: Algorithm 52.1].

52.2 Primary Goals

- Prevent Secondary Brain Injury: Secondary brain injury can result from hypoxia, hypotension, elevated ICP, seizures, and hyperthermia. Vigilant monitoring and immediate intervention are crucial to mitigate these risks.
- Maintain Oxygenation and Cerebral Perfusion: Ensure optimal oxygenation ($SpO_2 > 98\%$) and maintain cerebral perfusion pressure (CPP) between 60 and 70 mm Hg to preserve brain function. Blood pressure control is vital to sustain adequate cerebral perfusion without exacerbating intracranial hypertension.

52.3 Team Dynamics

- Effective Communication: Implement clear communication protocols within the trauma team to ensure timely and coordinated care.
- Role Distribution: Assign specific roles to team members to streamline interventions and reduce delays during acute management.

S. B. Mishra et al., *Mastering ICU Care*,
https://doi.org/10.1007/978-981-95-0179-3_52

52.4 Initial Assessment and Resuscitation (ABCDE Approach)

Airway (A)

- Airway Protection: Patients with a Glasgow Coma Scale (GCS) ≤8 or compromised airway reflexes require early intubation to prevent aspiration and ensure adequate oxygenation.
- Cervical Spine Precautions: Assume a cervical spine injury in all trauma patients until ruled out. Use the jaw-thrust maneuver to open the airway without moving the cervical spine.
- High-Flow Oxygen: Initiate 100% oxygen delivery to manage hypoxia and optimize oxygenation.

Breathing (B)

- Ventilation Management: Adjust ventilation to maintain $PaCO_2$ of approximately 35 mm Hg. Avoid hypercapnia (>45 mm Hg) and hypocapnia (<30 mm Hg), as both can adversely affect cerebral blood flow and ICP. A brief period of hyperventilation ($PaCO_2$ 25–30 mm Hg) may be used to manage immediate neurological deterioration, to buy time for other anti-ICP measures to be initiated.
- Oxygenation: Continuously monitor SpO_2 to maintain levels >98%.

Circulation (C)

- Blood Pressure Control: Maintain systolic blood pressure ≥ 100 mm Hg (for patients aged 50–69, aim for SBP ≥110 mm Hg or above for patients 15–49 or over 70 years) to ensure adequate CPP.
- Volume Resuscitation: Use isotonic fluids judiciously to correct hypotension while avoiding fluid overload that could increase ICP.
- Avoid Hypotension: Hypotension (SBP <100 mm Hg) can exacerbate secondary brain injury by reducing cerebral perfusion.

Disability (D)

- Neurological Assessment: Perform frequent GCS scoring and pupillary examinations to detect any neurological decline. Exclude confounding factors such as drugs, alcohol, other intoxicants, and injuries. Ensure normotension during neurological assessment. The best motor response elicited is a more accurate prognostic indicator than the worst response. The GCS score and pupillary examination must be completed before initiation of sedation or neuromuscular blockade.
- Monitor for Signs of Elevated ICP: Watch for changes in consciousness, pupil size/reactivity, and motor responses.

Exposure/Environmental Control (E)

- Temperature Management: Maintain normothermia (36–38 °C). Treat hyperthermia promptly, as fever can worsen neurological outcomes.
- Full-Body Examination: Expose the patient adequately to assess for other injuries while preventing hypothermia.

52.5 Imaging and Neurosurgical Consultation

- Head CT Scan: Obtain a non-contrast CT scan promptly once the patient is hemodynamically stable. This is critical for patients with a GCS ≤8 or focal neurological deficits.
- Neurosurgical Evaluation: Immediate consultation is necessary for any intracranial lesions requiring surgical intervention or if advanced monitoring is considered.
- Transfer Protocols: If neurosurgical services are not available, initiate transfer to an appropriate facility while stabilizing the patient.

52.6 ICP and CPP Management

ICP Monitoring

- Indications: Place an ICP monitor in patients with severe TBI (GCS ≤8) and an abnormal CT scan, or those with normal CT scans but with risk factors (age > 40, SBP <90 mm Hg, motor posturing).
- ICP Targets: Maintain ICP ≤20 mm Hg to reduce the risk of cerebral herniation.
- Advanced Cerebral Monitoring: Utilize tools like external ventricular drains (EVD) for both monitoring and therapeutic CSF drainage. Bedside transcranial doppler can also be done as an indirect method.

CPP Management

- CPP Targets: Maintain CPP between 60 and 70 mm Hg. Avoid CPP <60 mm Hg to prevent ischemia and CPP >70 mm Hg to reduce the risk of acute respiratory distress syndrome (ARDS).
- Blood Pressure Management: Use vasopressors if necessary to maintain adequate MAP while monitoring for potential increases in ICP. Maintain euvolemia.

52.7 Medical Management

52.7.1 Hyperosmolar Therapy

Mannitol

- Indications: Use for acute ICP spikes or sustained elevated ICP.
- Dosage: Administer 0.25–1 g/kg IV bolus. 1 g/kg over 5 min if a patient under observation develops a dilated pupil, has hemiparesis, or loses consciousness.
- Monitoring: Watch for hypotension, dehydration, and renal function.
- Contraindications: Active intracranial bleed, extradural hemorrhage, severe dehydration, severe pulmonary edema, severe renal disease and anuria.

Hypertonic Saline

- Indications: Alternative or adjunct to mannitol, especially in hypotensive patients.
- Dosage: 3% NaCl solution 250 mL over 30 min or continuous infusion.
- Monitoring: Check serum sodium levels to avoid hypernatremia and central pontine myelinolysis.

52.7.2 Controlled Hyperventilation

- Temporary Measure: A brief period of hyperventilation ($PaCO_2$ 35–40 mm Hg) may be used to manage immediate neurological deterioration, to buy time for other anti ICP measures to be initiated.
- Risks: Prolonged hyperventilation can cause cerebral vasoconstriction and ischemia. It should not be part of routine ICP management.

52.7.3 Sedation and Analgesia

- Medications: Use sedatives (e.g., propofol) and analgesics (e.g., fentanyl) to reduce metabolic demand and control ICP. High-dose barbiturates may be used to treat refractory raised ICP. Hypotension and delay in determining brain death are the factors that go against its regular use.
- Neuromuscular Blockade: Consider in patients with refractory ICP elevations.

52.7.4 Seizure Control

- Early Prevention: Administer anticonvulsants (e.g., phenytoin, levetiracetam) during the first week post-injury to prevent early post-traumatic seizures. It must be kept in mind that early anticonvulsant use does not change long-term traumatic seizure outcome. Prophylactic use of phenytoin or valproate is not recommended for preventing late post-traumatic seizures.
- Monitoring: Observe for side effects and therapeutic drug levels.

52.7.5 Temperature Management

- Normothermia: Actively prevent and treat fever using antipyretics and cooling devices.
- Hypothermia Therapy: Not routinely recommended but may be considered in refractory ICP cases, weighing potential systemic effects.

52.8 Monitoring and Maintenance

Neurological Monitoring

- Frequent Assessments: Regularly evaluate GCS, pupillary responses, and motor function to detect changes.
- Advanced Monitoring: Utilize cerebral oxygenation monitors or jugular venous oximetry when available.

Vital Signs and Laboratory Parameters

- Hemoglobin: Maintain ≥7 g/dL to ensure adequate oxygen delivery. Recent studies show that there is benefit in targeting.
- INR ≤ 1.4
- Blood Glucose: Keep levels between 80 and 180 mg/dL to avoid hypo- or hyperglycemia.
- Serum Sodium: Maintain between 135 and 145 mEq/L; monitor during hyperosmolar therapy.
- $PaCO_2$: Keep within 35–40 mm Hg to regulate cerebral blood flow.
- PaO_2: Ensure ≥100 mm Hg to prevent hypoxia.
- Pulse Oximetry: Maintain SpO_2 ≥98%.

pH 7.35–7.45.
Platelets $\geq 75 \times 10^3/\text{mm}^3$.

Infection Control

- Antibiotic Prophylaxis: Consider around neurosurgical procedures or in patients with CSF leaks.
- Aseptic Techniques: Strict adherence to prevent ventilator-associated pneumonia and line infections.

DVT Prophylaxis

- Mechanical Prophylaxis: Initiate with compression devices upon admission.
- Pharmacological Prophylaxis: Start low-dose anticoagulants once bleeding risks are controlled.

52.9 Surgical Intervention

52.9.1 Decompressive Craniectomy

Indications:

- Late Refractory ICP Elevation: Secondary decompressive craniectomy (DC) is recommended for patients with sustained ICP elevation (>25 mm Hg for 1–12 hours) refractory to maximal medical therapy, occurring within 10 days of injury.

- Early Refractory ICP Elevation: Routine use of DC for early refractory ICP elevation (>20 mm Hg for 15 min within a 1-hour period, within the first 72 hours) is not recommended to improve mortality and favorable outcomes.

Surgical Technique:

- Size of Craniectomy: A large frontotemporoparietal DC (not less than 12 × 15 cm or 15 cm in diameter) is recommended over smaller decompressions to reduce mortality and improve neurological outcomes.
- Procedure Selection: Choice between unilateral (hemicraniectomy) and bilateral (bifrontal craniectomy) decompression should be based on individual patient pathology and neurosurgical judgment.

Considerations:

- Outcome Expectations: While DC can reduce ICP and decrease the duration of intensive care, the relationship between these effects and long-term favorable outcomes is uncertain.
- Functional Prognosis: Discuss potential long-term functional outcomes and quality of life implications with the patient's family or surrogate decision-makers prior to surgery.

Complications: Be aware of risks such as surgical site infections, subdural hygromas, and syndrome of the trephined (neurological deterioration due to absence of bone flap).

Evidence Basis:

RESCUEicp Trial:

- Demonstrated that DC for late refractory ICP elevation improves mortality and increases favorable outcomes at 12 months.
- Patients who underwent DC had lower ICP and reduced ICU stays but experienced higher rates of some complications.

DECRA Trial:

- Showed that DC for early refractory ICP elevation did not improve mortality or favorable outcomes at 6 and 12 months.
- Patients had lower ICP and shorter ICU stays but worse functional outcomes compared to medical management.

Clinical Application:

- Individualized Decision-Making: Consider DC for patients with late refractory ICP elevation after exhaustive medical management.
- Avoid Routine Early DC: Do not use DC as an early intervention for ICP management without clear indications of refractory ICP unresponsive to initial therapies.
- Multidisciplinary Discussion: Engage neurosurgeons, intensivists, and ethical consultants when contemplating DC to ensure comprehensive patient-centered care [3].

52.9.2 Craniotomy

- Mass Lesions: Evacuate epidural or subdural hematomas causing mass effect or neurological deterioration promptly to prevent secondary injury.

52.9.3 Penetrating Injuries

- Object Removal: Do not remove impaled objects without imaging and surgical planning.
- Vascular Assessment: Evaluate for vascular injury before intervention.

52.10 Secondary Survey and Serial Assessments

- Comprehensive Evaluation: Perform a thorough secondary survey to identify other injuries that may contribute to hypoxia or hypotension.
- Serial Neurological Exams: Continue regular assessments to guide treatment adjustments.

52.11 Long-Term Care and Prognosis Considerations

52.11.1 Rehabilitation Planning

- Multidisciplinary Approach: Engage physical therapists, occupational therapists, speech therapists, and neuropsychologists early.
- Family Involvement: Include family members in care discussions and rehabilitation goals.

52.11.2 Complication Management

- Coagulopathy: Monitor coagulation profiles and correct abnormalities.
- Infections: Early detection and treatment of pneumonia, meningitis, or wound infections.
- Seizure Control: Adjust anticonvulsant therapy based on ongoing risk.

52.12 Conclusion

Effective ICU management of severe traumatic brain injury requires a systematic approach that incorporates early airway protection, meticulous monitoring of ICP and CPP, judicious use of medical therapies, and timely surgical interventions. Adhering to established guidelines and integrating multidisciplinary care can significantly improve patient outcomes. Preventing secondary injuries through vigilant monitoring, maintaining physiological homeostasis, and initiating early rehabilitation are essential steps in the recovery journey of patients with severe TBI.

Algorithm 52.1: Approach to head injury in the ICU

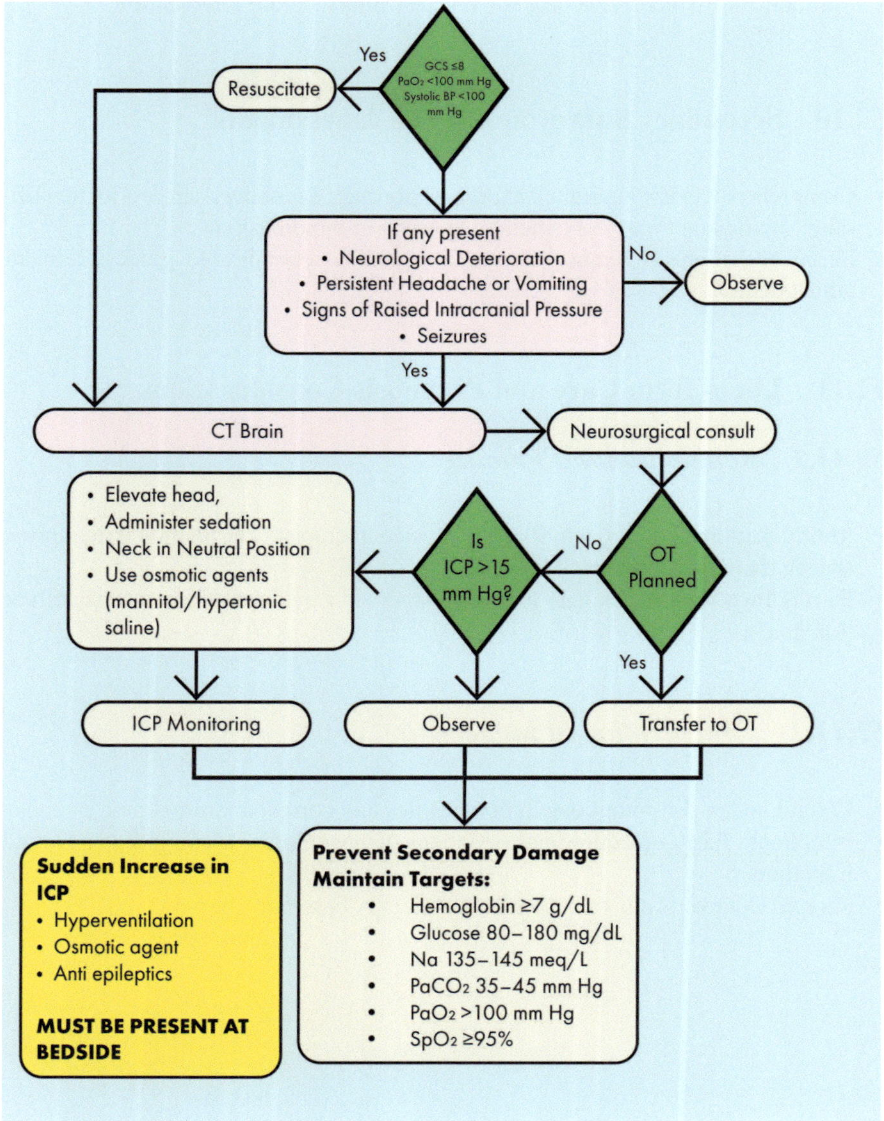

Bibliography

1. American College of Surgeons. Advanced trauma life support (ATLS): student course manual. 10th ed. Chicago: American College of Surgeons; 2018.
2. Brain Trauma Foundation. Guidelines for the management of severe traumatic brain injury. 4th ed. New York: Brain Trauma Foundation; 2016.
3. Hawryluk GWJ, Rubiano AM, Totten AM, O'Reilly C, Ullman JS, Bratton SL, et al. Guidelines for the management of severe traumatic brain injury: 2020 update of the decompressive craniectomy recommendations. Neurosurgery. 2020;87(3):427–34.

Chapter 53
Approach to Spinal Trauma in the ICU

53.1 Introduction

Spinal trauma in the ICU presents complex challenges requiring a systematic, multidisciplinary approach. The initial management prioritizes stabilization, airway protection, and the prevention of secondary injuries, particularly spinal cord damage. Adherence to Advanced Trauma Life Support (ATLS) protocols and careful spinal motion restriction (SMR) are essential during the early phase. Timely imaging, including MRI, plays a crucial role in diagnosing spinal cord injuries and guiding surgical decisions. Moreover, hemodynamic and respiratory support, along with vigilant neurological monitoring, are critical for optimizing outcomes. This chapter explores these key components in the management of spinal trauma in the ICU [Ref: Algorithm 53.1].

53.2 Initial Assessment and Stabilization and Screening

- ATLS Protocols and Multi-trauma Management: Rigorously apply Advanced Trauma Life Support (ATLS) protocols, especially in patients presenting with multiple injuries, to ensure comprehensive and systematic assessment. Prioritize airway, breathing, and circulation (ABC) management, focusing on preventing secondary spinal cord injury [1, 2].
- Spinal Motion Restriction (SMR): For hemodynamically stable patients, utilize SMR rather than full immobilization to avoid complications associated with prolonged rigid immobilization, such as pressure ulcers and respiratory compromise. Recent guidelines discourage the routine use of traditional rigid cervical collars and hard backboards in ABCDE-stable patients due to increased discomfort and secondary risks [3, 4].

S. B. Mishra et al., *Mastering ICU Care*,
https://doi.org/10.1007/978-981-95-0179-3_53

- Prehospital Spinal Stabilization Choices: In prehospital settings, consider vacuum mattresses as a safer alternative to rigid backboards for spinal stabilization. Vacuum mattresses provide effective motion restriction while minimizing discomfort and pressure-related complications.
- Thoracolumbar Trauma Considerations: For thoracolumbar trauma, avoid unnecessary fusion unless fracture instability or progressive neurologic deterioration is noted. Evidence increasingly supports the use of instrumentation without fusion for certain stable fractures. Percutaneous fixation is a minimally invasive option that can reduce recovery times and infection risks.

53.2.1 Screening

Cervical

- The presence of paraplegia or quadriplegia/tetraplegia is presumptive evidence of spinal instability.

Thoracolumbar

- The presence of paraplegia or a level of sensory loss on the chest or abdomen is presumptive evidence of spinal instability.

53.3 Airway Management in Cervical Spine Injuries

- Advanced Airway Techniques with Inline Stabilization: Secure the airway cautiously to prevent exacerbation of cervical spine injuries. Incorporate advanced airway techniques such as awake fiberoptic intubation or video laryngoscopy to maintain inline stabilization and minimize cervical spine movement.
- Avoidance of Cricoid Pressure: Updated guidelines from the Difficult Airway Society (DAS) and the American Osteopathic Association (AOA) advise against the use of cricoid pressure in cases where it might exacerbate cervical spine injuries. Cricoid pressure can potentially cause cervical spine displacement and should be avoided.

53.4 Imaging and Neurological Assessment

The bony level of injury refers to the specific vertebral level at which bony damage has occurred. The neurological level of injury describes the most caudal segment of the spinal cord that has normal sensory and motor function on both sides of the body. Any motor or sensory function below the injury level constitutes an incomplete injury and should be documented appropriately.

Central cord syndrome, anterior cord syndrome, and Brown-Sequard syndrome are the different injury patterns that are encountered in cases of spinal cord injury. Central cord syndrome is characterized by a disproportionately greater loss of motor strength in the upper extremities than in the lower extremities, with varying degrees of sensory loss. Anterior cord syndrome is characterized by paraplegia and a bilateral loss of pain and temperature sensation. Position, vibration, and deep pressure sense are preserved (dorsal columns sensations). Brown-Sequard syndrome consists of ipsilateral motor loss (corticospinal tract) and loss of position sense (dorsal column), associated with contralateral loss of pain and temperature sensation (spinothalamic tract). This is associated with penetrating injury.

Two commonly used scoring systems to decide whether a scan is warranted in cases of suspected cervical spinal trauma are the Canadian C-Spine Rule and the NEXUS (National Emergency X-Radiography Utilization Study) Criteria. Both are primarily used for cervical spine injuries in the emergency setting to determine the need for imaging in alert, stable patients.

53.4.1 Canadian C-Spine Rule

The Canadian C-Spine Rule is a decision-making tool to determine if cervical spine imaging is necessary in alert and stable trauma patients.

High-Risk Criteria (any of these mandates imaging):

- Age ≥ 65 years.
- Dangerous mechanism of injury (e.g., fall from height (1 m/5 stairs), axial load to head, high-speed motor vehicle accident (>100 km/h, rollover, ejection), motorized recreational collision, bicycle collision).
- Paresthesias in extremities.

Low-Risk Criteria (if any of these are present, further assessment can be considered before imaging):

- Simple rear-end motor vehicle accident.
- Sitting position in the emergency department.
- Ambulatory at any time since the injury.
- Delayed onset of neck pain.
- Absence of midline cervical spine tenderness.

Range of Motion Test:

- If low-risk criteria are met, ask the patient to rotate their neck 45 degrees left and right.
- Decision: If the patient can perform this rotation without pain, imaging may be safely avoided.

53.4.2 NEXUS Criteria (National Emergency X-Radiography Utilization Study)

The NEXUS criteria are another widely used set of rules to rule out cervical spine injury without imaging in alert, stable patients.

A patient can be cleared clinically without imaging if ***all*** the following criteria are met:

- No posterior midline cervical tenderness.
- No evidence of intoxication.
- Normal level of alertness (Glasgow Coma Scale score of 15).
- No focal neurological deficit.
- No painful distracting injuries (such as a long bone fracture or significant soft tissue injury).

Decision: If any of these criteria are not met, cervical spine imaging is recommended to rule out injury.

- Primary screening modality is multidetector CT (MDCT) from the occiput to T1 with sagittal and coronal reconstructions.
- MRI Importance and Timing: Perform imaging as early as possible, with MRI being critical for detecting soft tissue injuries and spinal cord damage. MRI should be done on a normal MDCT imaging to rule out occult instability (isolated ligamentous spine injury that results in instability without an associated fracture and/or subluxation). Early MRI aids in intervention planning, surgical decision-making, and provides reliable neuroprognostic information, particularly in determining rehabilitation goals.
- Standardized Neurological Assessments: Utilize standardized neurological assessment tools such as the American Spinal Injury Association (ASIA) Impairment Scale for consistent documentation of injury severity, baseline function, and progression assessment during the ICU stay. Daily ASIA assessments can monitor neurological changes and are crucial for revising long-term prognosis.

53.5 Hemodynamic and Respiratory Management

- Optimizing Hemodynamics: Maintain mean arterial pressure (MAP) goals generally above 85 mmHg to promote spinal cord perfusion during the acute phase of injury. Adjust this target in elderly patients or those with comorbidities and multi-trauma, where aggressive blood pressure management may pose risks. When fluids alone are insufficient to sustain adequate MAP, vasopressors (particularly norepinephrine, dopamine, and phenylephrine) are recommended. Avoid excessive fluid administration to minimize the risk of pulmonary edema.

Spinal shock patients usually do not respond much to fluid. Moreover, they are more likely to present with bradycardia in contrast to tachycardia in hypovolemic shock.

- Monitoring Respiratory Function: Vigilantly monitor respiratory function in patients with cervical and high thoracic injuries, as these can impair respiratory/intercostal muscles leading to respiratory failure. High cervical injury patients may require prolonged mechanical ventilation. In selected cases of lower cervical injuries, noninvasive ventilation support may be beneficial.

53.6 Surgical Interventions and Timing

- Early Surgical Decompression: Advocate for early surgical decompression, ideally within 24 hours, in cases of significant spinal cord compression to improve neurological outcomes. Early intervention can reduce secondary injury and enhance recovery potential [5, 6].
- Minimally Invasive Surgical Approaches: Utilize minimally invasive surgical techniques, including percutaneous fixation, when possible, to reduce recovery times and lower the risk of infection.
- Role of Fusion in Thoracolumbar Trauma: Avoid unnecessary fusion in thoracolumbar injuries unless there is fracture instability or progressive neurologic deterioration. Instrumentation without fusion is increasingly supported by evidence for certain stable fractures, preserving spinal mobility and reducing surgical morbidity.

53.7 Nonsurgical Management

For nonsurgical management of spinal trauma with confirmed injury but no surgical intervention planned, the following medical therapies are suggested based on the guidelines:

1. Pharmacological Management:

    - Steroids: The use of high-dose methylprednisolone for spinal cord injury was widely practiced in the past; however, its routine use is now controversial due to limited evidence of long-term benefit and potential adverse effects. Many guidelines no longer recommend steroids as a standard therapy, but some practitioners may still consider it in specific cases within the first 8 hours of injury, weighing risks and benefits [7, 8].
    - Blood Pressure Management: Maintaining a mean arterial pressure (MAP) >85 mmHg is critical for spinal cord perfusion, particularly in cervical injuries. Vasopressors like norepinephrine may be necessary if fluids alone do not achieve this target.

- Pain Management:
  - Neuropathic Pain: For neuropathic pain resulting from spinal cord injury, gabapentinoids (e.g., gabapentin, pregabalin) and tricyclic antidepressants are recommended. Combination therapy with selective serotonin and norepinephrine reuptake inhibitors may also be considered if monotherapy is ineffective.
  - Ketamine: As an adjunct for pain relief, ketamine has shown effectiveness in reducing neuropathic pain, particularly in the acute phase. It may be combined with opioids or other non-opioid analgesics in multimodal pain management.

2. Respiratory Support:
   - Tracheostomy and Respiratory Management: In cervical spine injuries, respiratory support is often required. Early tracheostomy (<7 days) may reduce complications related to prolonged intubation, especially in injuries above C5. For respiratory muscle support, positioning with abdominal binders or Trendelenburg positioning can help maintain ventilation in patients with compromised breathing.
3. Bladder and Bowel Management:
   - Proactive bladder management is critical due to the high risk of urinary retention and infection. A Foley catheter is generally placed initially to monitor urinary output and prevent bladder distension, while intermittent catheterization may be introduced later as needed.
4. Preventive Measures:
   - Pressure Ulcer Prevention: Patients with limited mobility due to spinal trauma are at risk of developing pressure ulcers. Regular repositioning, the use of pressure-relieving surfaces, and monitoring of skin integrity are essential in ICU care.
   - DVT Prophylaxis: Low-molecular-weight heparin or pneumatic compression devices are used to reduce the risk of deep vein thrombosis, given the high risk of thromboembolism in immobilized patients.
5. Rehabilitation Support:
   - Physical Therapy: Early passive and active physical therapy, focusing on range-of-motion exercises and respiratory muscle training, is crucial to prevent complications such as contractures and to support eventual functional recovery.

53.8 Postoperative Care and Monitoring

- Postoperative Vigilance: In the ICU, prioritize the early detection of complications such as respiratory compromise, infection, and thromboembolism. Implement prophylactic measures where appropriate, including thromboprophylaxis and infection control protocols.
- Ongoing Neurological Monitoring: Conduct daily ASIA assessments to monitor neurological changes, which are crucial for revising long-term prognosis and guiding rehabilitation strategies.
- Neuroprognostication and Family Communication: Engage in transparent discussions with patients and their families regarding neuroprognosis, incorporating MRI findings, injury levels, and severity to set realistic expectations about functional outcomes. This approach facilitates shared decision-making and helps in planning for rehabilitation and long-term care.

53.9 Rehabilitation and Long-Term Management

- Early Mobilization and Rehabilitation: Initiate rehabilitation as soon as the patient is medically stable, focusing on maximizing residual function, muscle strength, and developing adaptive techniques for daily activities. Early mobilization can improve outcomes and reduce complications such as muscle atrophy and joint contractures.
- Multidisciplinary Approach: Employ a multidisciplinary approach involving rehabilitation specialists, physical therapists, occupational therapists, and other relevant professionals. Evidence supports that such a comprehensive team significantly improves functional recovery and quality of life.

53.10 Conclusion

In conclusion, the approach to spinal trauma in the ICU requires a comprehensive, systematic method that prioritizes patient stabilization, early intervention, and continuous monitoring. Following protocols such as ATLS and utilizing appropriate spinal motion restriction techniques are essential to preventing secondary injury. Early surgical decompression, along with minimally invasive techniques, can improve outcomes, while careful respiratory and hemodynamic management is crucial for optimizing recovery. Regular neurological assessments guide clinical decisions, and rehabilitation, initiated early and supported by a multidisciplinary team, is key to enhancing long-term functional recovery. Effective communication with patients and families ensures informed decision-making and supports the overall care process.

Algorithm 53.1: Approach to spinal trauma in the ICU

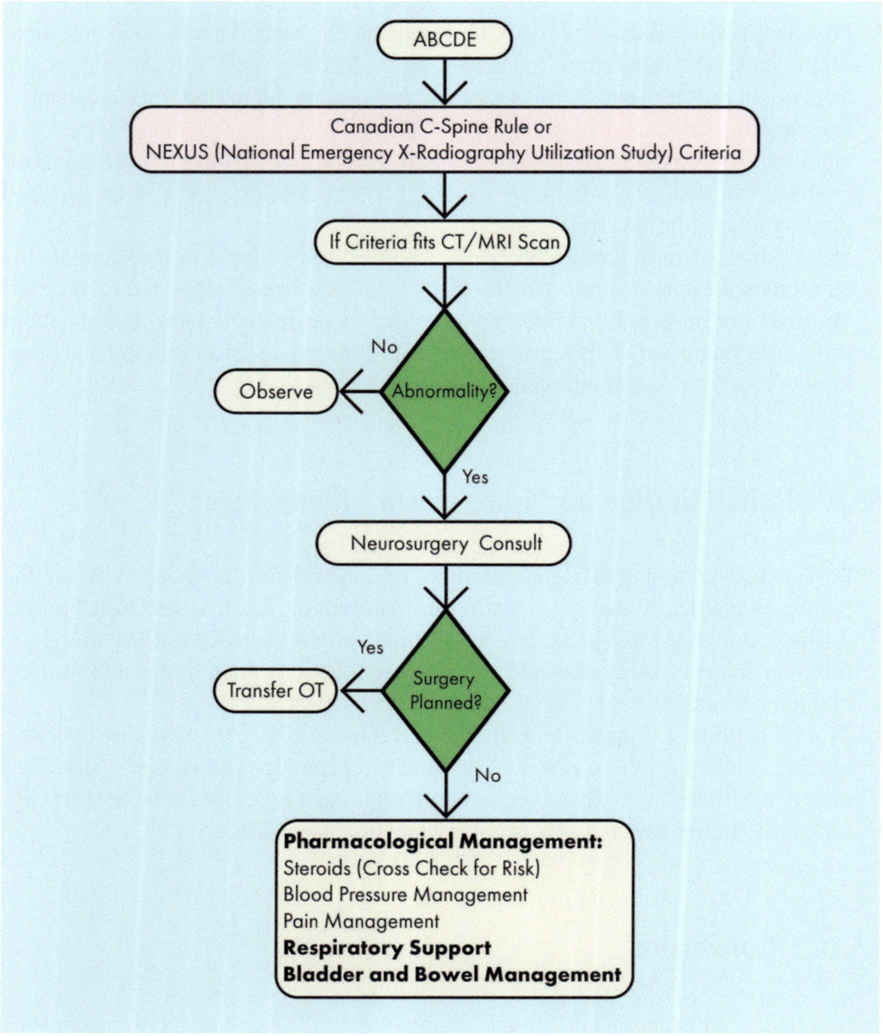

Bibliography

1. American College of Surgeons. Advanced trauma life support (ATLS): student course manual. 10th ed. Chicago: American College of Surgeons; 2018.
2. Roquilly A, Vigue B, Boutonnet M, Bouzat P, Buffenoir K, Cesareo E, et al. French recommendations for the management of patients with spinal cord injury or at risk of spinal cord injury. Anaesth Crit Care Pain Med. 2020;39(2):279–89.
3. Jain V, Chari R, Maslovitz S, Farine D, Maternal Fetal Medicine C, Bujold E, et al. Guidelines for the management of a pregnant trauma patient. J Obstet Gynaecol Can. 2015;37(6):553–74.
4. Chi JH, Eichholz KM, Anderson PA, Arnold PM, Dailey AT, Dhall SS, et al. Congress of neurological surgeons systematic review and evidence-based guidelines on the evaluation and treatment of patients with thoracolumbar spine trauma: novel surgical strategies. Neurosurgery. 2019;84(1):E59–62.
5. Maschmann C, Jeppesen E, Rubin MA, Barfod C. New clinical guidelines on the spinal stabilisation of adult trauma patients – consensus and evidence based. Scand J Trauma Resusc Emerg Med. 2019;27(1):77.
6. Mahanes D, Muehlschlegel S, Wartenberg KE, Rajajee V, Alexander SA, Busl KM, et al. Guidelines for neuroprognostication in adults with traumatic spinal cord injury. Neurocrit Care. 2024;40(2):415–37.
7. Yli-Hankala A, Chew MS, Olkkola KT, Rehn M, Sverrisson KO, Moller MH. Clinical practice guideline on spinal stabilisation of adult trauma patients: endorsement by the scandinavian society of anaesthesiology and intensive care medicine. Acta Anaesthesiol Scand. 2021;65(7):986–7.
8. Wiles MD, Iliff HA, Brooks K, Da Silva EJ, Donnellon M, Gardner A, et al. Airway management in patients with suspected or confirmed cervical spine injury: guidelines from the Difficult Airway Society (DAS), Association of Anaesthetists (AoA), British Society of Orthopaedic Anaesthetists (BSOA), Intensive Care Society (ICS), Neuro Anaesthesia and Critical Care Society (NACCS), Faculty of Prehospital Care and Royal College of Emergency Medicine (RCEM). Anaesthesia. 2024;79(8):856–68.

Chapter 54
Approach to Chest Trauma in the ICU

54.1 Introduction

Chest trauma represents a significant challenge in critical care, necessitating prompt recognition and management to reduce morbidity and mortality. The complexities of thoracic injuries require a comprehensive understanding of pathophysiology, evidence-based interventions, and coordinated interdisciplinary care. This chapter provides an in-depth, algorithmic approach to managing chest trauma in the Intensive Care Unit (ICU), integrating the latest guidelines, advanced diagnostic modalities, and evolving therapeutic techniques to optimize patient outcomes [1, 2] [Ref: Algorithm 54.1].

54.2 Pathophysiology of Chest Trauma

Chest trauma can be broadly categorized into blunt and penetrating injuries, each with distinct mechanisms and clinical implications. Blunt trauma, often resulting from motor vehicle collisions, falls, or crush injuries, involves a forceful impact that leads to compression, deceleration, or blast effects on the thoracic structures. These forces can cause rib fractures, pulmonary contusions, cardiac injuries, and great vessel tears. In contrast, penetrating trauma, such as stab wounds or gunshot injuries, involves the entry of foreign objects into the thoracic cavity, causing localized but potentially devastating damage to vital organs and structures like the lungs, heart, and major blood vessels.

The physiological responses to chest trauma are multifaceted. Hypoxia may occur due to impaired ventilation from collapsed lungs (pneumothorax) or accumulation of blood (hemothorax) within the pleural space. Hypovolemia is a concern in cases of significant blood loss from vascular injuries or massive hemothorax.

S. B. Mishra et al., *Mastering ICU Care*,
https://doi.org/10.1007/978-981-95-0179-3_54

Additionally, the body mounts an inflammatory response to injury, leading to edema and further compromising respiratory function. Understanding these pathophysiological processes is crucial for effective management and intervention.

54.3 Initial Assessment (Primary Survey)

A systematic and thorough initial assessment is paramount in managing chest trauma. Following the Advanced Trauma Life Support (ATLS) guidelines ensures that life-threatening conditions are identified and addressed promptly.

Airway: Assess the patency of the airway, looking for obstructions, facial injuries, or signs of inhalation injury. Look for evidence of air hunger, such as intercostal and supraclavicular muscle.

retractions, and look for any foreign body. Keep your ears open to a stridor or a marked change in the expected voice quality in patients who are able to speak. Look for tracheobronchial injury as patients may present with hemoptysis and severe breathlessness, cervical subcutaneous emphysema, tension pneumothorax, and/or cyanosis. Secure the airway early if there is any compromise, utilizing advanced airway management techniques as necessary. Treat the life-threatening conditions like airway obstruction, tracheobronchial tree injury, tension pneumothorax, open pneumothorax, massive hemothorax, and cardiac tamponade during the primary survey.

Breathing: Evaluate respiratory effort, chest wall movement after complete exposure of the chest and neck, and auscultate for breath sounds. Immediate intervention is required for conditions like tension pneumothorax, which necessitates needle decompression, or open pneumothorax, which requires occlusive dressings to prevent air entry into the pleural space.

Circulation: Assess hemodynamic status by checking pulses, blood pressure, and capillary refill. Look for signs of shock and control any external bleeding. Establish intravenous access (2 wide-bore IV cannula (14-16G) or central line) for fluid resuscitation and blood transfusions if indicated. Measure blood pressure and pulse pressure, and monitor the patient with electrocardiography and pulse oximetry. Look for mottling, pallor, and cyanosis.

Disability: Perform a quick neurological evaluation using the AVPU (Alert, Verbal, Pain, Unresponsive) scale to assess the level of consciousness. This step helps identify any neurological deficits that may result from hypoxia or hypoperfusion.

Exposure and Environment: Completely expose the patient to identify all injuries while taking measures to prevent hypothermia. Hypothermia can exacerbate coagulopathy and worsen patient outcomes.

54.4 Stabilization and Advanced Imaging

After the primary survey and initial stabilization, advanced imaging plays a critical role in diagnosing the extent of thoracic injuries.

Ultrasound (eFAST): The extended Focused Assessment with Sonography for Trauma (eFAST) is indispensable in unstable patients. It allows rapid bedside detection of pneumothorax, hemothorax, pericardial effusion/cardiac tamponade, and intra-abdominal bleeding without the need to move the patient.

Chest X-Ray (CXR): A portable chest X-ray should be obtained as soon as possible in a stable patient to identify pneumothorax, hemothorax, rib fractures, and mediastinal abnormalities. It provides a quick overview but may miss subtle or occult injuries.

Computed Tomography (CT) Scan: A CT scan of the chest offers a detailed evaluation of thoracic structures. It is particularly useful for detecting complex injuries, such as pulmonary contusions, tracheobronchial injuries, diaphragmatic tears, and vascular injuries. Dual-energy CT can enhance vascular assessment and is valuable in detecting aortic injuries.

Imaging Guidelines: In stable patients, a CT scan should follow initial imaging to ensure no injuries are missed. In contrast, unstable patients benefit from immediate bedside ultrasound and portable radiographs to guide urgent interventions [3, 4].

54.5 Resuscitation Measures

Effective resuscitation is crucial to address hypovolemia and hypoxia resulting from chest trauma.

Fluid Management: Begin with cautious administration of balanced crystalloids to maintain perfusion without exacerbating bleeding. In cases of significant hemorrhage, especially with penetrating trauma, early transfusion of blood products is essential. Implementing a massive transfusion protocol may be necessary, using balanced ratios of red blood cells, plasma, and platelets to address coagulopathy. IV fluids must be judiciously used as resuscitation without bleeding source control can lead to coagulopathy and poor outcomes.

Hemorrhage Control: Prompt insertion of chest tubes is required for pneumothorax or hemothorax to evacuate air or blood from the pleural space. For massive hemothorax, defined as the accumulation of more than 1500 mL of blood, large-bore (28–32 Fr) chest tubes are recommended to facilitate adequate drainage. Continuous monitoring of output guides the need for surgical intervention.

Massive Transfusion Protocols: It is defined as receiving 10 bags of packed red blood cells (pRBC) over 24 hours or 4 pRBC over 1 hour. These protocols are vital for patients with ongoing significant blood loss. Early and aggressive correction of coagulopathy, acidosis, and hypothermia—the lethal triad—is critical in improving survival rates. O group pRBC (packed red blood cells) and AB group plasma transfusions are preferred in emergency situations till cross-matching results are made available.

54.6 Pain Management

Adequate pain control is a cornerstone in the management of chest trauma, as pain can impede effective ventilation and lead to complications such as pneumonia.

Multimodal Analgesia: Employ a combination of systemic medications and regional anesthesia to optimize pain relief while minimizing side effects.

- Systemic Medications: Opioids remain the mainstay for severe pain but should be used judiciously due to the risk of respiratory depression. Non-opioid analgesics, including nonsteroidal anti-inflammatory drugs (NSAIDs) and acetaminophen, serve as adjuncts to reduce opioid requirements.

Regional Anesthesia:

- Epidural Analgesia: Particularly beneficial for patients with multiple rib fractures or flail chest. Epidurals provide superior pain control, facilitate deep breathing, and reduce pulmonary complications. Contraindications include coagulopathy and spinal injuries.
- Paravertebral Blocks: An alternative when epidural analgesia is contraindicated. This technique involves injecting local anesthetics near the spinal nerves supplying the thoracic wall, providing targeted pain relief.
- Intercostal Nerve Blocks: Suitable for patients with isolated rib fractures. While effective, they may require repeat dosing or the placement of a continuous catheter for sustained analgesia.

Evidence-Based Recommendations: Guidelines from the Trauma Anesthesiology Society and the Eastern Association for the Surgery of Trauma (EAST) support the use of regional anesthesia techniques. Clinicians should tailor analgesia plans based on individual patient factors, recognizing that responses may vary.

54.7 Specific Injury Management

Rib Fracture

- Non-Operative Management: Focuses on effective pain control and respiratory support through incentive spirometry and pulmonary hygiene to prevent atelectasis and pneumonia.
- Surgical Fixation: Indicated in cases of flail chest, severe displacement of rib fragments, or failure of conservative management leading to respiratory compro-

mise. Surgical stabilization of rib fractures has been shown to reduce ICU stay, decrease the duration of mechanical ventilation, and improve pain control.

Flail Chest

- Defined by segmental fractures of two or more adjacent ribs in two or more places, resulting in a free-floating chest wall segment and paradoxical movement during respiration. Management includes adequate pain control, ventilatory support—often requiring short duration mechanical ventilation. Proper analgesia may include multi-modal approach. Epidural analgesia along with nerve blocks with local anesthesia may help in alleviating the pain to a great extent.

Pneumothorax

- Tension Pneumothorax: A life-threatening condition requiring immediate needle decompression in the fifth intercostal space slightly anterior to mid-axillary line followed by chest tube placement. There are higher chances of decompression when using longer needles (8 cm) than shorter needles (5 cm).
- Simple Pneumothorax: Managed with chest tube insertion. Monitoring for lung re-expansion and resolution of air leaks is essential before considering chest tube removal.

Open Pneumothorax

- Large injury to chest wall that remains open to the atmosphere is known as open pneumothorax and is a medical emergency. For initial treatment, close the defect with a sterile occlusive dressing that covers the edges of the wound. The dressing must seal the wound from three sides, and one side (inferior) should be kept open for a flutter valve effect, so that air is not sucked in during inspiration and the extra pulmonary air is not trapped during expiration. Place a chest tube remote from the wound as soon as possible. Subsequent definitive surgical closure of the wound is frequently required.

Hemothorax

- Massive Hemothorax: Requires rapid drainage with large-bore chest tubes (28-32F) with simultaneous restoration of blood volume. Indications for emergent thoracotomy include initial chest tube output exceeding 1500 mL, persistent bleeding over 200 mL per hour for 2–4 hours, or ongoing transfusion requirements due to hemodynamic instability. Persistent need for blood transfusion is also an indication for emergency thoracotomy.

Cardiac and Great Vessel Injuries

- Recognition: High index of suspicion is necessary for patients with penetrating chest trauma or severe blunt force. Signs of cardiac tamponade include Beck's triad: hypotension, muffled heart sounds, and jugular venous distention.
- Management: Cardiac tamponade requires emergency pericardiocentesis or surgical intervention via thoracotomy. Great vessel injuries necessitate prompt surgical or endovascular repair to prevent exsanguination.

54.8 Advanced Interventions

Video-Assisted Thoracoscopic Surgery (VATS)

- Indications: VATS is increasingly utilized for the evacuation of retained hemothorax, repair of diaphragmatic injuries, management of persistent pneumothorax, and treatment of empyema.
- Benefits: The minimally invasive nature of VATS offers reduced postoperative pain, lower infection rates, shorter hospital stays, and quicker return to normal activities compared to open thoracotomy.

Thoracotomy

- Indications: Reserved for patients with life-threatening conditions unresponsive to less invasive measures, such as ongoing massive hemorrhage, cardiac tamponade not amenable to pericardiocentesis, or major airway injuries.
- Procedure: Requires a coordinated effort by an experienced surgical team, with rapid patient preparation and access to appropriate resources.

Emerging Technologies

- Endovascular Interventions: Offer less invasive options for managing vascular injuries, particularly in the aorta or major branches, using stent grafts and embolization techniques.
- Intrathoracic Vacuum-Assisted Closure Systems: Utilized for large thoracic wounds or infections, promoting wound healing and controlling contamination.

54.9 Monitoring and Secondary Survey

Frequent Reassessment: Continuous monitoring of vital signs, including respiratory rate, heart rate, blood pressure, and oxygen saturation, is essential. Serial laboratory tests, such as hemoglobin, hematocrit, and arterial blood gases, help assess the patient's response to treatment and detect complications.

Imaging Follow-Up: Repeat imaging studies are warranted based on clinical progression to monitor the resolution or progression of injuries.

Secondary Survey: A comprehensive head-to-toe examination aims to identify any additional injuries that may have been missed initially. Particular attention should be paid to potential spinal injuries, which can affect respiratory function and complicate management. Look for other significant injuries, namely, blunt esophageal rupture, subcutaneous emphysema, and diaphragmatic injury. Conditions like esophageal rupture and diaphragmatic injury need immediate surgical intervention. Subcutaneous emphysema may become worrisome in patients on positive pressure ventilation and may necessitate a thoracostomy.

54.10 ICU Management and Rehabilitation

Ventilatory Support: Mechanical ventilation may be necessary for patients with respiratory failure due to severe chest injuries. Strategies should focus on lung-protective ventilation to minimize ventilator-induced lung injury.

Pulmonary Hygiene: Implement measures such as chest physiotherapy, suctioning, and bronchodilators to maintain airway clearance and prevent atelectasis.

Early Mobilization: Initiating physical therapy as soon as feasible helps prevent muscle deconditioning, reduce the risk of deep vein thrombosis, and improve overall functional recovery.

Psychological Support: Recognize the psychological impact of traumatic injuries. Regular assessment for anxiety, depression, and post-traumatic stress disorder (PTSD) is important. Providing access to mental health professionals can aid in the patient's emotional recovery.

54.11 Infection Prevention and Control

Antibiotic Stewardship

- Prophylactic Antibiotics: The use of antibiotics should be guided by evidence-based protocols. Prophylactic antibiotics may be indicated in patients with open chest wounds or following tube thoracostomy in specific situations to prevent infectious complications like empyema.
- Empyema Prevention: Strict adherence to aseptic techniques during chest tube insertion and maintenance is critical. Regular monitoring for signs of infection, such as fever, elevated white blood cell count, and purulent drainage, allows for early intervention.

Chest Tube Management

- Insertion Technique: Employ sterile procedures and proper anatomical landmarks to minimize complications.
- Maintenance: Ensure that chest tubes remain patent and that drainage systems are functioning correctly. Regular dressing changes and site inspections are necessary.
- Removal Criteria: Chest tubes can be removed when there is no air leak, drainage is minimal (typically less than 200 mL over 24 hours), and imaging confirms lung re-expansion.

54.12 Patient-Centered Care

Individualized Plans: Management strategies should be tailored to each patient, taking into account factors such as age, comorbidities, and cultural or personal preferences. This individualized approach ensures that care aligns with the patient's values and needs.

Family Involvement: Engaging family members in the care process provides emotional support for the patient and can improve adherence to treatment plans. Providing clear communication about the patient's condition and prognosis fosters trust and collaboration.

54.13 Quality Improvement and Research

Monitoring Outcomes: Collecting data on patient outcomes, complications, and adherence to protocols is vital for continuous quality improvement. This information helps identify areas for improvement and measure the effectiveness of interventions.

Feedback Loops: Establish mechanisms for regular review of performance metrics and patient outcomes to refine clinical pathways and protocols.

Participation in Research: Encouraging involvement in clinical trials and registries contributes to the advancement of knowledge in chest trauma management. Identifying and addressing evidence gaps can lead to the development of new therapies and improved care standards.

54.14 Conclusion

Management of chest trauma in the ICU is complex and requires a multidisciplinary, evidence-based approach. By integrating advanced diagnostic techniques, adhering to updated guidelines for pain management and surgical interventions, and emphasizing the importance of coordinated care, healthcare professionals can significantly enhance patient outcomes. Continuous education, adherence to standardized protocols, and a commitment to patient-centered care are essential components in achieving the best possible results for patients suffering from thoracic injuries.

Algorithm 54.1: Approach to chest trauma in the ICU

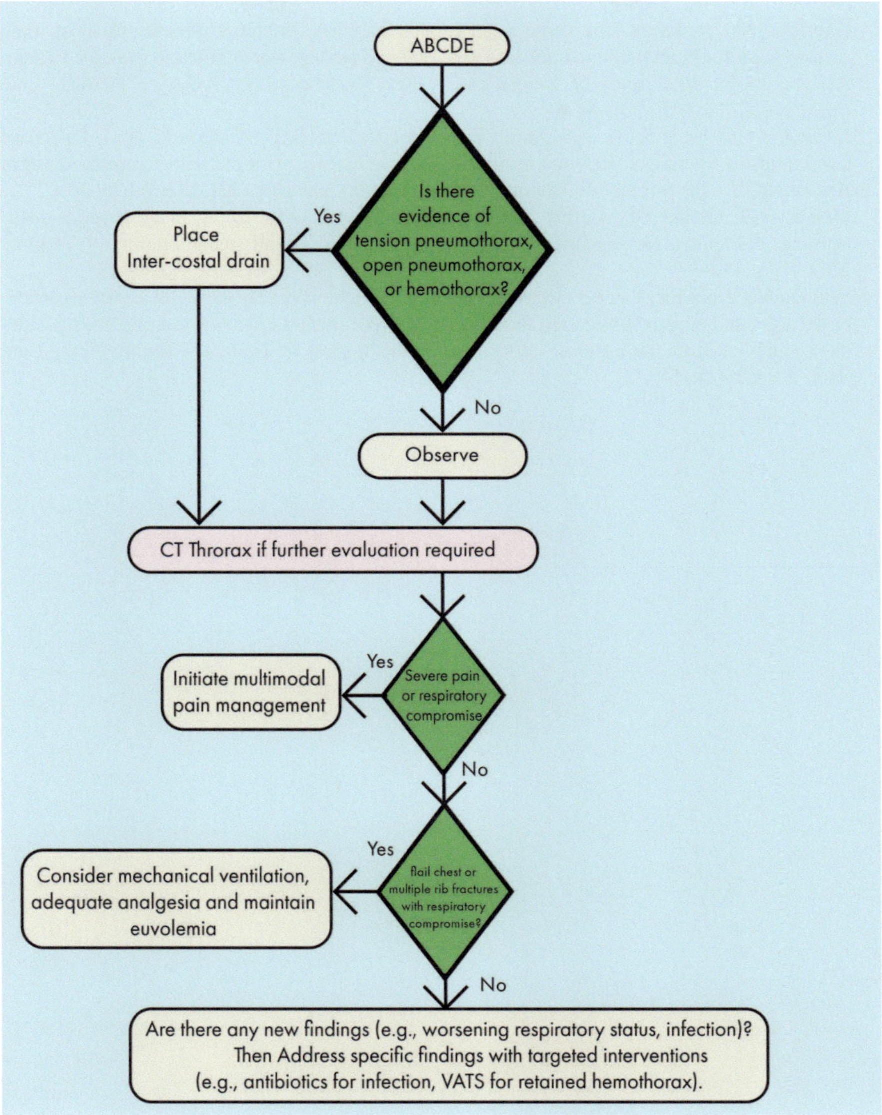

Bibliography

1. Galvagno SM Jr, Smith CE, Varon AJ, Hasenboehler EA, Sultan S, Shaefer G, et al. Pain management for blunt thoracic trauma: a joint practice management guideline from the Eastern Association for the Surgery of Trauma and Trauma Anesthesiology Society. J Trauma Acute Care Surg. 2016;81(5):936–51.
2. Kasotakis G, Hasenboehler EA, Streib EW, Patel N, Patel MB, Alarcon L, et al. Operative fixation of rib fractures after blunt trauma: a practice management guideline from the Eastern Association for the Surgery of Trauma. J Trauma Acute Care Surg. 2017;82(3):618–26.
3. Mowery NT, Gunter OL, Collier BR, Diaz JJ Jr, Haut E, Hildreth A, et al. Practice management guidelines for management of hemothorax and occult pneumothorax. J Trauma. 2011;70(2):510–8.
4. Seamon MJ, Haut ER, Van Arendonk K, Barbosa RR, Chiu WC, Dente CJ, et al. An evidence-based approach to patient selection for emergency department thoracotomy: a practice management guideline from the Eastern Association for the Surgery of Trauma. J Trauma Acute Care Surg. 2015;79(1):159–73.

Chapter 55
Approach to Abdominal Trauma in the ICU

55.1 Introduction

Abdominal trauma is a significant cause of morbidity and mortality worldwide, frequently leading to intensive care unit (ICU) admissions. The mechanisms of injury are diverse, encompassing blunt and penetrating trauma resulting from vehicle accidents, falls, sports injuries, assaults, domestic violence, and industrial accidents. In the United States, blunt abdominal trauma is more prevalent and often involves injuries to solid organs like the spleen, liver, and kidneys, as well as hollow viscera such as the intestines. Penetrating trauma, while less common, can be life-threatening and typically requires surgical intervention.

Epidemiological data indicate that abdominal trauma accounts for a substantial proportion of ICU admissions related to trauma, with high mortality rates, especially in cases involving multiple organ injuries or delayed diagnosis. The complexity of abdominal trauma is compounded by the risk of missed injuries and the subtlety of certain injury types, such as bowel and mesenteric injuries, which can complicate diagnosis and increase morbidity [1, 2] [Ref: Algorithm 55.1].

55.2 Initial Assessment

A prompt and structured approach to the initial assessment of abdominal trauma patients is critical. The Advanced Trauma Life Support (ATLS) guidelines recommend a systematic evaluation following the ABCDE (Airway, Breathing, Circulation, Disability, Exposure) protocol.

- Airway: Ensure airway patency while maintaining cervical spine precautions. Look for signs of airway obstruction or compromise.

S. B. Mishra et al., *Mastering ICU Care*,
https://doi.org/10.1007/978-981-95-0179-3_55

- Breathing: Assess ventilation and oxygenation status. Identify signs of respiratory distress, tension pneumothorax, hemothorax, or other thoracic injuries that may accompany abdominal trauma.
- Circulation: Evaluate hemodynamic status by checking pulse rate, blood pressure, and capillary refill. Initiate rapid fluid resuscitation if hypotension is present. Recognize signs of shock and control any external bleeding sources. Source control of hemorrhage and replacement of blood volume is necessary to maintain circulation. Mechanical stabilization of the pelvic ring and external counterpressure are necessary to reduce volume loss in case of pelvic injury. Pelvic binder can be used to temporarily fix the unstable pelvis if applied at level of greater trochanters of the femur.
- Disability: Perform a rapid neurological assessment using the Glasgow Coma Scale (GCS) to identify any brain injury or decreased level of consciousness.
- Exposure: Fully expose the patient to assess for additional injuries while preventing hypothermia. This involves removing clothing and conducting a thorough head-to-toe examination. Temperature management is essential, as hypothermia can exacerbate coagulopathy and shock.

In addition to the primary survey, early assessment of biomarkers such as lactate levels can provide insight into tissue perfusion and the severity of internal injuries. Elevated lactate may indicate hypoperfusion and is associated with increased morbidity. Procalcitonin levels can be considered, especially when there is a high suspicion of bowel or mesenteric trauma, as elevated levels may suggest bacterial translocation or infection.

55.3 Focused Abdominal Assessment

A detailed abdominal examination is crucial in identifying signs of internal injury.

- High-Risk Signs: Recognize specific external markers that correlate with serious internal injuries. The "seatbelt sign" (bruising across the abdomen from a seatbelt) is associated with an increased risk of bowel and mesenteric injuries. Cullen's sign (periumbilical ecchymosis) and Grey Turner's sign (flank ecchymosis) suggest retroperitoneal bleeding or pancreatic injury and warrant immediate investigation.
- Physical Examination: Look for tenderness, guarding, rigidity, distension, or bruising. Auscultate for bowel sounds, noting any absence that may indicate ileus or peritonitis.
- Dynamic Serial Examinations: Due to the possibility of delayed presentation of certain injuries, serial abdominal examinations are invaluable. Repeated assessments can detect evolving signs of peritoneal irritation or hemodynamic instability, particularly in hollow viscus or mesenteric injuries that may not be apparent initially.

55.4 Imaging and Diagnostic Tools

Imaging plays a pivotal role in the evaluation of abdominal trauma.

- E-FAST/eFAST (Extended Focused Assessment with Sonography for Trauma): An extension of the traditional FAST exam, E-FAST includes the thoracic cavity to detect pneumothorax and hemothorax, which is crucial in polytrauma patients. While E-FAST is rapid and noninvasive, it has limitations in detecting hollow viscus injuries and retroperitoneal bleeding. In case of unavailability of eFAST, diagnostic peritoneal lavage may be done by surgeons in hemodynamically unstable patients or in patients with multiple puncture wounds.
- Computed Tomography (CT) Scan: Contrast-enhanced CT scanning is the gold standard for stable patients. It provides detailed visualization of solid organ injuries and vascular damage and can suggest hollow viscus injuries through findings like free air or fluid without solid organ injury.
- Role of Repeat Imaging: In cases where initial imaging is inconclusive or the patient's clinical status changes, repeat imaging is essential. Guidelines recommend that for equivocal findings, repeat CT scans should be performed within a specific time frame (e.g., within 6 hours) to reassess and detect any progression of injuries.
- Limitations of Imaging: Be aware that certain injuries may not be detected on initial imaging studies. Hence, a high index of suspicion and clinical correlation are necessary.

55.5 Management Strategies

Management of abdominal trauma requires a tailored approach based on the patient's hemodynamic status and injury severity.

- Damage Control Surgery (DCS): In unstable patients with life-threatening injuries, DCS focuses on controlling hemorrhage and contamination with abbreviated surgical procedures. Definitive repair is deferred until physiological stabilization is achieved. This approach reduces operative time and allows for correction of coagulopathy, hypothermia, and acidosis.
- Nonoperative Management (NOM): Hemodynamically stable patients without peritoneal signs or other indications for immediate surgery may be managed non-operatively. Criteria for NOM include stable vital signs, controlled bleeding, and absence of hollow viscus injury. Close monitoring in an ICU setting with predefined thresholds for surgical intervention is critical, as delayed deterioration can occur.
- Angioembolization: In select stable patients with solid organ injuries, angioembolization can control bleeding and preserve organ function. It is less invasive than laparotomy and can be an effective alternative, especially for injuries to the spleen, liver, or kidneys.

55.6 Specific Injuries and Management

- Solid Organ Injuries: Management depends on the grade of injury and hemodynamic status. For liver and spleen injuries, nonoperative management is preferred in stable patients. Transitioning to operative management is indicated for ongoing bleeding, hemodynamic instability, or failure of conservative measures.
- Hollow Viscus Injuries: These injuries are challenging to diagnose and have a high risk of being missed. Signs such as free intraperitoneal air on imaging, unexplained peritoneal fluid, or persistent abdominal pain should raise suspicion. Surgical exploration is recommended when conservative measures fail or if there is evidence of perforation or peritonitis.
- Mesenteric Injuries: Mesenteric tears may not cause significant bleeding initially but can lead to ischemia and necrosis of bowel segments if untreated. Indications for surgical exploration include signs of mesenteric hematoma, devascularization of bowel segments on imaging, or clinical signs of ischemia.

55.7 Monitoring and Follow-Up

- Utilization of Biomarkers: Serial measurements of biomarkers like procalcitonin can aid in monitoring patients managed non-operatively. Rising levels may indicate infection or the development of bowel injury, prompting reevaluation.
- Importance of Reassessment: Frequent clinical reassessment is crucial. Changes in vital signs, abdominal examination findings, or laboratory results should prompt reevaluation. Guidelines suggest regular observation intervals and repeat imaging as necessary.

55.8 Complications and Prognosis

- Infection Prevention: There is a high risk of intra-abdominal infections, such as peritonitis and abscess formation, particularly with bowel injuries or delayed intervention. Early administration of appropriate antibiotics and close monitoring for signs of sepsis are essential components of management.
- Long-Term Outcomes: Despite advances in trauma care, patients with severe abdominal injuries face significant morbidity and mortality. Complications related to missed injuries, delayed interventions, and chronic conditions like adhesions, bowel obstruction, and postoperative infections can impact long-term outcomes.

55.9 Conclusion

Effective management of abdominal trauma in the ICU requires a structured, multi-disciplinary approach and adherence to established guidelines. Early recognition of injury patterns, prompt imaging, vigilant monitoring, and timely interventions are critical in reducing morbidity and mortality. By integrating clinical assessment with diagnostic tools and adopting individualized management strategies, healthcare providers can improve survival and outcomes for patients with abdominal trauma.

Algorithm 55.1: Approach to abdominal trauma in the ICU

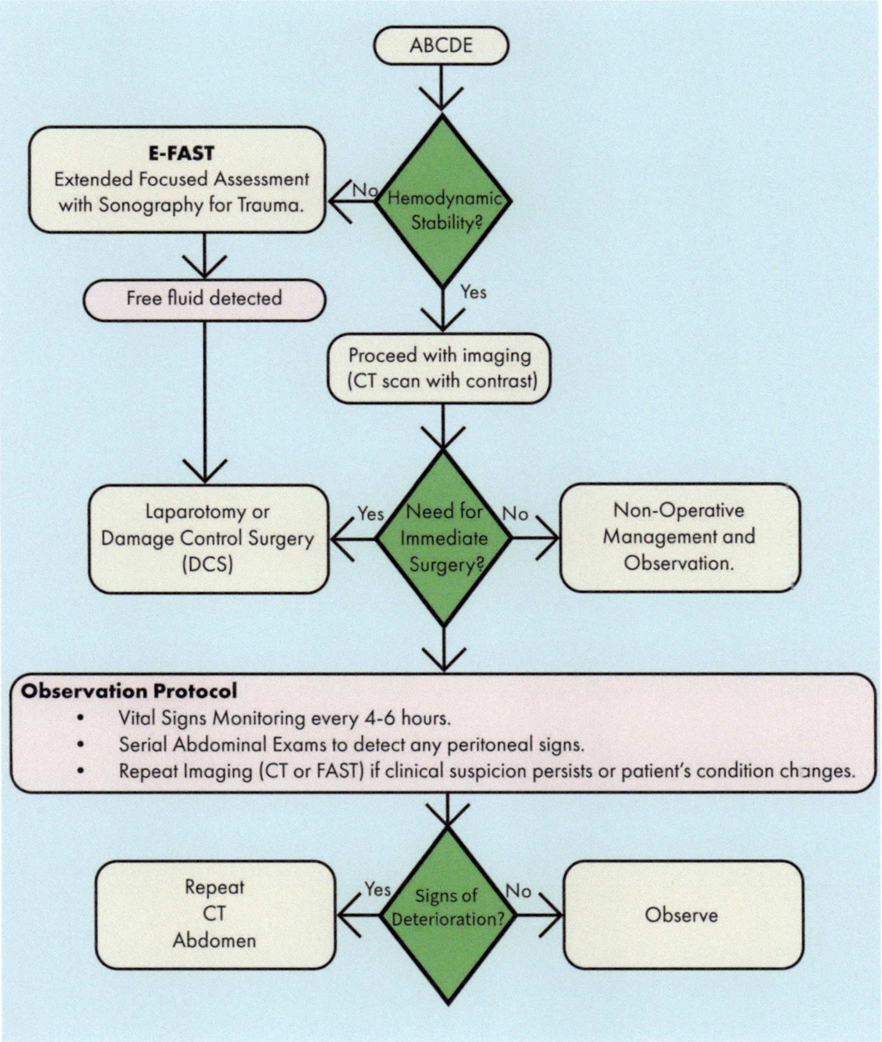

Bibliography

1. American College of Surgeons. Advanced Trauma Life Support (ATLS): student course manual. 10th ed. Chicago: American College of Surgeons; 2018.
2. Smyth L, Bendinelli C, Lee N, Reeds MG, Loh EJ, Amico F, et al. WSES guidelines on blunt and penetrating bowel injury: diagnosis, investigations, and treatment. World J Emerg Surg. 2022;17(1):13.

Chapter 56
Approach to Maxillofacial Trauma in the ICU

56.1 Introduction and Importance

Maxillofacial trauma presents significant challenges in airway management due to its close proximity to vital structures such as the airway and cervical spine. Injuries in this region can lead to altered pharyngeal reflexes, increasing the risk of aspiration and airway obstruction. The physiological impacts include compromised airway patency due to tissue swelling, bleeding, and displacement of anatomical structures. The potential for airway compromise is further heightened when cranial and spinal structures are involved, necessitating careful assessment and management.

Common complications such as trismus (inability to open the mouth fully) can hinder airway access, while pneumoencephalus (presence of air within the cranial cavity) may indicate severe cranial injury and necessitate careful neurological monitoring. Prompt and coordinated management is crucial to prevent airway compromise, control hemorrhage, and stabilize the cervical spine, especially in patients with multiple traumas. A multidisciplinary approach involving anesthesiologists, surgeons, emergency physicians, and critical care specialists is essential to address the complex needs of these patients effectively [1–3] [Ref: Algorithm 56.1].

56.2 Etiology and Mechanism of Injury

Maxillofacial injuries commonly result from road traffic accidents, assaults, falls, sports injuries, and industrial accidents. Alcohol and drug intoxication play a significant role in the etiology of these injuries, both as contributing factors to the incidents and as complicating factors in airway management. Intoxicated patients may have impaired consciousness and airway reflexes, increasing the risk of aspiration and making airway control more challenging.

S. B. Mishra et al., *Mastering ICU Care*,
https://doi.org/10.1007/978-981-95-0179-3_56

The mechanism of injury can be classified based on the impact force:

- High-Impact Trauma: Such as car accidents or falls from height, often result in complex fractures involving multiple facial bones.
- Low-Impact Trauma: Incidents like sports injuries or minor falls typically cause soft tissue damage without significant bony involvement.

Understanding the etiology and mechanism aids in anticipating the severity of injuries and potential complications.

56.3 Anatomy and Classification of Maxillofacial Injuries

56.3.1 Anatomy

The facial skeleton is structurally complex and can be divided into three regions:

- Upper Face: Frontal bone and sinus.
- Midface: Maxilla, zygomatic bones, nasal bones, ethmoid, lacrimal bones, and orbital structures.
- Lower Face: Mandible and temporomandibular joint.

56.3.2 Fracture Classification

56.3.2.1 Le Fort Fractures

These are classic patterns of midfacial fractures that help in assessing the extent of injury and planning management:

- Le Fort I: Horizontal fracture of the maxilla above the teeth (floating palate), separating the maxillary alveolar process from the rest of the midface.
- Le Fort II: Pyramidal fracture involving the maxilla and nasal bones, extending into the orbital floor (floating maxilla).
- Le Fort III: Craniofacial dissociation, where the entire midface is separated from the cranial base, involving the orbital walls and zygomatic arches (floating face).
- Le Fort IV: An extension of Le Fort III fractures into the frontal bone, involving both midface and cranial structures. This type includes frontal sinus involvement and may be associated with cranial injuries.

56.3.2.2 Other Fractures

- Mandibular Fractures: Can lead to airway obstruction due to posterior displacement of the tongue and soft tissues.

- Zygomaticomaxillary Complex Fractures: Affect the prominence of the cheek and the orbital floor, potentially impacting ocular function.

56.3.2.3 Associated Injuries

Certain fracture patterns, particularly Le Fort II, III, and IV, are associated with increased risk of cerebrospinal fluid (CSF) leaks, dural tears, and injuries to cranial nerves or the cervical spine. CSF leaks may present as rhinorrhea or otorrhea and indicate a breach in the cranial base, increasing the risk of meningitis. Understanding the correlation between fracture types and potential intracranial or spinal injuries is crucial for developing an effective management strategy and preventing complications.

56.4 Airway Management in Maxillofacial Trauma

56.4.1 Primary Concerns

Airway obstruction due to displaced fractures, bleeding, foreign bodies, soft tissue swelling, and impaired protective reflexes is the foremost concern. The potential for rapid airway compromise necessitates immediate assessment and intervention.

56.4.1.1 Airway Assessment

1. Assess the Ability to Speak and Protect Airway: Note any signs of airway compromise such as stridor, gurgling, or silence.
2. Visual Examination: Inspect the oral and nasal cavities for bleeding, foreign bodies, loose teeth, fractures, and soft tissue injuries.
3. Evaluate for Cervical Spine Injury: Cervical spine stabilization is mandatory to prevent additional injury.

56.4.1.2 Management Techniques

- Positioning: Position the patient to optimize airway patency and facilitate drainage of blood and secretions. Elevating the head or lateral positioning can be beneficial if cervical spine injury is ruled out.
- Suctioning: High-volume suction devices are essential for clearing the airway of blood, vomitus, and secretions. The suction-assisted laryngoscopy and airway decontamination (SALAD) technique can be employed to maintain a clear view during airway instrumentation in the presence of active bleeding.

- Adjuncts: Use of oropharyngeal and nasopharyngeal airways can assist in maintaining airway patency but must be used with caution or avoided in cases of suspected or confirmed skull base fractures due to the risk of intracranial placement.
- Advanced Airway Techniques: In situations where standard intubation is challenging due to anatomical distortion or profuse bleeding, consider alternate strategies such as video laryngoscopy with suction assistance or awake fiberoptic intubation if the patient's condition allows.

56.4.2 Surgical Airway Management

56.4.2.1 Timing

Early consideration for a surgical airway is crucial when airway obstruction is imminent or intubation attempts have failed.

56.4.2.2 Indications for Transition

- Inability to secure the airway through nonsurgical means after limited attempts.
- Significant facial trauma obstructing visualization of landmarks.
- Profuse bleeding or severe edema impeding intubation.

56.4.2.3 Early Tracheostomy

In the ICU setting, early tracheostomy may be indicated for patients who are expected to require prolonged ventilatory support, have severe maxillofacial injuries precluding oral or nasal intubation, or are at high risk of airway compromise due to progressive swelling.

56.5 Techniques for Airway Control

56.5.1 Nonsurgical Airway Options

- Orotracheal Intubation: Preferred method for securing the airway in most emergency situations. May be challenging due to facial deformities, bleeding, edema, or trismus.
- Nasotracheal Intubation: Considered when oral access is compromised but contraindicated in patients with suspected or confirmed skull base fractures due to the risk of intracranial tube placement and exacerbation of CSF leaks.

- Video Laryngoscopy: Provides improved visualization of the glottis in patients with difficult airways and distorted anatomy. Suction readiness is crucial to manage blood and secretions.
- Fiberoptic Intubation: Ideal for anticipated difficult airways and can be performed while the patient is awake, maintaining spontaneous ventilation. Limited by blood or secretions obstructing the scope.

56.5.2 Adjunctive Devices

- Oropharyngeal Airways (OPA): Help maintain airway patency in unconscious patients without a gag reflex. Care must be taken to avoid causing additional trauma.
- Nasopharyngeal Airways (NPA): Useful in maintaining airway patency in patients with trismus or limited mouth opening. Should be avoided in midface or skull base fractures.

56.5.3 Preoxygenation Strategies

- High-Flow Nasal Cannula (HFNC): Provides apneic oxygenation during airway management, prolonging safe apnea time.
- Non-rebreather Masks or Bag-Valve-Mask Devices: Adjuncts like two-person bag-valve-mask technique may improve efficacy when sealing is challenging.

56.5.4 Supraglottic Airway Devices

- Laryngeal Mask Airway (LMA), i-gel: Useful as rescue airways when intubation is unsuccessful. May not provide adequate protection against aspiration and can be difficult to insert in facial trauma.

56.5.5 Surgical Airway Options

- Cricothyrotomy: Recommended in "cannot intubate, cannot ventilate" scenarios due to speed and simplicity.
- Tracheostomy: Performed in a controlled setting, considered for prolonged mechanical ventilation or when other methods are contraindicated.

56.6 Hemorrhage and Circulatory Management

56.6.1 Hemorrhage Control

Maxillofacial injuries can result in significant hemorrhage due to the rich vascular supply, including branches of the external carotid artery.

56.6.2 Techniques for Hemorrhage Control

- Direct Pressure: Immediate application to bleeding sites.
- Nasal Packing and Tamponade: Effective for epistaxis from nasal or midface fractures.
- Hemostatic Agents: Topical agents like tranexamic acid, fibrin sealants, or absorbable hemostats promote clotting.
- Vascular Control Measures: Ligation or clamping of bleeding vessels during surgery.
- Embolization: Interventional radiology can perform embolization of bleeding vessels in intractable cases.

56.6.3 Circulation Management

- Monitoring for Hemorrhagic Shock: Assess vital signs, urine output, mental status, and skin perfusion.
- Fluid Resuscitation: Administer crystalloids and blood products as needed.

56.6.4 Monitoring for Coagulopathy

- Regular Monitoring: Check platelet count, PT/INR, aPTT, fibrinogen levels, and thromboelastography (TEG) when available.
- Correction of Coagulopathy: Early identification and management prevent exacerbation of bleeding.

56.6.5 ICU Preparedness

- Massive Transfusion Protocols: Be prepared to implement as needed.

- Maintain Normothermia and Correct Acidosis: Vital for managing coagulopathy.
- Collaboration with Hematology and Transfusion Services: Ensures optimal patient management.

56.7 Considerations for Cervical Spine Stability

56.7.1 Cervical Spine Immobilization

Patients with maxillofacial trauma have a high suspicion of cervical spine injuries.

56.7.2 Challenges with Rigid Collars

- May interfere with airway management by limiting mouth opening.
- Can increase intracranial pressure (ICP) due to jugular venous compression.
- May cause pressure ulcers with prolonged use.

56.7.3 Alternatives to Rigid Collars

- Manual In-Line Stabilization (MILS): Minimizes cervical spine movement during airway management.
- Vacuum Mattresses or Sandbags: Immobilize the patient without neck pressure.

56.7.4 Imaging for Cervical Spine Evaluation

- Computed Tomography (CT) Scan: Preferred for its rapid and detailed assessment of bony structures.
- Magnetic Resonance Imaging (MRI): Indicated for ligamentous injury, spinal cord injury, or unexplained neurological deficits.

56.7.5 Imaging Guidelines

- Follow protocols like the Canadian C-Spine Rule or NEXUS criteria.
- In unconscious or intubated patients, CT scanning of the entire cervical spine is recommended.

56.7.6 Implications for Management

- Early Identification: Prevents secondary spinal cord injury.
- Team Coordination: Involvement of trauma, radiology, and spine specialists is vital.

56.8 Secondary Survey and Comprehensive Assessment

56.8.1 Secondary Survey

Conduct a thorough head-to-toe examination to identify all injuries.

56.8.2 Ongoing Reassessment

- Monitor for Delayed Complications: Evolving hematomas, swelling, or infections.
- Regular Reassessment: Allows for early detection and intervention.

56.8.3 Neurological Monitoring

- Glasgow Coma Scale (GCS): Assess and monitor the level of consciousness.
- Serial Assessments: Detect deterioration indicating intracranial pathology.

56.8.4 Diagnostic Imaging

- Initial Imaging: CT scans of the head, face, and cervical spine.
- Repeat Imaging: Necessary to monitor known injuries or detect new developments.
- MRI: For detailed assessment of soft tissue injuries or unexplained deficits.

56.8.5 Monitoring Practices

- Vital Signs: Continuous monitoring of heart rate, blood pressure, respiratory rate, and oxygen saturation.

- Laboratory Assessments: Complete blood count, electrolytes, coagulation profile, arterial blood gases.
- Invasive Monitoring: Arterial lines, central venous catheters as needed.

56.8.6 Airway Vigilance

- Risk of Obstruction: Remain high due to swelling or hematoma expansion.
- Close Monitoring: Of airway patency and ventilatory parameters.

56.9 Conclusion and Key Takeaways

Maxillofacial trauma presents complex challenges that require a nuanced and adaptable approach to airway management and overall patient care.

56.9.1 Interdisciplinary Coordination

Effective management necessitates a coordinated, multidisciplinary effort involving anesthesiology, trauma surgery, maxillofacial surgery, otolaryngology, critical care, radiology, and nursing teams. Collaborative planning and communication are essential to address the evolving airway, hemodynamic, and neurological needs of these patients, ensuring timely interventions and optimizing outcomes.

56.9.2 Importance of Training and Protocols

Continuous education and training in advanced airway management techniques are critical for ICU providers. Simulation training in procedures such as cricothyrotomy, video-assisted laryngoscopy, and fiberoptic intubation enhances provider readiness for high-risk scenarios. Implementation of standardized protocols and checklists can improve team performance, reduce errors, and ensure that best practices are followed in the management of maxillofacial trauma.

Algorithm 56.1: Approach to maxillofacial trauma in the ICU

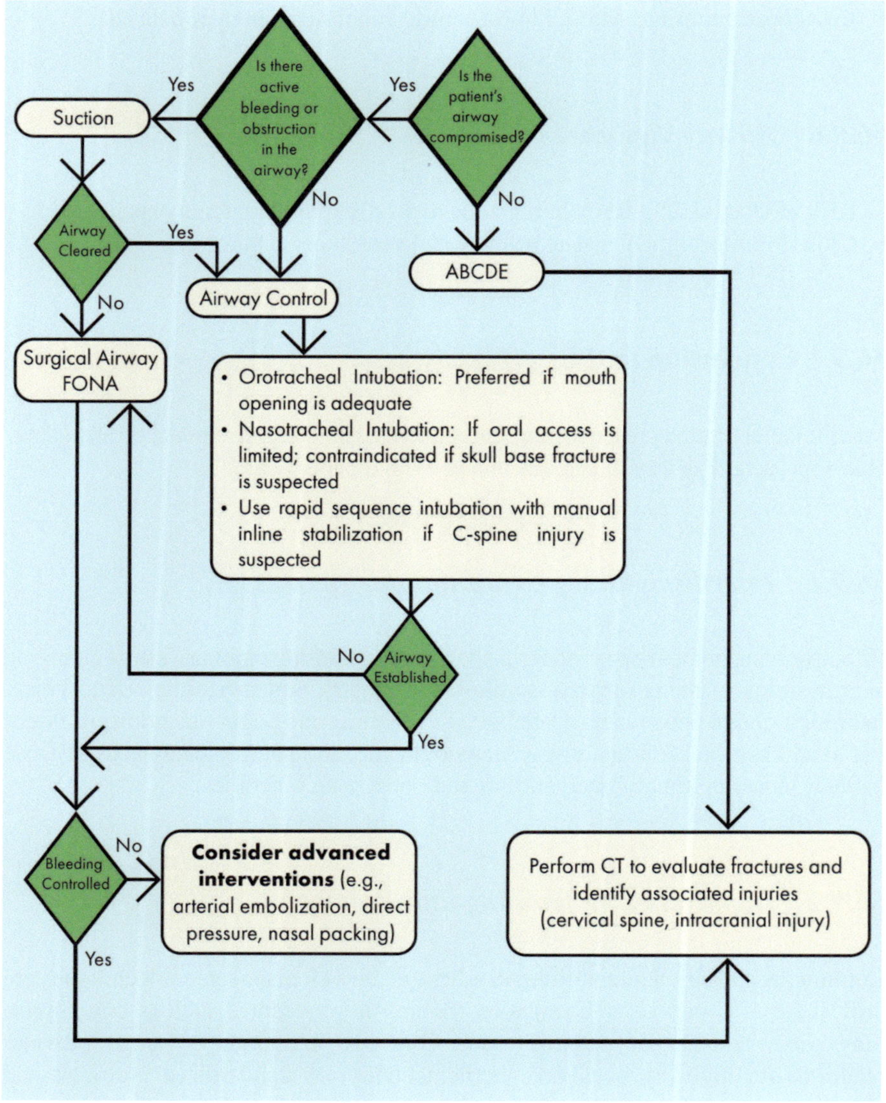

Bibliography

1. Jose A, Nagori SA, Agarwal B, Bhutia O, Roychoudhury A. Management of maxillofacial trauma in emergency: an update of challenges and controversies. J Emerg Trauma Shock. 2016;9(2):73–80.
2. Saini S, Singhal S, Prakash S. Airway management in maxillofacial trauma. J Anaesthesiol Clin Pharmacol. 2021;37(3):319–27.
3. Singh P, Mishra P, Tiwari T, Singh GP. Airway consideration in maxillofacial trauma. Traumaxilla. 2022;4(1–3):19–25.

Chapter 57
Approach to Crush Injury and Compartment Syndrome in the ICU

57.1 Introduction

Crush injuries and compartment syndrome are critical conditions frequently encountered in intensive care units (ICUs), particularly following natural disasters, vehicular accidents, industrial mishaps, and other traumatic events. A crush injury results from prolonged compression of muscle tissue, leading to significant morbidity and mortality if not promptly recognized and managed. When the force or duration of compression is substantial, it can progress to crush syndrome, a systemic condition characterized by severe metabolic disturbances and acute kidney injury due to rhabdomyolysis. Compartment syndrome, an emergency condition marked by elevated intra-compartmental pressure within muscle compartments, can lead to irreversible muscle and nerve damage, limb loss, or even death without timely intervention. This chapter provides a comprehensive overview of the pathophysiology, clinical presentation, diagnosis, and management strategies for crush injuries and compartment syndrome in the ICU setting, emphasizing the importance of early recognition and intervention to optimize patient outcomes [1, 2] [Ref: Algorithm 57.1]

57.2 Pathophysiology

57.2.1 Crush Injury and Crush Syndrome

A crush injury occurs when significant force compresses muscle tissue, causing direct cellular damage and disruption of the sarcolemma. This disruption leads to the release of intracellular contents—including potassium, myoglobin, creatine kinase (CK), phosphate, and other metabolites—into the systemic circulation. The sudden influx of potassium can result in hyperkalemia, posing a risk for

S. B. Mishra et al., *Mastering ICU Care*,
https://doi.org/10.1007/978-981-95-0179-3_57

life-threatening cardiac arrhythmias. Myoglobin, a heme-containing protein released from damaged muscle cells, can precipitate in the renal tubules, especially under acidic and hypovolemic conditions, leading to acute tubular necrosis and subsequent acute kidney injury (AKI), a phenomenon known as myoglobin-induced nephropathy.

Rhabdomyolysis, the breakdown of muscle fibers with the release of their contents into the bloodstream, is a hallmark of crush syndrome. In addition to hyperkalemia and AKI, metabolic acidosis develops due to the accumulation of lactic acid from anaerobic metabolism in ischemic tissues and the release of phosphate and sulfate from damaged cells. Hypocalcemia and hyperphosphatemia may also occur as phosphate binds calcium, reducing serum calcium levels. The massive fluid sequestration into damaged muscle compartments can lead to hypovolemia, exacerbating renal impairment and hemodynamic instability.

57.2.2 Compartment Syndrome

Compartment syndrome arises when increased pressure within a closed osteofascial compartment compromises circulation and function of the tissues within that space. Elevated intra-compartmental pressures exceed capillary perfusion pressure, leading to tissue ischemia and hypoxia. As ischemia progresses, cellular metabolism shifts to anaerobic pathways, producing lactic acid and resulting in metabolic acidosis. The increased vascular permeability associated with ischemia causes edema formation, further elevating intra-compartmental pressure and perpetuating a vicious cycle of worsening ischemia and tissue damage. If unrecognized or untreated, compartment syndrome can lead to irreversible muscle and nerve damage within hours, emphasizing the urgency of prompt diagnosis and intervention.

57.3 Etiology and Risk Factors

Crush injuries commonly result from events such as natural disasters (e.g., earthquakes), vehicular accidents, structural collapses, industrial accidents, and situations involving prolonged immobilization under heavy objects. Compartment syndrome is frequently associated with fractures, particularly of the tibia and forearm bones, tight casts or circumferential dressings that compress underlying tissues, burns leading to circumferential eschar formation, high-energy trauma causing significant soft tissue damage, and reperfusion injuries following the relief of arterial occlusion. Prolonged immobilization and constrictive bandages can also precipitate compartment syndrome. Understanding these risk factors is crucial for early identification and prevention of complications in high-risk patients.

57.4 Clinical Presentation

57.4.1 Crush Injury and Crush Syndrome

Patients with crush injuries may present with localized signs such as swelling, pain, bruising, and sensory or motor deficits in the affected area. Systemic manifestations include myoglobinuria, evidenced by dark brown urine, which indicates rhabdomyolysis. Laboratory findings often reveal hyperkalemia, hypocalcemia, hyperphosphatemia, elevated creatine kinase levels, and metabolic acidosis. Acute kidney injury may develop due to myoglobin-induced nephropathy, necessitating prompt recognition and management. The severity of symptoms correlates with the extent of muscle damage and the duration of compression.

57.4.2 Compartment Syndrome

The clinical hallmark of compartment syndrome is pain out of proportion to the injury, often described as deep, persistent, and poorly localized. Pain is exacerbated by passive stretching of the muscles within the compartment. Other symptoms include paresthesia (numbness or tingling), indicating nerve ischemia, and, in later stages, paralysis due to nerve and muscle dysfunction. Physical examination may reveal tense and swollen compartments that feel firm upon palpation. Pallor and diminished pulses may occur, but importantly, the presence of distal pulses does not exclude the diagnosis, as arterial blood flow may remain intact in the early stages. Reliance solely on the "5 P's" (pain, pallor, paresthesia, paralysis, pulselessness) can be misleading; therefore, a high index of suspicion and careful clinical assessment are essential.

57.5 Diagnosis

57.5.1 Crush Syndrome

The diagnosis of crush syndrome involves a combination of clinical assessment and laboratory investigations. Key laboratory tests include serum electrolytes, revealing elevated potassium levels (hyperkalemia), decreased calcium levels (hypocalcemia), and increased phosphate levels (hyperphosphatemia). Renal function tests often show elevated creatinine and urea levels, indicating impaired renal function. Creatine kinase levels are markedly elevated, reflecting muscle breakdown, with levels exceeding 5000 U/L suggestive of significant rhabdomyolysis. Myoglobin levels may also be elevated, although they are not routinely measured. Urinalysis showing myoglobinuria (positive dipstick for blood without red blood cells on microscopy) supports the diagnosis of rhabdomyolysis.

57.5.2 Compartment Syndrome

Compartment syndrome is primarily a clinical diagnosis, with emphasis on early recognition of symptoms. Intra-compartmental pressure measurement is a valuable adjunct when the clinical assessment is inconclusive, particularly in unresponsive or sedated patients. Pressures exceeding 30 mmHg are indicative of compartment syndrome. Alternatively, a differential pressure (diastolic blood pressure minus compartment pressure) less than 30 mmHg also supports the diagnosis. It is crucial to monitor intra-compartmental pressures in high-risk patients, even when clinical signs are subtle. Avoidance of regional anesthesia in suspected cases is important, as it can mask pain symptoms and delay diagnosis. Imaging studies are generally not helpful and can delay definitive treatment.

57.6 Management in the ICU

57.6.1 Immediate Stabilization

Initial management focuses on stabilizing airway, breathing, and circulation according to standard trauma protocols. Securing the airway and ensuring adequate oxygenation are essential, considering potential respiratory compromise from systemic effects. Rapid vascular access with large-bore intravenous lines is established to initiate aggressive fluid resuscitation. Isotonic saline is the fluid of choice, aiming to maintain a urine output of 100–200 mL/hour to prevent myoglobin-induced acute kidney injury. Potassium-containing fluids, such as lactated Ringer's solution, should be avoided due to the risk of exacerbating hyperkalemia.

57.6.2 Fluid Management

Aggressive intravenous hydration is critical to flush out nephrotoxic substances and preserve renal function. Isotonic saline is preferred to avoid introducing additional potassium into the circulation. Careful monitoring of fluid balance is necessary to prevent fluid overload or hypovolemia. Fluid resuscitation should be titrated based on hemodynamic parameters, urine output, and signs of volume status.

57.6.3 Electrolyte and Acid-Base Management

Hyperkalemia is a life-threatening complication that requires prompt treatment. Intravenous calcium gluconate is administered to stabilize cardiac membranes, followed by insulin with dextrose to facilitate the intracellular shift of potassium. Sodium bicarbonate may be used in cases of severe metabolic acidosis to further promote potassium uptake into cells and correct acidosis. Beta-2 agonists, such as nebulized salbutamol, can serve as adjunctive therapy to lower serum potassium levels. Hypocalcemia is corrected cautiously, typically only if symptomatic, to avoid the risk of arrhythmias due to rapid shifts in calcium levels. Continuous monitoring of electrolyte levels and acid-base status is essential to guide therapy.

57.6.4 Management of Compartment Syndrome

Prompt recognition and management of compartment syndrome are critical to prevent irreversible damage. Initial measures include removing any external constrictive devices, such as tight dressings or casts, and positioning the affected limb at the level of the heart to optimize venous return without compromising arterial flow. Elevation above heart level is avoided as it may decrease arterial perfusion.

Urgent surgical decompression via fasciotomy is indicated when clinical signs persist or intra-compartmental pressures exceed 30 mmHg. Fasciotomy involves longitudinal incisions to release all affected compartments, relieving pressure and restoring perfusion. The timing of fasciotomy is crucial, as delays can result in permanent tissue damage. All compartments at risk should be decompressed, and the incisions should be left open with appropriate wound management.

57.6.5 Postoperative Care

After fasciotomy, meticulous wound care is essential to prevent infection, a significant risk due to the open wounds created by the procedure. Regular inspection for signs of infection or necrosis is necessary, and repeated debridement may be required if necrotic tissue is present. Wound dressings should be maintained in a sterile manner, and appropriate antibiotic therapy initiated as prophylaxis against infection. Continuous reassessment of compartment pressures is important to detect any residual or recurrent compartment syndrome. Renal function should be monitored regularly, given the ongoing risk of myoglobin-induced nephropathy.

57.6.6 Renal Protection

Preventing acute kidney injury is a primary concern in crush syndrome management. Maintaining adequate urine output through aggressive hydration helps prevent myoglobin precipitation in renal tubules. Diuretics such as mannitol may be considered to promote diuresis but should be used cautiously and are not routinely recommended. Loop diuretics may be used in cases of fluid overload but are contraindicated in hypovolemic patients. Early initiation of renal replacement therapy, such as dialysis, is indicated if there is evidence of unresponsive renal failure or severe metabolic derangements.

57.6.7 Systemic Management

Pain control is a vital component of patient care but must be balanced against the need to monitor for signs of compartment syndrome. Opioid analgesics are administered judiciously, and regional anesthesia is avoided to prevent masking symptoms. Nutritional support with a high-protein diet is important to facilitate tissue repair and meet the increased metabolic demands of recovery. Infection control measures include prophylactic antibiotics post-fasciotomy and strict adherence to wound care protocols to prevent secondary infections.

57.6.8 Complications and Follow-Up

Patients with crush injuries and compartment syndrome are at risk for several complications. Acute kidney injury may progress to renal failure requiring dialysis. Systemic acidosis and persistent electrolyte imbalances, particularly hyperkalemia, can lead to hemodynamic instability and cardiac arrhythmias. Infection is a significant concern post-fasciotomy, necessitating vigilant wound care and appropriate antibiotic therapy. Delayed or inadequate treatment of compartment syndrome can result in irreversible muscle and nerve damage, leading to functional impairments.

Long-term follow-up includes regular assessment of limb function, wound healing, and renal function. Early involvement of rehabilitation services, such as physiotherapy and occupational therapy, is crucial to optimize functional recovery and assist patients in adapting to any residual deficits. Psychosocial support may be necessary to address the psychological impact of the injury and potential disability. Patient education on recognizing signs of complications and the importance of adherence to follow-up care is essential for optimal outcomes.

57.7 Conclusion

A structured and proactive approach to crush injury and compartment syndrome in the ICU is essential for optimizing patient outcomes. Early recognition of clinical signs, aggressive management of metabolic derangements, timely surgical intervention for compartment syndrome, and meticulous postoperative care are critical components in reducing morbidity and mortality. Interdisciplinary collaboration among critical care specialists, surgeons, nephrologists, and rehabilitation professionals is vital to provide comprehensive care and support to these patients. Through diligent monitoring and management, the risks of complications can be mitigated, limb function preserved, and survival rates improved.

Algorithm 57.1: Approach to crush injury and compartment syndrome in the ICU

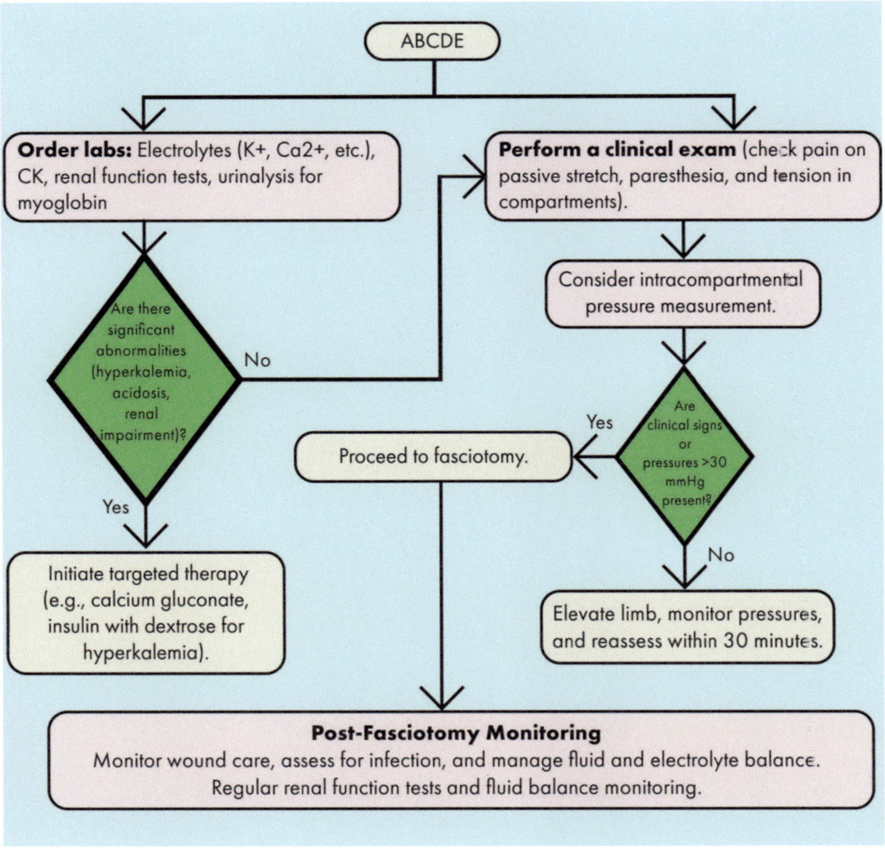

Bibliography

1. American College of Surgeons. Advanced Trauma Life Support (ATLS): student course manual. 10th ed. Chicago: American College of Surgeons; 2018.
2. Osborn CPM, Schmidt AH. Management of acute compartment syndrome. J Am Acad Orthop Surg. 2020;28(3):e108–e14.

Part VI
Cardiology

Chapter 58
Approach to Acute Severe Hypertension in the ICU

58.1 Introduction

Hypertension is a common condition encountered in acute care settings, particularly within the intensive care unit (ICU). While elevated blood pressure is frequent among critically ill patients, not all instances necessitate immediate intervention. Hypertension in the ICU can be reversible, often resulting from transient factors such as pain, anxiety, or agitation, or irreversible when linked to persistent pathological conditions. Understanding the nuances of hypertension in critically ill patients is essential for effective management and improving patient outcomes [1, 2]. [Ref: Algorithm 58.1].

58.2 Classification of Hypertension in the ICU

The classification of hypertension in the ICU is crucial for guiding management strategies. It is categorized based on blood pressure levels and the presence or absence of target-organ damage:

- Hypertensive Emergency: Characterized by severe elevations in blood pressure—typically a systolic blood pressure (SBP) exceeding 180 mm Hg or a diastolic blood pressure (DBP) over 110–120 mm Hg—accompanied by new or worsening target-organ damage. Immediate medical intervention is required to prevent morbidity and mortality.
- Asymptomatic Markedly Elevated Blood Pressure: Patients exhibit significantly elevated blood pressure (SBP/DBP >180/110–120 mm Hg) without any signs of target-organ damage. While immediate organ damage is not present, these patients require careful monitoring and intervention to prevent progression.

S. B. Mishra et al., *Mastering ICU Care*,
https://doi.org/10.1007/978-981-95-0179-3_58

- Asymptomatic Elevated Blood Pressure: Defined as SBP/DBP ≥130/80 mm Hg without evidence of organ involvement. Although less severe, sustained elevations can lead to long-term complications and warrant management.

It is important to note that target-organ damage can occur even at lower blood pressure thresholds, affecting vital organs such as the brain, heart, kidneys, arteries, and retina [3].

58.3 Malignant Hypertension

Malignant hypertension is a severe form of hypertension with distinct vascular pathology, including fibrinoid necrosis of arterioles and small arteries, particularly in the kidneys, and severe hypertensive retinopathy. This condition signifies advanced vascular damage and is associated with high morbidity and mortality. Prompt recognition and aggressive management are imperative to prevent irreversible organ damage.

58.4 Mechanisms and Triggers of Hypertensive Crises

Understanding the underlying mechanisms and triggers of hypertensive crises in the ICU is essential for prevention and management.

58.4.1 Pathophysiology and Triggers

Hypertensive crises may be precipitated by:

- Noncompliance with Antihypertensive Therapy: Sudden cessation or irregular intake of antihypertensive medications can lead to rebound hypertension.
- Use of Sympathomimetic Drugs: Substances like cocaine, amphetamines, or certain over-the-counter medications can induce severe hypertension.
- Acute Physical Stressors: Conditions such as infections, surgical procedures, pain, or agitation can elevate blood pressure due to increased sympathetic activity.

58.4.2 Pathogenesis of End-Organ Damage

In hypertensive emergencies, increased vascular wall stress leads to endothelial injury, initiating a cascade of pathological events:

- Endothelial Dysfunction: Mechanical stress damages the endothelium, disrupting its barrier function and promoting inflammation.
- Inflammatory Response: Endothelial injury triggers the release of inflammatory mediators, leading to leukocyte adhesion and further vascular damage.
- Increased Vascular Permeability: Damage to the endothelium increases permeability, resulting in edema and microhemorrhages within organs.
- Hypoperfusion and Ischemia: The combination of vasoconstriction and vascular injury leads to reduced blood flow and oxygen delivery to vital organs.
- Fibrinoid Necrosis: Particularly noted in malignant hypertension, fibrinoid necrosis involves the deposition of fibrin-like material in the vessel walls, leading to vessel obstruction and organ ischemia.

Understanding these mechanisms underscores the importance of prompt and effective blood pressure control to prevent irreversible organ damage.

58.5 Assessment of End-Organ Damage

A comprehensive evaluation of target-organ damage is critical in patients with hypertensive emergencies. The mnemonic BARKH serves as a useful tool to assess the affected organs:

- Brain: Assess for hypertensive encephalopathy, acute ischemic stroke (AIS), posterior reversible encephalopathy syndrome (PRES), and intracerebral hemorrhage (ICH).
- Arteries: Evaluate for aortic dissection, preeclampsia, eclampsia, and HELLP (hemolytic anemia, elevated liver enzymes, and low platelet) syndrome.
- Retina: Conduct fundoscopic examinations for signs of hypertensive retinopathy.
- Kidneys: Monitor for acute kidney injury (AKI) and thrombotic microangiopathy.
- Heart: Investigate for acute heart failure, pulmonary edema, and acute coronary syndromes (ACS).

58.6 Diagnostic Evaluation

Specific imaging and laboratory tests are essential to confirm end-organ involvement:

- Neurological Assessment: Utilize computed tomography (CT) or magnetic resonance imaging (MRI) to detect cerebral edema, infarcts, or hemorrhages.
- Cardiac Evaluation: Perform electrocardiograms (ECG) and measure cardiac biomarkers (e.g., troponin levels) to identify myocardial ischemia or infarction.

- Renal Function Tests: Assess serum creatinine, blood urea nitrogen (BUN), and perform urinalysis to evaluate kidney function.
- Ophthalmologic Examination: A fundoscopic exam can reveal retinal hemorrhages, exudates, or papilledema indicative of hypertensive retinopathy [4].

58.7 Target Blood Pressure Reduction Strategies

Effective management of hypertensive emergencies involves careful and controlled reduction of blood pressure to prevent further organ damage while avoiding hypoperfusion.

58.7.1 Organ-Specific Blood Pressure Goals

- Brain (e.g., Hypertensive Encephalopathy): Aim to reduce diastolic blood pressure to 100–110 mm Hg within the first few hours. This target helps stabilize cerebral perfusion while avoiding hypoperfusion-related injury.
  - AIS: Reduces MAP by 15%. SBP between 130 and 180 mm Hg.
  - ICH: Reduces MAP by 15% in the first hour.
  - PRES: MAP declines by 20–25% as early as possible.
- Aortic Dissection: Rapidly lower SBP to less than 120 mm Hg and heart rate below 60 beats per minute to minimize aortic wall stress.
  - Pulmonary Edema and ACS: Aim for an SBP of less than 140 mm Hg to decrease cardiac workload and improve oxygenation in. Target SBP < 180 mm Hg or reduce MAP by 25% in the first hour; target 160/100 mm Hg in next 2–6 hours if stable, then to normal in 24–48 hours in acute heart failure.
- Preeclampsia, HELLP, and Eclampsia: Reduce SBP to less than 160 mm Hg and DBP to less than 105 mm Hg to prevent maternal and fetal complications.
- Retina:
  - Target SBP <180 mm Hg/ MAP reduction by 15%.
  - Kidney:
  - Gradual reduction of MAP by 20–25%.

58.7.2 Caution Against Overly Rapid Reduction

Excessive and rapid lowering of blood pressure can lead to ischemic complications, particularly in the brain and heart. Cerebral autoregulation may be compromised, increasing the risk of cerebral hypoperfusion and subsequent infarction. Therefore, gradual reduction with close monitoring is essential.

58.8 Management Approach: Assess, Identify, Modify (AIM)

An effective management strategy can be encapsulated in the AIM framework:

- Assess: Obtain accurate blood pressure measurements and evaluate the severity of hypertension and presence of end-organ damage. Ensure correct reading, assess volume status, review home medications (e.g., abrupt stoppage of beta blockers) are some of the steps to be followed.
- Identify: Determine the underlying cause and affected organ systems through clinical evaluation and diagnostic testing.
- Modify: Implement appropriate pharmacological interventions and address modifiable factors contributing to hypertension.

58.9 Monitoring and Device Accuracy

In hypertensive emergencies, precise blood pressure monitoring is critical.

- Arterial Lines: Use intra-arterial lines for continuous and accurate measurements, which are essential for titrating intravenous antihypertensive medications.
- Noninvasive Monitoring: For patients without arterial lines, blood pressure should be measured every 15–30 min initially. Utilize automated blood pressure devices with appropriate cuff sizes, and confirm readings manually to ensure accuracy, especially in critically unstable patients.

58.10 Drug Titration

Careful titration of antihypertensive medications is crucial to achieve target blood pressure goals without causing rapid reductions that may lead to hypoperfusion.

- Start Low, Go Slow: Initiate therapy with lower doses and adjust gradually based on the patient's response and tolerability.
- Frequent Monitoring: Reassess blood pressure at appropriate intervals (e.g., every 5–15 min during titration) to guide dosage adjustments.
- Individualized Approach: Consider patient-specific factors such as age, comorbidities, and the presence of organ dysfunction when titrating medications [5].

58.11 Drug Choices Based on Organ Impact

Selection of antihypertensive agents should be tailored to the patient's specific clinical scenario and target-organ involvement.

58.11.1 Brain-Related Crises

Labetalol: An intravenous beta-blocker that offers controlled reduction of blood pressure without significant effects on cerebral blood flow.

- Dosage and Titration: Start with 20 mg IV over 2 min. Additional doses of 20–80 mg can be administered every 10 min until target blood pressure is achieved, or a continuous infusion of 1–8 mg/min can be used. Monitor blood pressure every 5–10 min during titration to avoid rapid drops. (European) Initial 0.3–1.0-mg/kg dose (maximum 20 mg), slow IV injection every 10 min or 0.4–1.0-mg/kg/h IV infusion up to 3 mg/kg/h. Adjust rate up to total cumulative dose of 300 mg. This dose can be repeated every 4–6 h. (AHA 2017).

Nicardipine: A calcium channel blocker effective in lowering blood pressure with the advantage of preserving cerebral autoregulation.

- Dosage and Titration: Initiate at 5 mg/hour IV infusion, increasing by 2.5 mg/hour every 5–15 min as needed, up to a maximum of 15 mg/hour. Adjust titration intervals carefully to prevent overshooting the target blood pressure.

58.11.2 Heart-Related Crises

Nitroglycerin (NTG): Ideal for patients with ACS or pulmonary edema, as it reduces preload and afterload, improving myocardial oxygen supply and decreasing cardiac workload.

- Dosage and Titration: Start at 5 mcg/min IV infusion, increasing by 5 mcg/min every 3 to 5 min until desired blood pressure or symptom relief is achieved, to a maximum of 20 mcg/min. Frequent monitoring is necessary due to its rapid onset and short duration of action.

Avoidance of Nitroprusside: Due to risks of cyanide toxicity and potential worsening of renal function, nitroprusside is generally avoided, especially in patients with renal impairment. However, it can be used for acute pulmonary edema. Initial 0.3–0.5 mcg/kg/min; increase in increments of 0.5 mcg/kg/min to achieve BP target; maximum dose 10 mcg/ kg/min; duration of treatment as short as possible. For infusion rates ≥4–10 mcg/kg/min or duration >30 min, thiosulfate can be co-administered to prevent cyanide toxicity.

Esmolol: is also the agent of choice along with NTG for ACS.

- Dosage and titration: Loading dose 500–1000 mcg/kg/min over 1 min followed by a 50-mcg/kg/min infusion. For additional dosing, the bolus dose is repeated and the infusion increased in 50-mcg/kg/min increments as needed to a maximum of 200 mcg/kg/min.
- Caution: Avoid in bradycardia, heart block, decompensated heart failure.

58.11.3 Preeclampsia and Eclampsia Management

In pregnant patients with hypertensive crises:
Magnesium Sulfate: First-line therapy for the prevention and treatment of eclampsia seizures.

- Dosage: Administer a loading dose of 4–6 grams IV over 15–20 min, followed by a maintenance infusion of 1–2 grams per hour.

Blood Pressure Control: Use hydralazine or labetalol for acute blood pressure management.

- Hydralazine Dosage: Start with 5–10 mg IV over 2 min, repeat every 20–30 min as needed. Initial 10 mg via slow IV infusion (maximum initial dose 20 mg); repeat every 4–6 h as needed. Unpredictable response and long duration of action go against its use as a first-line agent.
- Labetalol Dosage: Begin with 20 mg IV over 2 min, followed by doses of 40 mg and then 80 mg at 10-min intervals if needed, up to a total of 220 mg. Initial 0.3–1.0-mg/kg dose (maximum 20 mg), slow IV injection every 10 min or 0.4–1.0-mg/kg/h IV infusion up to 3 mg/kg/h. Adjust rate up to a total cumulative dose of 300 mg. This dose can be repeated every 4–6 h.
- Agents to Avoid: ACE inhibitors and ARBs are contraindicated due to teratogenic risks and adverse effects on fetal renal development.

58.11.4 Renal Protection

In patients with renal compromise:

- Preferred Agents: Labetalol and nicardipine are safer options due to minimal nephrotoxicity.
- Agents to Avoid: Nitroprusside should be avoided because its metabolites (thiocyanate and cyanide) can accumulate in renal failure, leading to toxicity.

58.11.5 Alternative Medications for Special Cases

Clevidipine: An ultra-short-acting dihydropyridine calcium channel blocker suitable for rapid titration and blood pressure control, especially when beta-blockers are contraindicated.

- Dosage and Titration: Start at 1–2 mg/hour IV infusion, doubling the dose at short intervals (90 s) initially, then increasing by less than double every 5–10 min as needed. Maximum recommended dose is 32 mg/hour.

Esmolol: A short-acting beta-blocker beneficial in situations requiring quick onset and offset of action, such as in perioperative hypertension or tachyarrhythmias.

- Dosage and Titration: Begin with a 500 mcg/kg IV bolus over 1 min, followed by an infusion of 50 mcg/kg/min. Adjust infusion rate by 25–50 mcg/kg/min every 5–10 min as needed, up to a maximum of 300 mcg/kg/min.

58.11.6 Patient-Specific Considerations

- Chronic Obstructive Pulmonary Disease (COPD): Beta-blockers may exacerbate bronchospasm; thus, agents like nicardipine or clevidipine are preferred.
- Chronic Kidney Disease (CKD): Drugs with minimal renal metabolism and excretion are favored to prevent accumulation and toxicity.
- Heart Failure with Reduced Ejection Fraction (HFrEF): Avoid negative inotropic agents; consider ACE inhibitors or angiotensin receptor blockers (ARBs).
- Heart Failure with Preserved Ejection Fraction (HFpEF): Focus on controlling blood pressure and relieving symptoms without compromising diastolic filling.
- Pregnancy: Use labetalol or hydralazine for blood pressure control; avoid ACE inhibitors and ARBs due to teratogenic risks.

Tables summarizing medications, dosages, and special considerations for various organ systems can provide quick reference for clinicians (Tables 58.1 and 58.2).

Table 58.1 Medications for rapid blood pressure control in organ crises

Organ system	Preferred medications	Dosage guidelines
Brain (e.g., intracerebral hemorrhage)	Labetalol, nicardipine	Labetalol: 20 mg IV over 2 min; repeat every 10 min or infusion 1–8 mg/min. Nicardipine: Start at 5 mg/h, increase by 2.5 mg/h every 5–15 min
Heart (ACS, pulmonary edema)	Nitroglycerin, labetalol	Nitroglycerin: Start at 5mcg/min, increase by 5 mcg/min every 3–5 min. Labetalol: 20 mg IV, may repeat every 10 min based on response
Arteries (aortic dissection)	Esmolol, labetalol	Esmolol: 500 mcg/kg bolus, then 50 mcg/kg/min infusion, titrate as needed. Labetalol: Similar dosages as in brain crises. Beta blockade should precede vasodilator use if any needed (nicardipine/nitroprusside)
Kidneys (AKI)	Labetalol, nicardipine	As per brain crisis dosages; avoid agents with nephrotoxic potential
Retina (hypertensive retinopathy)	Nicardipine, labetalol	Follow brain crisis dosing to prevent worsening retinopathy
Pregnancy (severe preeclampsia, eclampsia)	Labetalol, hydralazine, magnesium sulfate	Labetalol: 20 mg IV over 2 min; repeat as needed. Hydralazine: 5–10 mg IV over 2 min; may repeat every 20–30 min. Magnesium sulfate: Loading dose of 4–6 g IV over 15–20 min, maintenance 1–2 g/h

Table 58.2 Special considerations in comorbid conditions

Condition	Preferred agents	Agents to avoid
COPD	Nicardipine, clevidipine	Beta-blockers due to risk of bronchospasm
Chronic kidney disease (CKD)	Labetalol, nicardipine	Nitroprusside (risk of thiocyanate/cyanide toxicity)
Heart failure with reduced ejection fraction (HFrEF)	ACE inhibitors, ARBs	Calcium channel blockers due to negative inotropy
Heart failure with preserved ejection fraction (HFpEF)	Diuretics, ACE inhibitors	Avoid negative inotropic agents like beta-blockers
Pregnancy	Labetalol, hydralazine	ACE inhibitors, ARBs, due to fetal toxicity

58.12 Conclusion

Managing hypertension in the ICU requires a comprehensive and systematic approach that prioritizes patient safety and optimal outcomes. By focusing on accurate assessment, individualized treatment strategies, and careful monitoring, healthcare providers can effectively address hypertensive crises. Incorporating organ-specific management plans, providing detailed titration guidance, and ensuring proper transition to post-acute care are essential components of high-quality care. Including practical case scenarios enhances understanding and application of these principles. Adherence to the latest clinical guidelines and evidence-based practices will improve patient outcomes and reduce the risk of long-term complications associated with hypertension. By integrating these refinements, the chapter provides ICU clinicians with a precise, actionable guide for managing hypertensive crises, balancing rapid intervention with careful titration to avoid complications.

Algorithm 58.1: Approach to acute severe hypertension in the ICU

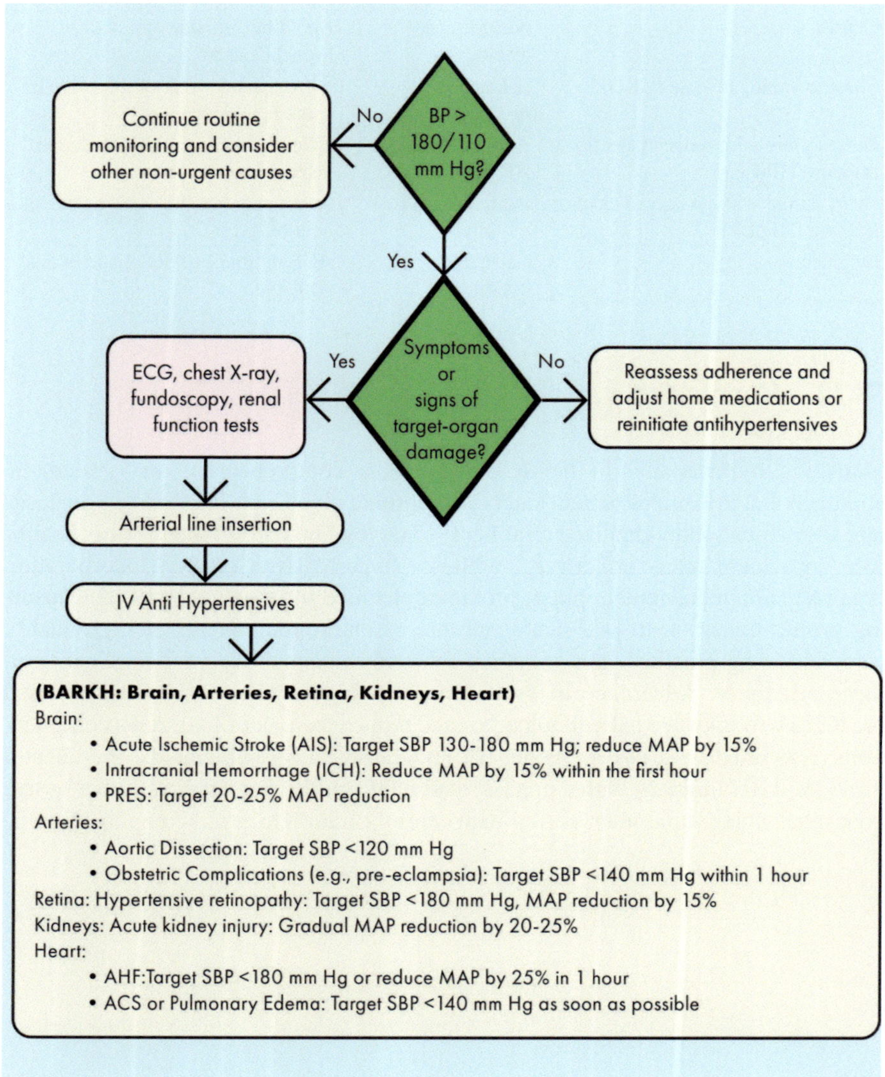

Bibliography

1. Kreutz R, Brunstrom M, Burnier M, Grassi G, Januszewicz A, Muiesan ML, et al. 2024 European Society of Hypertension clinical practice guidelines for the management of arterial hypertension. Eur J Intern Med. 2024;126:1–15.
2. McEvoy JW, McCarthy CP, Bruno RM, Brouwers S, Canavan MD, Ceconi C, et al. 2024 ESC guidelines for the management of elevated blood pressure and hypertension. Eur Heart J. 2024;45(38):3912–4018.
3. Kulkarni S, Glover M, Kapil V, Abrams SML, Partridge S, McCormack T, et al. Management of hypertensive crisis: British and Irish hypertension society position document. J Hum Hypertens. 2023;37(10):863–79.
4. Stabile E, Muiesan ML, Ribichini FL, Sangiorgi G, Taddei S, Versaci F, et al. Italian Society of Interventional Cardiology (GISE) and Italian Society of Arterial Hypertension (SIIA) position paper on the role of renal denervation in the management of the difficult-to-treat hypertension. Minerva Cardiol Angiol. 2024;72(4):313–28.
5. Unger T, Borghi C, Charchar F, Khan NA, Poulter NR, Prabhakaran D, et al. 2020 International Society of Hypertension Global Hypertension Practice Guidelines. Hypertension. 2020;75(6):1334–57.

Chapter 59
Approach to Bradycardia in the ICU

59.1 Introduction

Bradycardia is defined as a heart rate originating from the sinus node at less than 60 beats per minute. It can be physiological, as seen in well-trained athletes or pathological, indicating underlying cardiac or systemic issues. While asymptomatic and physiological bradycardia generally does not require intervention, symptomatic bradycardia demands immediate attention to prevent potential catastrophic outcomes such as syncope, heart failure, or sudden cardiac death. New-onset bradycardia, especially when accompanied by symptoms like dizziness, fatigue, or chest pain, often signals underlying cardiac pathology and necessitates prompt evaluation and management [1–3] [Ref: Algorithm 59.1].

59.2 Pathophysiology and Etiology

Bradycardia results from impaired impulse generation in the sinoatrial (SA) node, impaired conduction through the atrioventricular (AV) node, or both. The causes of bradycardia are diverse and can be categorized into several groups:

59.2.1 Drug-Induced Bradycardia

Medications are a common cause of bradycardia. Drugs such as beta-blockers, calcium channel blockers, digoxin, antiarrhythmic agents, and certain antiepileptics can depress SA node activity or AV node conduction. Overdose of these medications can lead to severe bradycardia requiring emergency intervention.

S. B. Mishra et al., *Mastering ICU Care*,
https://doi.org/10.1007/978-981-95-0179-3_59

[α-2 agonist (clonidine, dexmedetomidine), α-blocker (prazosin), cholinergic agents (neostigmine), beta blockers (metoprolol, bisoprolol, labetalol, carvedilol), antiarrhythmics (amiodarone, diltiazem, verapamil, flecainide), ivabradine, digoxin, and rarely anti-seizure medicines (carbamazepine, lacosamide, phenytoin), Propofol, Lithium].

59.2.2 Metabolic and Endocrine Causes

Metabolic disturbances like hyperkalemia, hypokalemia, hypocalcemia, and hypoxia can affect cardiac conduction. Hypothyroidism slows metabolic processes and can lead to bradycardia. Hypothermia also decreases heart rate by slowing the rate of depolarization in cardiac pacemaker cells. Uremia, advanced liver disease, hypermagnesemia, hypercapnia, and acidemia are the other metabolic causes that can lead to bradycardia.

59.2.3 Cardiovascular Causes

Intrinsic cardiac diseases such as acute myocardial infarction (especially inferior wall MI), anterior wall myocardial infarction, myocarditis, acute hypertension, and infiltrative diseases like amyloidosis, hemochromatosis, and sarcoidosis can damage the conduction system. AV blocks of varying degrees can result from ischemia or fibrosis of the conduction pathways.

59.2.4 Infections and Inflammatory Conditions

Infections such as Lyme disease, endocarditis, and viral myocarditis can involve the cardiac conduction system. Systemic inflammatory diseases like systemic lupus erythematosus and scleroderma may also affect cardiac conduction.

59.2.5 Increased Vagal Tone and Other Causes

Conditions that increase vagal tone, such as vasovagal syncope or increased intracranial pressure, can lead to bradycardia. Sleep apnea is another important cause, particularly in patients experiencing nocturnal bradycardia. Sudden pain, sick sinus, acute stressful vomiting, coughing, straining, micturition (Valsalva), surgeries, and raised intra-cranial pressure (tumor, traumatic brain injury, intracranial hemorrhage, large acute ischemic stroke, and chronic liver disease) can also lead to bradycardia.

59.3 Clinical Presentation

Patients with bradycardia may present with a variety of symptoms, ranging from mild fatigue and dizziness to syncope and heart failure. Symptoms are often a result of decreased cardiac output due to the slow heart rate. Key clinical features include:

- Dizziness or lightheadedness.
- Syncope or near-syncope.
- Fatigue.
- Shortness of breath.
- Chest pain.
- Confusion or altered mental status.

59.4 Evaluation

59.4.1 Immediate Assessment and Stabilization

A rapid and systematic approach is essential in evaluating a patient with bradycardia. Look for hypotension, acute onset altered mentation, signs of shock, ischemic discomfort, and acute heart failure as these signs mandate immediate treatment.

59.4.2 ABCDE Assessment

- Airway and Breathing: Ensure the airway is open and assess breathing. Provide supplemental oxygen to maintain adequate oxygenation.
- Circulation: Assess hemodynamic status by checking blood pressure, heart rate, and peripheral perfusion. Aim to maintain a mean arterial pressure (MAP) greater than 65 mm Hg.
- Disability: Evaluate neurological status, including level of consciousness and signs of stroke.
- Exposure: Fully expose the patient to assess for any signs of trauma, rash, or other physical findings that may indicate the cause of bradycardia.

Vital Sign Monitoring: Continuous monitoring of vital signs is crucial. Place the patient on cardiac monitors to observe electrocardiogram (ECG) rhythms, measure blood pressure (BP) regularly, and monitor oxygen saturation (SpO_2).

59.4.3 Identification of Reversible Causes

It is important to identify and correct reversible causes promptly. A checklist of potential factors includes:

- Hypoxia.
- Electrolyte imbalances (e.g., hyperkalemia, hypokalemia).
- Hypothermia.
- Toxins or drug overdose.
- Cardiac tamponade.
- Tension pneumothorax.
- Thrombosis (pulmonary or coronary).
- Trauma.

59.5 History and Physical Examination

A thorough history and physical examination help identify potential causes.

59.5.1 History

- Review medications, including recent changes or overdoses.
- Ask about chest pain, dyspnea, palpitations, or syncope.
- Inquire about recent infections, trauma, or exposure to toxins.
- Explore family history of cardiac conditions.
- Assess sleep patterns to evaluate for sleep apnea.

59.5.2 Physical Examination

- Observe general appearance for signs of distress.
- Check for cyanosis or pallor.
- Auscultate the heart for murmurs or gallops.
- Assess lung fields for crackles or rales, indicating heart failure.
- Examine for peripheral edema.
- Perform a neurological assessment.

59.6 Investigations

59.6.1 Electrocardiogram (ECG)

A 12-lead ECG is essential to evaluate the type of bradycardia and identify conduction abnormalities.

- Sinus Bradycardia: Normal P waves with a rate less than 60 bpm.
- First-Degree AV Block: Prolonged PR interval (>200 ms) without dropped beats.
- Second-Degree AV Block Type I (Mobitz I/Wenckebach): Progressive prolongation of PR interval until a QRS complex is dropped.
- Second-Degree AV Block Type II (Mobitz II): Constant PR intervals with intermittent dropped QRS complexes.
- Third-Degree AV Block: Complete dissociation between atrial and ventricular activity.
- Left Bundle Branch Block (LBBB): Widened QRS complexes with specific patterns; requires further evaluation.
- Junctional Rhythm/Escape: Constant RR interval with rate < 60 (around 40), retrograde P-waves may be seen.
- Ventricular Escape: Wide QRS with rate of 30–40 beats per minute.

59.6.2 Laboratory Tests

- Complete Blood Count (CBC).
- Basic Metabolic Panel: Electrolytes (Na^+, K^+, Ca^{2+}, Mg^{2+}), renal function, glucose.
- Thyroid Function Tests: To assess for hypothyroidism.
- Cardiac Enzymes: Troponin levels to evaluate for myocardial infarction
- Arterial Blood Gas (ABG): To assess oxygenation and acid-base status.
- Drug Levels: If overdose is suspected.
- Genetic Testing: In cases of suspected inherited arrhythmias.

59.6.3 Imaging and Advanced Diagnostics

- Chest X-ray: To assess for cardiac enlargement or pulmonary pathology.
- Echocardiography: Especially important in patients with LBBB or suspected structural heart disease to evaluate ventricular function and structural abnormalities.

- Ambulatory ECG Monitoring (Holter Monitor): For patients with intermittent symptoms to detect transient arrhythmias.
- Sleep Studies: In patients with nocturnal bradycardia or suspected sleep apnea.

59.7 Management

- Management of bradycardia focuses on symptomatic relief, stabilization, and addressing the underlying cause.

59.7.1 General Measures

- Ensure Airway and Breathing: Provide oxygen and support ventilation if necessary.
- Establish IV Access: For medication administration.
- Continuous Monitoring: ECG, blood pressure, and SpO_2.

59.7.2 Pharmacological Treatment

59.7.2.1 Atropine

Atropine is the first-line medication for symptomatic bradycardia.

- Dosage: Administer 1 mg IV bolus.
- Repeat: Every 3–5 minutes as needed.
- Maximum Dose: Do not exceed a total of 3 mg.

59.7.2.2 If Atropine Is Ineffective

When atropine fails to improve the heart rate, consider the following:
Dopamine Infusion.

- Dosage: Start at 5–20 mcg/kg/min.
- Titration: Adjust based on patient response.
- Tapering: Slowly reduce the dose as the patient's condition stabilizes.

Epinephrine Infusion.

- Dosage: Administer 2–10 mcg/min.
- Adjustment: Titrate according to clinical response.

59.7.2.3 Second-Line Medications

Aminophylline.

- Used in refractory cases where standard agents are ineffective.

Glucagon.

- Especially useful for bradycardia induced by beta-blocker or calcium channel blocker overdose.
- Dosage: Initial bolus followed by an infusion as needed. 50 micrograms/kg iv loading dose, followed by a continuous infusion of 1–15 mg/h

Isoproterenol.

- Considered when bradycardia is due to drug toxicity and pacing is unavailable.
- Caution: Use with care due to potential arrhythmogenic effects.

59.7.3 Pacing

- Pacing is indicated when pharmacological therapy is ineffective or contraindicated.

59.7.3.1 Transcutaneous Pacing

- Indication: Symptomatic high-degree AV blocks (second or third degree) unresponsive to atropine.
- Procedure: Apply pacing pads and initiate pacing while preparing for transvenous pacing if necessary.
- Analgesia and Sedation: Consider for patient comfort.

59.7.3.2 Transvenous Pacing

- Indication: Persistent bradyarrhythmias not responsive to medications or transcutaneous pacing.
- Procedure: Insertion of a pacing catheter into the right ventricle.
- Monitoring: Continuous ECG and hemodynamic monitoring.

59.7.3.3 Permanent Pacing

- Indication: Patients with recurrent or severe symptoms, or irreversible causes of bradycardia.

- Device: Implantation of a permanent pacemaker.
- Considerations: Evaluate patient's suitability and preference.

59.7.3.4 Advanced Pacing Options

His-Bundle Pacing

- Targets the His-Purkinje conduction system to maintain physiological ventricular activation.
- Reduces the risk of pacing-induced cardiomyopathy associated with right ventricular pacing.

Cardiac Resynchronization Therapy (CRT)

- Beneficial for patients with heart failure and intraventricular conduction delays.
- Improves ventricular synchrony and cardiac output.

59.7.4 Management of Conduction Delays

Patients with LBBB on ECG require special attention:

- Echocardiography.
- Early assessment of left ventricular function.
- Identifies structural heart disease.
- Consider Advanced Pacing.
- His-bundle pacing or CRT to minimize dysynchrony and preserve cardiac function.

59.7.5 Addressing Underlying Causes

- Medication Review.
- Discontinue or adjust medications contributing to bradycardia.
- Electrolyte Correction.

Normalize levels of potassium, calcium, and magnesium.

- Manage Hypothyroidism.

Initiate thyroid hormone replacement therapy.

- Treat Infections.

Appropriate antimicrobial therapy for conditions like Lyme disease or endocarditis.

- Manage Sleep Apnea

Referral for sleep studies and initiation of continuous positive airway pressure (CPAP) therapy if indicated.

59.8 Patient-Centered Care

- Effective management of bradycardia involves engaging the patient in decision-making.

59.9 Shared Decision-Making

- Discussion of Options.
- Explain the benefits and risks of pharmacological therapy versus pacing.
- Patient Preferences.
- Consider the patient's quality of life, occupation, and personal goals.
- Informed Consent.
- Essential before initiating temporary or permanent pacing procedures.

59.10 Conclusion

Bradycardia can range from a benign finding to a life-threatening condition requiring immediate intervention. A systematic approach that includes rapid assessment, identification of reversible causes, appropriate pharmacological therapy, and pacing interventions is essential. Advanced diagnostics and therapies, including His-bundle pacing and CRT, offer improved outcomes for patients with structural heart disease. Engaging patients in their care through shared decision-making enhances adherence and satisfaction with treatment. Recognizing and managing bradycardia effectively can prevent serious complications and improve patient quality of life.

Algorithm 59.1: Approach to bradycardia in the ICU

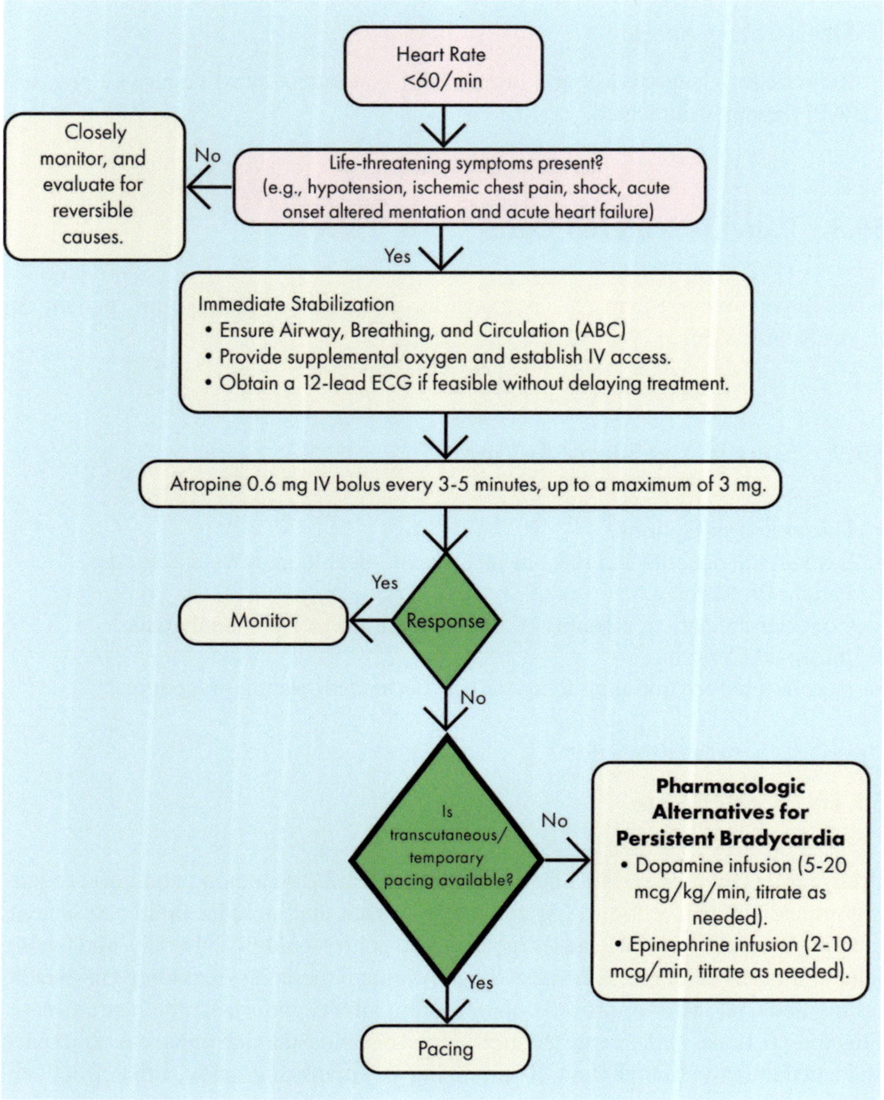

Bibliography

1. Kusumoto FM, Schoenfeld MH, Barrett C, Edgerton JR, Ellenbogen KA, Gold MR, et al. 2018 ACC/AHA/HRS guideline on the evaluation and Management of Patients with Bradycardia and Cardiac Conduction Delay: a report of the American College of Cardiology/American Heart Association task force on clinical practice guidelines and the Heart Rhythm Society. Circulation. 2019;140(8):e382–482.
2. Glikson M, Nielsen JC, Kronborg MB, Michowitz Y, Auricchio A, Barbash IM, et al. 2021 ESC guidelines on cardiac pacing and cardiac resynchronization therapy. Eur Heart J. 2021;42(35):3427–520.
3. Lattell J, Upadhyay GA. Bradyarrhythmias and physiologic pacing in the ICU. J Intensive Care Med. 2022;37(5):595–610.

Chapter 60
Approach to Tachycardia in the ICU

60.1 Introduction

Tachycardia, defined as a heart rate exceeding 100 beats per minute (bpm), is a common occurrence in the intensive care unit (ICU). It can range from a benign physiological response to a manifestation of life-threatening arrhythmias. Rapid identification and appropriate management are crucial to prevent hemodynamic compromise and adverse outcomes [1, 2] [Ref: Algorithm 60.1].

60.2 Initial Evaluation and Assessment

When a patient presents with tachycardia in the ICU, the first step is a thorough evaluation to determine the presence of life-threatening symptoms such as hypotension, ischemic chest pain, dyspnea, altered mental status, or signs of shock. These symptoms suggest that the tachycardia may be compromising cardiac output and end-organ perfusion.

Immediate assessment should focus on airway, breathing, and circulation (ABCs). Ensure the airway is patent, provide supplemental oxygen to maintain oxygen saturation (SpO_2) of at least 94%, and establish continuous monitoring of heart rhythm, blood pressure, and SpO_2. Intravenous access should be secured promptly to facilitate the administration of medications or fluids as needed. A 12-lead electrocardiogram (ECG) is essential for rhythm analysis and aids in identifying the specific type of tachycardia.

Identifying and correcting reversible causes is paramount. Common contributors include hypoxia, electrolyte imbalances (such as hypo- or hyperkalemia, hypomagnesemia, hypocalcemia), acid-base disturbances, hypovolemia, pain, anxiety, and

S. B. Mishra et al., *Mastering ICU Care*,
https://doi.org/10.1007/978-981-95-0179-3_60

fever. Addressing these factors can often alleviate tachycardia without the need for advanced interventions [3].

A thorough physical examination has to be done. Look for fever, anemia, and dehydration (dry mucosa).

All systems must be thoroughly examined.

CNS: Look for fever, seizure, delirium, headache, and other reversible causes. NCCT brain may be done to look for SAH or stroke. Meningitis, traumatic brain injury, stroke, and autonomic dysfunction can also cause tachycardia. Inadequate sedation of ventilated patients can also lead to tachycardia. Hypoglycemia may also cause tachycardia.

CVS: ECG should be done to know the type of tachyarrhythmia. Chest pain, AMI, and hypotension can also cause tachycardia.

RS: Bronchospasm, dyspnea due to pneumonia, pneumothorax, massive pleural effusion, pulmonary edema, or respiratory distress due to any cause can also cause tachycardia. Endotracheal tube block due to secretions or mucus plug can also cause tachycardia. Ventilator dysynchrony and endotracheal tube in situ can also lead to tachycardia. Pulmonary embolism, diffuse alveolar hemorrhage, and hemoptysis should also be kept in consideration.

Abdomen: Pain abdomen due to any cause can also lead to tachycardia, e.g., appendicitis, cholecystitis, pancreatitis, gastritis, colitis, esophageal spasm, perforation, peritonitis, and intestinal obstruction. Acute gastroenteritis leading to severe fluid loss is also a cause for the same.

Genitourinary: Renal and ureteric stones can lead to pain and thus tachycardia. Cystitis and acute urinary retention can also cause tachycardia.

Peripheral: Peripheral vascular diseases, thrombophlebitis, and deep vein thrombus can lead to pain and thus tachycardia.

Endocrinology: Thyroid and adrenal disorders can also lead to tachycardia. Hypoglycemia can also cause tachycardia.

Sepsis: Infection and sepsis has to be looked for. It can lead to SIRS and cause tachycardia. Source of sepsis should be looked for.

Electrolytes: Potassium, Calcium, and magnesium abnormalities can lead to tachyarrhythmias.

Drugs: Drug abuse, bronchodilators, thyroid medicines, and vasopressors (adrenaline, noradrenaline), dobutamine, dopamine, and methylxanthines.

Others: Neuroleptic malignant syndrome, malignant hyperthermia, and phechromocytoma.

60.2.1 Rhythm Analysis

Accurate rhythm analysis is critical for determining the appropriate management strategy. The ECG should be assessed for QRS complex width and rhythm regularity:

- QRS Width:
  - Narrow QRS Complex (<120 ms): Indicates that ventricular depolarization is occurring via the normal His-Purkinje system, suggesting a supraventricular origin.
  - Wide QRS Complex (≥120 ms): May indicate ventricular tachycardia (VT) or supraventricular tachycardia (SVT) with aberrant conduction (e.g., bundle branch block or preexcitation).
- Rhythm Regularity:
  - Regular Rhythm: Consistent R-R intervals.
  - Irregular Rhythm: Variable R-R intervals.

60.3 Differential Diagnosis of Tachycardias

- Narrow QRS Complex Tachycardias.
  - Regular Rhythm.

Sinus tachycardia is characterized by a gradual onset and termination, with heart rates typically less than 150 bpm. It is often a physiological response to stressors such as pain, hypovolemia, or hypoxia. Management focuses on treating the underlying cause rather than the tachycardia itself.

Atrioventricular nodal reentrant tachycardia (AVNRT) and atrioventricular reentrant tachycardia (AVRT) present with sudden onset and termination, with heart rates ranging from 150 to 250 bpm. Initial management includes vagal maneuvers to stimulate the vagus nerve and slow conduction through the atrioventricular (AV) node. If these are ineffective, adenosine is administered as a rapid intravenous bolus (starting with 6 mg, followed by 12 mg if necessary). Beta-blockers or calcium channel blockers, such as verapamil, may be used if adenosine is contraindicated or ineffective. Synchronized cardioversion should be done in hemodynamically unstable patients (50–100 joules) [4].

  - Irregular Rhythm.

Atrial fibrillation (AF) is identified by the absence of discernible P waves and an irregularly irregular rhythm. Management focuses on rate control and anticoagulation. Beta-blockers (e.g., esmolol) or calcium channel blockers (e.g., diltiazem) are used to control the ventricular rate. In patients with heart failure or contraindications to these medications, digoxin or amiodarone may be considered. Anticoagulation is essential for stroke prevention, especially if the duration of AF exceeds 48 hours. The choice between novel oral anticoagulants (NOACs) and traditional agents like warfarin depends on patient-specific factors, including renal function and potential drug interactions. Synchronized cardioversion should be done in hemodynamically unstable patients.

Atrial flutter presents with characteristic sawtooth flutter waves on ECG and an atrial rate around 300 bpm. Management is similar to that of AF, with a focus on rate control and anticoagulation. Synchronized cardioversion may be more effective in atrial flutter and can be considered at lower energy levels (50–100 joules).

- Wide QRS Complex Tachycardias.
  - Regular Rhythm.

Ventricular tachycardia (VT) with pulse is a life-threatening arrhythmia characterized by wide QRS complexes and a regular rhythm. Features suggestive of VT include AV dissociation, fusion beats, capture beats, QRS morphology consistent with ventricular origin, and extreme axis deviation. Immediate management involves the administration of antiarrhythmic medications such as amiodarone (150 mg IV over 10 minutes) or procainamide (10–15 mg/kg IV over 30 minutes). If the patient is hemodynamically unstable or if pharmacological therapy is ineffective, synchronized cardioversion starting at 100 joules is indicated.

SVT with Aberrancy can mimic VT but is due to supraventricular impulses conducted aberrantly through the ventricles, often because of preexisting bundle branch block patterns. Differentiating SVT with aberrancy from VT is crucial, as the management differs. Criteria such as the Brugada algorithm or Vereckei criteria may aid in differentiation. If SVT with aberrancy is confirmed, management is similar to that of narrow QRS complex SVT.

  - Irregular Rhythm.

Polymorphic VT, such as torsades de pointes, is characterized by varying QRS amplitude and axis on the ECG and is often associated with a prolonged QT interval. Management includes the administration of magnesium sulfate (2 grams IV over 10 minutes) and correction of electrolyte abnormalities. Overdrive pacing may be necessary if the arrhythmia is refractory to medical therapy.

Atrial fibrillation with preexcitation occurs in patients with accessory pathways (e.g., Wolff-Parkinson-White syndrome) and presents as an irregular wide-complex tachycardia. AV node blocking agents are contraindicated as they may enhance conduction through the accessory pathway and precipitate ventricular fibrillation. Procainamide is the preferred agent to stabilize the rhythm in this scenario.

60.4 Mechanisms of Tachyarrhythmias

Understanding the underlying mechanisms of tachyarrhythmias aids in predicting recurrence and tailoring interventions:

- Increased Automaticity: Enhanced spontaneous depolarization of pacemaker cells, leading to arrhythmias such as sinus tachycardia.

- Reentry Circuits: Occur when a propagating impulse fails to extinguish itself and reenters and reactivates myocardial tissue, causing arrhythmias like AVNRT, AVRT, and VT.
- Triggered Activity: Results from after depolarizations that reach threshold potential, leading to arrhythmias such as torsades de pointes.

Proarrhythmic substrates include structural heart diseases that predispose patients to arrhythmias:

- Myocardial Scar Tissue: Post-myocardial infarction scarring can create reentrant circuits leading to VT.
- Hypertrophic Cardiomyopathy: Disorganized myocardial architecture increases the risk of ventricular arrhythmias and sudden cardiac death.

60.5 Management of Sinus Tachycardia

Differentiating between physiological and inappropriate sinus tachycardia is essential:

- Physiological sinus tachycardia is a normal response to stressors. Management involves treating the underlying cause without specific cardiac interventions.
- Inappropriate sinus tachycardia is characterized by an elevated heart rate at rest without an identifiable cause. Management may require beta-blockers or calcium channel blockers to control the heart rate. Conditions like postural orthostatic tachycardia syndrome (POTS) should be considered, and management tailored accordingly [5]

60.6 Treatment Strategies and Advanced Therapies

60.6.1 Acute Management Flowcharts

Utilizing flowcharts can streamline decision-making in acute settings by guiding clinicians through treatment choices based on QRS width, rhythm regularity, and hemodynamic stability. These visual aids enhance efficiency in time-sensitive situations.

60.6.2 Advanced Therapies

For patients with persistent or recurrent tachyarrhythmias despite optimal medical therapy, advanced interventions may be necessary:

- Catheter Ablation: Recommended for certain SVTs and VT, as per AHA guidelines, to eliminate the arrhythmogenic focus or pathway.
- Implantable Cardioverter-Defibrillator (ICD): Considered in patients at high risk of sudden cardiac death, such as those with significant left ventricular dysfunction or previous cardiac arrest, following the 2017 AHA/ACC/HRS guidelines.

60.6.3 Anticoagulation in Atrial Fibrillation

Patients with AF, especially those with prolonged arrhythmia duration or high thromboembolic risk, require anticoagulation:

- Risk Assessment: Use the CHA_2DS_2-VASc score to evaluate stroke risk.
- Anticoagulant Options:
  - Novel Oral Anticoagulants (NOACs): Such as apixaban and rivaroxaban, are preferred due to their predictable pharmacokinetics and ease of use.
  - Warfarin: May be used in patients with contraindications to NOACs or with mechanical heart valves.
  - Considerations in Critically Ill Patients: Renal function, potential drug interactions, and bleeding risks must be carefully assessed when initiating anticoagulation.

60.7 Prognostic Insights and Long-Term Management

Tachycardia episodes in the ICU have significant prognostic implications:

- Recurrence Rates: High in patients with underlying heart disease or persistent triggers.
- Progression to Sustained Arrhythmias: Early identification and management can prevent deterioration to more severe arrhythmias requiring long-term interventions.
- Outcomes: Vary depending on the arrhythmia type, underlying cause, and timeliness of management.

60.8 Conclusion

Effective management of tachycardia in the ICU requires a systematic and comprehensive approach that prioritizes rapid assessment, identification of the arrhythmia type, and prompt initiation of appropriate therapy. Incorporating the latest ESC and AHA/ACC/HRS guidelines ensures that care aligns with current standards and evidence-based practices.

Emphasizing the correction of reversible causes and providing early systemic support are crucial steps in optimizing patient outcomes. Understanding the mechanisms of tachyarrhythmias aids in predicting recurrence and tailoring interventions. Advanced therapies should be considered for patients with refractory or recurrent arrhythmias.

Algorithm 60.1: Approach to tachycardia in the ICU

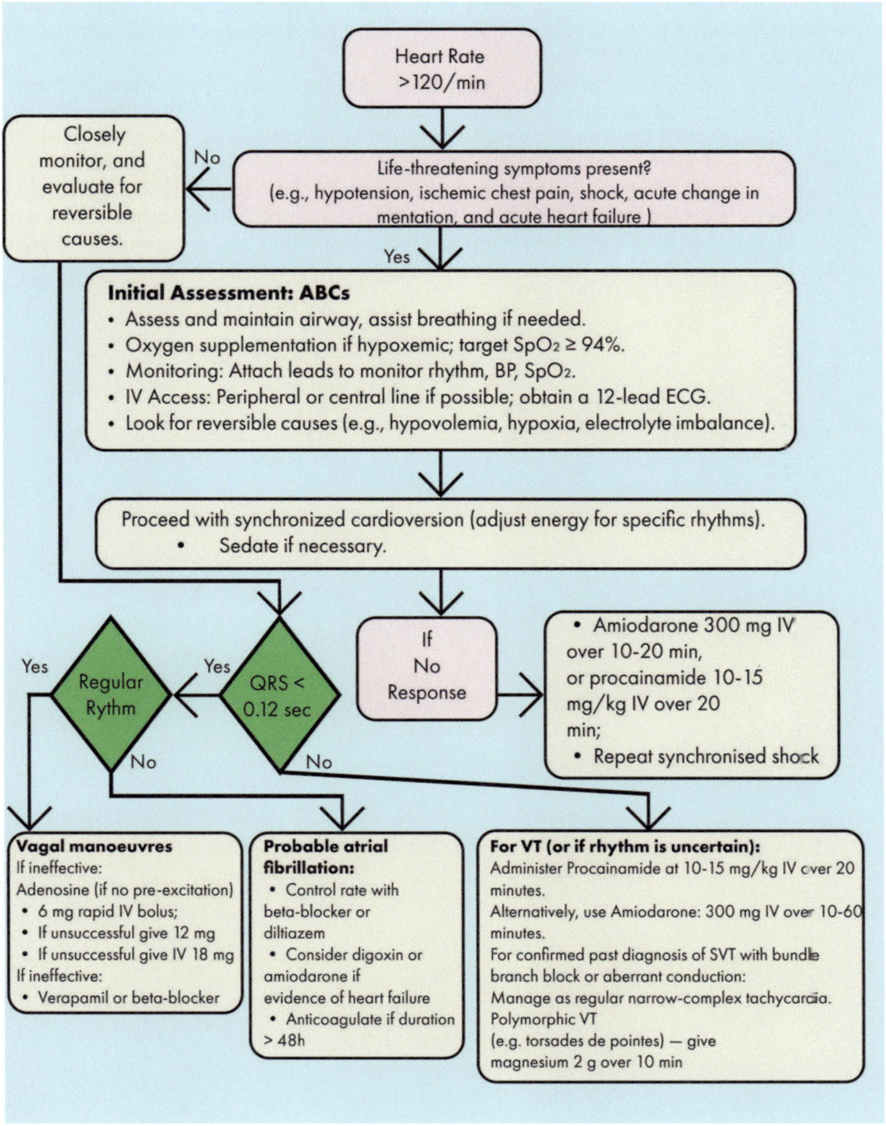

Bibliography

1. Gordon P, Kerton M. Cardiac arrhythmias in the critically ill. Anaesth Intensive Care Med. 2021;22(5):301–12.
2. Senaratne JM, Sandhu R, Barnett CF, Grunau B, Wong GC, van Diepen S. Approach to ventricular arrhythmias in the intensive care unit. J Intensive Care Med. 2021;36(7):731–48.
3. Boriani G, Fauchier L, Aguinaga L, Beattie JM, Blomstrom Lundqvist C, Cohen A, et al. European Heart Rhythm Association (EHRA) consensus document on management of arrhythmias and cardiac electronic devices in the critically ill and post-surgery patient, endorsed by Heart Rhythm Society (HRS), Asia Pacific Heart Rhythm Society (APHRS), Cardiac Arrhythmia Society of Southern Africa (CASSA), and Latin American Heart Rhythm Society (LAHRS). Europace. 2019;21(1):7–8.
4. Brugada J, Katritsis DG, Arbelo E, Arribas F, Bax JJ, Blomstrom-Lundqvist C, et al. 2019 ESC guidelines for the management of patients with supraventricular tachycardia the task force for the management of patients with supraventricular tachycardia of the European Society of Cardiology (ESC). Eur Heart J. 2020;41(5):655–720.
5. Page RL, Joglar JA, Caldwell MA, Calkins H, Conti JB, Deal BJ, et al. 2015 ACC/AHA/HRS guideline for the management of adult patients with supraventricular tachycardia: a report of the American College of Cardiology/American Heart Association task force on clinical practice guidelines and the Heart Rhythm Society. Circulation. 2016;133(14):e506–74.

Chapter 61
Approach to Shock in the ICU

61.1 Introduction

Shock is a life-threatening condition frequently encountered in the intensive care unit (ICU), characterized by inadequate tissue perfusion and oxygenation. Early recognition and prompt management are crucial to prevent progression to multi-organ dysfunction and death. Patients often present with undifferentiated shock, where the cause is not immediately apparent. To address this challenge, systematic assessment protocols like the "MINUTES" bundle have been developed to streamline initial management [1]. The MINUTES acronym stands for:

- Maintain ABCs (airway, breathing and circulation).
- Infuse vasopressors/fluids.
- Investigate.
- Ultrasound.
- Treat etiology.
- Evaluate for stabilization.

Understanding the progressive stages of shock—pre-shock, shock, and end-organ dysfunction—is essential. Early-stage shock is often reversible with timely intervention, highlighting the importance of rapid diagnosis and treatment [Ref: Algorithm 61.1].

S. B. Mishra et al., *Mastering ICU Care*,
https://doi.org/10.1007/978-981-95-0179-3_61

61.2 Step-by-Step Explanation of the Algorithm

61.2.1 Initial Assessment: Hypotension Criteria

The first step in approaching a patient suspected of being in shock is the assessment of hypotension. Hypotension is defined by a mean arterial pressure (MAP) of less than 65 mmHg or a systolic blood pressure below 90 mmHg. Recognizing hypotension is crucial, as it is a hallmark of shock and indicates inadequate perfusion pressure. Immediate recognition prompts further evaluation and intervention to prevent deterioration.

61.2.2 Evaluate for Signs of Shock

After identifying hypotension, clinicians should evaluate the patient for signs of shock, which include tachycardia, altered mental status, decreased urine output, cold, clammy skin, reduced capillary perfusion, and skin mottling. If these signs are absent, the patient should be monitored closely for any changes (see next section). However, if signs of shock are present, immediate stabilization is necessary. Early detection of these clinical signs allows for prompt intervention before irreversible organ damage occurs.

Capillary perfusion/refill time (CRT) steps:

1. Moderate pressure is applied to the nail bed until it turns white (usually 5–10 seconds), then pressure is removed and the time it takes for the nail to return to pink is measured.
2. Ideally, measure at room temperature (20–25 °C).
3. Capillary refill time > 5 seconds is said to be abnormal.

61.2.3 If no Shock Signs: Monitor

In patients without overt signs of shock but with hypotension, continuous monitoring is essential. Key parameters to monitor include urine output, mental status, and skin temperature and perfusion. Monitoring these parameters helps detect subtle changes that may indicate deterioration, allowing for timely intervention if the patient's condition worsens.

61.2.4 *If Shock Signs Present: Stabilization (MINUTES BUNDLE)*

61.2.4.1 M (Maintain ABCs)

For patients exhibiting signs of shock, immediate stabilization is imperative. This involves maintaining airway, breathing, and circulation—the "M" in the MINUTES bundle. Ensure the airway is patent and consider intubation if necessary. Provide supplemental oxygen and monitor oxygen saturation to support breathing. Establish intravenous access to manage circulation effectively.

61.2.4.2 IN (Infuse)

Next, infuse vasopressors and fluids—the "IN" in MINUTES. Administer 1 liter of crystalloid fluids rapidly and initiate a norepinephrine infusion, even through a peripheral line if central access is not yet established. Norepinephrine is considered the first-line vasopressor for septic and distributive shock due to its efficacy and safety profile. Immediate stabilization supports circulatory function and maintains perfusion while further assessments are conducted [2].

IN (Investigate)

The "IN" in MINUTES stands for investigate, emphasizing the need for prompt diagnostic evaluations. Laboratory tests should include blood gas analysis to assess oxygenation, ventilation, and acid-base status, as well as serum lactate levels, which serve as a marker of tissue hypoperfusion. A complete blood count, electrolytes, and renal and liver function tests provide additional information about the patient's physiological state. If cardiogenic shock is suspected, cardiac enzymes should be measured.

Imaging studies are also crucial. A chest X-ray should be performed within the first 10 minutes to identify potential causes such as pneumothorax, pulmonary edema, or a widened mediastinum. Early investigations provide critical insights into the underlying etiology of the shock, guiding further management.

61.2.4.3 U (ultrasound)

The "U" in MINUTES stands for ultrasound, highlighting the role of point-of-care ultrasound (POCUS) in the rapid assessment of patients in shock. Cardiac ultrasound can assess for pericardial effusion, evaluate ventricular function, and detect signs of cardiac tamponade. Lung ultrasound is useful for detecting pneumothorax, pleural effusions, or pulmonary edema. Assessment of the inferior vena cava (IVC) collapsibility can help estimate the patient's volume status.

Critical care echocardiography (CCE) further enhances hemodynamic assessment by measuring parameters such as the left ventricular outflow tract velocity time integral (LVOT VTI) to estimate cardiac output and assessing right atrial pressure to evaluate preload status. Ultrasound aids in rapidly differentiating shock types and identifying conditions that require immediate intervention.

61.2.4.4 TE (Treat Etiology/underlying cause)

Based on the findings from investigations and ultrasound, targeted management should be initiated—the "T" in MINUTES. The treatment approach varies depending on the type of shock identified.

S (Stabilize organ perfusion) - see later section.

Diagnosis involves obtaining a history of recent bleeding, vomiting, diarrhea, or other fluid losses. Physical examination may reveal signs of dehydration. A positive Passive Leg Raise (PLR) test indicates fluid responsiveness. Management focuses on restoring circulating volume by continuing crystalloid infusion and considering blood products if hemorrhage is present. Controlling fluid loss is essential, requiring surgical or medical intervention to address bleeding sources. Caution must be exercised to avoid over-resuscitation and prevent fluid overload.

Steps of Passive Leg Raise Test:

1. Start from the semi-recumbent position with their head at a 45° angle.
2. Lower the patient's upper body until it's horizontal.
3. Passively raise the patient's legs to a 45° angle (by tilting bed, not the legs directly).
4. Direct measurement of cardiac output is to be done and not by the simple measurement of blood pressure. The technique used to measure cardiac output during PLR must be able to detect short-term and transient changes since the PLR effects may vanish after 1 minute.
5. Cardiac output must be measured not only before and during PLR but also after PLR when the patient has been moved back to the semi-recumbent position, in order to check that it returns to its baseline.
6. Avoid confounding factors (pain, cough, discomfort, and awakening could provoke adrenergic stimulation).

Diagnosis is based on electrocardiogram (ECG) findings of ischemic changes or arrhythmias, echocardiography revealing reduced ejection fraction or regional wall motion abnormalities, and elevated cardiac biomarkers such as troponin levels. Management includes initiating inotropic agents like dobutamine to improve cardiac output and consulting cardiology for potential revascularization procedures, such as percutaneous coronary intervention or thrombolysis. Fluids should be used cautiously to avoid exacerbating pulmonary edema. Monitoring for arrhythmias and worsening heart failure is critical. Target a MAP of 65 mm Hg and a urine output of 0.5 ml/kg/hr. Avoid higher doses of noradrenaline and MAP as they lead to increased afterload and oxygen consumption by the failing myocardium. Milrinone can also be used in specific cases.

Diagnosis relies on POCUS findings. In tension pneumothorax, absent lung sliding is observed; pericardial tamponade presents with pericardial effusion and diastolic collapse of the right heart chambers; pulmonary embolism may show right ventricular dilation. Management involves relieving the mechanical obstruction to restore circulation. Tension pneumothorax requires immediate needle decompression followed by chest tube placement. Pericardial tamponade necessitates urgent pericardiocentesis. Pulmonary embolism is treated with thrombolytics or surgical embolectomy.

Diagnosis includes a history of infections, allergic reactions, or spinal injury, and physical examination may reveal warm, flushed skin and low systemic vascular resistance. Management depends on the specific cause:

- Septic Shock: Administer broad-spectrum antibiotics within the first hour after drawing necessary culture and continue norepinephrine infusion, adding vasopressin if needed. Fluid resuscitation should be guided by PLR and hemodynamic monitoring. Source control should be achieved.
- Anaphylactic Shock: Immediate intramuscular epinephrine is essential (0.5 mg, 1:1000), with antihistamines and corticosteroids as adjunctive therapy.
- Neurogenic Shock: Requires fluids and vasopressors to maintain MAP, along with stabilization of any spinal injury.

Careful monitoring is necessary to prevent fluid overload and adjust vasopressor doses based on response.

61.2.4.5 S (Stabilize organ perfusion)

The final steps in the MINUTES bundle are to evaluate for stabilization. Assess the patient's response to treatment by continuously monitoring vital signs, including heart rate, blood pressure, respiratory rate, and oxygen saturation. Urine output should be closely observed, aiming for greater than 0.5 mL/kg/hour as an indicator of renal perfusion. Serial lactate measurements can help assess the adequacy of tissue perfusion.

Advanced monitoring techniques may be employed to guide ongoing management. Insertion of an arterial line allows for continuous blood pressure monitoring and frequent blood gas sampling. A central venous catheter facilitates central venous pressure monitoring and administration of medications. Cardiac output monitoring, using pulse contour analysis or thermodilution techniques, provides valuable information about the patient's hemodynamic status. The venous excess ultrasound (VExUS) examination can be used to evaluate for venous congestion. These measures ensure that interventions are effective and allow for adjustments to treatment as necessary.

61.3 Conclusion

Managing shock in the ICU requires a structured and rapid approach. The MINUTES bundle provides a practical framework for early recognition and intervention, crucial in the reversible stages of shock. Incorporating point-of-care ultrasound (POCUS) and critical care echocardiography (CCE) enhances diagnostic accuracy, allowing for timely and targeted therapy. Recognizing the characteristics of each shock type guides appropriate management while avoiding potential pitfalls, such as fluid overload in cardiogenic shock. Early and aggressive treatment of specific etiologies—like antibiotics for septic shock or decompression for tension pneumothorax—can significantly improve patient outcomes. Continuous evaluation and advanced monitoring ensure that therapy is effective and adjusted to the patient's evolving condition, ultimately reducing the risk of multi-organ failure and mortality.

Algorithm 61.1: Approach to shock in the ICU

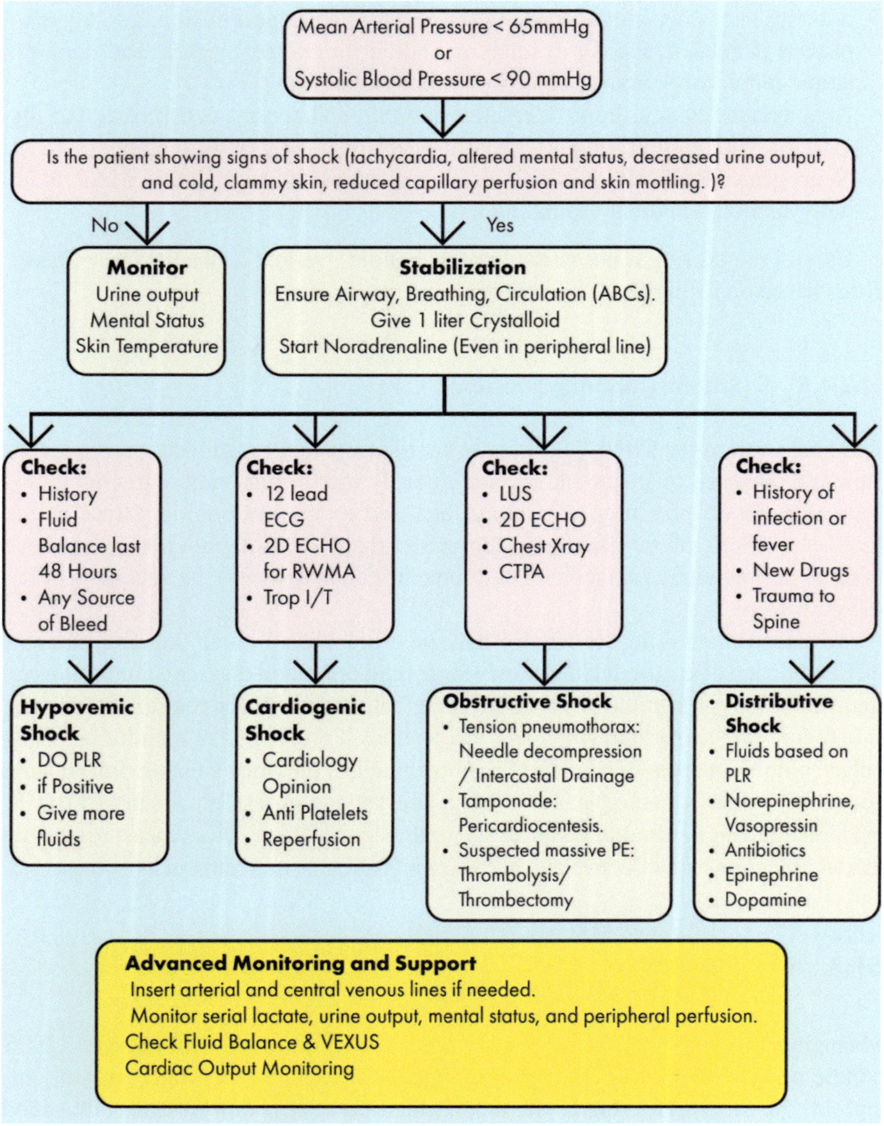

Bibliography

1. Hasanin A, Sanfilippo F, Dunser MW, Ahmed HM, Zieleskiewicz L, Myatra SN, et al. The MINUTES bundle for the initial 30 min management of undifferentiated circulatory shock: an expert opinion. Int J Emerg Med. 2024;17(1):96.
2. Salinas P, Sohn J, Diaz-Gomez JL. Critical care echocardiography-a driven approach to undifferentiated shock. Tex Heart Inst J. 2023;50(5)

Chapter 62
Approach to Chest Pain in the ICU

62.1 Introduction

Chest pain in the intensive care unit (ICU) is a critical symptom that demands a swift and systematic approach to identify potentially life-threatening conditions. Differentiating between cardiac and noncardiac causes is of paramount importance, and utilizing structured assessment tools can significantly enhance diagnostic accuracy. The pain can be visceral or somatic. Visceral pain is usually dull and over a larger area without any localization; whereas somatic pain is usually sharp, stabbing, and localized to a specific spot/area (dermatomal distribution). Importantly, clinicians must recognize that chest pain presentations can vary across different populations. Women, for instance, may experience symptoms beyond chest pain, such as nausea, fatigue, or shortness of breath, which can lead to underdiagnosis. Older adults often present with atypical symptoms like shortness of breath or confusion rather than chest pain alone. This chapter presents a comprehensive algorithm for evaluating chest pain in the ICU, incorporating current international guidelines, risk stratification methods, and considerations for diverse populations to ensure prompt and appropriate management [1, 2]. [Ref: Algorithm 62.1].

62.2 Primary Assessment (ABCDE Approach)

The initial step in managing a patient with chest pain in the ICU is the primary assessment using the Airway, Breathing, Circulation, Disability, and Exposure (ABCDE) approach. This systematic method aims to stabilize the patient and address any immediate life-threatening issues. Clinicians should assess vital signs and oxygenation status promptly, initiating resuscitation measures if necessary. In unstable patients, point-of-care ultrasound (POCUS) can be invaluable for rapidly evaluating conditions such as pneumothorax, pleural effusion, or cardiac tamponade.

S. B. Mishra et al., *Mastering ICU Care*,
https://doi.org/10.1007/978-981-95-0179-3_62

62.3 Initial Evaluation and Risk Stratification

Following stabilization, a detailed evaluation of the chest pain is essential. Employing the SOCRATES mnemonic—Site, Onset, Character, Radiation, Alleviating/Aggravating Factors, Timing, Exacerbating Factors, and Severity—provides a structured framework for characterizing the pain. Determining the exact location and nature of the pain, noting when and how it started, and identifying any radiation to other areas like the arm or jaw are crucial steps. Understanding what alleviates or aggravates the pain, whether it is constant or intermittent, and any triggers or activities that worsen it can offer vital clues. Quantifying the pain intensity using a severity scale aids in assessing the patient's condition.

62.3.1 Gender-Specific Considerations

It is important to recognize that women may present with symptoms beyond chest pain, such as nausea, fatigue, indigestion, or shortness of breath. These nonspecific symptoms can often lead to underdiagnosis of acute coronary syndromes (ACS) in women. Clinicians should maintain a high index of suspicion and consider cardiac causes even when chest pain is not the predominant symptom in female patients.

62.3.2 Age-Related Assessment

Older adults may present with atypical symptoms such as shortness of breath, confusion, syncope, or weakness rather than classic chest pain. Cognitive impairment and communication difficulties in this population may further obscure the clinical picture. A comprehensive evaluation, including collateral history from caregivers when necessary, is essential to avoid missing critical diagnoses in older patients who are at higher risk for ACS.

62.3.3 Risk Stratification Pathways

To categorize the patient's risk level for cardiac events, clinicians should apply validated risk stratification scores recommended by current guidelines, such as the HEART, EDACS, or TIMI scores. These clinical decision pathways are designed to streamline the diagnostic process and are adaptable to various settings, including the emergency department and outpatient clinics. Utilizing these tools helps in identifying patients who require urgent intervention versus those who can be managed conservatively.

62.4 Electrocardiogram (ECG) Evaluation

A 12-lead ECG should be performed within 10 min of the patient's presentation. The ECG is instrumental in detecting signs of ischemia or infarction, such as ST-segment changes, T-wave inversions, or new-onset left bundle branch block. New-onset ST elevation (in two or more contiguous leads) indicates STEMI (ST elevation myocardial infarction) and new-onset left bundle branch block. ST depression and pathological q waves signify non-ST-elevated myocardial infarction (NSTEMI). If the ECG indicates STEMI, immediate reperfusion therapy is indicated. For NSTEMI or unstable angina, further cardiac evaluation and management are necessary. It is important to note that a normal or nondiagnostic ECG does not rule out cardiac ischemia; therefore, continued evaluation is warranted.

62.5 Biomarker Assessment

High-sensitivity troponin testing is a cornerstone in the assessment of patients with chest pain. Initial troponin levels should be obtained promptly, with repeat measurements at appropriate intervals—typically around −3–4 h—to detect rising trends indicative of myocardial injury. Serial measurements enhance diagnostic accuracy, particularly in low-risk patients where initial levels may be normal.

62.6 Imaging and Additional Diagnostic Tests

Chest radiography is a valuable tool for identifying noncardiac causes of chest pain, such as pneumothorax, pneumonia, or aortic anomalies. Advanced imaging modalities should be selected based on the clinical scenario and the most probable diagnoses. Coronary computed tomography (CT) angiography may be considered for low- to intermediate-risk patients with possible cardiac chest pain and normal ECG and troponin results. Echocardiography is useful for evaluating structural heart diseases, wall motion abnormalities, or pericardial effusion.

For patients with symptoms suggestive of pulmonary embolism, a ventilation-perfusion (V/Q) scan or CT pulmonary angiography should be performed. In cases where aortic dissection is suspected—particularly in patients presenting with sudden, severe chest or back pain—aortic imaging with CT or magnetic resonance imaging (MRI) is essential for diagnosis.

62.7 Management Based on Identified Cause

62.7.1 Cardiac Causes

Acute Coronary Syndrome (ACS): Management of ACS involves both medical therapy and possible revascularization. Medical management includes initiation of oxygen therapy to target saturation levels >94%, administration of antiplatelet agents such as aspirin (160–325 mg orally chewable/dispersible) and P2Y12 inhibitors (Clopidogrel 300 mg orally), or Ticagrelor 180 mg orally if immediate percutaneous coronary intervention (PCI) or coronary arterial bypass graft (CABG) is not planned in next few hours. Heparin bolus of 60 U/kg (maximum 4000 U) followed by an initial infusion of 12 U/kg per hour (maximum 1000 U/hr) adjusted to maintain activated partial thromboplastin time (aPTT) at 1.5–2.0 times control (approximately 50–70 seconds) must be given intravenously to patients undergoing reperfusion therapy with alteplase, reteplase, or tenecteplase. LMWH might be considered as an acceptable alternative to UFH as ancillary therapy for patients less than 75 years of age who are receiving fibrinolytic therapy, provided that significant renal dysfunction (serum creatinine greater than 2.5 mg/dL in men or 2.0 mg/dL in women) is not present. Enoxaparin (30 mg IV bolus followed by 1.0 mg/kg subcutaneous injection every 12 h until hospital discharge) can be used alternatively in combination with full-dose tenecteplase. Sublingual NTG (Nitroglycerine) 0.4 mg or IV infusion (5–200 mcg/min) can be used for chest pain. However, it must be avoided if systolic blood pressure is below 90 mm Hg. Morphine can be used for pain at a dose of 2–4 mg IV followed by 1–2 mg IV every 15 min. Other opioids like fentanyl may also be used for pain relief. Beta-blockers to reduce myocardial oxygen demand and statins for lipid management are other supportive managements to be started along with antiplatelets and analgesia. Urgent percutaneous coronary intervention (PCI) is indicated for patients with STEMI. For those with NSTEMI, the decision to pursue PCI or continue with medical management is guided by risk stratification and patient stability.

Pericardial Tamponade: In cases of pericardial tamponade, prompt pericardiocentesis is required to relieve pressure on the heart and restore normal hemodynamics.

62.7.2 Noncardiac Causes

Pulmonary Embolism (PE): Management of PE depends on the patient's stability. Stable patients should receive anticoagulation therapy to prevent further clot formation. In unstable patients, where there is hemodynamic compromise, thrombolytic therapy or surgical embolectomy may be necessary.

Aortic Dissection: Treatment of aortic dissection is determined by the location of the dissection. Type A dissections, involving the ascending aorta, require emergency surgical repair. Type B dissections, involving the descending aorta, are typically managed medically with strict blood pressure control, with surgery reserved for complications or persistent pain.

Pneumothorax: In the event of a large or tension pneumothorax, insertion of a chest tube is required to re-expand the lung and alleviate symptoms.

Gastrointestinal Causes: For suspected gastroesophageal reflux disease (GERD), administration of proton pump inhibitors or gastrointestinal (GI) cocktails may provide symptom relief. However, clinicians should be cautious, as symptom relief does not confirm the diagnosis, and further evaluation may be necessary to rule out cardiac causes.

62.8 Conclusion

A systematic approach to chest pain in the ICU is essential for the rapid identification and management of life-threatening conditions. By utilizing structured assessment tools like SOCRATES for history taking, applying risk stratification scores such as HEART, EDACS, or TIMI, and adhering to current international guidelines, clinicians can improve diagnostic accuracy and patient outcomes. Recognizing the variations in chest pain presentations among women, older adults, and diverse populations is crucial to avoid underdiagnosis and ensure equitable care. Incorporating patient-centered care, shared decision-making, and patient education further enhances the therapeutic relationship and ensures that management strategies align with the patient's values and preferences.

Flowchart Summary: Approach to Chest Pain in the ICU

1. Primary Assessment (ABCDE) and Stabilization
    - Secure airway, support breathing, ensure adequate circulation.
    - Assess vital signs and hemodynamic stability.
    - Use POCUS if indicated for rapid assessment.
2. Initial Evaluation
    - Conduct a thorough history using the SOCRATES mnemonic.
    - Be attentive to gender-specific and age-related symptoms.
    - Apply risk stratification tools (HEART, EDACS, TIMI) as per guidelines.
    - Address cultural and language barriers to obtain accurate history.
3. ECG Evaluation
    - Perform an ECG within 10 min of presentation.
    - Interpret ECG findings promptly to guide management.

4. Biomarker Assessment
    - Obtain high-sensitivity troponin levels.
    - Repeat measurements to detect rising trends.
5. Further Diagnostic Testing
    - Select imaging modalities based on clinical suspicion.
    - Use echocardiography, coronary CT angiography, V/Q scan, CT pulmonary angiography, or CT/MRI as appropriate.
6. Management
    - Tailor treatment to the identified cause following current guidelines.
    - Initiate ACS protocols, manage noncardiac causes accordingly.

Key Points to Remember

- Prioritize Life-Threatening Conditions: Always address immediate threats to life and stabilize the patient before proceeding with further evaluation.
- Structured Assessment Tools: Utilize tools like SOCRATES and guideline-recommended risk stratification scores to enhance diagnostic accuracy.
- Consider Population-Specific Presentations: Be aware of gender-specific, age-related, and culturally influenced variations in symptom presentation to avoid underdiagnosis.
- Timely ECG and Biomarker Testing: Early ECG and troponin assessments are critical in diagnosing acute coronary syndromes.
- Selective Imaging Modalities: Choose imaging studies based on clinical suspicion to identify or rule out specific conditions efficiently.
- Cause-Specific Management: Follow current guidelines to tailor treatment to the identified cause, whether cardiac or noncardiac.

Algorithm 62.1: Approach to chest pain in the ICU

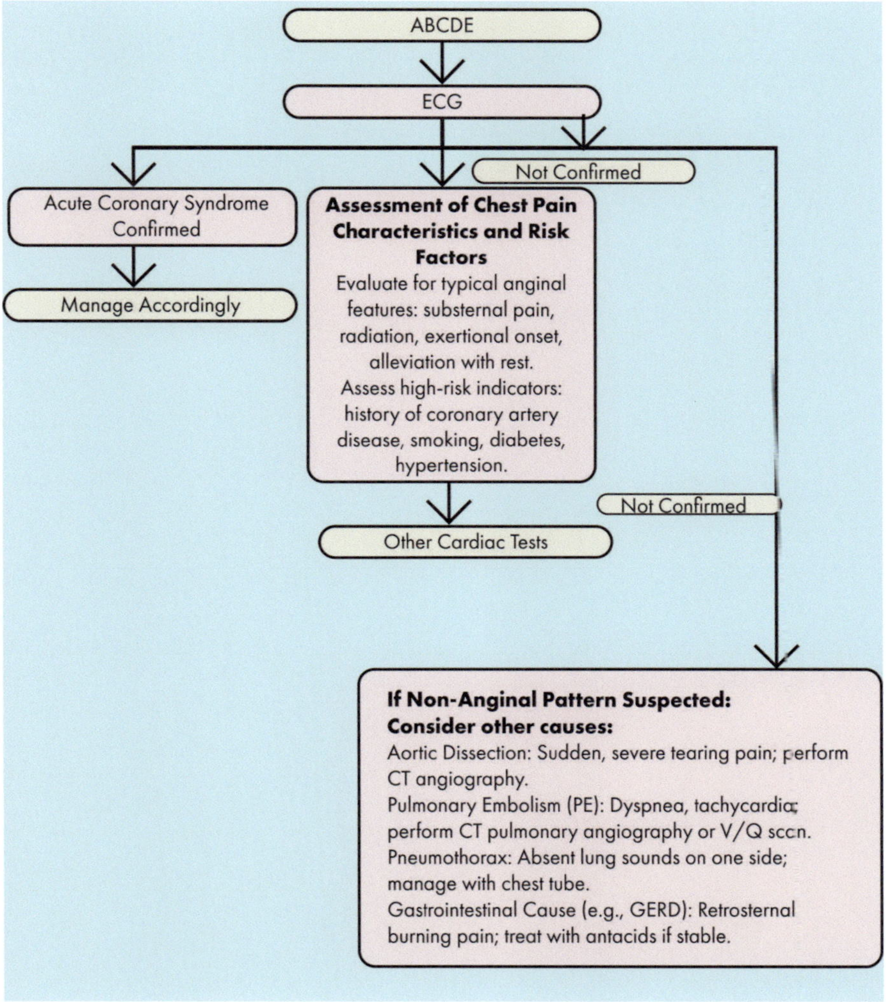

Bibliography

1. Gulati M, Levy PD, Mukherjee D, Amsterdam E, Bhatt DL, Birtcher KK, et al. 2021 AHA/ACC/ASE/CHEST/SAEM/SCCT/SCMR guideline for the evaluation and diagnosis of CHEST pain: a report of the American College of Cardiology/American Heart Association joint committee on clinical practice guidelines. Circulation. 2021;144(22):e368–454.
2. Ng IKS, Chia YW, See KC, Teo DBS. Approach to acute chest pain and acute coronary syndrome in adults. Singapore Med J. 2024;65(2):111.

Chapter 63
Approach to STEMI in the ICU

63.1 Introduction

ST-elevation myocardial infarction (STEMI) is a critical form of acute coronary syndrome resulting from a complete occlusion of a coronary artery, leading to significant myocardial ischemia and necrosis. Rapid recognition and immediate intervention are paramount to minimize myocardial damage, preserve cardiac function, and improve survival rates. This chapter delineates a comprehensive approach to STEMI management, integrating current guidelines to optimize care from initial presentation through post-reperfusion and secondary prevention phases [1, 2] [Ref: Algorithm 63.1].

63.2 Management

The prompt administration of a loading dose of aspirin—typically 300 mg (162–325 mg)—is recommended immediately upon STEMI diagnosis, unless contraindicated. Aspirin inhibits platelet aggregation, reducing thrombus formation and limiting myocardial damage, and should be continued indefinitely as part of long-term management.

Upon presentation, swiftly establishing eligibility for reperfusion therapy is crucial to avoid delays.. Early stratification using clinical assessment and diagnostic tools, such as a 12-lead electrocardiogram (ECG), helps determine the most appropriate reperfusion strategy. ST-elevation in specific leads correlates with the infarct location and guides subsequent interventions.

S. B. Mishra et al., *Mastering ICU Care*,
https://doi.org/10.1007/978-981-95-0179-3_63

63.3 Reperfusion Therapy Decision-Making

The choice between primary percutaneous coronary intervention (PCI) and fibrinolytic therapy is a critical decision in the management of STEMI, significantly impacting patient outcomes. This decision hinges on several factors, including the timing of symptom onset, the availability and proximity of PCI-capable facilities, patient-specific contraindications, and logistical considerations that may affect treatment delays.

63.4 Timing Since Symptom Onset

Guidelines universally emphasize the importance of time in myocardial salvage—the adage "time is myocardium" underscores that delays in reperfusion increase the extent of myocardial necrosis and worsen clinical outcomes. For patients presenting within 12 h of symptom onset, reperfusion therapy is strongly recommended unless contraindicated. Early intervention within this window maximizes the potential for myocardial salvage and improves survival rates.

63.5 Primary PCI Within 120 min

Primary PCI is the preferred reperfusion strategy. Factors favoring primary PCI include:

- Symptom Onset within 12 h: Patients presenting early benefit most from PCI.
- High-Risk Features: Hemodynamic instability, cardiogenic shock, severe heart failure, or arrhythmias.
- Diagnosis Uncertainty: PCI allows for definitive diagnosis and treatment.
- Late Presentation: Patients presenting between 12 and 24 h after symptom onset may still benefit from PCI, especially if there is evidence of ongoing ischemia.

63.6 Logistical Considerations

The total ischemic time should remain within the 120-minute window. If anticipated delays exceed this timeframe, alternative strategies should be considered.

63.7 Fibrinolytic Therapy

If primary PCI cannot be performed within 120 min, immediate initiation of fibrinolytic therapy is recommended, ideally within 30 min of diagnosis of STEMI. Commonly used fibrinolytics include tenecteplase, alteplase, or reteplase are administered to dissolve the thrombus occluding the coronary artery (Table 63.1). Tenecteplase is often preferred due to its ease of administration (single bolus) and fibrin specificity.

63.8 Criteria for Fibrinolysis

- Symptom Onset within 12 h: Greatest benefit when administered early.
- PCI Delay: When PCI cannot be achieved within the recommended timeframes.
- No Contraindications to Fibrinolysis: Absence of bleeding disorders, recent surgeries, or history of hemorrhagic stroke.
- Contraindications to Fibrinolysis:
  - Absolute: Any prior ICH known structural cerebral vascular lesion (e.g., AVM), Known malignant intracranial neoplasm (primary or metastatic), ischemic stroke within 3 months EXCEPT acute ischemic stroke within 3 h, suspected aortic dissection, active bleeding or bleeding diathesis (excluding menses), significant closed head or facial trauma within 3 months.
  - Relative: History of chronic severe, poorly controlled hypertension, severe uncontrolled hypertension on presentation (SBP greater than 180 mm Hg or DBP greater than 110 mm Hg), history of prior ischemic stroke greater than 3 months, dementia, or known intracranial pathology not covered in contraindications, Traumatic or prolonged (greater than 10 min) CPR or major surgery (less than 3 weeks), recent (within 2–4 weeks) internal bleeding, noncompressible vascular punctures, For streptokinase/anistreplase: prior exposure (more than 5 days ago) or prior allergic reaction to these agents, pregnancy, active peptic ulcer.

Table 63.1 Dosing regimens for common fibrinolytic agents used in STEMI management

Drug	Dose
Streptokinase	1.5 million U over 30–60 min IV
Reteplase (rPA)	10 U IV bolus initially, followed by 10 U IV bolus 30 minute after
Alteplase (tPA)	Bolus 15 mg IV, followed by infusion 0.75 mg/kg for 30 min (up 50 mg) and then 0.5 mg/kg for 60 min (up to 35 mg)
Tenecteplase (TNK-tPA)	Single IV bolus with 30 mg for 60 kg; 35 mg for 60–69 kg;40 mg for 70–79 kg; 45 mg for 80–89 kg; 50 mg for ≥ 90 kg

63.9 Monitoring and Follow-Up

After fibrinolysis, patients should be closely monitored for signs of reperfusion, such as resolution of chest pain, reduction of ST-segment elevation by ≥50% within 60–90 min, and the occurrence of reperfusion arrhythmias. Failure to achieve reperfusion criteria necessitates immediate rescue PCI.

63.10 Pharmacologic Support in PCI

Antithrombotic therapy is a cornerstone of STEMI management during and after PCI, aiming to prevent thrombotic complications while minimizing bleeding risks. The selection of specific agents and dosing regimens should consider individual patient factors, access site, and concomitant therapies.

63.11 Anticoagulant Therapy (Up to 8 Days/ until Revascalurization)

- Unfractionated Heparin (UFH): UFH is widely used due to its rapid onset and ease of monitoring. The recommended dosing during PCI is 70–100 IU/kg when GPIs are not used and 50–70 IU/kg when GPIs are administered. Activated clotting time (ACT) should be monitored to guide dosing.
- Bailout Glycoprotein IIb/IIIa Inhibitors (GPIs): Agents such as abciximab, tirofiban, or eptifibatide may be used selectively in cases of large thrombus burden, slow-flow/no-reflow phenomena, or other thrombotic complications during PCI. Their use requires careful consideration due to increased bleeding risk.
- Bivalirudin: A direct thrombin inhibitor, bivalirudin is an alternative to UFH, particularly beneficial when femoral arterial access is used. It has a lower risk of bleeding complications compared to UFH with GPIs. The recommended dosing is a bolus of 0.75 mg/kg followed by an infusion of 1.75 mg/kg/h during the procedure.
- LMWH might be considered an acceptable alternative to UFH as ancillary therapy for patients less than 75 years of age who are receiving fibrinolytic therapy, provided that significant renal dysfunction (serum creatinine greater than 2.5 mg/dL in men or 2.0 mg/dL in women) is not present. Enoxaparin (30 mg IV bolus followed by 1.0 mg/kg subcutaneous injection every 12 h until hospital discharge) used in combination with full-dose tenecteplase is the most comprehensively studied regimen in patients less than 75 years of age.

Patients who fail thrombolysis (ST segments fail to decrease by 50%) should undergo rescue PCI (if available) or may be shifted to a center that is equipped for PCI.

63.12 Antiplatelet Therapy

- Aspirin: A loading dose of 162–325 mg orally (or 75–250 mg IV) should be administered followed by a maintenance dose of 75–162 mg daily indefinitely.
- P2Y12 Inhibitors:
  - Prasugrel: Recommended for patients undergoing primary PCI who are not on oral anticoagulants and have no history of stroke or transient ischemic attack. Loading dose is 60 mg orally, followed by 10 mg daily. Prasugrel is associated with a faster onset of action and greater platelet inhibition compared to clopidogrel but with an increased bleeding risk.
  - Clopidogrel: Preferred in patients on oral anticoagulants or with contraindications to prasugrel. Loading dose is 300–600 mg orally, followed by 75 mg daily. It has a slower onset and variable antiplatelet effect due to genetic polymorphisms affecting metabolism.
  - Ticagrelor: An alternative to prasugrel and clopidogrel, ticagrelor has a rapid onset and potent platelet inhibition. Loading dose is 180 mg orally, followed by 90 mg twice daily. Caution is advised in patients with a history of intracranial hemorrhage or severe hepatic impairment.

63.13 Individual Patient Factors

- Renal Function: Adjust dosing of anticoagulants in patients with renal impairment. Bivalirudin infusion rate should be reduced in severe renal dysfunction.
- Bleeding Risk: Assess bleeding risk using scoring systems (e.g., CRUSADE score) to guide antithrombotic therapy choices.
- Drug Interactions and Allergies: Review medications to avoid adverse interactions and consider allergies to antiplatelet agents or anticoagulants.

63.14 Post-PCI Antithrombotic Therapy

- Dual Antiplatelet Therapy (DAPT): Continue DAPT for at least 12 months unless contraindicated. Duration may be adjusted based on bleeding risk and stent type.
- Anticoagulation: Generally discontinued after PCI unless there is an indication for long-term anticoagulation (e.g., atrial fibrillation), in which case triple therapy strategies should be carefully managed to minimize bleeding.

63.15 Considerations for High Bleeding Risk Patients

Patients with a high risk of bleeding present a therapeutic challenge, requiring a delicate balance between preventing thrombotic events and minimizing hemorrhagic complications. Risk factors for bleeding include advanced age, low body weight, renal insufficiency, history of bleeding, anemia, and use of other anticoagulant or antiplatelet medications.

63.16 Risk Stratification

- Bleeding Risk Scores: Utilize tools like the HAS-BLED or CRUSADE scores to quantify bleeding risk and guide therapy.
- Patient Assessment: Comprehensive evaluation of patient history, comorbid conditions, and concomitant medications is essential.

63.17 Antiplatelet Therapy Modifications

Choice of P2Y12 Inhibitor:

- Clopidogrel: Often favored in high bleeding risk patients due to its lower bleeding risk profile compared to prasugrel and ticagrelor.
- Ticagrelor: May be considered, but with caution, as it carries an intermediate bleeding risk.
- Prasugrel: Generally avoided in high bleeding risk patients due to increased hemorrhagic complications.

Aspirin Monotherapy: In patients with very high bleeding risk or significant contraindications to DAPT, aspirin monotherapy may be considered after careful evaluation. However, this approach may increase the risk of stent thrombosis and should be reserved for exceptional cases.

63.18 Duration of Dual Antiplatelet Therapy

- Shortened DAPT Duration: Recent guidelines allow for a shorter duration of DAPT (e.g., 3–6 months) in high bleeding risk patients, particularly with the use of newer-generation drug-eluting stents that have lower rates of stent thrombosis.
- De-escalation Strategies: Transitioning from a potent P2Y12 inhibitor to clopidogrel after an initial period may reduce bleeding without significantly increasing ischemic risk.

63.19 Anticoagulant Therapy Adjustments

- Reduced Dosing: Consider lower doses of anticoagulants like UFH during PCI, guided by ACT measurements.
- Avoid GPIs: Omit routine use of GPIs unless absolutely necessary, as they significantly increase bleeding risk.
- Bivalirudin Use: May be advantageous due to its reversible action and lower bleeding risk compared to UFH with GPIs.

63.20 Bleeding Management Protocols

- Preparedness: Have protocols in place for the prompt recognition and management of bleeding complications.
- Transfusion Strategies: Judicious use of blood transfusions, balancing the risks of anemia and transfusion-related complications.

63.21 Post-reperfusion Care

After reperfusion, comprehensive post-procedural management is crucial to address potential complications and prevent recurrent events. Mandatory assessment of left ventricular function should be conducted to stratify the risk of heart failure and other adverse outcomes. Echocardiography is the preferred modality for evaluating ventricular performance and detecting mechanical complications.

If ongoing ischemia persists after reperfusion attempts, guidelines recommend follow-up angiography to assess for residual stenosis or reocclusion. For patients with multivessel disease who are stable and not in cardiogenic shock, complete revascularization during the same hospital admission is advised. This approach has been shown to improve long-term outcomes but may pose increased risks in patients with hemodynamic instability or shock.

Secondary Prevention Measures Long-term management following STEMI is aimed at reducing recurrent ischemic events, preventing heart failure, and improving survival.

Evidence-based pharmacologic and lifestyle interventions form the cornerstone of secondary prevention:

- Beta-blockers: Recommended unless contraindicated, to reduce myocardial oxygen demand, prevent arrhythmias, and improve survival.
- ACE inhibitors/ARBs/ARNI: Initiated early, particularly in patients with LV dysfunction, diabetes, hypertension, or anterior MI, to improve ventricular remodeling and long-term outcomes.

- Statins: High-intensity statin therapy (e.g., atorvastatin 40–80 mg, rosuvastatin 20–40 mg) should be started as soon as possible to achieve LDL-C reduction and plaque stabilization.
- Mineralocorticoid receptor antagonists: Indicated in patients with LV ejection fraction ≤40% with heart failure symptoms or diabetes, provided renal function and potassium levels are adequate.
- Lifestyle Modifications: Smoking cessation, dietary changes (low-salt, low-saturated fat), weight control, and structured exercise or cardiac rehabilitation programs.
- Follow-up: Regular outpatient follow-up for optimization of therapy, adherence monitoring, and risk factor control.

63.22 Conclusion

Managing STEMI requires a multifaceted approach that begins with rapid recognition and immediate initiation of evidence-based interventions. Early administration of aspirin and prompt determination of reperfusion eligibility are critical initial steps. The choice between primary PCI and fibrinolysis depends on timing, availability, and patient-specific factors. Antithrombotic therapy must be tailored to balance efficacy and bleeding risk. Post-reperfusion care, including left ventricular function assessment and consideration of complete revascularization, plays a pivotal role in optimizing outcomes.

Algorithm 63.1: Approach to STEMI in the ICU

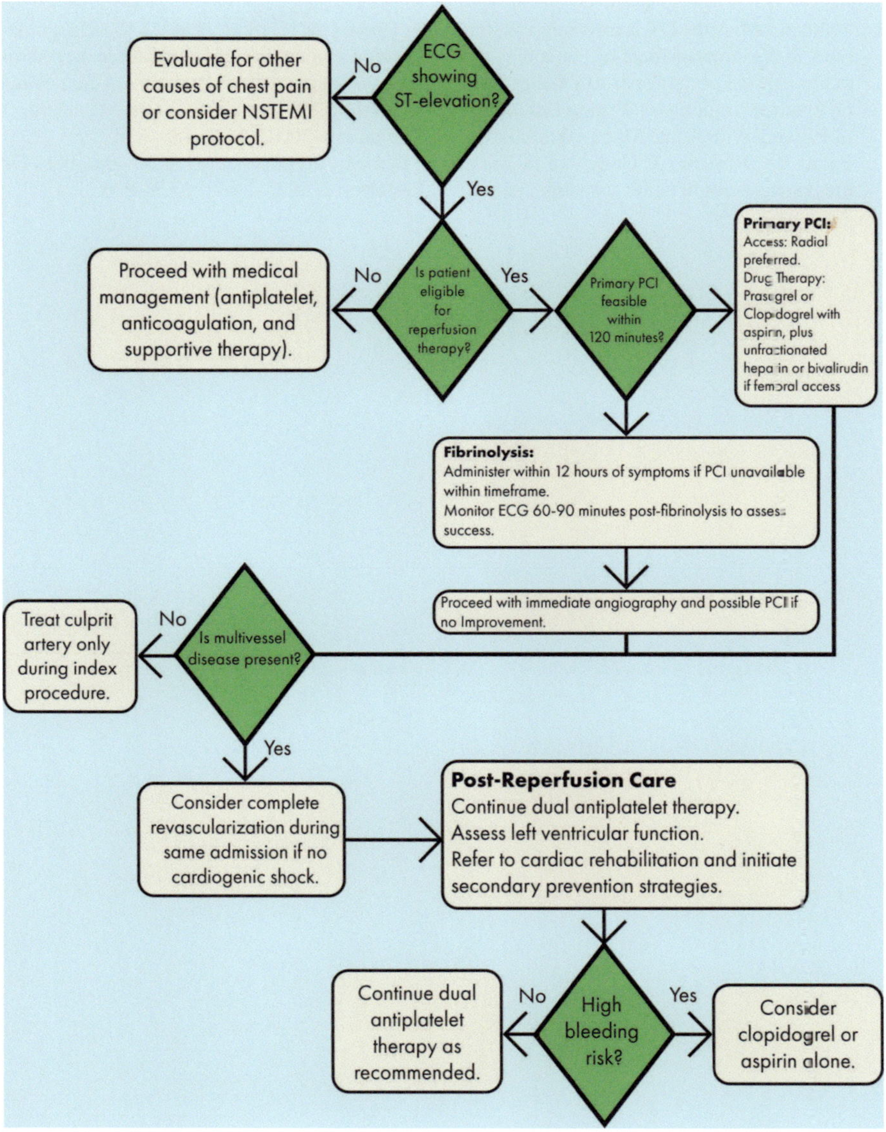

Bibliography

1. Antman EM, Anbe DT, Armstrong PW, Bates ER, Green LA, Hand M, et al. ACC/AHA guidelines for the management of patients with ST-elevation myocardial infarction–executive summary: a report of the American College of Cardiology/American Heart Association Task Force on Practice Guidelines (Writing Committee to Revise the 1999 Guidelines for the Management of Patients With Acute Myocardial Infarction). Circulation. 2004;110(5):588–636.
2. Byrne RA, Rossello X, Coughlan JJ, Barbato E, Berry C, Chieffo A, et al. ESC guidelines for the management of acute coronary syndromes. Eur Heart J. 2023;44(38):3720–826.

Chapter 64
Approach to NSTEMI in the ICU

64.1 Introduction

NSTEMI, a variant of acute coronary syndrome (ACS), presents with myocardial damage evidenced by elevated troponins, yet lacks the hallmark ST-segment elevation on ECG. The pathophysiology of NSTEMI involves a mismatch between myocardial oxygen supply and demand. This imbalance is often due to partial occlusion of a coronary artery by a thrombus superimposed on a disrupted atherosclerotic plaque. However, other mechanisms such as plaque instability, vasospasm, myocarditis, or even non-atherosclerotic causes like pulmonary embolism can also precipitate NSTEMI. Understanding these varied etiologies is crucial for distinguishing NSTEMI from other forms of ACS and tailoring appropriate management strategies [1–3] [Ref: Algorithm 64.1].

64.2 Detailed Pathophysiology

The fundamental issue in NSTEMI is the insufficient oxygen delivery to meet the myocardial metabolic demands. Plaque instability leads to endothelial disruption, exposing subendothelial collagen and initiating platelet aggregation and thrombus formation. This process can result in transient or incomplete occlusion of the coronary artery, leading to ischemia and myocardial injury. Vasospasm, often induced by endothelial dysfunction or exposure to vasoconstrictive substances, can further reduce coronary blood flow. Non-atherosclerotic causes, such as myocarditis or pulmonary embolism, can mimic NSTEMI by causing myocardial strain or injury through inflammatory processes or increased right ventricular workload, respectively.

S. B. Mishra et al., *Mastering ICU Care*,
https://doi.org/10.1007/978-981-95-0179-3_64

64.3 Risk Stratification

Accurate risk assessment is essential for guiding both therapeutic choices and prognostic conversations in patients with NSTEMI. The GRACE (Global Registry of Acute Coronary Events) score remains a widely validated tool for estimating six-month mortality, incorporating parameters such as patient age, heart rate, systolic blood pressure, serum creatinine, cardiac arrest on arrival, ST-segment shifts, elevated cardiac biomarkers, and Killip classification. Nevertheless, exclusive reliance on GRACE may overlook specific clinical subtleties.

To enhance clinical decision-making, additional scoring systems like TIMI (Thrombolysis In Myocardial Infarction) and HEART (History, ECG, Age, Risk factors, Troponin) are often employed. The TIMI score includes variables such as patient age, history of coronary artery disease, recent aspirin use, frequency of angina, ECG changes, and biomarker elevation. In contrast, the HEART score evaluates a combination of clinical history, electrocardiographic findings, patient age, traditional risk factors, and troponin levels, categorizing patients into low, moderate, or high risk for adverse cardiac outcomes.

By combining these scoring systems, clinicians can better identify patients who may benefit from early invasive strategies versus those who might be managed conservatively. For example, a patient with a low GRACE score but high TIMI or HEART scores might warrant more aggressive intervention than initially anticipated.

Bleeding risk assessment is equally crucial, particularly in older adults, patients with renal dysfunction, or those with a history of bleeding disorders. The CRUSADE score evaluates factors such as hematocrit levels, creatinine clearance, heart rate, systolic blood pressure, signs of congestive heart failure, and sex to predict the likelihood of in-hospital major bleeding. The ARC-HBR (Academic Research Consortium-High Bleeding Risk) criteria provide a standardized definition of high bleeding risk, incorporating clinical and laboratory parameters.

Balancing ischemic and bleeding risks is essential when selecting antithrombotic therapies. Overlooking bleeding risk can lead to severe complications, including intracranial hemorrhage or gastrointestinal bleeding, which can be as detrimental as ischemic events. Therefore, a dual assessment of both ischemic and bleeding risks ensures a more tailored and safer therapeutic approach.

64.4 Management Strategies

Management of NSTEMI in the ICU should be individualized based on the patient's overall risk profile, comorbidities, and preferences. For low-risk patients—those with low scores on risk stratification tools and no significant hemodynamic instability—a conservative management approach may be appropriate. This strategy includes pharmacotherapy aimed at stabilizing the plaque, preventing thrombus propagation, and alleviating symptoms.

Oxygen Therapy: Supplemental oxygen is indicated for patients whose arterial oxygen saturation drops below 90%, those in respiratory distress, or when clinical signs suggest hypoxemia.

Pain Management: For patients with non-ST-elevation acute coronary syndromes experiencing persistent ischemic chest discomfort, sublingual nitroglycerin (0.3–0.4 mg) may be administered at five-minute intervals, up to three doses. If chest pain continues and there are no contraindications, intravenous nitroglycerin may be considered. When further analgesia is required, intravenous morphine (1–5 mg) can be used cautiously with close monitoring of blood pressure, with repeat dosing every 5–30 mins as necessary.

Beta-Blockers: Oral beta-blockers should be initiated within the first 24 h in clinically stable patients who do not show evidence of heart failure, reduced cardiac output, elevated risk of cardiogenic shock, or any other contraindications. Options include metoprolol succinate, carvedilol, or bisoprolol.

Calcium Channel Blockers (CCBs): In cases where beta-blockers are unsuitable, non-dihydropyridine CCBs like verapamil or diltiazem may be employed, provided the patient has preserved left ventricular function and no high-risk features such as significant AV block, prolonged PR interval, or predisposition to shock.

Statins: High-intensity statin therapy should be initiated or continued in all patients diagnosed with NSTE-ACS unless there is a specific contraindication.

ACE Inhibitors: These agents are recommended for long-term therapy in patients with reduced left ventricular ejection fraction (<40%), hypertension, diabetes, or stable chronic kidney disease, provided there are no contraindications to their use. Aldosterone receptor blockers (ARBs): In cases where ACE inhibitors are contraindicated or not tolerated, ARBs can be considered as an appropriate alternative.

64.5 Antiplatelet Therapy

Aspirin continues to serve as the foundation of antiplatelet treatment in acute coronary syndromes. It is typically initiated with a loading dose of 162–325 mg, followed by a daily maintenance dose ranging from 75–100 mg. Dual antiplatelet therapy (DAPT), involving the addition of a second agent, enhances platelet inhibition and is recommended for up to 12 months in patients with NSTE-ACS.

The choice among $P2Y_{12}$ inhibitors—clopidogrel, ticagrelor, and prasugrel—should consider bleeding risk, drug interactions, and coexisting conditions. Ticagrelor is preferred in many cases due to its rapid onset and reversible action, though it may not be ideal in patients with reactive airway disease or bradycardia. Prasugrel, while potent, is generally not recommended for individuals over 75 years or those with a history of cerebrovascular events due to increased bleeding risk.

- Clopidogrel: Loading dose of 300–600 mg, followed by 75 mg once daily.
- Ticagrelor: Loading dose of 180 mg, followed by 90 mg twice daily.

64.6 Anticoagulation

Anticoagulants work synergistically with antiplatelet agents by inhibiting the coagulation cascade.

Unfractionated heparin (UFH) is a commonly used agent, particularly in patients with renal dysfunction, because of its short half-life and the ability to reverse its effects with protamine.

- Dose: Start with 60 IU/kg (max 4000 IU) as an IV bolus, followed by 12 IU/kg/hour (max 1000 IU/hour) as continuous infusion, adjusted based on aPTT levels. Therapy is usually maintained for 48 h or until PCI is completed.

Low molecular weight heparin (enoxaparin) provides more stable pharmacokinetics but requires renal dose adjustment.

- Dose: 1 mg/kg subcutaneously every 12 h; reduce to once daily if creatinine clearance is below 30 mL/min. A 30 mg IV loading dose may be administered initially in select patients.

Fondaparinux, a selective factor Xa inhibitor, is associated with a lower bleeding risk and is suitable for many NSTE-ACS patients, except during PCI where catheter thrombosis risk necessitates adjunctive UFH or bivalirudin.

- Dose: 2.5 mg subcutaneously once daily until PCI or hospital discharge.

Bivalirudin is reserved for patients undergoing early invasive strategies.

- Dose: Begin with a 0.10 mg/kg IV bolus, followed by infusion at 0.25 mg/kg/hour, maintained until angiography or PCI. Glycoprotein IIb/IIIa inhibitors are used selectively alongside DAPT in this context.

For intermediate to high-risk patients, timely invasive strategies are crucial. Hemodynamically unstable patients—those with persistent chest pain, arrhythmias, heart failure, or signs of cardiogenic shock—should undergo immediate coronary angiography followed by revascularization as appropriate. Stable patients with elevated risk scores but without ongoing ischemia may benefit from an early invasive approach within 24–72 h. This timing allows for optimization of medical therapy, correction of modifiable risk factors, and thorough patient assessment.

Balancing the urgency of invasive procedures with the patient's bleeding risk is essential. Strategies to minimize bleeding include using radial artery access during PCI, selecting appropriate antithrombotic regimens, and careful monitoring of anticoagulation levels. Multidisciplinary discussions involving cardiologists, intensivists, and pharmacists can help tailor the best approach for each patient.

64.7 Biomarker Utility and Diagnostic Algorithms

The advent of high-sensitivity cardiac troponin (hs-cTn) assays has significantly improved the early diagnosis of NSTEMI. These assays can detect minute elevations in troponin levels within hours of myocardial injury, enabling rapid rule-in or rule-out protocols. Early detection allows for prompt initiation of therapy, which is critical in reducing myocardial damage and improving outcomes.

In practice, a serial measurement protocol is often employed. Troponin levels are measured at presentation and repeated after 1–3 h. A significant rise or fall in troponin levels supports the diagnosis of acute myocardial injury. This dynamic assessment is particularly valuable in patients with chronic elevations of troponin due to renal failure or other chronic conditions.

Dynamic ECG monitoring complements biomarker assessment. Transient ST-segment changes, T-wave inversions, or new bundle branch blocks can provide evidence of ongoing ischemia, even when initial ECGs are inconclusive. Continuous ECG monitoring in the ICU allows for the detection of arrhythmias or ischemic episodes that might otherwise go unnoticed.

In patients with suspected ACS but nondiagnostic initial findings, combining hs-cTn assays with risk scores like TIMI or HEART can improve diagnostic accuracy. For example, a low HEART score combined with negative serial hs-cTn measurements can safely identify patients at low risk, potentially reducing unnecessary hospital admissions and invasive procedures.

Advanced imaging modalities, such as echocardiography or cardiac MRI, can further aid in diagnosis. Echocardiography can detect wall motion abnormalities indicative of ischemia, while cardiac MRI can assess myocardial viability and detect areas of infarction or inflammation.

Incorporating these diagnostic tools into a systematic algorithm enhances the clinician's ability to stratify risk accurately, initiate appropriate therapy promptly, and improve patient outcomes.

64.8 Monitoring and Secondary Prevention

Assessing left ventricular function before discharge is crucial for prognostication and guiding long-term therapy. Echocardiography provides valuable information on ventricular function, regional wall motion abnormalities, and potential complications like heart failure or valvular dysfunction. Routine imaging, especially in high-risk patients, can identify secondary complications that may require additional interventions.

Beyond left ventricular function assessment, secondary prevention is critical to reduce recurrence and improve survival:

- Beta-blockers: Unless contraindicated, to lower oxygen demand and arrhythmia risk.
- ACE inhibitors/ARBs: For LVEF ≤40%, diabetes, hypertension, or CKD.
- Statins: High-intensity therapy for all, aiming for LDL-C ≤55 mg/dL and ≥ 50% reduction.

MRAs (Mineralocorticoid receptor antagonists): For LVEF ≤40% with HF or diabetes, if renal function permits.

- Antiplatelet therapy: Continue DAPT up to 12 months, then lifelong aspirin. Lifestyle: Smoking cessation, diet, exercise, and cardiac rehabilitation.

64.9 Interprofessional Care Coordination

Effective management of NSTEMI necessitates a coordinated interprofessional approach. Collaboration among cardiologists, intensivists, nurses, pharmacists, and rehabilitation specialists ensures that care pathways are standardized and that diagnostics and management are timely. Such coordination enhances patient outcomes by ensuring continuity of care from the ICU to discharge and beyond.

64.10 Conclusion

Managing NSTEMI in the ICU requires a comprehensive approach that encompasses detailed pathophysiological understanding, meticulous risk stratification, tailored therapeutic interventions, and robust secondary prevention strategies. By integrating various risk assessment tools, clinicians can fine-tune treatment plans to balance ischemic and bleeding risks effectively. Advances in biomarker assays and diagnostic algorithms have improved early detection and management decisions. Ongoing monitoring and interprofessional collaboration are essential for optimizing patient outcomes and preventing recurrent events. Timely risk stratification, appropriate use of antithrombotic therapy, and coordinated multidisciplinary care are central to improving NSTEMI outcomes in critically ill patients.

Algorithm 64.1: Approach to NSTEMI in the ICU

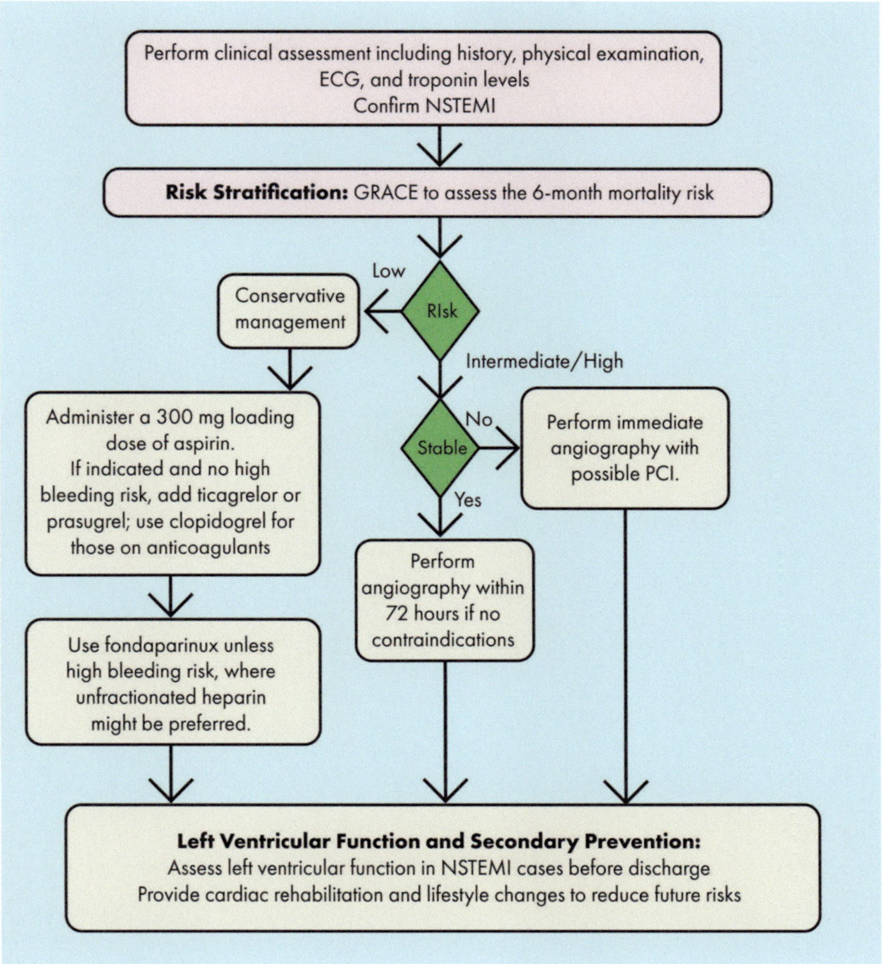

Bibliography

1. Amsterdam EA, Wenger NK, Brindis RG, Casey DE Jr, Ganiats TG, Holmes DR Jr, et al. AHA/ACC guideline for the management of patients with non-ST-elevation acute coronary syndromes: a report of the American College of Cardiology/American Heart Association Task Force on Practice Guidelines. Circulation. 2014;130(25):e344–426.
2. Collet JP, Thiele H, Barbato E, Barthelemy O, Bauersachs J, Bhatt DL, et al. 2020 ESC Guidelines for the management of acute coronary syndromes in patients presenting without persistent ST-segment elevation. Eur Heart J. 2021;42(14):1289–367.
3. Byrne RA, Rossello X, Coughlan JJ, Barbato E, Berry C, Chieffo A, et al. ESC Guidelines for the management of acute coronary syndromes. Eur Heart J. 2023;44(38):3720–826.

Chapter 65
Approach to Cardiogenic Shock in the ICU

65.1 Introduction

Cardiogenic shock (CS) is a life-threatening condition characterized by inadequate tissue perfusion due to severe impairment of cardiac function. It results from a significant reduction in cardiac output, commonly caused by acute myocardial infarction (AMI), severe valvular disease, or mechanical complications. Despite advances in management, CS continues to have a high mortality rate. Early recognition and a multidisciplinary approach in the ICU are essential for improving patient outcomes. This chapter provides a comprehensive approach to managing cardiogenic shock, emphasizing staging, detailed pathophysiology, innovative management strategies, and long-term considerations [1, 2] [Ref: Algorithm 65.1].

65.2 Multidisciplinary Shock Teams

Effective management of cardiogenic shock necessitates the involvement of a multidisciplinary shock team. This team typically includes cardiologists, intensivists, cardiac surgeons, emergency physicians, nurses, and other specialists. Collaborative decision-making enhances patient outcomes by integrating diverse expertise, leading to more comprehensive and timely care plans. The formation of such teams is emphasized in recent consensus statements, highlighting their role in improving survival rates and optimizing resource utilization [3].

S. B. Mishra et al., *Mastering ICU Care*,
https://doi.org/10.1007/978-981-95-0179-3_65

65.3 Pathophysiology

Understanding the complex pathophysiology of cardiogenic shock is crucial for effective management. The body initiates several compensatory mechanisms in response to decreased cardiac output:

- Sympathetic Activation: The sympathetic nervous system responds by increasing heart rate and systemic vasoconstriction to maintain blood pressure and perfusion to vital organs.
- Renin-Angiotensin-Aldosterone System (RAAS): Activation of the RAAS leads to sodium and water retention, increasing preload in an attempt to augment cardiac output.
- Inflammatory Cascades: In severe cases, systemic inflammation can lead to vasodilation and capillary leakage, exacerbating hypotension and tissue hypoperfusion. Nitric oxide, interleukins, and tumor necrosis factor alpha (TNF-α) are the mediators.

These compensatory mechanisms can become maladaptive over time, contributing to worsening cardiac function and progression of shock.

65.4 Comprehensive Classification

65.4.1 SCAI Shock Staging

The Society for Cardiovascular Angiography and Interventions (SCAI) has developed a staging system ranging from A to E to classify the severity of cardiogenic shock:

- Stage A (At risk): Patients are at risk of developing shock but are hemodynamically stable.
- Stage B (Beginning shock): Early signs of shock with mild hemodynamic compromise.
- Stage C (Classic shock): Hypotension with signs of hypoperfusion requiring interventions.
- Stage D (Deteriorating shock): Failure to respond to initial therapies; worsening hemodynamics.
- Stage E (Extremis): Critical condition with severe hypotension and hypoperfusion despite maximal support.

This dynamic staging aids in guiding treatment decisions and monitoring patient progression or improvement.

65.4.2 *Phenotypic Classifications*

Identifying the phenotype of cardiogenic shock helps tailor therapy:

- Cardiorenal Syndrome: Characterized by renal impairment due to decreased renal perfusion; management focuses on optimizing volume status and renal function.
- Cardiometabolic Shock: Associated with metabolic disturbances like hyperglycemia and acidosis; requires metabolic stabilization alongside hemodynamic support.

Recognizing these phenotypes enables clinicians to address specific underlying mechanisms contributing to shock.

65.5 Etiological Diversity

While AMI is the most common cause, other etiologies should be considered:

- Fulminant Myocarditis: Acute inflammation of the myocardium leading to severe ventricular dysfunction.
- Takotsubo Cardiomyopathy: Stress-induced cardiomyopathy presenting with transient left ventricular apical ballooning.
- Septic Cardiomyopathy: Cardiac dysfunction resulting from severe sepsis and systemic inflammation.

Recognizing these conditions is important, as management may differ from typical ischemic causes.

65.6 Clinical Signs and Symptoms

Patients with cardiogenic shock generally have altered mental status, hypotension, arrhythmia, diminished pulses, breathlessness/dyspnea, peripheral edema, jugular venous distension, and orthopnea. They mostly have cool extremities and signs of pulmonary congestion. This is generally termed as "cold and wet" and is generally associated with reduced cardiac index (CI), increased systemic vascular resistance (SVR), and pulmonary capillary wedge pressure (PCWP), whereas patients with normal PCWP are euvolemic and as termed "cold and dry." The "wet and warm" types are usually underrecognized and have high mortality. This is an inflammatory response to acute cardiac injury and has low CI, low to normal SVR, and elevated PCWP.

Investigations:

1. Cardiac catheterization is the definitive diagnostic investigation, and it also helps guide the intervention in cardiogenic shock.
2. ECG: Within 10 min of presentation, if shock is suspected to be of cardiac origin.
3. Complete blood counts and metabolic panel (blood gas analysis, electrolytes, renal function tests, and liver function tests): Should be obtained every 12–24 h to gather information about oxygenation, organ failure, and electrolyte status.
4. Echocardiography: Helps detect complications and the site of failure (right or left ventricle) and also gives an idea about the vessel involved (regional wall motion abnormality).

65.7 Stabilization

Maintain airway, breathing, and oxygenation. Target blood saturation levels above 90%. Use supplemental oxygen. Noninvasive ventilation can also be tried. If inadequate, go for invasive ventilation targeting lung-protective ventilation (5–7 ml/kg). Low tidal volume helps in blood flow between pulmonary and parenchymal vasculature.

Fluid resuscitation is challenging in CS as it may lead to congestion. Right heart catheterization helps guide fluid therapy in right ventricular failure if the patient is hypovolemic. Conservative boluses of 250–500 ml may be used.

65.8 Early Intervention Protocols

Implementing protocols for early invasive hemodynamic assessment and intervention is crucial. Standardized protocols ensure prompt recognition of cardiogenic shock and initiation of appropriate therapies, potentially preventing disease progression. These protocols typically include:

- Rapid bedside echocardiography.
- Early placement of arterial and central venous lines.
- Timely initiation of inotropes and vasopressors.
- Immediate consultation with the multidisciplinary shock team.

Vasopressor support (norepinephrine) should be initiated and titrated to a mean arterial pressure (MAP) of 65 mm Hg. Vasopressin may be more beneficial in acute right ventricular failure due to lower pulmonary vasoconstriction. Other agents that can be used are phenylephrine, epinephrine, dopamine, dobutamine, and levosimendan. Nitric oxide, milrinone, prostacyclin, and dobutamine are the vasoactive agents within the pulmonary circuit.

65.9 Early Hemodynamic Monitoring

Continuous blood pressure monitoring must be done using an arterial line. Early insertion of pulmonary artery catheters (PACs) or utilization of advanced noninvasive monitoring techniques is recommended for precise hemodynamic assessment. Real-time data on cardiac output, pulmonary pressures, and systemic vascular resistance guide therapeutic interventions and adjustments. SvO_2 (mixed venous oxygen saturation) must be measured. Low SvO_2 indicates reduced cardiac output, anemia, hypoxemia, or increased oxygen consumption. It can also help assess response to therapy. It should be done every 4 h in the early stages of shock. PACs also offer therapeutic advantages via continuous monitoring of cardiac output during inotrope and pulmonary vasodilator titration.

65.10 Innovative Management Strategies

65.10.1 Temporary Mechanical Circulatory Support (tMCS) Devices

For patients not responding adequately to pharmacologic therapy, temporary mechanical circulatory support devices offer hemodynamic stabilization:

- Intra-aortic Balloon Pump (IABP): Augments diastolic pressure to improve coronary perfusion; suitable for patients with less severe hemodynamic compromise.
- Impella Devices: Microaxial flow pumps providing forward blood flow; ideal for left ventricular support.
- Tandem Heart: Provides left atrial to femoral arterial bypass; used in severe left ventricular failure.
- Extracorporeal Membrane Oxygenation (ECMO): Offers both cardiac and respiratory support; used in profound shock with multi-organ failure.

The choice of device depends on the patient's hemodynamic profile, severity of shock, and specific clinical scenario.

65.11 Management Framework

Acute MI-Associated Cardiogenic Shock (AMI-CS)

1. Urgent Revascularization: Primary percutaneous coronary intervention (PCI) is the gold standard.
2. Pharmacologic Support: Initiate inotropes (e.g., dobutamine) and vasopressors (e.g., norepinephrine) to stabilize hemodynamics.

3. Antiplatelet and Anticoagulant Therapy: Administer as per guidelines to prevent further thrombotic events.
4. Mechanical Support: Consider tMCS devices if there is inadequate response to pharmacologic therapy.

Non-AMI Cardiogenic Shock

1. Identify Underlying Cause: Utilize imaging and laboratory studies to diagnose conditions like valvular disorders, tamponade, or ventricular septal defects.
2. Definitive Management:
   - Valvular Disease: Surgical or transcatheter valve repair/replacement.
   - Tamponade: Urgent pericardiocentesis.
   - Mechanical Complications: Surgical repair of ventricular ruptures or defects.
3. Supportive Care: Optimize preload, afterload, and contractility with appropriate medications.

65.12 Prognostic Insights

Biomarkers

- Lactate Levels: Elevated lactate indicates tissue hypoperfusion; trends in lactate clearance are useful prognostic indicators.
- Other Biomarkers: Elevated troponins, B-type natriuretic peptide (BNP), and inflammatory markers provide additional prognostic information.

Monitoring these biomarkers aids in assessing the severity of shock and the effectiveness of interventions.

Step-by-Step Algorithm

1. Confirmation of Cardiogenic Shock.
   - Clinical Assessment: Hypotension (SBP <90 mm Hg), signs of hypoperfusion (cold extremities, altered mental status).
   - Diagnostic Tools: Bedside echocardiography, ECG, laboratory tests (elevated lactate, troponins, BNP).
2. SCAI Staging Assessment.
   - Determine the shock stage (A to E) to guide urgency and level of intervention.
3. Multidisciplinary Team Activation.
   - Involve the shock team early for collaborative decision-making.
4. Monitoring and Initial Workup.
   - For Stage A-B patients:
   - Close hemodynamic monitoring.
   - Routine workup to identify reversible factors.

5. Initiation of Pharmacologic Support and Hemodynamic Monitoring.
   - For Stage C-E patients:
   - Start inotropes and vasopressors.
   - Initiate advanced hemodynamic monitoring (e.g., pulmonary artery catheter).
6. Assessment for Acute Myocardial Infarction (AMI).
   - Yes:
   - Proceed with urgent revascularization (PCI or CABG).
   - No:
   - Evaluate for mechanical complications or other etiologies.
7. Management of Mechanical Complications.
   - Valvular Disease: Surgical or transcatheter intervention.
   - Tamponade: Pericardiocentesis.
   - Ventricular Rupture: Emergency surgical repair.
8. Evaluating Response to Support.
   - Adequate Response:
   - Gradual weaning from support under close monitoring.
   - Inadequate Response:
   - Escalate to tMCS devices.
9. Consider Mechanical Circulatory Support (tMCS).
   - Select an appropriate device based on hemodynamic needs.
10. Transfer to Specialized Cardiac Center if Lack of Improvement.
    - For advanced therapies or interventions not available at the current facility.

65.13 Conclusion

Management of cardiogenic shock in the ICU requires a structured, multidisciplinary approach that encompasses early recognition, detailed understanding of pathophysiology, comprehensive classification, and innovative management strategies. Incorporating protocols for early intervention, utilizing advanced hemodynamic monitoring, and considering etiological diversity are essential steps. Prognostic insights from biomarkers and implementing regionalized systems of care further enhance patient management. Attention to long-term outcomes, including prevention of recurrent shock and management of chronic heart failure, is crucial for improving survival and quality of life. Familiarity with this comprehensive approach enables clinicians to make informed decisions, ultimately leading to better patient outcomes in this high-stakes environment.

Algorithm 65.1: Approach to cardiogenic shock in the ICU

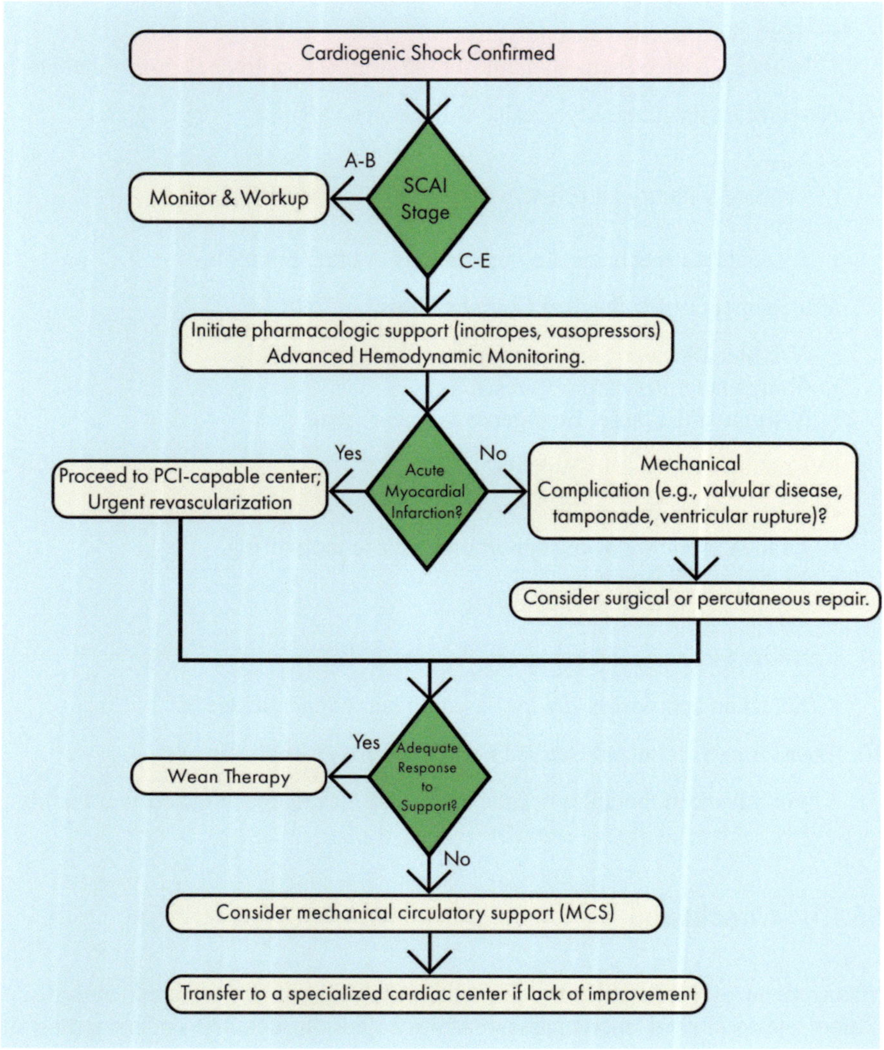

Bibliography

1. Alkhunaizi FA, Smith N, Brusca SB, Furfaro D. The Management of Cardiogenic Shock from Diagnosis to devices: a narrative review. CHEST. Crit Care. 2024;2(2)
2. Baran DA, Billia F, Randhawa V, Cowger JA, Barnett CM, Chih S, et al. Consensus statements from the International Society for Heart and Lung Transplantation consensus conference: heart failure-related cardiogenic shock. J Heart Lung Transplant. 2024;43(2):204–16.
3. Vahdatpour C, Collins D, Goldberg S. Cardiogenic shock. J Am Heart Assoc. 2019;8(8):e011991.
4. Laghlam D, Benghanem S, Ortuno S, Bouabdallaoui N, Manzo-Silberman S, Hamzaoui O, et al. Management of cardiogenic shock: a narrative review. Ann Intensive Care. 2024;14(1):45.

Chapter 66
Approach to Cardiac Tamponade in the ICU

66.1 Introduction

Cardiac tamponade is a life-threatening condition resulting from the accumulation of fluid, blood, pus, or gas within the pericardial sac, leading to increased intrapericardial pressure. This pressure impedes normal cardiac filling, reduces stroke volume, and can precipitate severe hemodynamic instability. Rapid recognition and intervention are paramount, as untreated tamponade can swiftly progress to cardiac arrest. This chapter provides an evidence-based approach to diagnosing and managing cardiac tamponade in the intensive care unit (ICU), emphasizing timely assessment, diagnostic strategies, and interprofessional collaboration to optimize patient outcomes [1] [Ref: Algorithm 66.1].

66.2 Etiology

Etiology: Can be infectious or noninfectious

Infectious: Viral pericarditis (Echovirus, coxsackievirus, parvovirus B 19, and human herpes virus 6) tubercular

Noninfectious: Autoimmune disorders, uremia, malignancy, metabolic disorders, mediastinal radiation, post-traumatic pericarditis, aortic diseases, medications, idiopathic

The noninfectious effusion is mostly due to the imbalance between hydrostatic and colloid osmotic pressures.

S. B. Mishra et al., *Mastering ICU Care*,
https://doi.org/10.1007/978-981-95-0179-3_66

66.3 Classification

- Based on size
  - Mild: End diastolic echo-free space diameter less than 1 cm (around 100 ml)
  - Moderate: End diastolic echo-free space diameter > 1 cm but <2 cm (100–500 ml)
  - Large: End diastolic echo-free space diameter > 2 cm
- Based on duration
  - Acute: Effusions lasting <1 week
  - Subacute: Effusions lasting 1 week to 3 months
  - Chronic: Effusions present for >3 months

66.4 Acute vs Chronic Fluid Accumulation

The development of cardiac tamponade depends not only on the volume of pericardial fluid but also on the rate of accumulation:

- Acute Accumulation: Rapid fluid accumulation, such as from trauma or ventricular rupture, can lead to tamponade with as little as 100–200 mL of fluid. The pericardium lacks time to stretch, resulting in a swift rise in intrapericardial pressure.
- Chronic Accumulation: Slow fluid accumulation, often seen in malignancy, uremia, or autoimmune disorders, allows the pericardium to adapt and stretch over time. Patients may tolerate larger effusions (up to 1–2 liters) before tamponade physiology develops.

66.5 Role of Pericardial Compliance

Pericardial compliance is crucial in tamponade development:

- Low Compliance: In acute settings, the stiff pericardium cannot accommodate sudden increases in volume, leading to rapid pressure escalation.
- High Compliance: In chronic conditions, gradual stretching increases compliance, delaying tamponade onset despite larger effusion volumes.

The interplay between fluid volume, accumulation rate, and pericardial compliance determines the hemodynamic impact on the heart.

66.6 Clinical Features

Variations in Presentation

Clinical manifestations of cardiac tamponade can vary based on underlying conditions:

- Typical Symptoms: Dyspnea, chest pain, tachycardia, hypotension, and anxiety.
- Low-Pressure Tamponade: In uremic or hypovolemic patients, tamponade may occur with lower pericardial pressures, presenting with subtle signs due to decreased intravascular volume.

66.7 Physical Examination Findings

- Beck's Triad: Hypotension, muffled heart sounds, and elevated jugular venous pressure (JVP).
- Pulsus Paradoxus: An inspiratory drop in systolic blood pressure greater than 10 mmHg. However, it may be absent or less pronounced in:
- Aortic Regurgitation: Due to constant forward flow during diastole.
- Severe Shock: When arterial pressures are critically low.
- Right Ventricular Hypertrophy: Where right-sided pressures are elevated.
- Ewart's Sign: Dullness to percussion, bronchial breath sounds, and egophony at the left infrascapular area due to compression of the left lower lobe by a large pericardial effusion.

66.8 Diagnostic Strategies

Advanced Echocardiographic Findings

Echocardiography is the cornerstone of tamponade diagnosis:

- Chamber Collapse: Diastolic collapse of the right atrium and right ventricle indicates elevated pericardial pressures exceeding intracardiac pressures.
- Doppler Assessment:
- Respiratory Variations: Exaggerated (>25%) respiratory variations in mitral and tricuspid inflow velocities reflect interventricular dependence characteristic of tamponade.
- Inferior Vena Cava (IVC) Distension: A plethoric IVC with minimal respiratory variation suggests elevated right atrial pressures.

Other Imaging Modalities

- Computed Tomography (CT)
  - Utility: Provides detailed anatomical information, useful in complex cases or when echocardiographic windows are poor.
  - Limitations: Requires patient stability and transportation, may delay intervention.
- Magnetic Resonance Imaging (MRI)
  - Utility: Offers high-resolution images, beneficial in chronic pericardial diseases.
  - Limitations: Limited availability and contraindications in unstable patients.

66.9 Indications and Approaches for Pericardiocentesis

Detailed Contraindications

Pericardiocentesis is generally safe but contraindicated in specific scenarios:

- Aortic Dissection: Draining the pericardial sac may remove the tamponade effect on a ruptured aorta, worsening hemorrhage.
- Ventricular Free Wall Rupture: Common post-myocardial infarction; surgical repair is preferred to prevent exacerbating bleeding.

66.10 Imaging-Guided Techniques

Enhancing procedural safety through imaging:

- Echocardiography-Guided Pericardiocentesis:
  - Real-Time Visualization: Guides needle insertion away from vital structures.
  - Site Selection: Determines the optimal access point based on effusion size and location.
- Fluoroscopy-Guided Pericardiocentesis:
  - Contrast Injection: Assists in visualizing the pericardial space.
  - Limitations: Requires fluoroscopy suite availability and may expose patients to radiation.

Approaches to Pericardiocentesis

- Subxiphoid Approach:
  - Advantages: Avoids injury to coronary arteries and lungs.
  - Technique: Needle insertion below the xiphoid process angled towards the left shoulder.

- Apical Approach:
  - Advantages: Direct access in patients with large left-sided effusions.
  - Technique: Needle insertion at the left ventricular apex under imaging guidance.
- Parasternal Approach:
  - Advantages: Useful for anterior effusions.
  - Technique: Needle insertion adjacent to the left sternal border.

66.11 Post-procedural Management

Monitoring Re-accumulation
Hemodynamic Monitoring: Continuous assessment for signs of recurrent tamponade.

- Follow-Up Imaging:
  - Echocardiography: Repeated studies to assess effusion size.
  - Chest X-ray: Evaluates catheter position and detects complications like pneumothorax.

Catheter Management
- Pericardial Catheters:
  - Indications: Left in place for ongoing drainage in cases with high reaccumulation risk.
  - Care: Maintain sterile technique to prevent infection.
    Management of Complications
- Infection:
  - Prevention: Aseptic technique during insertion and maintenance.
  - Treatment: Antibiotics and possible catheter removal if infection occurs.
- Myocardial Injury:
  - Detection: Monitor for arrhythmias or changes in cardiac enzymes.
  - Management: Immediate cessation of the procedure and supportive care.

66.12 Treatment Variations

Surgical Options

- Pericardial Window Creation:
  - Indications: Recurrent, loculated, or purulent effusions not amenable to pericardiocentesis.
  - Procedure: Surgical creation of an opening in the pericardium to allow continuous drainage into the pleural or peritoneal cavity.

- Pericardiectomy:
  - Indications: Constrictive pericarditis or refractory effusions.
  - Outcome: Complete removal of the pericardium relieves constriction but carries a higher surgical risk.

66.13 Interprofessional Collaboration

Effective management requires a coordinated approach:

- ICU Team:
  - Role: Provides hemodynamic support, monitors for clinical deterioration, and manages ventilatory status.
  - Communication: Ensures timely updates among team members.
- Cardiologists:
  - Role: Perform diagnostic echocardiography, guide pericardiocentesis, and manage medical therapy.
  - Consultation: Essential for complex cases requiring advanced interventions.
- Cardiothoracic Surgeons:
  - Role: Evaluate for and perform surgical procedures like pericardial window or pericardiectomy.
  - Collaboration: Early involvement improves outcomes in cases requiring surgery.
- Additional Specialists:
  - Oncologists: Manage malignancy-related effusions.
  - Nephrologists: Address uremic pericarditis and dialysis needs.
  - Infectious Disease Experts: Guide therapy for purulent pericardial infections.

66.14 Prognostic Insights

Outcomes Based on Etiology

- Malignancy-Associated Tamponade:
  - Prognosis: Generally poorer due to advanced disease; high recurrence rates.
  - Management: May require pericardial window or sclerosis agents.

- Traumatic Tamponade:
  - Prognosis: Prompt surgical intervention can be life-saving.
  - Considerations: Often part of complex injuries requiring multidisciplinary care.
- Uremic Tamponade:
  - Prognosis: Favorable with aggressive dialysis and drainage.
  - Management: Pericardiocentesis combined with initiation or intensification of dialysis.

Mortality and Morbidity

- Early Recognition and Intervention: Critical for improving survival rates.
- Recurrent Effusions: Associated with higher morbidity; necessitate long-term management strategies.

66.15 Conclusion

Managing cardiac tamponade in the ICU demands rapid identification, decisive intervention, and seamless inter-professional collaboration. Understanding the nuances of clinical presentation, especially in atypical or low-pressure scenarios, is essential. Advanced diagnostic strategies, particularly echocardiographic techniques, enhance detection and guide safe pericardiocentesis. Post-procedural care focuses on preventing reaccumulation and managing complications. Recognizing when surgical interventions are warranted ensures comprehensive care. Ultimately, tailored management based on etiology and patient-specific factors improves prognostic outcomes in this critical condition.

Algorithm 66.1: Approach to cardiac tamponade in the ICU

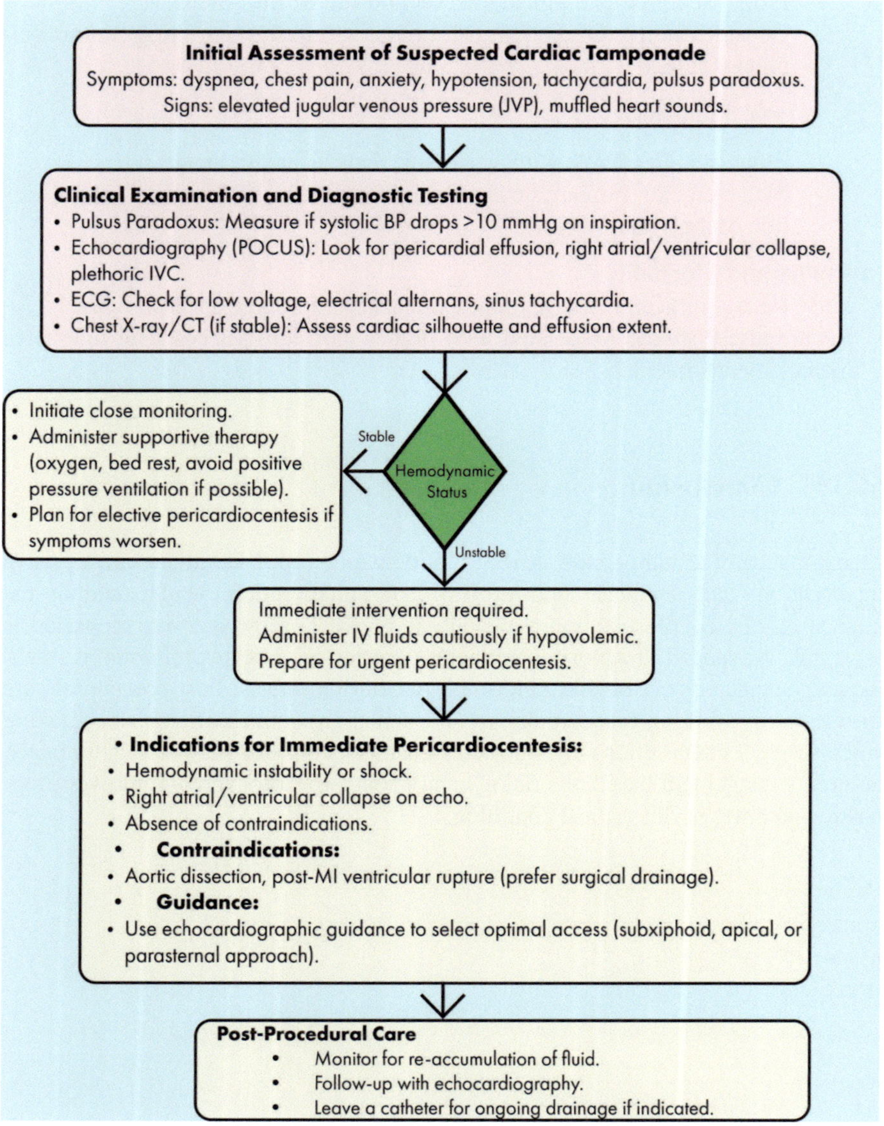

Bibliography

1. Little WC, Freeman GL. Pericardial disease. Circulation. 2006;113(12):1622–32.

Chapter 67
Approach to Left Ventricular Failure in the ICU

67.1 Introduction

Left ventricular failure (LVF) frequently presents in critical care settings and reflects the heart's diminished capacity to sustain effective forward flow, leading to systemic hypoperfusion and pulmonary congestion. Patients may complain of breathlessness during exertion or sleep, and physical assessment might reveal cold limbs, neck vein distension, and lung crackles. A structured ICU strategy for LVF involves not only stabilizing the acute episode but also mitigating modifiable triggers and concurrent diseases to reduce recurrent admissions and improve survival [1–3] [Ref: Algorithm 67.1].

67.2 Definition

Heart failure is a multifaceted clinical syndrome characterized by signs and symptoms arising from structural or functional abnormalities that impair the heart's ability to fill with or eject blood effectively. This does not include asymptomatic structural heart diseases or cardiomyopathies.

67.3 Stages of Heart failure

Heart failure progression is typically categorized to guide therapy:

- Stage A: Individuals at high risk (e.g., with hypertension, diabetes, or a family history) but without structural heart disease or symptoms.

S. B. Mishra et al., *Mastering ICU Care*,
https://doi.org/10.1007/978-981-95-0179-3_67

- Stage B: Patients with cardiac structural changes (e.g., low EF, ventricular hypertrophy) or elevated cardiac biomarkers, yet asymptomatic.
- Stage C: Symptomatic individuals with known heart disease, whether symptoms are new or recurrent.
- Stage D: Refractory heart failure with frequent decompensation requiring advanced support or frequent hospitalization.

Even if a patient with symptomatic heart failure (stage C) becomes asymptomatic with appropriate treatment, they remain classified as having stage C heart failure due to their clinical history.

Stage C heart failure can be further subclassified into the following categories:

- **New-onset (de novo) HF:** First presentation of heart failure symptoms in a patient with no prior history of the condition.
- **Resolution of symptoms:** Patients whose symptoms have improved or resolved with therapy but who still meet criteria for stage C due to underlying structural heart disease.
- **Persistent HF:** Ongoing symptoms despite medical management.
- **Worsening HF:** Clinical deterioration or exacerbation of symptoms in a patient with previously stable heart failure.

Classification of Heart Failure Based on Left Ventricular Ejection Fraction (LVEF):

- **HFrEF (Heart Failure with Reduced Ejection Fraction):** Defined by an LVEF ≤40%.
- **HFimpEF (Heart Failure with Improved Ejection Fraction):** Refers to patients with a previously documented LVEF ≤40% that has improved to >40% on subsequent evaluation.
- **HFmrEF (Heart Failure with Mildly Reduced Ejection Fraction):** LVEF ranging between 41% and 49%, accompanied by evidence of elevated left ventricular filling pressures—either at rest or during stress—such as increased natriuretic peptide levels or abnormal hemodynamic findings via noninvasive or invasive assessments.
- **HFpEF (Heart Failure with Preserved Ejection Fraction):** Characterized by an LVEF ≥50% along with evidence of elevated left ventricular filling pressures, demonstrated through raised natriuretic peptide concentrations or supportive findings from imaging or invasive hemodynamic studies.

67.4 Etiology and Risk Factors

Risk factors: Hypertension, obesity, diabetes, atherosclerotic cardiovascular disease.

Etiology:

Cardiac: Ischemic heart disease and myocardial infarction, hypertension and valvular heart disease, familial or genetic cardiomyopathies; amyloidosis, heart rhythm–related (e.g., tachycardia-mediated, PVCs, RV pacing).

Noncardiac causes: Several extracardiac conditions can lead to or worsen left ventricular failure. These include toxic exposure (e.g., chemotherapeutic or cardiotoxic medications), metabolic and endocrine disorders such as thyroid dysfunction, acromegaly, or pheochromocytoma, and systemic diseases like diabetes or obesity. Inflammatory or infectious myocarditis, substance abuse (notably alcohol, methamphetamines, or cocaine), and stress-induced cardiomyopathy (e.g., Takotsubo) are also implicated abuse (e.g., alcohol, cocaine, methamphetamine), stress cardiomyopathy (Takotsubo).

Understanding and addressing modifiable risk factors is crucial in the prevention and management of LVF. Hypertension and coronary artery disease are primary contributors to the development of LVF. Early detection and aggressive management of these conditions can prevent the progression to heart failure.

67.5 Comprehensive Patient Evaluation

1. Patient Presentation.
   - Initial evaluation involves identifying symptoms and signs indicative of LVF, including dyspnea, orthopnea, and paroxysmal nocturnal dyspnea.
   - Physical examination should assess for signs of hypoperfusion (e.g., cold extremities) and congestion (e.g., elevated JVP, pulmonary rales).
2. Immediate Vital Signs and Advanced Diagnostics.
   - Monitor vital signs closely.
   - Perform a bedside echocardiogram to determine left ventricular EF.
   - Utilize advanced imaging modalities like cardiac MRI to assess myocardial fibrosis and viability.
   - Order laboratory tests (complete blood count, urinalysis, serum electrolytes, blood urea nitrogen, serum creatinine, glucose, lipid profile, liver function tests, iron studies, and thyroid function tests), including BNP/NT-proBNP to distinguish acute heart failure from other causes of dyspnea, troponins for myocardial injury. A 12-lead ECG should be obtained. BNP levels are useful for diagnosis or exclusion of HF and to establish prognosis.
3. Assessment of Comorbid Conditions.
   - Evaluate and manage comorbidities such as diabetes, anemia, chronic kidney disease, iron deficiency, and atrial fibrillation, as they significantly affect LVF prognosis.

67.6 Imaging

A chest radiograph serves as a helpful initial investigation to assess for heart enlargement, pulmonary vascular congestion, or interstitial and alveolar fluid accumulation. It can also point toward alternative diagnoses contributing to respiratory symptoms. Despite its utility, transthoracic echocardiography (TTE) is generally the preferred first-line modality for a detailed evaluation of cardiac anatomy and performance. When more information is required, advanced imaging such as cardiac MRI, nuclear techniques like SPECT or radionuclide ventriculography, PET scans, cardiac CT, or coronary angiography may be employed to provide additional structural or perfusion data.

67.7 Management Based on Hemodynamic Status

Effective management of left ventricular failure (LVF) necessitates a clear understanding of the patient's hemodynamic status, which reflects how efficiently the heart is pumping blood and whether there is excess fluid accumulation in the body. Patients are typically classified into four categories based on their signs and symptoms: warm and dry (compensated), warm and wet (congestion), cold and dry (hypoperfusion), and cold and wet (congestion with hypoperfusion). Each category requires specific management strategies to address the underlying issues and improve patient outcomes.

1. Warm and Dry (Compensated)

Warm and dry patients have adequate blood flow to bodily tissues, indicated by warm skin, and no significant fluid buildup in the lungs or tissues. This state suggests that the heart is compensating well despite underlying dysfunction. The primary goal for these patients is to optimize long-term treatment to prevent the progression of heart failure.

Management involves initiating or adjusting Guideline-Directed Medical Therapy (GDMT):

- ACE Inhibitors or ARBs (e.g., lisinopril, enalapril, losartan, valsartan): These agents reduce afterload by dilating blood vessels, ease cardiac workload, and limit disease progression by mitigating adverse remodeling.
- ARNIs (e.g., sacubitril/valsartan): A combination of neprilysin inhibition with ARB action, these drugs enhance natriuretic peptide activity and improve both symptoms and prognosis in HFrEF.
- Beta-Blockers (e.g., metoprolol, carvedilol): These reduce myocardial oxygen demand and blunt the effects of sympathetic overactivity, thereby improving survival and reducing hospitalization rates.
- MRAs (e.g., spironolactone, eplerenone): These inhibit aldosterone, promoting natriuresis while preventing myocardial fibrosis and adverse remodeling.

- SGLT2 Inhibitors (e.g., empagliflozin, dapagliflozin): Initially developed for diabetes, these agents now have proven benefit across heart failure phenotypes by promoting osmotic diuresis and improving cardiovascular outcomes.

2. Warm and Wet (Congestion)

In the warm and wet category, patients have adequate blood flow to tissues but experience excess fluid accumulation, leading to symptoms like shortness of breath and swelling (edema). The primary focus for these patients is to remove excess fluid to relieve symptoms and prevent complications.

Management Strategies Include

- Administering intravenous diuretics like furosemide (Lasix) to promote the excretion of excess fluid through increased urine production.
- Implementing sodium restriction to reduce further fluid retention. This approach is particularly important for patients with heart failure with preserved ejection fraction (HFpEF).
- Monitoring fluid balance carefully by tracking fluid intake and output, and conducting daily weight measurements to detect fluid retention early.
- Considering ultrafiltration if diuresis is inadequate. Ultrafiltration mechanically removes excess fluid from the blood when diuretics are insufficient.
- Employing conservative diuretic protocols for patients at risk of kidney dysfunction to prevent worsening renal function. This involves using the lowest effective diuretic dose and closely monitoring kidney function.

3. Cold and Dry (Hypoperfusion)

Patients categorized as Cold and Dry exhibit reduced blood flow to tissues, indicated by cool extremities, but do not have significant fluid overload. The management goal is to improve blood flow to organs while ensuring adequate blood volume.

Management Involves:

- Assessing Volume Status to check for dehydration, as low blood volume can further reduce blood pressure and perfusion.
- Administering a Fluid Bolus if Hypovolemic, which involves giving intravenous fluids to increase blood volume.
- Initiating Inotropic Support if needed with medications like dobutamine or milrinone that strengthen the heart's contractions and improve its ability to pump blood.
- Monitoring for Signs of Ischemia or Arrhythmias because inotropes can increase the heart's oxygen demand, potentially leading to chest pain or irregular heart rhythms. Continuous cardiac monitoring is essential during inotropic therapy.

Key Points highlight the importance of balancing fluid administration to avoid overloading the patient, which could lead to congestion. Frequent assessments are necessary to adjust treatment promptly based on the patient's response.

4. Cold and Wet (Congestion with Hypoperfusion)

The cold and wet category is the most severe, with patients experiencing poor blood flow to tissues and excess fluid accumulation. Aggressive treatment is required to improve heart function and remove excess fluid.

Management Strategies Include:

- Using a combination of inotropes and vasodilators:
  - Inotropes like dobutamine or milrinone enhance the strength of the heart's contractions.
  - Vasodilators such as nitroglycerin or nitroprusside relax blood vessels, reducing resistance and easing the heart's workload.
  - Ensuring adequate blood pressure since vasodilators can lower blood pressure, and excessively low levels can compromise blood flow to vital organs. Medications should be titrated carefully, with close monitoring of blood pressure.
- Considering mechanical circulatory support devices if pharmacological interventions are insufficient:
  - Intra-aortic balloon pump (IABP) assists the heart by increasing blood flow to the coronary arteries and decreasing the heart's workload.
  - Ventricular assist devices (VADs) take over some or all of the heart's pumping function.
  - Extracorporeal membrane oxygenation (ECMO) provides both cardiac and respiratory support by oxygenating the blood outside the body.

Key points stress that urgent intervention is critical to prevent organ damage. A multidisciplinary approach involving cardiologists, intensivists, and surgeons may be necessary to manage these complex cases effectively.

67.8 Advanced Therapies and Mechanical Support

When standard medical treatments are insufficient, advanced therapies can be life-saving options for patients with severe heart failure. These interventions aim to improve survival rates and quality of life.

67.8.1 Cardiac Resynchronization Therapy (CRT)

Purpose: CRT aims to improve heart efficiency by helping the ventricles beat in sync, enhancing the coordination of heart contractions. A specialized pacemaker sends electrical impulses to both ventricles simultaneously, improving symptoms and potentially increasing survival.

Considerations:
Ideal Candidates: Patients with HFrEF who have a prolonged QRS duration on electrocardiogram (indicating electrical delay) and persistent symptoms despite optimal medical therapy.

67.8.2 Ventricular Assist Devices (VADs)

Purpose: VADs support a failing heart by assisting in pumping blood throughout the body.

Use Cases:
- Bridge to Transplantation: Keeps patients stable while awaiting a heart transplant.
- Destination Therapy: Provides a long-term solution for patients who are not candidates for transplantation.

Function: A VAD is a mechanical pump surgically implanted to take over some or all of the left ventricle's pumping functions.

Considerations:
- Risks: Potential complications include infection, blood clots, and device malfunction.

Lifestyle Impact: Patients must adapt to significant lifestyle changes and require ongoing medical care.

67.8.3 Heart Transplantation

Purpose: Heart transplantation is considered for patients with end-stage heart failure unresponsive to all other treatments, offering a chance for extended survival and improved quality of life.

Considerations:
- Eligibility: Patients must meet strict criteria, including overall health status, absence of other significant diseases, and the ability to adhere to lifelong immunosuppressive therapy.

Post-Transplant Care: Requires lifelong medications to prevent organ rejection and frequent medical evaluations to monitor for complications.

67.9 Assess for Reversible Causes

Identifying and treating underlying issues can improve heart function or even reverse heart failure in some cases. Addressing these reversible causes is a critical component of comprehensive heart failure management.

67.9.1 Ischemia (Reduced Blood Flow to the Heart)

Action Steps:

- Diagnosis: Utilize tests such as electrocardiograms (ECG), stress tests, or coronary angiography to detect blockages in the coronary arteries.
- Treatment:
  - Medications: Prescribe anti-anginal drugs and antiplatelet agents to improve blood flow and prevent clot formation.
  - Procedures: Perform angioplasty with stenting or coronary artery bypass grafting (CABG) to restore adequate blood flow to the heart muscle.

67.9.2 Arrhythmias (Abnormal Heart Rhythms)

Action Steps:

- Diagnosis: Continuous ECG monitoring is essential to detect irregular heart rhythms like atrial fibrillation, which can exacerbate heart failure symptoms.
- Treatment:
  - Medications: Use antiarrhythmic drugs to control heart rate and rhythm.
  - Procedures: Consider electrical cardioversion or catheter ablation therapy to restore normal rhythm.

67.9.3 Valvular Disease

Action Steps:

- Diagnosis: Perform echocardiography to assess the structure and function of heart valves.
- Treatment:
  - Medications: Manage symptoms with appropriate pharmacotherapy.
  - Procedures: Surgical repair or replacement of the faulty valve may be necessary. Minimally invasive techniques like trans-catheter aortic valve replacement (TAVR) can be options for select patients.

67.9.4 Infection

Action Steps:

- Diagnosis: Conduct blood tests, imaging studies, and cultures to identify infections such as endocarditis.

- Treatment:
  - Antibiotics: Administer appropriate antimicrobial therapy based on the identified organism.
  - Supportive Care: Manage fever and other systemic symptoms to reduce cardiac workload.

67.10 Monitoring and Fluid Management

Continuous assessment and timely adjustments are crucial for effective heart failure management. Proper monitoring helps in detecting changes early and modifying treatment to prevent deterioration.

67.10.1 Daily Monitoring

Fluid Balance:
- Intake and Output Charts: Keep detailed records of all fluids consumed and excreted to maintain appropriate fluid balance.
- Urine Output: Monitor as an indicator of kidney function and effectiveness of diuretic therapy.

Weight Monitoring:
- Daily Weights: Weigh the patient at the same time each day, preferably in the morning after urination, to detect fluid retention promptly.

Electrolyte Levels:
Regular Blood Tests: Check levels of sodium, potassium, and kidney function markers to identify imbalances that may require intervention.

67.10.2 Adjust Therapy

Based on Clinical Response:
- Symptoms: Monitor for worsening shortness of breath, increased swelling, fatigue, or other signs of heart failure exacerbation.
- Vital Signs: Regularly assess blood pressure, heart rate, and oxygen saturation to guide therapy adjustments.

Based on Laboratory Results:
- Kidney Function: Adjust diuretic doses if there is evidence of renal impairment.

Electrolyte Imbalances: Supplement or modify medications to correct abnormalities.

67.10.3 Fluid Management

Individualized Strategies:

- Fluid Restriction: Limit total daily fluid intake based on the patient's condition and risk of fluid overload.
- Diuretic Adjustments: Modify doses according to the patien's response and kidney function, aiming for optimal fluid removal without causing dehydration.

Sodium Restriction:

- Dietary Changes: Educate patients on consuming low-sodium foods and understanding food labels to reduce sodium intake.

Goal: Typically, sodium intake is limited to less than 2000 mg per day to prevent fluid retention.

67.11 Conclusion

A systematic and comprehensive approach to managing left ventricular failure in the ICU is essential for improving patient outcomes. This includes not only acute stabilization but also addressing modifiable risk factors, comorbidities, and implementing evidence-based therapies. Advances in pharmacological treatments and mechanical support devices have expanded the options available for patients with LVF. Ongoing monitoring and adjustment of therapy, along with patient education, play a critical role in the successful management of this complex condition.

Algorithm 67.1: Approach to left ventricular failure in the ICU

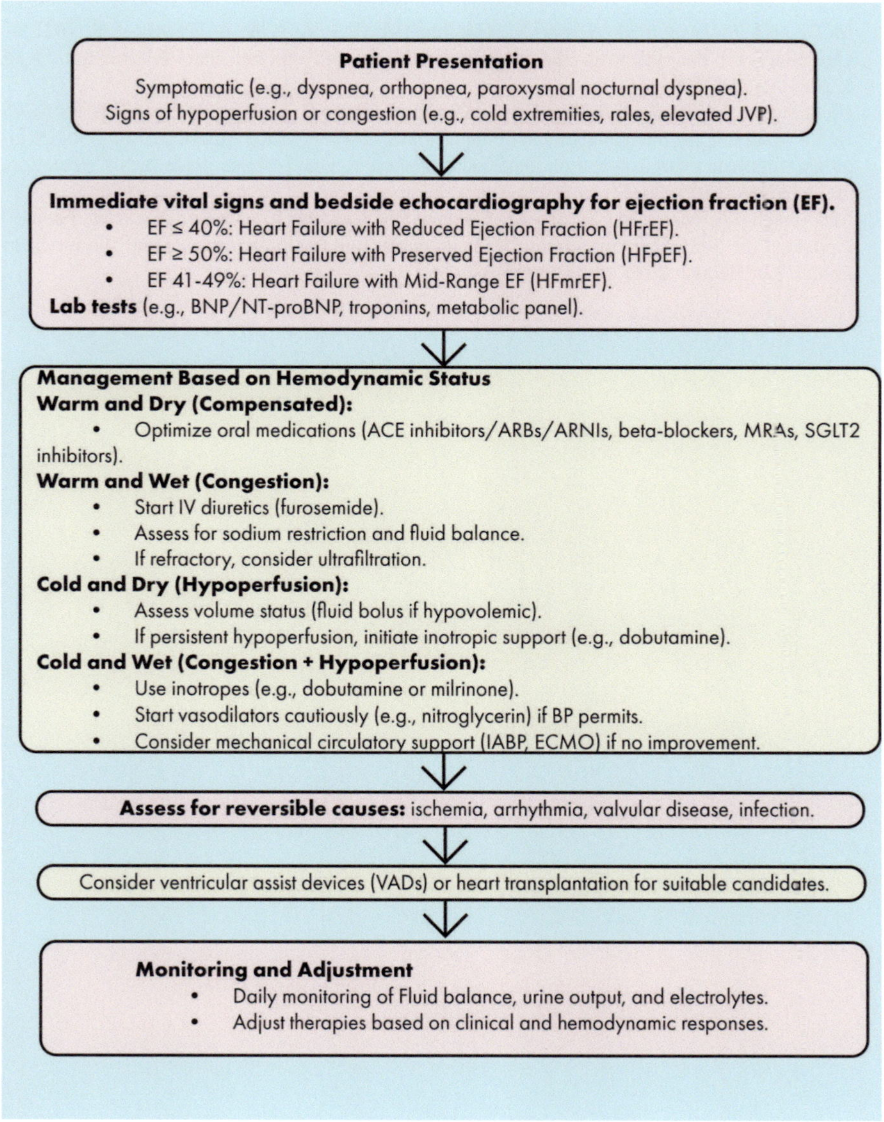

Bibliography

1. McDonagh TA, Metra M, Adamo M, Gardner RS, Baumbach A, Bohm M, et al. 202ESC Guidelines for the diagnosis and treatment of acute and chronic heart failure. Eur Heart J. 2021;42(36):3599–726.
2. Heidenreich PA, Bozkurt B, Aguilar D, Allen LA, Byun JJ, Colvin MM, et al. AHA/ACC/HFSA guideline for the management of heart failure: a report of the American college of cardiology/American heart association joint committee on clinical practice guidelines. Circulation. 2022;145(18):e895–e1032.
3. McDonagh TA, Metra M, Adamo M, Gardner RS, Baumbach A, Bohm M, et al. Focused Update of the 2021 ESC Guidelines for the diagnosis and treatment of acute and chronic heart failure. Eur Heart J. 2023;44(37):3627–39.

Chapter 68
Approach to Right Ventricular Failure in the ICU

68.1 Introduction

Right ventricular failure (RVF) in the intensive care unit (ICU) is a critical condition that requires prompt and comprehensive management. The right ventricle (RV) possesses unique anatomical and physiological characteristics, making it particularly sensitive to changes in afterload and ventricular interdependence. RVF can result from various etiologies, including acute events like pulmonary embolism and chronic conditions such as pulmonary hypertension. Understanding the distinctions between acute and chronic RVF, as well as the underlying pathophysiology, is essential for effective intervention. This chapter provides an in-depth approach for assessing, diagnosing, and treating RVF in the ICU, incorporating advanced diagnostic tools, therapeutic strategies, and interdisciplinary management principles [1, 2] [Ref: Algorithm 68.1].

Causes of RVF

Acute RVF

- Volume Overload: Acute left heart failure
- Pressure Overload: Acute pulmonary embolism, acute chest syndrome in sickle cell disease
- Decreased Contractility: Acute myocardial ischemia, fulminant myocarditis, pericardial tamponade

Chronic RVF

- Chronic Pulmonary Hypertension
- Constrictive Pericarditis
- Exacerbation of Chronic Lung Disease
- Cardiomyopathies
- Congenital Heart Disease (atrial septal defect, ventricular septal defect)

S. B. Mishra et al., *Mastering ICU Care*,
https://doi.org/10.1007/978-981-95-0179-3_68

68.2 Diagnosis

Accurate recognition of RVF requires a combination of clinical assessment, laboratory tests, echocardiography and invasive hemodynamic monitoring.

68.3 Advanced Diagnostic Tools and Techniques

Cardiac Imaging

Echocardiography: Bedside transthoracic echocardiography remains the first-line diagnostic tool for evaluating RV size, function, and interventricular septal motion.

- TAPSE < 17 mm
- TR peak velocity > 2.8 m/s
- RV dilation
- RV end diastolic diameter/LV end diastolic diameter > 1
- D-shaped LV
- IVC > 21 mm, inspiratory collapse < 50%

However, echocardiography can sometimes be inconclusive due to poor acoustic windows or complex anatomy.

- Cardiac Magnetic Resonance Imaging (MRI): Offers superior spatial resolution and is considered the gold standard for quantifying RV volumes, mass, fibrosis, and ejection fraction. MRI is particularly useful for detailed evaluation of RV morphology and function when echocardiography is insufficient.
- Nuclear Imaging: Techniques such as radionuclide ventriculography can assess RV function and myocardial perfusion, aiding in the detection of ischemia or scarring.

Invasive Hemodynamic Monitoring

- Right Heart Catheterization: Provides comprehensive assessment of intracardiac pressures, pulmonary artery pressures, and cardiac output. It is especially valuable in complex cases where precise hemodynamic measurements guide therapeutic decisions.
- RV-Pulmonary Artery (PA) Coupling: Measurement of RV-PA coupling using pressure-volume loops can help tailor interventions based on the efficiency of RV ejection into the pulmonary circulation.

68.4 Differentiating Chronic vs. Acute RV Failure

Pathophysiological Differences

- Acute RVF: Often results from sudden increases in afterload (e.g., massive pulmonary embolism) or acute loss of contractility (e.g., RV myocardial infarction). The RV is unable to adapt quickly, leading to rapid hemodynamic deterioration.
- Chronic RVF: Develops over time due to conditions like pulmonary hypertension or rheumatic heart disease. The RV undergoes adaptive remodeling but eventually decompensates.

Management Strategies

- Acute RVF: Requires immediate reduction of RV afterload and support of RV function. Thrombolysis for pulmonary embolism or revascularization for RV infarction is critical intervention.
- Chronic RVF: Focuses on managing the underlying disease process, such as optimizing pulmonary vasodilator therapy in pulmonary hypertension and addressing valvular lesions in rheumatic heart disease.

68.5 Expanded Pathophysiological Insights

Unique RV Characteristics

- Anatomy and Function: The RV has a crescent shape and thinner free wall compared to the left ventricle (LV), making it more compliant but less tolerant to increased afterload.
- Sensitivity to Afterload: The RV is highly sensitive to changes in pulmonary vascular resistance. Even modest increases can significantly impair RV output.
- Interventricular Interdependence: The RV and LV share the interventricular septum and pericardial space. Changes in RV size and pressure can affect LV filling and function.

Impact on LV Filling and Cardiac Output

- Ventricular Interdependence: In acute RVF, RV dilation shifts the interventricular septum toward the LV, reducing LV diastolic compliance and preload, leading to decreased cardiac output.
- Systemic Effects: Reduced LV output exacerbates systemic hypotension, further compromising coronary perfusion and perpetuating RV ischemia.

Etiological Spectrum

- Pulmonary Embolism
- Pulmonary Hypertension
- Right Ventricular Infarction
- Myocarditis
- Congenital Heart Defects: Such as atrial septal defects or tetralogy of Fallot, which is more prevalent in certain regions and can lead to chronic RV overload

- Rheumatic Heart Disease: Common in developing countries, affecting the mitral and tricuspid valves and leading to RVF

68.6 Advanced Therapeutics

Pharmacological Interventions

- Preload Optimization: diuretics, RRT.
- Pulmonary Vasodilators: Inhaled nitric oxide and prostacyclin analogs reduce pulmonary vascular resistance, decreasing RV afterload.
- Phosphodiesterase Inhibitors: Medications like milrinone enhance RV contractility and cause pulmonary vasodilation, improving RV output.
- Inotropes: Dobutamine and dopamine can be used to augment RV contractility but should be carefully titrated.

Mechanical Support Devices

- Impella RP: A percutaneous right ventricular assist device that supports RV function by directly unloading the RV and improving cardiac output.
- Extracorporeal Membrane Oxygenation (ECMO): Veno-arterial ECMO provides both cardiac and respiratory support. RV-specific configurations can be tailored to the patient's needs.
- Evidence of Efficacy: Recent studies have demonstrated improved outcomes with early implementation of mechanical support in severe RVF.

Outcome Metrics and Prognostication

- Mortality and Morbidity Statistics: Acute RVF has a high in-hospital mortality rate, ranging from 25% to 50%, depending on the etiology and severity. Chronic RVF also carries significant morbidity, impacting quality of life and long-term survival.
- Prognostic Indicators: Elevated biomarkers (e.g., BNP), hemodynamic parameters from right heart catheterization, and imaging findings can help predict outcomes.
- Importance of Early Intervention: Timely recognition and management of RVF are critical in improving survival rates and reducing complications.

68.7 Future Directions

Emerging Research

- Pharmacological Therapies: Investigating drugs targeting RV-specific molecular pathways, such as agents that modulate RV metabolism or fibrosis.
- Gene and Stem Cell Therapy: Potential to repair damaged myocardium and improve RV function.
- Biomarkers: Development of novel biomarkers for early detection and monitoring of RVF progression.

Technological Advances

- Improved Imaging Techniques: Enhanced MRI protocols and 3D echocardiography for better RV assessment.
- Wearable Hemodynamic Monitors: Allow for continuous monitoring of RV function in high-risk patients.

68.8 Conclusion

Managing right ventricular failure in the ICU demands a comprehensive understanding of its unique pathophysiology, etiological diversity, and the interplay between the RV and pulmonary circulation. Advanced diagnostic tools, including cardiac MRI and right heart catheterization, provide detailed insights necessary for tailored interventions. Differentiating between acute and chronic RVF guides specific management strategies, emphasizing the need for prompt treatment in acute cases and ongoing management in chronic conditions. Incorporating advanced therapeutics, such as pulmonary vasodilators and mechanical support devices like Impella RP and ECMO, can significantly impact patient outcomes. An interdisciplinary approach ensures comprehensive care, addressing all aspects of the patient's condition. Ongoing research and future innovations hold promise for improving prognostication and developing targeted therapies for RVF.

Algorithm 68.1: Approach to right ventricular failure in the ICU

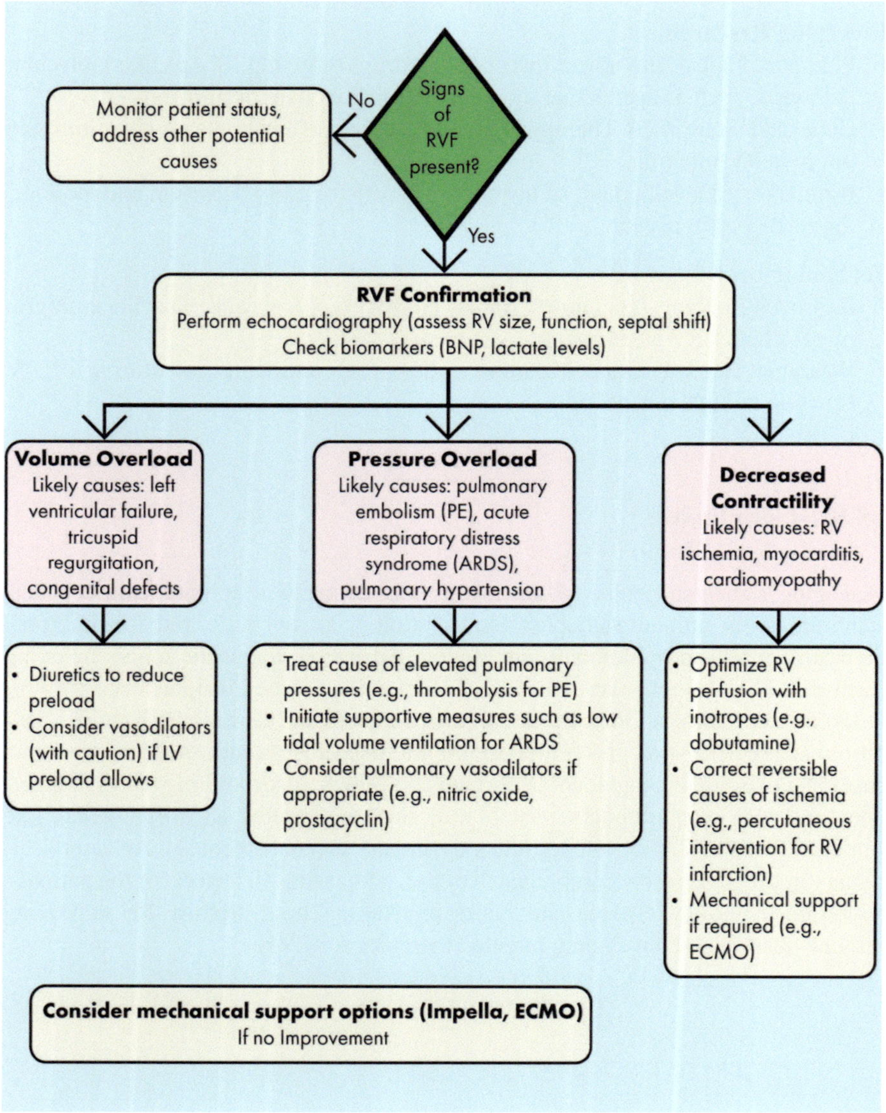

Bibliography

1. Monteagudo-Vela M, Tindale A, Monguio-Santin E, Reyes-Copa G, Panoulas V. Right ventricular failure: Current strategies and future development. Front Cardiovasc Med. 2023;10:998382.
2. Arrigo M, Price S, Harjola VP, Huber LC, Schaubroeck HAI, Vieillard-Baron A, et al. Diagnosis and treatment of right ventricular failure secondary to acutely increased right ventricular afterload (acute cor pulmonale): a clinical consensus statement of the Association for Acute CardioVascular Care of the European Society of Cardiology. Eur Heart J Acute Cardiovasc Care. 2024;13(3):304–12.

Chapter 69
Approach to Diastolic Heart Failure (HFpEF) in the ICU

69.1 Introduction

Heart failure with preserved ejection fraction (HFpEF), previously known as diastolic heart failure, is becoming increasingly prevalent, particularly in aging populations and among individuals with comorbidities such as obesity, diabetes mellitus, and hypertension. As these conditions become more common, HFpEF has emerged as a significant contributor to cardiovascular morbidity and mortality worldwide.

69.2 Pathophysiology

Unlike heart failure with reduced ejection fraction (HFrEF), HFpEF is characterized by symptoms of heart failure despite a preserved left ventricular ejection fraction (LVEF $\geq$ 50%). The pathophysiology involves elevated left ventricular filling pressures due to impaired relaxation and increased myocardial stiffness, without significant systolic dysfunction.

69.3 Diagnosis

Diagnosing HFpEF poses substantial challenges in the ICU setting because of the lack of definitive diagnostic tests and the potential for misdiagnosis. Symptoms like dyspnea and edema are nonspecific and can overlap with other conditions common in critically ill patients [1] [Ref: Algorithm 69.1].

1. Monitor Patient Status and Address Potential Causes

S. B. Mishra et al., *Mastering ICU Care*,
https://doi.org/10.1007/978-981-95-0179-3_69

- Initial Monitoring: Begin with vigilant monitoring of the patient's clinical status, including vital signs, respiratory function, and cardiac parameters. Common symptoms include dyspnea, fatigue, and signs of fluid overload like peripheral edema.
- Identify and Exclude Alternative Causes: Before focusing on HFpEF, rule out other potential causes of the patient's symptoms. Employ a systematic framework to consider conditions such as pulmonary embolism, chronic obstructive pulmonary disease, pneumonia, anemia, and renal insufficiency. This step is crucial to prevent misdiagnosis and ensure appropriate management.

2. Integrate Scoring Systems for Structured Diagnosis

   - Utilize H2FPEF and HFA-PEFF Scoring Systems: Implement the H2FPEF and HFA-PEFF algorithms to assess the probability of HFpEF systematically.

H2FPEF Score Components:

- Heavy (BMI > 30 kg/m^2): Obesity contributes to HFpEF and can affect natriuretic peptide levels.
- Hypertensive (≥2 antihypertensive medications): Indicates the burden of hypertension.
- Atrial Fibrillation: Common in HFpEF and affects diastolic filling.
- Pulmonary Hypertension (estimated pulmonary artery systolic pressure > 35 mm Hg): Suggests elevated left-sided filling pressures.
- Elder (age > 60 years): Age-related changes in myocardial compliance.
- Filling Pressure (E/e' > 9): Direct measure of diastolic dysfunction.

HFA-PEFF Algorithm: Combines functional (echocardiographic parameters), morphological (left atrial enlargement, left ventricular hypertrophy), and biomarker domains (natriuretic peptides) to provide a comprehensive assessment.

- Address Limitations of Natriuretic Peptides: Recognize that natriuretic peptide levels may be lower in obese patients, potentially leading to underdiagnosis. Use BMI-corrected thresholds or consider additional biomarkers like ST2 or galectin-3 to improve diagnostic accuracy.
- Differential Diagnosis for Dyspnea and Edema: Employ a framework to rule out HFpEF mimics such as restrictive cardiomyopathies, constrictive pericarditis, and high-output heart failure. Advanced imaging modalities and hemodynamic studies can aid in differentiation.

3. Perform Comprehensive Echocardiographic Evaluation

   - Echocardiography: Conduct a detailed echocardiogram to assess:
   - Left Ventricular Ejection Fraction (LVEF): Confirm preservation of systolic function (LVEF ≥ 50%).
   - Diastolic Function: Evaluate parameters like E/A ratio, E/e' ratio, deceleration time, and left atrial volume index.
   - Left Atrial Size: Enlargement suggests chronic diastolic dysfunction.

- Right Ventricular Function: Assess for involvement that may affect prognosis.
- Pulmonary Artery Pressures: Elevated pressures can indicate pulmonary hypertension secondary to left heart disease.

4. Interpretation Based on Echocardiographic Findings

- If LVEF < 50% or Findings Are Unclear:
- Reevaluate Differential Diagnosis: Consider alternative diagnoses like HFrEF, hypertrophic cardiomyopathy, or infiltrative diseases (e.g., amyloidosis).
- Further Diagnostic Testing: Utilize cardiac MRI, right heart catheterization, or endomyocardial biopsy if indicated.
- If LVEF ≥ 50% with Evidence of Diastolic Dysfunction:
- Confirm HFpEF Diagnosis: Elevated left ventricular filling pressures and diastolic dysfunction support the diagnosis. Elevated natriuretic peptide levels further corroborate, using adjusted thresholds for BMI if necessary.

5. Identify and Assess Comorbidities

- Comorbidity Evaluation: Systematically assess for conditions contributing to HFpEF:
- Hypertension: Common and modifiable risk factor.
- Diabetes Mellitus: Contributes to microvascular dysfunction.
- Obesity: Leads to systemic inflammation and increased cardiac workload.
- Atrial Fibrillation: Affects diastolic filling and hemodynamics.
- Chronic Kidney Disease: Alters volume status and electrolyte balance.
- Anemia: Reduces oxygen delivery, exacerbating cardiac stress.

Comorbidity Management:

- Hypertension: Aim for strict blood pressure control using ACE inhibitors, ARBs, or calcium channel blockers.
- Diabetes: Optimize glycemic control with medications that have cardiovascular benefits, like SGLT2 inhibitors.
- Atrial Fibrillation: Implement rate control with beta-blockers or calcium channel blockers; consider rhythm control strategies.
- Anemia: Investigate and treat underlying causes; consider transfusion if indicated.

6. Check for Acute Decompensation Triggers

Identification of Acute Triggers: Evaluate for factors precipitating decompensation:

- Infections: Pneumonia, urinary tract infections.
- Arrhythmias: New-onset or uncontrolled atrial fibrillation.
- Anemia: Acute blood loss or chronic deficiencies.
- Renal Dysfunction: Acute kidney injury or worsening chronic kidney disease.
- Medication Noncompliance: Missed doses of diuretics or other heart failure medications.
- Fluid Overload: Excessive intravenous fluids or dietary indiscretion.

Specific Protocols for Acute Triggers:
- Infections: Initiate prompt antimicrobial therapy based on suspected pathogens.
- Arrhythmias: Employ rate control agents or electrical cardioversion if hemodynamically unstable.
- Anemia: Transfuse packed red blood cells if hemoglobin levels are critically low.
- Renal Dysfunction: Adjust medications accordingly and consider renal replacement therapy if indicated.

69.4 Management Strategies

Guideline-Directed Medical Therapy (GDMT) and Non-pharmacological Strategies
- Angiotensin Receptor-Neprilysin Inhibitors (ARNIs)/ARBs:
- Evidence: PARAGON-HF trial indicates that sacubitril/valsartan may benefit certain HFpEF patients.
- Recommendation: Use in patients with elevated natriuretic peptides and structural heart disease.
- Comorbidity Optimization: Continue aggressive management of hypertension, diabetes, and other contributing conditions.

8. Practical Recommendations for Volume Management

Diuretics:
- Loop Diuretics: Use furosemide or torsemide to manage congestion, adjusting doses based on urine output and renal function.
- Thiazide Diuretics: Add in cases of diuretic resistance.
- Monitoring: Regularly assess electrolytes, renal function, and weight.

Invasive Hemodynamic Monitoring:
- Indication: In patients with refractory symptoms or uncertain volume status.
- Technique: Use pulmonary artery catheterization to guide diuretic therapy and assess cardiac output.

69.5 Use of Advanced Imaging and Monitoring

- Routine Echocardiography:
  - Purpose: Monitor disease progression, assess response to therapy, and evaluate for complications like pulmonary hypertension.
  - Frequency: As clinically indicated, especially after significant changes in symptoms.
- Pulmonary Artery Pressure Monitoring:

  - High-Risk Patients: Consider implantable devices like the CardioMEMS for continuous monitoring.
  - Benefits: Early detection of pressure changes allows for timely intervention, reducing hospitalizations.
- Advanced Imaging:
  - Cardiac MRI: Provides detailed tissue characterization, identifying fibrosis or infiltrative diseases.
  - Nuclear Imaging: Assists in differentiating between ischemic and nonischemic causes.

69.6 Conclusion

Managing HFpEF in the ICU setting demands a comprehensive, multidisciplinary approach due to its complex pathophysiology and the prevalence of comorbidities. Utilizing structured diagnostic algorithms like H2FPEF and HFA-PEFF enhances diagnostic accuracy and guides targeted therapy. Addressing limitations in diagnostic tools, such as adjusting natriuretic peptide thresholds for BMI, helps prevent misdiagnosis, especially in obese patients. Guideline-directed medical therapy, including the use of SGLT2 inhibitors, MRAs, and ARNIs/ARBs, forms the cornerstone of pharmacological management. Non-pharmacological strategies and aggressive management of comorbidities are equally important.

A multidisciplinary team approach ensures comprehensive care, leveraging the expertise of various specialists. Advanced imaging and monitoring techniques facilitate ongoing assessment and timely interventions. By systematically addressing each aspect of HFpEF, clinicians can improve symptom control, reduce hospitalizations, and enhance the quality of life for critically ill patients.

Algorithm 69.1: Approach to diastolic heart failure (HFpEF) in the ICU

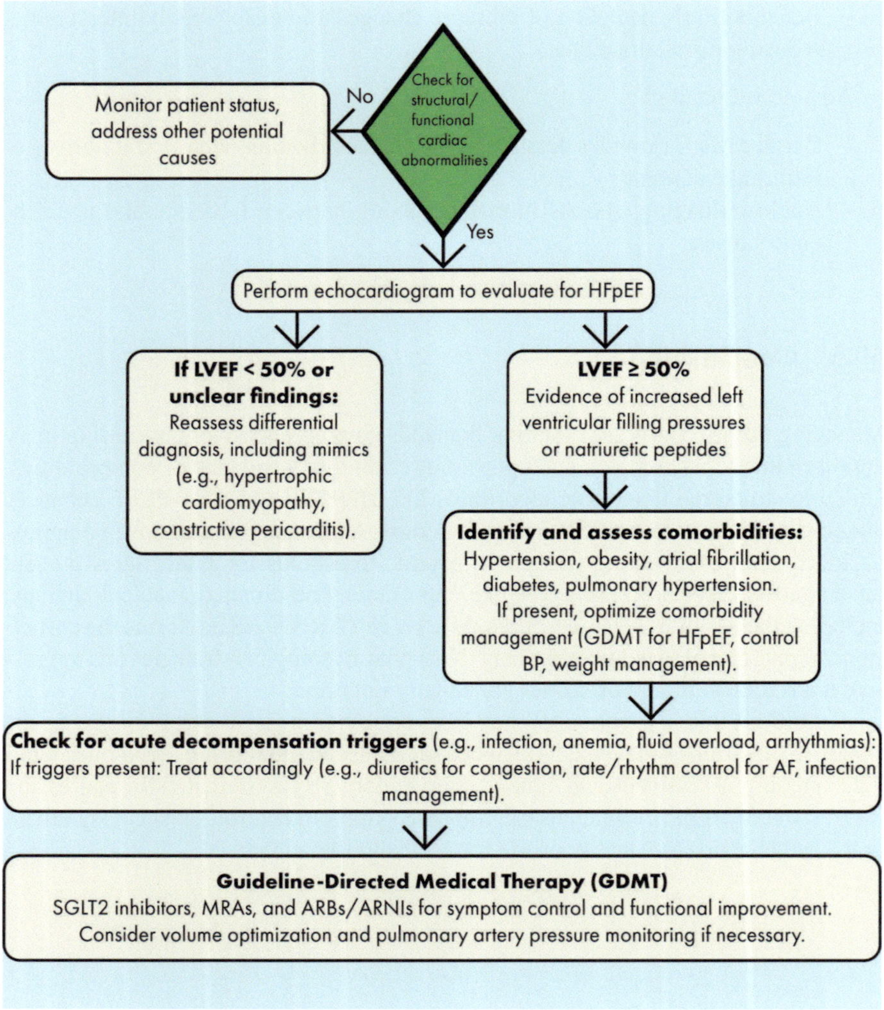

Bibliography

1. Kittleson Michelle M, Panjrath Gurusher S, Amancherla K, Davis Leslie L, Deswal A, Dixon Dave L, et al. ACC expert consensus decision pathway on management of heart failure with preserved ejection fraction. J Am Coll Cardiol. 2023;81(18):1835–78.

Chapter 70
Approach to Infective Endocarditis in the ICU

70.1 Introduction

Infective endocarditis (IE) is a severe, life-threatening infection of the endocardial surface of the heart, primarily affecting the heart valves. IE in the intensive care unit (ICU) often presents with diagnostic ambiguity, frequently mimicking other systemic infections. Early bedside suspicion and coordination with microbiology and cardiology teams are essential. Risk factors include prosthetic heart valves, previous history of endocarditis, intravenous drug use, immunosuppression, and recent healthcare exposure. Early recognition and initiation of appropriate diagnostics and treatment are essential for improving patient outcomes. This chapter provides ICU clinicians with a structured approach for assessing and managing suspected infective endocarditis [1, 2] [Ref: Algorithm 70.1].

70.2 Diagnosis Initial Suspicion

- Clinical Features: IE may present with a variety of symptoms, including fever, new or changing heart murmurs, embolic events (e.g., stroke, limb ischemia), sepsis, and peripheral manifestations like Janeway lesions, Osler nodes, Roth spots, or splinter hemorrhages. These findings should raise suspicion, particularly if multiple features are present.
- Risk Factors: Patients with prosthetic heart valves, previous endocarditis, and congenital heart disease, a history of intravenous drug use, immunosuppression, or recent healthcare exposure (such as surgery or invasive procedures) are at heightened risk. Awareness of these risk factors can prompt early evaluation for IE.

S. B. Mishra et al., *Mastering ICU Care*,
https://doi.org/10.1007/978-981-95-0179-3_70

- Microbial Shifts: There is an increased prevalence of healthcare-associated infections with methicillin-resistant *Staphylococcus aureus* (MRSA) and other resistant pathogens, reflecting current epidemiological trends. This shift necessitates vigilance in both diagnosis and empirical therapy selection.

1. Suspicion for Infective Endocarditis

   - Assess the likelihood of IE based on clinical presentation and risk factors. If IE is not considered likely, evaluate other possible causes of the symptoms, such as other infectious or inflammatory conditions.

2. Diagnostic Evaluation

   - Blood Cultures: Obtain at least three separate blood cultures from different venipuncture sites before initiating antibiotics with the first and last samples drawn at least 1 hour apart. In cases of suspected blood culture-negative endocarditis, consider serological and molecular diagnostic techniques to detect fastidious organisms like *Coxiella burnetii* or *Bartonella* species.
   - Echocardiography:
   - Transthoracic Echocardiography (TTE): Initiate diagnostic imaging with TTE, which is noninvasive and can provide initial evidence of vegetations, abscesses, or valve dysfunction.
   - Transesophageal Echocardiography (TEE): If TTE is inconclusive or if the patient has prosthetic valves, TEE should be performed due to its higher sensitivity and specificity.
   - Advanced Imaging Techniques: In cases where TEE is inconclusive or in prosthetic valve endocarditis, consider advanced imaging modalities like positron emission tomography-computed tomography (PET-CT) or cardiac magnetic resonance imaging (MRI). These techniques can detect occult infections and embolic phenomena.

70.2.1 Modified Duke Criteria: Clinical Framework for Diagnosing Infective Endocarditis

The Modified Duke Criteria provide a structured, evidence-based method to support the diagnosis of infective endocarditis by integrating clinical features, microbiological data, and imaging findings.

1. Definite Infective Endocarditis

   - Pathological Confirmation: Diagnosis is established when microorganisms are directly isolated from cardiac tissue, such as vegetations or abscesses, through culture or histological examination. Alternatively, microscopic features consistent with endocarditis in excised cardiac material also fulfill this criterion.

- Clinical Combination-Based Diagnosis: Can be made when any of the following are met:
  - Two major criteria
  - One major and three minor criteria
  - Five minor criteria

2. Possible Infective Endocarditis
   - Supported by:
   - One major and one minor criterion
   - Three minor criteria

3. Major Diagnostic Criteria
   - Microbiological evidence:
     - Two or more blood cultures positive for typical IE pathogens
     - A single positive culture or high-titer serology (e.g., *Coxiella burnetii* with anti-phase I IgG ≥1:800) also qualifies
   - Evidence of endocardial involvement:
     - Findings on echocardiography include:
       - Mobile intracardiac mass attached to valves, supporting structures, or device leads
       - Perivalvular abscess formation
       - Prosthetic valve dehiscence
       - Newly developed valvular regurgitation (excluding simple murmur changes)

4. Minor Diagnostic Criteria
   - Presence of known cardiac abnormalities or IV drug use
   - Temperature ≥ 38 °C
   - Vascular complications such as emboli, infarcts, aneurysms, or peripheral lesions (e.g., Janeway)
   - Immunological signs like Osler nodes, Roth spots, glomerulonephritis, or positive rheumatoid factor
   - Microbiological findings that don't fulfill major criteria (e.g., single positive culture or atypical

70.3 Management

70.3.1 Empirical Therapy (Table 70.1)

Empiric antibiotic therapy generally includes intravenous vancomycin combined with ceftriaxone or ampicillin to cover common organisms like *Staphylococcus*, *Streptococcus*, and *Enterococcus* species (Table 70.1 and 70.2).

Table 70.1 Native Valve Endocarditis

Organism	Antibiotic	Dose	Duration	Remarks
Viridans streptococci or *streptococcus gallolyticus* strains with confirmed sensitivity to penicillin	Ceftriaxone or	2 g IV once daily	4 weeks	
	Penicillin G or	Penicillin G at 12 to 18 million units daily, infused continuously or intermittently in 4 to 6 divided doses	4 weeks	
	Ampicillin or	A total of 12 grams per day administered intravenously in 4 to 6 separate doses	4 weeks	
	Ceftriaxone + gentamicin or	Ceftriaxone 2 grams IV once per day combined with gentamicin at 3 mg/kg IV given once daily	2 weeks	
	Vancomycin	Administer 30 mg/kg per day intravenously, divided into 2 doses	4 weeks	Desired trough levels 10 and 15 μg/mL
Viridans streptococci and *S. Gallolyticus* strains demonstrating intermediate or reduced susceptibility to penicillin	Penicillin G + Gentamicin	24 million U IV in 4–6 equally divided doses +3 mg/kg IV once daily	Penicillin 4 weeks Gentamicin 2 weeks	Use ceftriaxone if ceftriaxone sensitive
	Ampicillin + gentamicin	12 g/day IV in 4–6 divided doses +3 mg/kg IV once daily	Ampicillin 4 weeks + gentamicin 2 weeks	
	Vancomycin	30 mg/kg IV in 2 divided doses	4 weeks	Only for patients unable to tolerate penicillin or ceftriaxone

(continued)

Table 70.1 (continued)

Organism	Antibiotic	Dose	Duration	Remarks
Enterococcus	Penicillin G + gentamicin Or	18–30 million U IV in 4–6 equally divided doses +3 mg/kg IV in 3 divided doses	4–6 weeks	When symptoms have been present for less than 3 months, a 4-week antibiotic regimen is advised; if symptoms exceed 3 months, a 6-week duration is recommended for native valve endocarditis
	Ampicillin Or	Administer a total of 12 grams per day intravenously, divided into 4 to 6 doses	4–6 weeks	Same as above
	Vancomycin + gentamicin Or	Administer vancomycin 30 mg/kg per day intravenously in 2 doses, along with gentamicin 3 mg/kg per day IV split into 3 equal administrations	6 weeks	Beta-lactamase producer
	Ampicillin + ceftriaxone	Administer ampicillin 2 grams intravenously every 4 hours, along with an additional ceftriaxone 2 grams IV every 12 hours	6 weeks	In renal failure who can't tolerate gentamicin
	Linezolid	Administer 600 mg either intravenously or orally every 12 hours	6 weeks	In cases where the pathogen exhibits resistance to penicillin, aminoglycosides, and vancomycin
Staphylococci	Nafcillin or oxacillin (sensitive)	Administer a total of 12 grams intravenously over 24 hours, divided into 4 to 6 equal doses	6 weeks	A full treatment course is required for left-sided endocarditis and complicated right-sided cases, while a shorter 2-week regimen may be sufficient for uncomplicated right-sided infections

(continued)

Table 70.1 (continued)

Organism	Antibiotic	Dose	Duration	Remarks
	Cefazolin	Administer a total of 6 grams intravenously per day, split into 3 equal doses	6 weeks	
	Vancomycin	Administer 30 mg per kg of body weight per day, split into 2 equal intravenous doses	6 weeks	
	Daptomycin	At least 8 mg per kg per dose	6 weeks	
HACEK	Ceftriaxone or	2 g IV once daily	4 weeks	
	Ampicillin or	12 g/day IV in 4–6 divided doses		
	Ciprofloxacin	400 mg IV twice daily or 500 mg orally twice daily	6 weeks	If unable to tolerate cephalosporin
Non-HACEK gram-negative	Penicillin G/ ampicillin/ ceftriaxone/ carbapenem + gentamicin/ ciprofloxacin			Along with surgery
Fungal	Amphotericin B followed by lifelong oral azole		6 weeks	Along with surgery

70.3.2 Prognostic Scoring and Risk Assessment

- EuroSCORE II: Incorporate prognostic tools like EuroSCORE II at admission to assess surgical risk and aid in decision-making. This scoring system evaluates factors such as patient age, comorbidities, and hemodynamic status to predict operative mortality.

70.3.3 Clinical Stability

- Assessment: Monitor the patient's response to empirical therapy, focusing on fever resolution, hemodynamic stability, and symptom progression.

Table 70.2 Prosthetic valve endocarditis

Organism	Antibiotic	Dose	Duration	Remarks
Viridans group streptococci and *streptococcus gallolyticus* strains confirmed to be sensitive to penicillin	Ceftriaxone ± gentamicin or	Ceftriaxone 2 g IV once daily, with or without gentamicin at 3 mg/kg per day administered as a single IV or IM dose	Ceftriaxone 6 weeks Gentamicin 2 weeks	Extend gentamicin therapy to 6 weeks when the minimum inhibitory concentration (MIC) exceeds 0.12 μg/mL for the identified pathogen
	Penicillin G or	Penicillin G at a total daily dose of 24 million units, administered intravenously either as a continuous infusion or in 4 to 6 evenly spaced doses	6 weeks	
	Vancomycin or	Vancomycin at a total daily dose of 30 mg/kg IV, administered in 2 equal doses over 24 hours	6 weeks	
	Ampicillin	Administer ampicillin 2 grams intravenously every 4 hours	6 weeks	
Strains of VGS and *S. Gallolyticus* exhibiting partial resistance to penicillin	Ceftriaxone + gentamicin or	Ceftriaxone 2 g IV once daily combined with gentamicin 3 mg/kg per day, administered as a single IV or IM dose	Ceftriaxone 6 weeks Gentamicin 2 weeks	Extend gentamicin therapy to 6 weeks when the minimum inhibitory concentration (MIC) exceeds 0.12 μg/mL for the identified pathogen
	Vancomycin or	30 mg/kg per 24 h IV in 2 equally divided doses	6 weeks	
	Ampicillin	2 g IV every 4 h	6 weeks	
Staphylococci	Nafcillin or oxacillin (sensitive) + rifampin + gentamicin	2 g/24 h IV in 4–6 equally divided doses + 900 mg per 24 h IV or orally in 3 equally divided doses + 3 mg/kg per 24 h IV or IM in 2 or 3 equally divided doses	Oxacillin ≥6 weeks Rifampin ≥6 weeks Gentamicin 2 weeks	If oxacillin sensitive

(continued)

Table 70.2 (continued)

Organism	Antibiotic	Dose	Duration	Remarks
	Vancomycin + rifampin + gentamicin	30 mg/kg 24 h in 2 equally divided doses + 900 mg per 24 h IV or orally in 3 equally divided doses + 3 mg/kg per 24 h IV or IM in 2 or 3 equally divided doses	≥6 weeks	If oxacillin resistant, maintain trough concentration of 10–20 μg/mL. Rifampin is included to target biofilm-associated pathogens on prosthetic material
Enterococci	Same as native valve endocarditis (usually always 6 weeks)			
HACEK	Same as native valve endocarditis (duration of therapy: 6 weeks)			
Non-HACEK gram-negative	Same as native valve endocarditis (antibiotics + surgery)			
Fungal	Same as native valve endocarditis (amphotericin B + surgery)			

- Stable Patients: If the patient is clinically stable, continue antimicrobial therapy tailored to culture results and monitor for complications.
- Unstable Patients: If the patient remains unstable or deteriorates, proceed to urgent multidisciplinary evaluation.

70.3.4 Multidisciplinary Care and Cardiothoracic Surgery Review

- Endocarditis Team: Establish a dedicated "Endocarditis Team" involving infectious disease specialists, cardiologists, cardiac surgeons, microbiologists, and other relevant experts. This team approach has been shown to improve patient outcomes.
- Surgical Timing and Indications:
  - Persistent Bacteremia: Ongoing bacteremia despite adequate antibiotic therapy suggests uncontrolled infection requiring surgical intervention.
  - Valve Dysfunction: Severe valve dysfunction leading to heart failure may necessitate urgent valve repair or replacement.
  - Large Vegetations: Vegetations larger than 10 mm, especially those with prior embolic events, increase the risk of further embolism.
  - Abscess Formation or Fungal Infection: Intracardiac abscesses and fungal endocarditis often require surgical debridement due to poor response to medical therapy alone.
  - Neurological Complications: Careful timing of surgery is critical in patients with recent cerebral emboli or hemorrhage; collaboration with neurologists is essential [3].

70.3.5 *Management of Complications*

Neurological:

- Embolic Stroke: Implement neuroimaging if neurological signs arise. Manage strokes according to standard protocols, considering the risks and benefits of anticoagulation.
- Mycotic Aneurysms: Monitor for cerebral mycotic aneurysms, which may require neurosurgical intervention.

Cardiac:

- Heart Failure: Optimize medical management and consider mechanical support if necessary.
- Arrhythmias: Monitor and treat arrhythmias promptly.

Systemic Embolism:

- Splenic Abscess: Suspect in patients with left upper quadrant pain; management may include antibiotics and possible surgical intervention.
- Renal Infarction: Monitor renal function and manage accordingly.
- Peripheral Emboli: Assess limbs for ischemia; surgical or endovascular interventions may be required.

70.4 Emerging Evidence and Research Trends

- Minimally Invasive Surgical Techniques: Research into less invasive surgical options aims to reduce operative risk and improve recovery times.
- Molecular Diagnostics: Advances in molecular techniques may enhance the detection of fastidious organisms and guide more precise antimicrobial therapy.

70.5 Conclusion

The management of infective endocarditis in the ICU is complex and requires a multidisciplinary, systematic approach for diagnosis, treatment, and prevention of complications. Early recognition, comprehensive diagnostic evaluation—including advanced imaging and microbiological techniques—and prompt initiation of appropriate antimicrobial therapy are crucial. The involvement of an Endocarditis Team facilitates coordinated care, optimizing both medical and surgical interventions. By integrating prognostic assessments, patient-centered education, and awareness of emerging evidence, ICU clinicians can significantly improve patient outcomes in this challenging condition.

Algorithm 70.1: Approach to infective endocarditis in the ICU

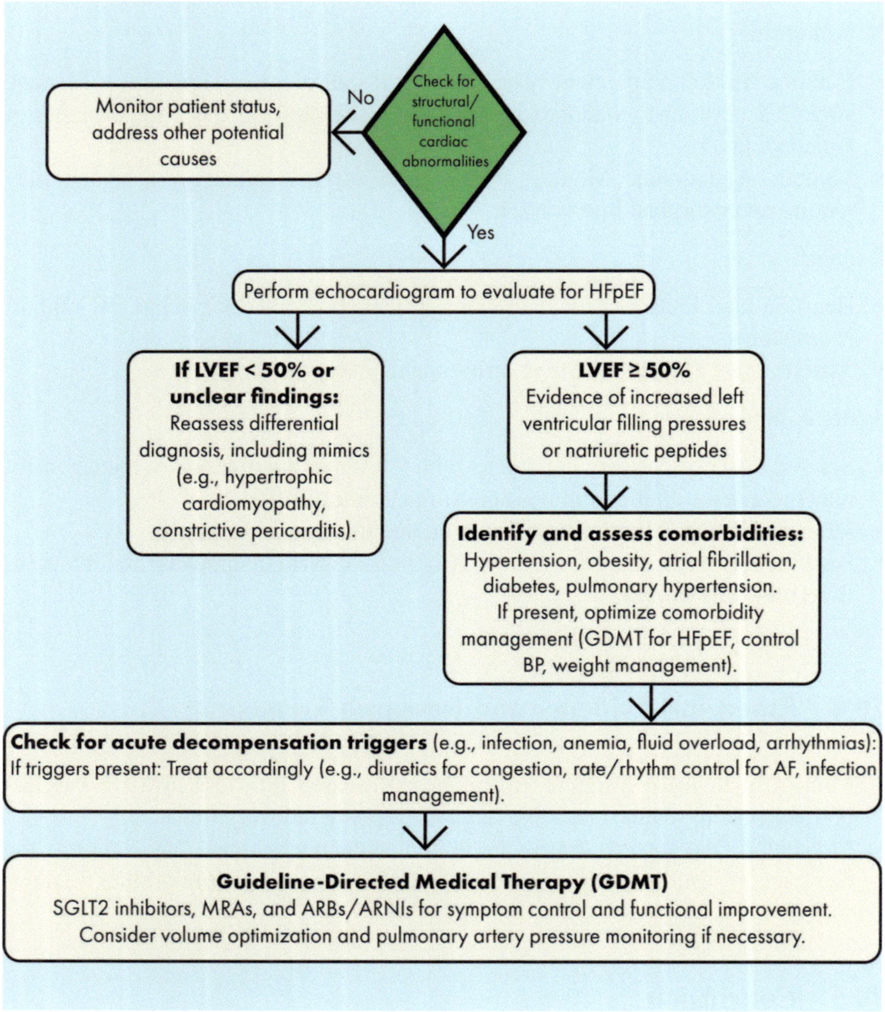

Bibliography

1. Delgado V, Ajmone Marsan N, de Waha S, Bonaros N, Brida M, Burri H, et al. ESC guidelines for the management of endocarditis. Eur Heart J. 2023;44(39):3948–4042.
2. McDonald EG, Aggrey G, Tarik Aslan A, Casias M, Cortes-Penfield N, Dong MQD, et al. Guidelines for diagnosis and management of infective endocarditis in adults: a WikiGuidelines group consensus statement. JAMA Netw Open. 2023;6(7):e2326366.
3. Baddour LM, Wilson WR, Bayer AS, Fowler VG Jr, Tleyjeh IM, Rybak MJ, et al. Infective endocarditis in adults: diagnosis, antimicrobial therapy, and Management of Complications: a scientific statement for healthcare professionals from the American Heart Association. Circulation. 2015;132(15):1435–86.

Chapter 71
Approach to Myocarditis in the ICU

71.1 Introduction

Myocarditis is an inflammatory disease of the myocardium that poses significant diagnostic and therapeutic challenges in the intensive care unit (ICU). Its clinical presentation can mimic other cardiac conditions, such as acute coronary syndromes, making timely and accurate diagnosis crucial. Advances in diagnostic criteria, imaging modalities, and understanding of its diverse etiologies have improved patient management [1] [Ref: Algorithm 71.1].

71.2 Diagnostic Approach

71.2.1 Enhanced Diagnostic Criteria

Accurate diagnosis of myocarditis requires a combination of clinical suspicion and advanced diagnostic tools. The Lake Louise Criteria, established for cardiac magnetic resonance imaging (CMR), serve as a standardized approach to differentiate myocarditis from other cardiac conditions. These criteria focus on the detection of myocardial edema, hyperemia, and necrosis or fibrosis through specific CMR sequences.

In complex cases where CMR findings are inconclusive, combining CMR with endomyocardial biopsy (EMB) enhances diagnostic accuracy. EMB allows for histological examination and immunohistochemical analysis, providing definitive evidence of myocarditis and aiding in identifying specific etiologies.

S. B. Mishra et al., *Mastering ICU Care*,
https://doi.org/10.1007/978-981-95-0179-3_71

71.2.2 Advanced Imaging Modalities

Beyond CMR, positron emission tomography (PET) imaging has emerged as a valuable tool in detecting myocardial inflammation. PET imaging, especially when combined with CMR, improves diagnostic sensitivity and specificity. Additionally, emerging biomarkers such as microRNAs are being investigated for their potential to provide noninvasive diagnostic information and to monitor disease progression [2].

71.3 Etiological Classification

Understanding the underlying cause of myocarditis is essential for targeted therapy. The etiologies of myocarditis are diverse and include:

- Viral Myocarditis
  - Viruses are the most common cause of myocarditis. Common viral agents include Coxsackievirus B, Parvovirus B19, Adenovirus, and Human Herpesvirus 6. Molecular techniques like polymerase chain reaction (PCR) on EMB samples can detect viral genomes, guiding antiviral therapy.
- Autoimmune Myocarditis
  - Autoimmune processes can lead to myocarditis either as a primary cardiac manifestation or secondary to systemic autoimmune diseases such as systemic lupus erythematosus or sarcoidosis. Identification of autoimmune etiology is critical, as it alters the management approach towards immunosuppressive therapy.
- Drug-Induced and Hypersensitivity Myocarditis
  - Certain medications and hypersensitivity reactions can induce myocarditis. Offending agents include some antibiotics, antiepileptics, and chemotherapeutic agents. Early recognition and discontinuation of the causative drug are vital.
- Rare Causes
  - Immune Checkpoint Inhibitor-Associated Myocarditis: With the increasing use of immune checkpoint inhibitors in oncology, myocarditis has emerged as a rare but severe adverse effect. Early detection is essential due to its high mortality rate.
  - Genetic Predispositions: Genetic mutations affecting cardiac proteins can predispose individuals to myocarditis. Understanding genetic factors may guide future personalized therapies [3].

71.4 Clinical Presentations

Myocarditis presents with a spectrum of clinical manifestations:

1. Arrhythmias and Conduction Abnormalities

   - Patients may develop arrhythmias ranging from premature ventricular contractions to life-threatening ventricular tachyarrhythmias. Conduction abnormalities, including atrioventricular block, are also common.

2. Fulminant Cardiogenic Shock

   - Fulminant myocarditis is characterized by sudden and severe heart failure leading to cardiogenic shock. It requires immediate recognition and aggressive management in the ICU..

3. Pediatric Considerations

   - Pediatric myocarditis often presents differently from adults, with infants and children exhibiting symptoms such as irritability, poor feeding, and respiratory distress. Management strategies may differ due to variations in etiology and disease progression in the pediatric population.

71.5 Management Strategies

71.5.1 Risk Stratification and Personalized Treatment

Management of myocarditis is tailored based on the severity of the presentation:

Stable Patients

- Supportive Care: Includes monitoring for arrhythmias, managing heart failure symptoms, and restricting physical activity to reduce cardiac stress.
- Medical Therapy: Standard heart failure medications such as ACE inhibitors, beta-blockers, and diuretics may be used cautiously.

Fulminant Myocarditis

- Hemodynamic Support: Inotropes may be necessary to support cardiac output.
- Mechanical Circulatory Support: Devices such as intra-aortic balloon pumps, ventricular assist devices, or extracorporeal membrane oxygenation (ECMO) may be life-saving.
- Immunosuppressive Therapy: Early initiation may be considered, especially in autoimmune etiologies.

Specific Therapies

- Immunosuppressive Therapy: Indicated for autoimmune myocarditis. Corticosteroids and other immunosuppressive agents can reduce myocardial inflammation.
- Antiviral Therapy: While the role of antiviral therapy remains limited, it may be considered in cases with confirmed viral etiology, particularly with replicating viruses.

71.5.2 Integration of Immunophenotyping

Emerging techniques like immunophenotyping of EMB samples help identify specific inflammatory pathways involved in myocarditis. This approach allows for the development of targeted therapies, potentially improving outcomes by addressing the underlying immunological mechanisms.

71.5.3 Prognostic Markers

Biomarkers play a significant role in assessing prognosis:

- Troponins: Elevated levels indicate myocardial injury and are associated with worse outcomes.
- N-terminal pro-B-type Natriuretic Peptide (NT-proBNP): Elevated levels reflect ventricular dysfunction and correlate with disease severity and prognosis.

71.6 Conclusion

Myocarditis in the ICU demands a comprehensive and nuanced approach, integrating advanced diagnostic criteria, understanding of diverse etiologies, and personalized management strategies. Incorporating standardized criteria like the Lake Louise Criteria and utilizing advanced imaging modalities enhance diagnostic accuracy. Recognizing rare causes and pediatric differences ensures that all patient populations receive appropriate care. Risk stratification and the integration of immunophenotyping pave the way for targeted therapies, improving patient outcomes. Through this systematic approach, ICU clinicians can effectively navigate the complexities of myocarditis, providing optimal care for this challenging condition.

Algorithm 71.1: Approach to myocarditis in the ICU

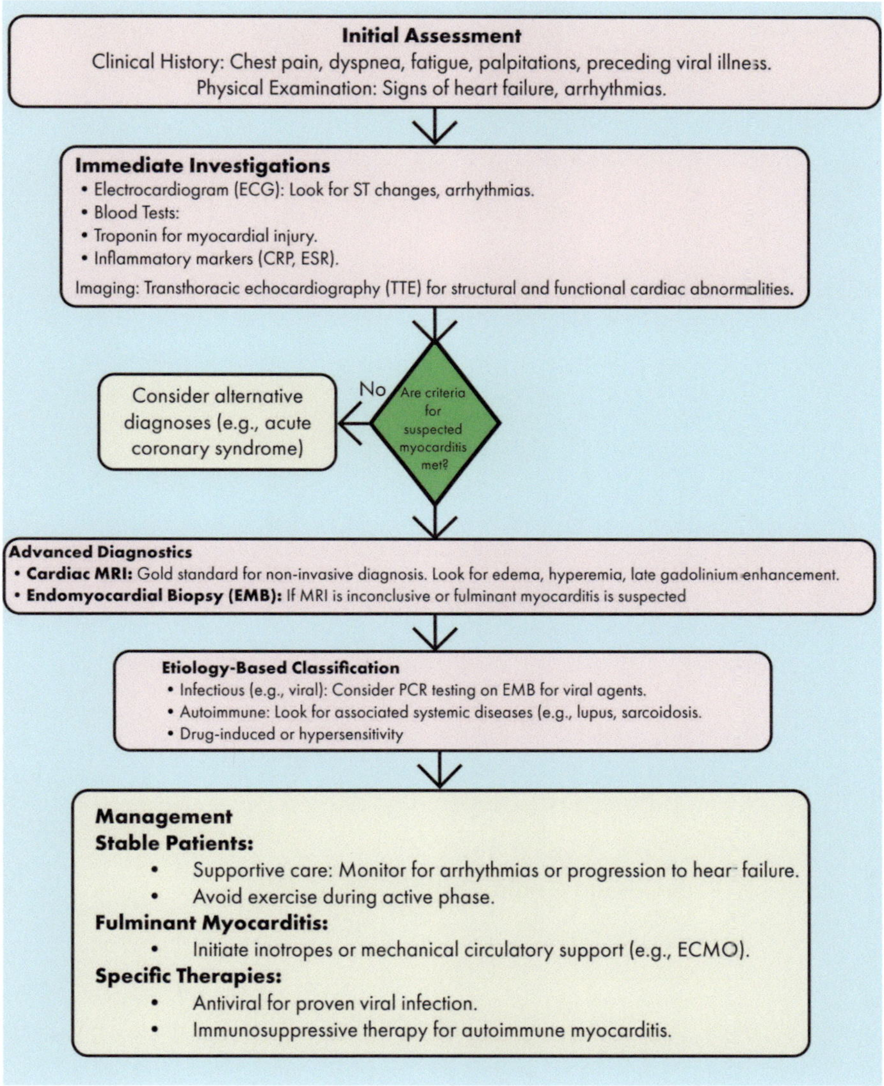

Bibliography

1. Nagai T, Inomata T, Kohno T, Sato T, Tada A, Kubo T, et al. JCS 2023 guideline on the diagnosis and treatment of myocarditis. Circ J. 2023;87(5):674–754.
2. Chabior A, Tyminska A, Pawlak A, Giordani A, Caforio A, Grabowski M, et al. Advances in myocarditis management in the light of the latest research and recent guidelines of the European Society of Cardiology. Cardiol J. 2024;31(2):342–51.
3. Lampejo T, Durkin SM, Bhatt N, Guttmann O. Acute myocarditis: aetiology, diagnosis and management. Clin Med (Lond). 2021;21(5):e505–e10.

Chapter 72
Approach to Aortic Dissection in the ICU

72.1 Introduction

Aortic dissection, the most common of the acute aortic syndrome, is a life-threatening condition that demands prompt diagnosis and management in the intensive care unit (ICU). It occurs when a tear in the intimal layer of the aorta allows blood to enter the medial layer, creating a false lumen that compromises blood flow and weakens the vessel wall. This can result in catastrophic complications such as aortic rupture, aortic regurgitation, myocardial ischemia, cardiac tamponade, acute stroke, malperfusion of critical organs, or death. Early identification and treatment are crucial to improve patient outcomes [1] [Ref: Algorithm 72.1].

72.2 Definition

Aortic dissection is defined as acute if it is during the first 2 weeks after symptom onset or chronic if it is beyond the second week. It has also been divided into four temporal types by the International Registry of Acute Aortic Dissection (IRAD): hyperacute (<24 h), acute (2–7 d), subacute (8–30 d), and chronic (>30 d).

In similar lines the Society of Thoracic Surgeons and Society for Vascular Surgery have also categorized aortic dissection into four temporal types: hyperacute (<24 h), acute (1–14 d), subacute (15–90 d), and chronic (>90 d).

S. B. Mishra et al., *Mastering ICU Care*,
https://doi.org/10.1007/978-981-95-0179-3_72

72.3 Risk Stratification

72.3.1 Classification Systems

Aortic dissections are classified to guide management strategies and predict outcomes. The two primary classification systems are the Stanford and DeBakey systems.

Stanford Classification:
- Type A: Involves the ascending aorta and may extend to the arch and descending aorta
- Type B: Involves only the descending aorta distal to the left subclavian artery, without involvement of the ascending aorta

DeBakey Classification:
- Type I: Originates in the ascending aorta, involves the arch, and often extends beyond the arch distally
- Type II: Confined to the ascending aorta
- Type III: Originates in the descending aorta and extends distally (type IIIa is limited to the thoracic aorta; type IIIb extends below the diaphragm)

Including both classifications provides additional granularity, particularly useful in surgical planning and prognostication.

72.3.2 Risk Factors and Genetic Predispositions

Identifying risk factors is essential for clinical suspicion and early diagnosis.

- Hypertension: The most common risk factor, contributing to intimal tearing due to increased shear stress.
- Genetic Predispositions:
- Marfan Syndrome: A connective tissue disorder caused by mutations in the FBN1 gene, leading to cystic medial necrosis and weakening of the aortic wall.
- Loeys-Dietz Syndrome and Ehlers-Danlos Syndrome Type IV: Other connective tissue disorders associated with aortic dissection.
- Bicuspid Aortic Valve (BAV): Patients with BAV have a higher incidence of aortopathy due to abnormal aortic wall stress.
- Familial Thoracic Aortic Aneurysm and Dissection (FTAAD): Genetic mutations (e.g., in ACTA2, MYH11 genes) increase susceptibility.

Understanding these predispositions is crucial, as the ACC/AHA guidelines recommend lower thresholds for surgical intervention in patients with these conditions due to their higher risk of dissection at smaller aortic diameters.

72.4 Management

72.4.1 *Consider Other Differential Diagnoses*

- Description: Rule out other life-threatening causes of acute chest or back pain, such as myocardial infarction, pulmonary embolism, or acute pericarditis.
- Rationale: Misdiagnosis can delay critical treatment. Clinical signs such as tearing pain, malperfusion, or syncope may increase suspicion of aortic dissection, but an electrocardiogram (ECG), cardiac biomarkers, chest X-ray, and D-dimer can help exclude alternative diagnoses.
- Key Consideration: Initiating anticoagulation in suspected acute coronary syndrome (ACS) without recognizing aortic dissection could worsen the condition, potentially leading to fatal hemorrhage.

72.4.2 *Assess Symptoms of Aortic Dissection*

- Key Question: Does the patient have sudden, severe chest or back pain with a “tearing” or “ripping” quality or signs of malperfusion?
- Description: Classic symptoms include acute, severe pain radiating to the back, abdomen, or legs, and malperfusion syndromes such as limb ischemia, renal failure, mesenteric ischemia, or neurological deficits.
- Rationale: These symptoms are characteristic of aortic dissection and should prompt immediate evaluation. Absence of typical pain does not exclude the diagnosis, especially in patients with risk factors [2].

72.4.3 *Evaluate Risk Factors*

- Key Risk Factors: Hypertension, connective tissue disorders (e.g., Marfan syndrome), bicuspid aortic valve, familial history of aortic disease, previous cardiac surgery, or a history of aortic aneurysm.

72.4.4 *Perform Advanced Imaging*

- Bedside Transesophageal Echocardiography (TEE):
- When Indicated: Immediate bedside TEE is the preferred diagnostic modality as it allows rapid, detailed visualization of the proximal aorta, aortic valve, and pericardial space, and can confirm the diagnosis without requiring patient transport.
- Aortic diameter measurements should be obtained perpendicular to the long axis of the aorta at specified segmental locations, with measurements also taken at the locations of any abnormalities.

- Computed Tomography Angiography (CTA):
  - CTA of the chest, abdomen, and pelvis is the gold standard for diagnosing aortic dissection as it provides high-resolution, three-dimensional imaging of the entire aorta, allowing precise localization of the dissection, evaluation of branch vessel involvement, and differentiation between Type A and Type B dissections. However, it requires iodinated contrast and radiation exposure. Thus, one must ensure that the renal function is adequate.
- Magnetic Resonance Imaging (MRI):
  - MRI is an alternative for patients with contraindications to iodinated contrast or when radiation exposure is a concern. Drawbacks of MRI are limited availability, longer scan times, and contraindications in patients with certain implants or unstable conditions.
- 4D Flow MRI:
  - Provides time-resolved, three-dimensional imaging of blood flow dynamics within the aorta as it offers insights into flow patterns that may contribute to dissection progression or aneurysm formation.
- Automated Aortic Measurement Systems:
  - Utilize artificial intelligence algorithms to assess aortic dimensions accurately. It enhances detection of subtle changes in aortic size, aiding in early diagnosis and surveillance.

It is neither specific nor sensitive to diagnose aortic dissection. However, there are some findings that may raise suspicion. Mediastinal widening, disruption of the normally distinct contour of the aortic knob, "Calcium sign," which appears as a separation of the intimal calcification from the aortic wall of >5 mm, double density appearance within the aorta, tracheal deviation to the right, and deviation of the nasogastric tube to the right are few findings that are suggestive of aortic dissection.

72.4.5 Classify the Dissection

- Stanford and DeBakey Classifications: Use both systems to determine the extent and location of the dissection.

72.5 Aortic Dissection Risk Scoring System

Acute aortic dissection risk scoring systems (e.g., aortic dissection detection risk score [AAD-RS] or aorta simplified score [AORTAs]) can aid in the diagnostic evaluation of patients presenting with aortic dissection.

Table 72.1 Acute aortic dissection detection risk score (ADD-RS) components

High-risk conditions	High-risk pain features	High-risk examination features
Marfan syndrome or other connective tissue disease	Chest, back, or abdominal pain described as: Abrupt onset, severe in intensity, ripping or tearing in quality	Pulse deficit or systolic blood pressure differential
Family history of aortic disease		Focal neurologic deficit (with pain)
Known aortic valve disease		Murmur of aortic regurgitation (new, with pain)
Recent aortic manipulation		Hypotension or shock state
Known thoracic aortic aneurysm		

Table 72.2 AORTAs simplified pretest probability score for aortic dissection

Clinical item	Points
Hypotension/shock	2
Aneurysm	1
Pulse deficit	1
Neurologic deficit	1
Severe pain	1
Sudden-onset pain	1

AAD-RS: For each risk category, 1 point is assigned if ≥1 risk factors are present. Consequently, the total ADD-RS will range from 0 to 3. An ADD-RS of 0 points is low risk; 1 point is moderate risk; and 2 to 3 points is high risk (Table 72.1).

Aorta Simplified Score (AORTAs) Pretest Probability Assessment Score: The points are summed, and a total score of 0 to 1 point is low-probability of aortic dissection, where a total of ≥2 points is high probability (Table 72.2).

72.6 Management Based on Classification

1. Type A Dissection (Ascending Aorta Involved)
   - Urgency: Type A dissections are surgical emergencies due to the risk of aortic rupture, pericardial tamponade, acute aortic regurgitation, and coronary artery involvement.
   - Treatment:
     - Hemodynamic Stabilization: Arterial line insertion for continuous blood pressure (BP) monitoring.
     - Blood Pressure Control: Target systolic BP <120 mmHg and heart rate 60–80 beats per minute using intravenous beta-blockers (e.g., esmolol, labetalol). If beta-blockers are contraindicated (e.g., acute AR, heart block,

or bradycardia), consider calcium channel blockers (verapamil/diltiazem). Add intravenous vasodilators if BP is not controlled by beta blockers alone.
  - Pain Management: Administer analgesics (e.g., morphine) to reduce sympathetic stimulation. Avoid ketorolac as it may cause hypertension.
  - Surgical Intervention: Type A is associated with high risk of life-threatening complications. Thus, it is prudent to go for surgical intervention if there is a proven or suspicion of Type A dissection. Type A dissection presenting with malperfusion syndrome is an absolute indication for immediate surgical intervention.
    - Emergent Surgery: Open surgical repair involving resection of the intimal tear, obliteration of the false lumen, and restoration of aortic continuity.
    - Considerations: Involvement of the aortic valve or coronary arteries may necessitate additional procedures (e.g., aortic valve replacement, coronary artery bypass grafting).
- If Surgery Is Not Feasible:
  - Medical Management: Reserved for patients with prohibitive surgical risk; involves strict blood pressure control and close monitoring.
  - Palliative Care: Focuses on symptom management and quality of life when neither surgery nor medical therapy is appropriate.
- Management in Specific Populations:
  - Pregnant Patients: Requires a multidisciplinary team involving obstetricians, cardiothoracic surgeons, and anesthesiologists. Early surgical intervention during the first and second trimester is often recommended, with consideration of fetal viability and maternal health. In the third trimester, urgent cesarean section followed by aortic surgery is recommended.

2. Type B Dissection (Descending Aorta Only)
   Uncomplicated Type B Dissections:
   - Medical Management:
     - Blood Pressure Control: Achieve target systolic BP <120 mmHg and heart rate 60–80 bpm using intravenous beta-blockers. Vasodilators (e.g., nitroprusside) may be added if blood pressure remains elevated.
     - Monitoring: Close hemodynamic monitoring and serial imaging to assess for complications.

Complicated Type B Dissections:
- Indications for Intervention: Evidence of malperfusion syndromes (renal failure, mesenteric ischemia, limb ischemia), aortic rupture, rapid expansion, or persistent/refractory pain.
- Endovascular Repair (Endovascular stent grafting) and TEVAR (Thoracic endovascular aortic repair).
  - Description: Placement of a stent graft to cover the intimal tear and redirect blood flow into the true lumen.

  - Advantages: Less invasive than open surgery, shorter recovery times, and reduced perioperative morbidity and mortality.
  - Considerations: Requires suitable vascular anatomy; long-term durability is still under investigation.

- Surgical Intervention: Open repair may be necessary if TEVAR is contraindicated or not feasible due to anatomical considerations.
- Emerging Recommendations:
  - Early TEVAR: Recent studies suggest benefits of early TEVAR even in uncomplicated Type B dissections to promote aortic remodeling and reduce long-term complications.
- Special Considerations:
  - Pregnant Patients: Management is predominantly medical, balancing maternal and fetal risks. TEVAR is generally avoided due to radiation exposure [3].

72.7 Incorporate Advanced Pharmacological Guidelines

- Beta-Blocker Therapy:
  - Nuances: Select agents with rapid onset and short half-life (e.g., esmolol) for titration; consider nonselective beta-blockers for additional vasodilatory effects.
  - Contraindications: In patients with asthma or severe bradycardia, use calcium channel blockers (e.g., diltiazem) as alternatives.
- Vasodilators:
  - Usage: Add vasodilators (e.g., nitroprusside, nicardipine) if blood pressure remains elevated despite beta-blockade.
  - Monitoring: Watch for reflex tachycardia; beta-blockers should be initiated first to prevent this effect.
- Considerations for Complicated Cases:
  - Malperfusion Syndromes: Inotropes may be necessary to support end-organ perfusion but should be balanced against increased aortic wall stress.

72.8 Focus on Complication Mitigation

1. Malperfusion Syndromes
   - Renal Ischemia:
     - Management: Revascularization via TEVAR or surgical fenestration; renal replacement therapy if necessary.

- Limb Ischemia:
  - Management: Surgical or endovascular intervention to restore perfusion; fasciotomy if compartment syndrome develops.
- Mesenteric Ischemia:
  - Management: Emergent intervention due to high mortality; requires prompt revascularization.

2. Stroke Prevention
   - Risk Factors: Extension of the dissection into carotid arteries or hypotension leading to cerebral hypoperfusion.
   - Management: Blood pressure optimization; surgical repair if dissection involves cerebral vessels.
3. Aortic Rupture
   - Emergency: Immediate surgical or endovascular repair is required.
   - Prevention: Strict blood pressure control and timely intervention for high-risk dissections.

72.9 New Insights from Recent Guidelines

1. Reduced Thresholds for Intervention
   - Indexed Aortic Diameter: Intervention thresholds may be lower for patients with smaller body size or genetic predispositions.
   - ACC/AHA Recommendations: Surgery may be considered at an aortic diameter of 5.0 cm or even smaller in patients with Marfan syndrome or other high-risk features.
2. Acute Aortic Syndrome Spectrum
   - Intramural Hematoma:
     - Description: Hemorrhage within the aortic wall without intimal tear.
     - Management: Similar to aortic dissection; Type A requires surgery; Type B may be managed medically or with TEVAR.
   - Penetrating Atherosclerotic Ulcer:
     - Description: Ulceration of atherosclerotic plaque penetrating the internal elastic lamina.
     - Management: Depends on symptoms and size; TEVAR may be indicated for symptomatic or enlarging ulcers.

72.10 Conclusion

The management of aortic dissection in the ICU demands a structured and comprehensive approach centered on early diagnosis, prompt imaging, accurate classification, and appropriate intervention. Understanding the nuances of risk stratification, including genetic predispositions and the use of both Stanford and DeBakey classification systems, guides clinical decision-making.

Type A dissections require emergent surgical repair due to the high risk of mortality, while Type B dissections may be managed medically or with endovascular techniques depending on the presence of complications. Strict blood pressure control is pivotal in all cases to prevent progression or rupture. Long-term surveillance and management, including regular imaging and blood pressure optimization, are essential to prevent re-dissection and other complications. Incorporating the latest guidelines and leveraging a multidisciplinary team approach enhance patient care and outcomes. By staying abreast of emerging diagnostic tools and evolving management strategies, clinicians can improve the prognosis for patients with this critical condition.

Algorithm 72.1: Approach to aortic dissection in the ICU

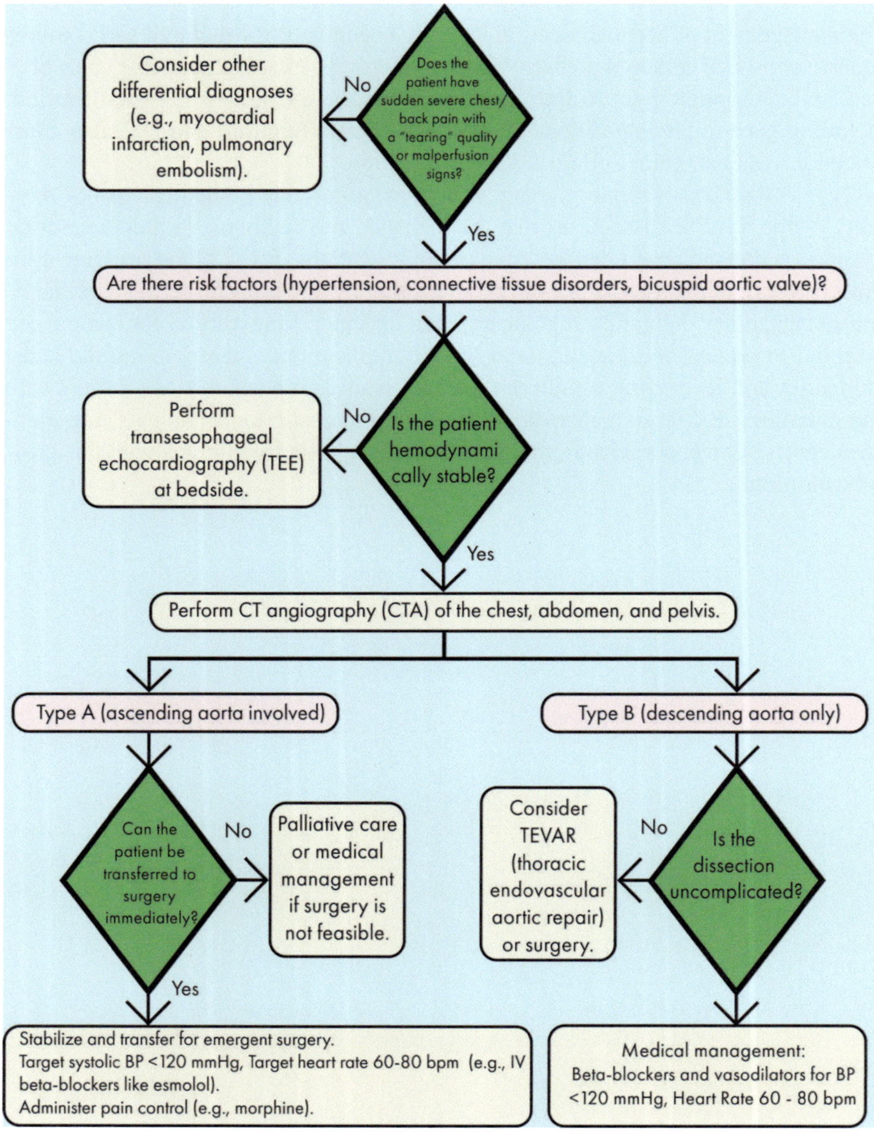

Bibliography

1. Isselbacher EM, Preventza O, Hamilton Black J, Augoustides JG, Beck AW, Bolen MA, et al. ACC/AHA guideline for the diagnosis and Management of Aortic Disease: a report of the American Heart Association/American College of Cardiology Joint Committee on clinical practice guidelines. Circulation. 2022;146(24):e334–482.
2. Erwin Iii JP, Committee ACCSSO, Cibotti-Sun M, Elma M. Aortic disease guideline-at-a-glance. J Am Coll Cardiol. 2022;80(24):2348–52.
3. Force M, Czerny M, Grabenwoger M, Berger T, Aboyans V, Della Corte A, et al. EACTS/STS guidelines for diagnosing and treating acute and chronic syndromes of the aortic organ. Ann Thorac Surg. 2024;118(1):5–115.
4. Mazzolai L, Teixido-Tura G, Lanzi S, Boc V, Bossone E, Brodmann M, et al. ESC guidelines for the management of peripheral arterial and aortic diseases. Eur Heart J. 2024;45(36):3538–700.

Part VII
Pulmonary

Chapter 73
Approach to Pulmonary Embolism in the ICU

73.1 Introduction

Pulmonary embolism (PE) is a potentially life-threatening condition resulting from the obstruction of the pulmonary arteries, most commonly due to thromboemboli originating from deep vein thrombosis (DVT). In the intensive care unit (ICU), prompt recognition and appropriate management are essential to reduce mortality and morbidity. This chapter provides a comprehensive approach for diagnosing and managing PE in critically ill patients, integrating the latest clinical guidelines, evidence-based recommendations, and special considerations for various patient populations [1, 2] [Ref: Algorithm 73.1].

73.2 Clinical Presentation and Risk Factors

PE often presents with nonspecific symptoms such as acute dyspnea, chest pain—which may be pleuritic or tachycardia, hypoxemia, syncope, and sometimes hemoptysis. Recognizing these symptoms in the context of risk factors is crucial for early suspicion. Key risk factors include recent surgery, major trauma, lower limb fracture, spinal cord injury, prolonged immobilization, myocardial injury, metastatic cancer, pregnancy, hormonal therapy, prior thromboembolism, obesity, smoking, and inherited thrombophilias. In the ICU setting, where patients may already be critically ill with overlapping symptoms, a high index of suspicion is necessary.

S. B. Mishra et al., *Mastering ICU Care*,
https://doi.org/10.1007/978-981-95-0179-3_73

73.3 Diagnostic Approach

73.3.1 Clinical Prediction Rules

To stratify patients based on the likelihood of PE, clinical prediction tools such as the Wells Score and the Geneva Score are utilized. These tools consider various clinical variables to categorize patients into low, intermediate, or high pretest probability for PE. An important advancement in this area is the use of age-adjusted D-dimer cut-offs. For patients over 50 years old, the D-dimer threshold is adjusted by multiplying the patient's age by 10 μg/L, improving specificity and reducing unnecessary imaging in older adults.

73.3.2 D-Dimer Testing

In patients categorized as low probability, D-dimer testing serves as a valuable diagnostic tool due to its high sensitivity. A negative D-dimer result effectively rules out PE in these patients, allowing clinicians to consider alternative diagnoses without subjecting patients to imaging studies. Point-of-care D-dimer assays are particularly beneficial in resource-constrained ICU settings, enabling rapid decision-making.

73.3.3 Imaging Studies

For patients with intermediate to high pretest probability or a positive D-dimer test, imaging studies are the next step. Computed tomography pulmonary angiography (CTPA) is the gold standard for diagnosing PE, offering direct visualization of emboli within the pulmonary arteries. Alternative imaging modalities include ventilation-perfusion (V/Q) scans, which are especially useful when CTPA is contraindicated due to contrast allergies or renal insufficiency. A high-probability V/Q scan confirms the diagnosis of PE, while a normal scan effectively excludes it. PE is diagnosed with high probability V/Q scan. Normal V/Q scan rejects the diagnosis of PE. Compression ultrasound of the lower extremities can help detect deep vain thrmbosis (DVT) when imaging for pulmonary embolism(such as CTPA or V/Q scan) is not feasible. In pregnant patients, modified imaging protocols are employed to minimize fetal radiation exposure while ensuring accurate diagnosis. When CTPA is not feasible, bedside transthoracic echocardiography should be done [3].

73.3.4 Echocardiography

In suspected high-risk PE, absence of echocardiographic signs of RV dysfunction excludes PE as the cause of hemodynamic instability. And when immediate CTPA is not feasible in suspected high-risk PE, the unequivocal echocardiographic signs of RV pressure overload, with specific findings such as 60/60 sign, McConnell sign, or presence of right-heart thrombi, justify emergency reperfusion treatment for PE.

73.4 Risk Stratification and Clinical Assessment

Upon confirmation of PE, risk stratification is vital to guide management decisions. The Pulmonary Embolism Severity Index (PESI) and its simplified version (sPESI) are validated tools combining clinical variables to predict 30-day mortality risk. Patients are classified into low-risk (PESI Class I-II or sPESI score of 0) or higher-risk categories based on these scores [4].

73.4.1 Hemodynamic Stability

Assessing hemodynamic status is a critical component of risk stratification. Hemodynamically unstable patients, defined by sustained hypotension (systolic blood pressure < 90 mmHg) or shock, are considered to have high-risk PE (massive PE) and require immediate reperfusion therapy. Stable patients without signs of shock are further evaluated for right ventricular (RV) dysfunction and elevated biomarkers to determine the risk of adverse outcomes.

73.4.2 Intermediate Risk Stratification

Stable patients are subcategorized into intermediate-high and intermediate-low risk based on the presence of RV dysfunction and elevated cardiac biomarkers such as troponins and B-type natriuretic peptide (BNP) or N-terminal pro-BNP. Intermediate-high risk patients exhibit both RV dysfunction and biomarker elevation, indicating a higher risk of deterioration and necessitating closer monitoring and management with anticoagulation. Intermediate-low risk patients have either RV dysfunction or elevated biomarkers and are managed with standard anticoagulation therapy while being vigilantly observed for any signs of clinical worsening [5].

73.4.3 Role of Biomarkers

Biomarkers play a significant role in the risk stratification and management of PE. Elevated cardiac troponins reflect myocardial injury due to RV strain, while elevated BNP or N-terminal pro-BNP levels indicate RV dysfunction. These biomarkers help identify patients at higher risk of adverse outcomes and guide decisions regarding the intensity of monitoring and the need for potential escalation of therapy. In low-risk patients with normal biomarker levels, early discharge and outpatient management may be considered, provided that adequate home support is available.

73.4.4 Therapeutic Management

Oxygen therapy should be started when $SaO_2 < 90\%$.
Noninvasive ventilation or high-flow nasal cannula should be preferred.

When invasive mechanical ventilation is used positive end-expiratory pressure should be applied with caution as it may reduce venous return and worsen the low cardiac output due to RV failure.

For hypotension, judicious volume loading should be done when there is absence of elevated filling pressure as assessed by ultrasound imaging of inferior vena cava, and vasopressor should be started early.

73.4.5 Anticoagulation Therapy

Anticoagulation is the cornerstone of PE management. Direct oral anticoagulants (DOACs), such as apixaban and rivaroxaban, are preferred as first-line agents due to their ease of use, predictable pharmacokinetics, and favorable safety profiles. They eliminate the need for routine laboratory monitoring and have fewer dietary restrictions compared to vitamin K antagonists like warfarin. In patients with contraindications to DOACs, such as severe renal impairment or antiphospholipid syndrome, low molecular weight heparin (LMWH), fondaparinux, or unfractionated heparin (UFH) may be used. Special populations, such as pregnant women, require careful consideration; LMWH is the anticoagulant of choice during pregnancy, as DOACs cross the placenta and are contraindicated [6].

73.4.6 Advanced Interventional Therapies

For patients with massive PE and hemodynamic instability, immediate reperfusion therapy is indicated. Systemic thrombolysis with agents like alteplase is strongly recommended, as it rapidly dissolves the thrombus, restores pulmonary perfusion, and reduces RV afterload. UFH infusion is to be continued during infusion of alteplase. Catheter-directed thrombolysis is an alternative that delivers thrombolytics directly to the site of the clot at lower doses, minimizing systemic bleeding risks. Mechanical thrombectomy, including catheter-assisted and surgical embolectomy, is considered in patients with contraindications to thrombolysis or when thrombolytic therapy has failed. The utilization of pulmonary embolism response teams (PERT) facilitates rapid, multidisciplinary decision-making, integrating expertise from critical care, cardiology, pulmonology, hematology, and interventional radiology to tailor the best therapeutic approach for each patient. Drugs used for the management of PE with doses are shown in Table 73.1.

73.4.7 Special Considerations

73.4.7.1 Pregnancy

Managing PE during pregnancy presents unique challenges. Diagnostic imaging must balance the need for accurate detection with minimizing radiation exposure to the fetus. Modified protocols for V/Q scans or the use of MRI are considered.

Table 73.1 Table drugs for pulmonary embolism management

Drug name	Dose	Indications	Contraindications
Apixaban	10 mg BID for 7 days, then 5 mg BID	Treatment of acute PE and prevention of recurrence	Severe renal impairment (CrCl <15 mL/min)
Rivaroxaban	15 mg BID for 21 days, then 20 mg once daily	Treatment of acute PE and prevention of recurrence	Severe renal impairment (CrCl <15 mL/min)
Dabigatran	150 mg BID (after 5–10 days of parenteral anticoagulation)	Treatment of acute PE and prevention of recurrence	Severe renal impairment (CrCl <30 mL/min)
Edoxaban	60 mg once daily (after 5–10 days of parenteral anticoagulation)	Treatment of acute PE and prevention of recurrence	Severe renal impairment (CrCl <15 mL/min)
Warfarin	Dose adjusted to maintain INR between 2.0–3.0	Long-term anticoagulation for PE	Pregnancy, significant bleeding risk
Enoxaparin	1 mg/kg BID or 1.5 mg/kg once daily (adjust for renal function)	Preferred anticoagulant in pregnancy and cancer-associated thrombosis	Active bleeding, severe thrombocytopenia
Dalteparin	200 IU/kg once daily (max 18,000 IU/day)	Preferred anticoagulant in pregnancy and cancer-associated thrombosis	Active bleeding, severe thrombocytopenia
Heparin (UFH)	80 units/kg IV bolus, then 18 units/kg/hour infusion	Immediate anticoagulation in unstable patients	Active bleeding, severe thrombocytopenia
Alteplase (tPA)	100 mg IV over 2 hours	High-risk PE with hemodynamic instability	Active bleeding, recent intracranial hemorrhage
Tenecteplase	Weight-based bolus (e.g., 0.5 mg/kg)	High-risk PE with hemodynamic instability	Active bleeding, recent intracranial hemorrhage

LMWH remains the anticoagulant of choice due to its safety profile in pregnancy. Collaborative care involving obstetrics, maternal-fetal medicine, and critical care specialists is essential to optimize outcomes for both the mother and the fetus.

73.4.7.2 Outpatient Management

Selected low-risk patients with PE may be candidates for outpatient management. Criteria include hemodynamic stability, low PESI or sPESI scores, absence of severe comorbidities, and the availability of reliable home support systems. Outpatient management involves initiating anticoagulation therapy, providing thorough patient education on medication adherence and symptom monitoring, and arranging prompt outpatient follow-up.

73.4.7.3 Risk of Overuse in Diagnostics

While the prompt diagnosis of PE is crucial, there is a risk of overutilization of imaging studies, particularly in low-risk patients. Unnecessary exposure to radiation and contrast agents can be avoided by adhering to validated clinical prediction rules and using D-dimer testing judiciously. Clinicians are encouraged to apply careful clinical judgment, integrating patient history, physical examination findings, and pretest probability assessments before proceeding to imaging.

73.4.7.4 Long-Term Follow-Up and Complications

PE can have long-term sequelae, underscoring the importance of ongoing follow-up. Chronic thromboembolic pulmonary hypertension (CTEPH) is a serious complication resulting from persistent pulmonary artery obstruction, leading to increased pulmonary vascular resistance and right heart failure. Additionally, patients may develop post-PE syndrome, characterized by persistent dyspnea, reduced exercise capacity, and impaired quality of life. Regular follow-up visits should include clinical assessments, echocardiography, and functional tests to detect these complications early. Management strategies may involve pulmonary hypertension therapies, pulmonary endarterectomy for CTEPH, and rehabilitation programs to improve functional status.

73.4.7.5 Evidence-Based Recommendations

This chapter aligns with current guidelines from leading organizations such as the American Heart Association (AHA) and the European Society of Cardiology (ESC). Strong recommendations include the use of systemic thrombolysis for patients with high-risk (massive) PE and hemodynamic instability, and the preference for DOACs in anticoagulation therapy for most patients without contraindications. Conditional recommendations, based on individual patient factors and emerging evidence, guide the use of catheter-directed therapies and the consideration of outpatient management for low-risk patients.

73.5 Conclusion

The management of PE in the ICU requires a multifaceted approach that encompasses timely diagnosis, accurate risk stratification, and the implementation of appropriate therapeutic interventions. Incorporating age-adjusted D-dimer cut-offs and clinical prediction rules enhances diagnostic accuracy while reducing unnecessary imaging. Risk stratification models like PESI and sPESI inform treatment decisions and help identify patients suitable for outpatient management. Advanced interventional therapies and the formation of multidisciplinary teams, such as PERT, enhance the care of high-risk patients. Special considerations for pregnancy and the emphasis on long-term follow-up address the unique needs of specific patient populations and potential chronic complications. Adherence to evidence-based guidelines ensures optimal outcomes, improves resource utilization, and advances the standard of care for patients with PE in the ICU setting.

Algorithm 73.1: Approach to pulmonary embolism (PE) in the ICU

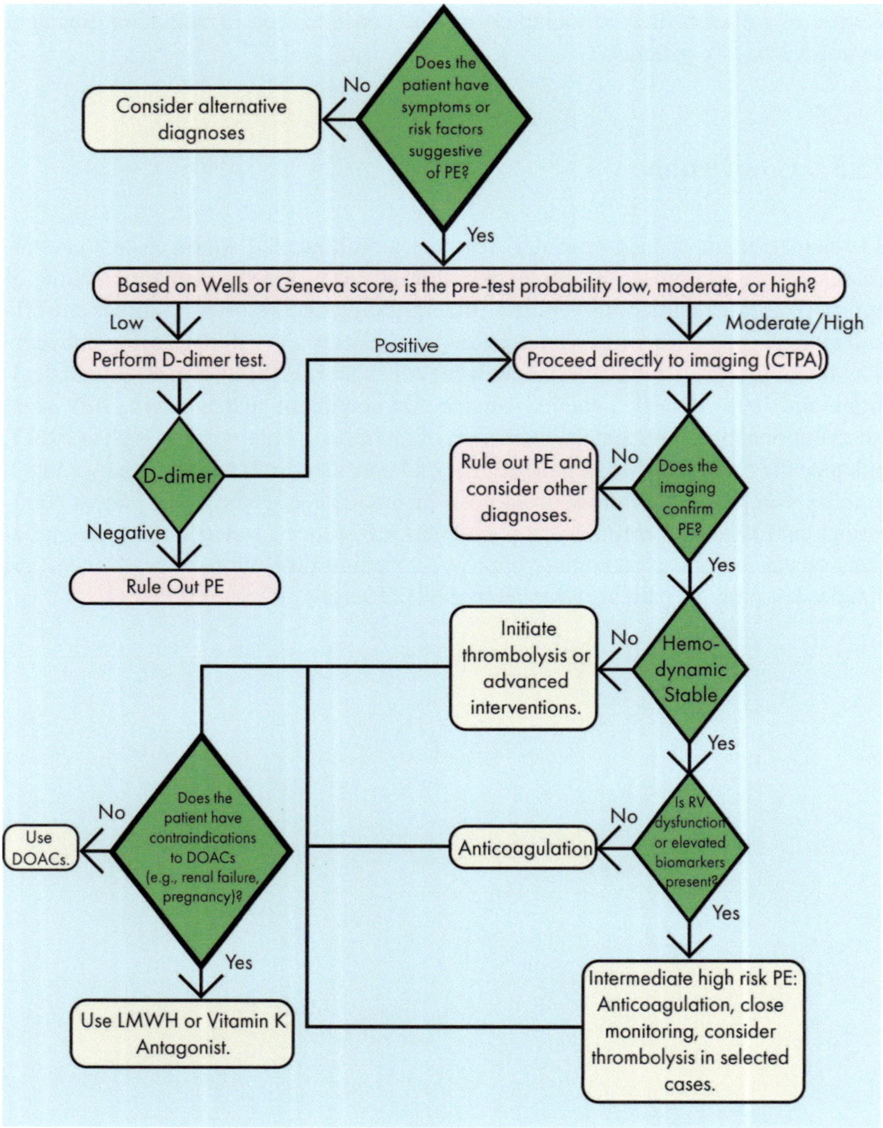

Bibliography

1. Erythropoulou-Kaltsidou A, Alkagiet S, Tziomalos K. New guidelines for the diagnosis and management of pulmonary embolism: key changes. World J Cardiol. 2020;12(5) 161–6.
2. Ortel TL, Neumann I, Ageno W, Beyth R, Clark NP, Cuker A, et al. American Society of Hematology 2020 guidelines for management of venous thromboembolism: treatment of deep vein thrombosis and pulmonary embolism. Blood Adv. 2020;4(19):4693–738.
3. Konstantinides SV, Meyer G, Becattini C, Bueno H, Geersing GJ, Harjola VP, et al. ESC guidelines for the diagnosis and management of acute pulmonary embolism developed in collaboration with the European Respiratory Society (ERS). Eur Heart J. 2020;41(4):543–603.
4. Kahn SR, de Wit K. Pulmonary embolism. N Engl J Med. 2022;387(1):45–57.
5. Jaff MR, McMurtry MS, Archer SL, Cushman M, Goldenberg N, Goldhaber SZ, et al. Management of massive and submassive pulmonary embolism, iliofemoral deep vein thrombosis, and chronic thromboembolic pulmonary hypertension: a scientific statement from the American Heart Association. Circulation. 2011;123(16):1788–830.
6. Stevens SM, Woller SC, Kreuziger LB, Bounameaux H, Doerschug K, Geersing GJ, et al. Antithrombotic therapy for VTE disease: second update of the CHEST guideline and expert panel report. Chest. 2021;160(6):e545–608.

Chapter 74
Approach to Respiratory Failure in the ICU

74.1 Introduction

Respiratory failure is a critical and life-threatening condition frequently encountered in the intensive care unit (ICU). It is characterized by the respiratory system's inability to maintain adequate gas exchange, leading to hypoxemia (low arterial oxygen), hypercapnia (elevated arterial carbon dioxide), or a combination of both. Patients may present with tachypnea, dyspnea, altered mental status, or overt signs of respiratory distress. Rapid identification of the underlying cause and prompt initiation of targeted interventions are essential to improve outcomes [1, 2].

Advancements in bedside diagnostic tools, particularly lung ultrasound (LUS), have revolutionized the assessment of respiratory failure in critically ill patients. Algorithms integrating LUS, arterial blood gas (ABG) analysis, and other diagnostic modalities, such as the bedside lung ultrasound in emergency (BLUE) protocol, provide a structured approach to differential diagnosis and management [Ref: Algorithm 74.1].

74.2 Algorithmic Approach to Respiratory Failure

74.2.1 Initial Assessment and Bedside Lung Ultrasound (LUS)

A. Role of LUS in Differential Diagnosis

LUS is a rapid, noninvasive tool that can be performed at the bedside to assess lung pathology. It is more accurate than chest X-rays and can significantly reduce diagnostic time.

S. B. Mishra et al., *Mastering ICU Care*,
https://doi.org/10.1007/978-981-95-0179-3_74

- Pleural Sliding and Lung Point Identification
- Presence of Lung Sliding (Seashore Sign on M-mode): Indicates that the visceral and parietal pleura are apposed, effectively ruling out pneumothorax at that site.
- Absence of Lung Sliding (Barcode or Stratosphere Sign on M-mode): Suggests a possible pneumothorax. Identifying the lung point, the exact location where normal lung sliding meets absent sliding, confirms the diagnosis of pneumothorax with high specificity. Prompt intervention with chest tube insertion is typically indicated.
- A-lines and B-lines Pattern Recognition
- A-lines: Horizontal reverberation artifacts indicating normally aerated lung or hyperinflated lung (e.g., COPD, asthma).
- B-lines: Vertical, comet-tail artifacts originating from the pleural line, indicating interstitial syndrome due to various pathologies such as pulmonary edema, pneumonia, or ARDS.
- Advanced Techniques
- PLAPS (Posterolateral Alveolar and/or Pleural Syndrome): Involves scanning posterior lung zones to detect alveolar consolidation or pleural effusion, aiding in diagnosing pneumonia, pleural effusions, or pulmonary edema [3].

B. Monitoring Response to Treatment

LUS can be used to monitor the effectiveness of therapeutic interventions:

- PEEP Titration and Recruitment Maneuvers: LUS can assess changes in aeration patterns, guiding optimal PEEP settings to improve oxygenation.
- Mechanical Ventilation Weaning: Monitoring the resolution of B-lines and consolidation can inform readiness for weaning from mechanical ventilation [4].

74.2.2 Arterial Blood Gas (ABG) Analysis and Interpretation

ABG analysis provides critical information about oxygenation, ventilation, and acid-base status.

A. Evaluation of the Alveolar-arterial (A-a) Gradient

- Calculating the A-a Gradient: The A-a gradient helps identify the cause of hypoxemia. An increased A-a gradient indicates problems with gas exchange due to V/Q mismatch, shunt, or diffusion impairment.
- Example Calculation:
- $PAO_2 = FiO_2 \times (Patm - PH_2O) — (PaCO_2 / R)$
  where FiO_2 is the fraction of inspired oxygen, Patm is atmospheric pressure, PH_2O is water vapor pressure, $PaCO_2$ is arterial CO_2, and R is the respiratory quotient (~0.8).
- Normal A-a Gradient: Increases with age; approximate normal value is (Age/4) + 4.

B. Causes of Increased A-a Gradient

- V/Q Mismatch: Conditions like pulmonary embolism, pneumonia, or COPD exacerbation.
- Diffusion Impairment: Interstitial lung diseases, pulmonary fibrosis.

C. Hypercapnia (Elevated $PaCO_2$)

- Indicates hypoventilation due to central, neuromuscular, or mechanical causes [5].

74.2.3 *Differential Diagnosis Based on LUS and ABG Findings*

A. Hypoxemic Respiratory Failure (Type I)

- Characterized by $PaO_2 < 60$ mmHg with normal or low $PaCO_2$.

Normal LUS finding:

- Pulmonary embolism

Diffuse B-line Pattern on LUS:

- Pulmonary Edema:
- Cardiogenic: Left ventricular dysfunction; confirm with echocardiography showing reduced ejection fraction.
- Non-cardiogenic (ARDS): Increased permeability pulmonary edema.

Berlin Definition of ARDS:

- Timing: Within one week of a known clinical insult.
- Chest Imaging: Bilateral opacities not fully explained by effusions, lobar/lung collapse, or nodules.
- Origin of Edema: Respiratory failure not fully explained by cardiac failure or fluid overload.
- Oxygenation: $PaO_2/FiO_2 \leq 300$ mmHg with PEEP ≥ 5 cm H_2O.

Early Identification and Management:

- Low Tidal Volume Ventilation: 6 mL/kg predicted body weight to prevent ventilator-induced lung injury.
- PEEP Optimization: To prevent alveolar collapse and improve oxygenation.
- ARDS Risk Prediction Tools: Use of scores like APACHE II for risk stratification.
- Interstitial Lung Disease: Chronic conditions presenting with diffuse B-lines and increased A-a gradient.

Focal B-line Pattern on LUS:

Pneumonia:

- LUS Findings: Consolidations with dynamic air bronchograms, shred sign.
- Management: Antibiotic therapy and source control.

Pulmonary Embolism:

- LUS Findings: May show normal lung patterns; consider in unexplained hypoxemia with elevated A-a gradient.
- BLUE Protocol Application: Specific LUS signs can aid in diagnosis [6].

B. Hypercapnic Respiratory Failure (Type II)

- Characterized by $PaCO_2 > 45$ mmHg, indicating hypoventilation.

A-line Pattern on LUS (Normal Lung Findings):
Central Hypoventilation:

- Neurological Causes: Brainstem lesions, drug overdose.

Neuromuscular Disorders:

- Examples: Guillain-Barré syndrome, myasthenia gravis, amyotrophic lateral sclerosis.

Chest Wall Disorders:

- Examples: Severe obesity (Pickwickian syndrome), kyphoscoliosis, diaphragmatic paralysis.

Management:

- Ventilatory Support: Noninvasive ventilation (NIV) or invasive mechanical ventilation.
- Treat Underlying Cause: Address neurological or neuromuscular conditions.

B-line Pattern on LUS:
Obstructive Lung Diseases:
COPD Exacerbation, Asthma:

- Hyperinflated lungs may show A-lines, but B-lines can be present due to associated conditions.
- Management: Bronchodilators, steroids, NIV.

74.2.4 Ventilation Strategies and Therapeutic Escalation

A. Noninvasive Ventilation (NIV) and High-Flow Nasal Cannula (HFNC)

Indications:

- Mild to Moderate Respiratory Failure: When the patient is hemodynamically stable and can protect their airway.
- HFNC: Provides heated, humidified oxygen at high flow rates, improving oxygenation and reducing work of breathing.

B. Invasive Mechanical Ventilation

Indications:

- Failure of NIV or HFNC: Worsening gas exchange, inability to protect airway.
- Severe ARF or ARDS: Requires lung-protective ventilation strategies.

C. Advanced Therapies

Prone Positioning:

- Benefits: Improves ventilation-perfusion matching, reduces mortality in severe ARDS.
- Implementation: At least 16 hours per day in prone position.

Extracorporeal Membrane Oxygenation (ECMO):

- Indications: Refractory hypoxemia despite optimal conventional therapy.
- Considerations: Requires specialized centers and resources [7].

A. Monitoring and Weaning

- Use of LUS in Ventilation Management:
- Semiquantification of Lung Aeration: Guides adjustments in ventilatory settings.
- Weaning Decisions: Resolution of pathological LUS findings can support readiness for weaning.

74.2.5 Comprehensive Diagnostic Tools

A. SpO_2/FiO_2 Ratio

- Utility: Provides an estimate of oxygenation status when ABG is not available, useful in resource-limited settings.
- Interpretation: Lower ratios indicate more severe hypoxemia.

74.3 Pathophysiological Insights and Systemic Considerations

A. Distinguishing Hypoxemic vs. Hypercapnic Respiratory Failure

- Hypoxemic (Type I): Due to V/Q mismatch, shunt, diffusion impairment.
- Hypercapnic (Type II): Due to alveolar hypoventilation.

B. Impact of Systemic Inflammatory Processes

- Sepsis-Induced ARF:
- Mechanisms: Increased capillary permeability, alveolar flooding.
- Management: Treat underlying infection, supportive care.

74.4 Evidence-Based Outcomes

- Effectiveness of LUS:
- Improved Diagnostic Accuracy: Superior to chest X-rays in detecting pneumothorax, pleural effusion, consolidation.
- Reduced Mortality in ARDS: Early intervention guided by LUS and adherence to lung-protective strategies reduces mortality.

74.5 Algorithm Refinements and BLUE Protocol Integration

A. BLUE Protocol Application

- Structured Approach: Uses LUS findings to rapidly diagnose acute respiratory failure etiologies.
- Diagnostic Markers: Combines pleural sliding, A/B-lines, lung point, PLAPS for accurate diagnosis.

B. Semiquantification of Lung Aeration

- Scoring Systems: Quantifies B-lines and consolidations to guide therapy.
- Ventilatory Adjustments: Helps in optimizing PEEP and tidal volumes.

74.6 Therapeutic Escalation Framework

- Stepwise Approach:
- Initial Oxygen Supplementation: Nasal cannula, face mask.
- Escalation to HFNC or NIV: Based on patient response and severity.
- Invasive Mechanical Ventilation: If noninvasive methods fail or are contraindicated.
- Advanced Support (ECMO): For refractory cases.

74.7 Conclusion

Managing respiratory failure in the ICU requires a systematic and evidence-based approach. Bedside lung ultrasound has become an indispensable tool, offering rapid, accurate diagnostics that guide targeted interventions. Integrating detailed ABG interpretation, understanding pathophysiological mechanisms, and applying structured protocols like the BLUE protocol enhance diagnostic precision. Early identification and management of conditions like ARDS, strategies such as low tidal volume ventilation and prone positioning have been shown to reduce mortality. A comprehensive understanding of ventilation approaches, from noninvasive methods to advanced support like ECMO, allows for appropriate therapeutic escalation based on patient needs. By incorporating these advanced techniques and evidence-based practices into a cohesive algorithm, clinicians can improve outcomes for patients experiencing respiratory failure in the ICU.

Algorithm 74.1: Approach to respiratory failure in the ICU

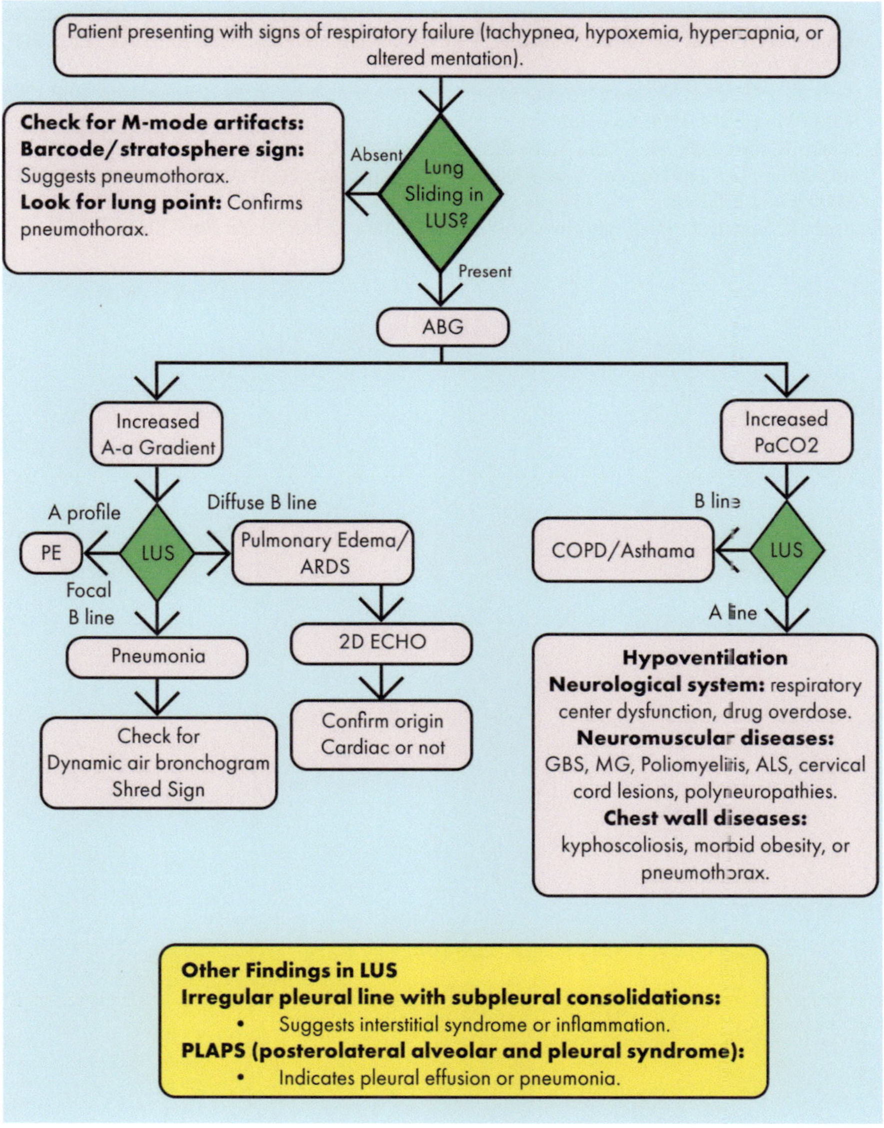

Bibliography

1. Mojoli F, Bouhemad B, Mongodi S, Lichtenstein D. Lung ultrasound for critically ill patients. Am J Respir Crit Care Med. 2019;199(6):701–14.
2. Islam M, Levitus M, Eisen L, Shiloh AL, Fein D. Lung ultrasound for the diagnosis and Management of Acute Respiratory Failure. Lung. 2020;198(1):1–11.
3. Lichtenstein DA, Meziere GA. Relevance of lung ultrasound in the diagnosis of acute respiratory failure: the BLUE protocol. Chest. 2008;134(1):117–25.
4. Zapata L, Blancas R, Conejo-Marquez I, Garcia-de-Acilu M. Role of ultrasound in acute respiratory failure and in the weaning of mechanical ventilation. Med Intensiva (Engl Ed). 2023;47(9):529–42.
5. Janz DR, Ware LB. Approach to the patient with the acute respiratory distress syndrome. Clin Chest Med. 2014;35(4):685–96.
6. Linko R, Okkonen M, Pettila V, Perttila J, Parviainen I, Ruokonen E, et al. Acute respiratory failure in intensive care units. FINNALI: a prospective cohort study. Intensive Care Med. 2009;35(8):1352–61.
7. Scala R, Heunks L. Highlights in acute respiratory failure. Eur Respir Rev. 2018:27(147).

Chapter 75
Approach to Acute Exacerbation of Chronic Obstructive Pulmonary Disease in the ICU

75.1 Introduction

Acute exacerbation of chronic obstructive pulmonary disease (AECOPD) is a critical and potentially life-threatening event characterized by a sudden worsening of respiratory symptoms beyond normal day-to-day variations. According to the Global Initiative for Chronic Obstructive Lung Disease (GOLD) 2024 guidelines, AECOPD is defined by acute symptoms such as dyspnea, cough, and sputum production that worsen in <14 days and necessitate a change in regular medication. A key feature emphasized in the updated guidelines is dynamic hyperinflation, resulting from airflow limitation and air trapping, which significantly contributes to increased dyspnea and the work of breathing during exacerbations. Common triggers include respiratory infections (viral or bacterial) and environmental factors like air pollution and exposure to toxic gases [1–3] [Ref: Algorithm 75.1].

Risk stratification is a cornerstone of effective management and prognosis in patients with acute exacerbations of chronic obstructive pulmonary disease (AECOPD). It helps identify the severity of the disease, determine the likelihood of future exacerbations, and tailor the intensity of interventions required. The process begins with a detailed evaluation of the patient's exacerbation history. This includes analyzing the frequency of past exacerbations—mild, moderate, or severe—and their impact on the patient's overall health. Severe exacerbations requiring hospitalization or intensive care admission carry a higher risk of morbidity and mortality, making this historical information critical for guiding care.

To systematically quantify symptom burden and functional impairment, validated tools such as the Modified Medical Research Council (mMRC) Dyspnea Scale and the COPD Assessment Test (CAT) are widely used. The mMRC Dyspnea Scale focuses on the degree of breathlessness experienced by the patient during daily activities, ranging from mild breathlessness with strenuous exercise (Grade 0) to dyspnea preventing the patient from leaving the house or occurring even at rest

S. B. Mishra et al., *Mastering ICU Care*,
https://doi.org/10.1007/978-981-95-0179-3_75

(Grade 4). The CAT, on the other hand, is a broader measure, assessing the impact of COPD on the patient's overall health, including symptoms like cough, sputum production, chest tightness, activity limitations, and sleep disturbances, with scores ranging from minimal (≤ 10) to very severe impact (≥ 30).

These tools offer a snapshot of the current disease state and help predict the disease's trajectory. For instance, patients with higher mMRC or CAT scores often exhibit more severe symptoms, more significant functional limitations, and a higher risk of exacerbations. Integrating these scores into the stratification process allows clinicians to classify patients into low-risk or high-risk categories, directly influencing management decisions. For example, high-risk patients—those with frequent exacerbations (two or more per year) or a history of hospitalization—may benefit from more aggressive therapies, including inhaled corticosteroids (ICS) or dual bronchodilator therapy with long-acting beta-agonists (LABAs) and long-acting muscarinic antagonists (LAMAs), alongside closer monitoring and early intervention for future exacerbations.

75.2 Initial Presentation and Assessment

- Clinical Evaluation: Patients may present with increased dyspnea, cough, sputum volume or purulence, wheezing, chest tightness, and fatigue. Assess for signs of respiratory distress, including tachypnea, use of accessory muscles, and cyanosis.
- Risk Stratification: Utilize the patient's exacerbation history, mMRC Dyspnea Scale, and CAT score to assess the severity of the current exacerbation and the risk of future events.
- Identify Triggers: Determine potential precipitating factors such as infections or environmental exposures.

75.3 Diagnostic Workup

- Laboratory Tests:
- Complete Blood Count (CBC): Evaluate for leukocytosis indicating infection or anemia contributing to dyspnea.
- Blood Eosinophil Count: Helps determine the likelihood of response to inhaled corticosteroids (ICS) therapy during exacerbations.
- Arterial Blood Gas (ABG):
- Assess oxygenation (PaO_2), carbon dioxide retention ($PaCO_2$), and acid-base status (pH). It is essential for detecting hypercapnic respiratory failure.
- Imaging Studies:
- Chest X-ray: Rule out alternative diagnoses such as pneumonia, pneumothorax, or pulmonary edema.

- Advanced Imaging: Consider chest CT scans for suspected complications or alternative diagnoses. Incidental lung findings can aid in COPD screening.
- Spirometry (Post-Stabilization):
- Essential for confirming COPD diagnosis and assessing the degree of airflow obstruction once the patient is stable.
- Microbiological Tests:
- Sputum Culture: Particularly in cases with frequent exacerbations or suspected antibiotic resistance.

75.4 Confirming AECOPD Diagnosis

- Based on the clinical presentation and diagnostic findings, confirm if the symptoms are consistent with AECOPD.
- Differential Diagnosis: Exclude other potential causes such as heart failure exacerbation, pulmonary embolism, or pneumonia.

75.5 Management

75.5.1 Oxygen Therapy

- Supplemental Oxygen:
- Administer oxygen to maintain target SpO_2 between 88% and 92% to prevent hypoxemia while minimizing the risk of CO_2 retention due to hypoventilation.
- Monitoring:
- Closely monitor for signs of hypercapnia (e.g., altered mental status) and adjust oxygen therapy accordingly.

75.5.2 Assessing Acid-Base Status and Respiratory Failure

- ABG Interpretation:
- A pH < 7.35 with elevated $PaCO_2$ indicates respiratory acidosis.
- Determine the severity of hypercapnic respiratory failure to guide ventilation strategies.

75.5.3 Non-Invasive Ventilation (NIV)

- Early Initiation:

NIV should be started when at least one of the following applies:

- Respiratory acidosis (pH $\leq$ 7.35 and $PaCO_2 \geq$ 45 mmHg)
- Severe dyspnea
- Persistent hypoxemia despite supplemental oxygen therapy

- Benefits:
- NIV improves gas exchange, reduces work of breathing, decreases intubation rates, and has been shown to improve survival.
- Predictors of Success:
- pH > 7.25, alert mental status, and hemodynamic stability are associated with better NIV outcomes.
- Once patient improves and tolerates 4 h of unassisted breathing, NIV can be discontinued directly
- Contraindications:
- Include hemodynamic instability, inability to protect the airway, severe agitation, or facial abnormalities preventing mask fitting.
- Management:
- Use a full-face mask for better tolerance.
- Monitor for improvement in respiratory rate, work of breathing, and ABG parameters.

75.5.4 Escalation to Invasive Mechanical Ventilation

- Indications:
- Failure of NIV (worsening acidosis, hypoxemia, or mental status), respiratory or cardiac arrest, or severe hemodynamic instability.
- Ventilation Strategies:
- Mode: Volume-control or pressure-control ventilation.
- Tidal Volume (V_t): 6–8 mL/kg of ideal body weight to minimize the risk of volutrauma.
- Respiratory Rate: Set to allow sufficient expiratory time, typically 8–12 breaths per minute.
- Inspiratory to Expiratory Ratio (I: E Ratio): Prolong expiratory time (e.g., 1:3 or longer) to reduce air trapping.
- Positive End-Expiratory Pressure (PEEP):
- Apply external PEEP cautiously (usually 80% of intrinsic PEEP) to reduce the work of breathing and assist in alveolar emptying.
- FiO_2: Adjust to maintain SpO_2 at 88–92%.
- Plateau Pressure: Keep $\leq$30 cm H_2O to prevent barotrauma.

75.5.5 Managing Auto-PEEP and Dynamic Hyperinflation

- Auto-PEEP Identification:
- Recognize signs such as difficulty triggering breaths, hyperinflated lungs, and hemodynamic compromise.
- Adjustments to Ventilator Settings:
- Tidal Volume: Reduce to lower inspiratory volumes.
- Respiratory Rate: Decrease to extend expiratory time.
- Expiratory Time: Lengthen to allow complete exhalation and reduce air trapping.
- Flow Rates: Increase inspiratory flow rates to shorten inspiratory time.
- Heart-Lung Interactions:
- Be aware that dynamic hyperinflation can impair venous return and reduce cardiac output. Monitor hemodynamics closely.

75.5.6 Pharmacological Management

- Bronchodilators:
- Short-Acting Beta-Agonists (SABA): Administer nebulized albuterol for rapid bronchodilation.
- Short-Acting Anticholinergics: Ipratropium bromide may be added for additional bronchodilatory effect.
- Systemic Corticosteroids:
- Administer prednisone 40 mg daily for 5 days to reduce airway inflammation.
- Long-Term Use: Long-term oral corticosteroids are discouraged due to significant side effects unless necessary.
- Inhaled Corticosteroids (ICS):
- Consider adding ICS in patients with elevated blood eosinophil counts or frequent exacerbations despite optimal bronchodilator therapy.
- Be cautious of potential side effects like pneumonia risk.
- Combination Therapy:
- Long-acting beta-agonist (LABA)/Long-Acting Muscarinic Antagonist (LAMA): Preferred maintenance therapy for reducing exacerbations and improving lung function.
- Adjust maintenance medications accordingly during hospitalization and ensure continuity post-discharge.
- Antibiotics:
- Indicated if there is increased sputum purulence, volume, or signs of bacterial infection. Duration of antibiotic therapy is 5–7 days.
- Choose antibiotics based on local resistance patterns and patient history.

75.5.7 Supportive Care and Monitoring

- Fluid Management:
- Avoid fluid overload; monitor for signs of right heart failure.
- Nutrition:
- Assess nutritional status; provide interventions for malnourished patients to improve outcomes.
- Thromboembolism Prophylaxis
- Monitoring:
- Regularly reassess respiratory status, ABGs, and hemodynamics.
- Monitor for complications such as infections, thromboembolic events, or arrhythmias.

75.5.8 Prevention Strategies

- Vaccinations:
- Ensure vaccination against influenza, pneumococcal infections, and respiratory syncytial virus (RSV) as appropriate.
- Smoking Cessation:
- Provide counseling and support for smoking cessation, as it is the most effective intervention for slowing disease progression.
- Environmental Modifications:
- Advise on reducing exposure to pollutants and occupational irritants.

75.5.9 Pulmonary Rehabilitation

- Post-Exacerbation:
- Early initiation of pulmonary rehabilitation programs post-discharge can reduce readmissions, improve exercise capacity, and enhance quality of life.
- Components:
- Includes exercise training, education, nutritional advice, and psychosocial support.

75.5.10 *Monitoring and Discharge Planning*

- Discharge Criteria:
- Clinical stability with improved symptoms, stable ABGs, and the ability to use inhaled medications.
- Follow-Up Recommendations:
- Arrange follow-up appointments within 4 weeks post-discharge.
- Assess adherence to therapy, inhaler technique, and symptom control.
- Medication Adjustments:
- Optimize long-term maintenance therapy, including LABA/LAMA combinations.
- Reassess the need for ICS and adjust accordingly.
- Telehealth Services:
- Utilize telehealth for remote monitoring, education, and support to enhance adherence and early detection of exacerbations.
- Education:
- Provide comprehensive education on disease management, recognizing early signs of exacerbation, and when to seek medical attention.

75.6 Conclusion

The management of acute exacerbation of COPD in the ICU requires a multifaceted approach that includes prompt recognition, thorough assessment, and the implementation of evidence-based interventions. Early initiation of noninvasive ventilation can significantly improve outcomes in hypercapnic respiratory failure. Individualized mechanical ventilation strategies are essential for patients requiring intubation, with careful adjustments to prevent dynamic hyperinflation and minimize the impact on cardiac function.

Pharmacological management should be updated to reflect current guidelines, emphasizing the use of combination bronchodilator therapy and cautious use of corticosteroids. Preventive measures, including vaccinations and smoking cessation, are crucial for reducing the frequency of exacerbations and improving long-term outcomes. Incorporating nutritional support and pulmonary rehabilitation can enhance recovery and quality of life.

Effective discharge planning, including patient education and follow-up care, is vital to prevent readmissions and ensure sustained management of COPD. Emerging tools like telehealth can augment traditional care models, providing additional support to patients in managing their condition.

Algorithm 75.1: Approach to acute exacerbation of chronic obstructive pulmonary disease (AECOPD) in the ICU

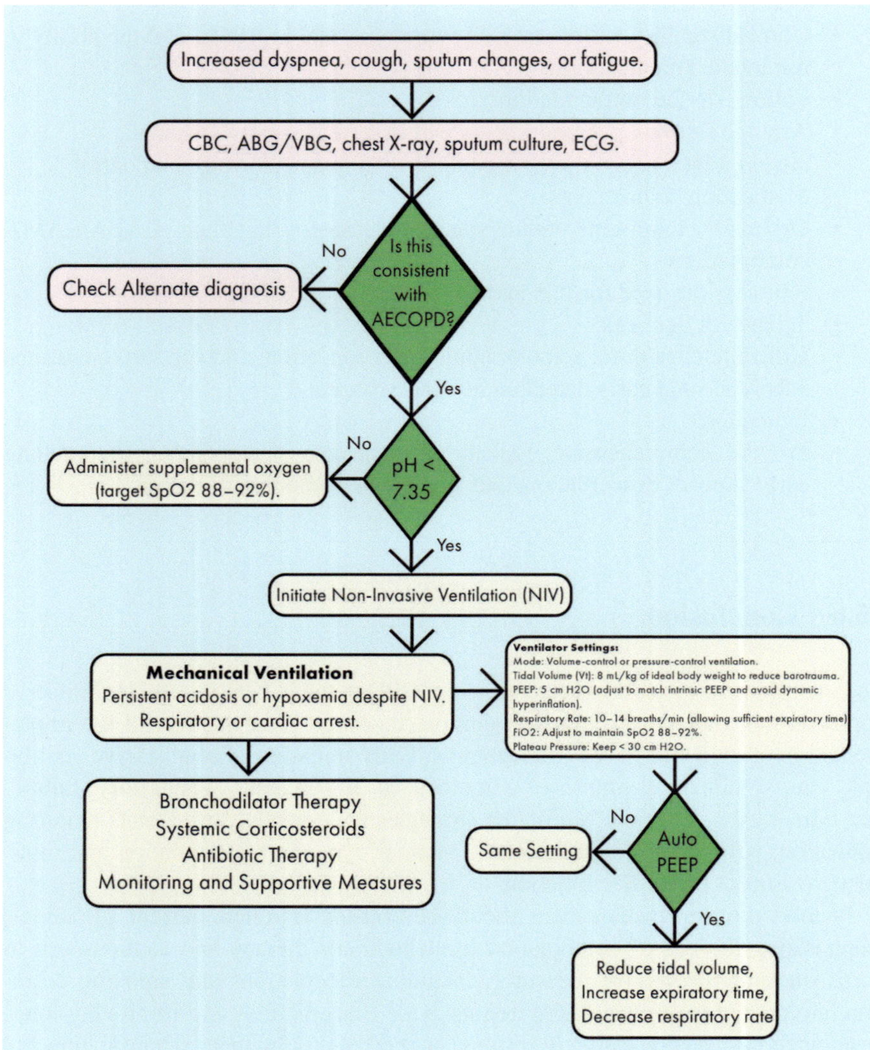

Bibliography

1. Global Initiative for Chronic Obstructive Lung Disease (GOLD). Global Strategy for the Diagnosis, Management, and Prevention of Chronic Obstructive Pulmonary Disease. 2024 Report. GOLD; 2023.
2. Demoule A, Brochard L, Dres M, Heunks L, Jubran A, Laghi F, et al. How to ventilate obstructive and asthmatic patients. Intensive Care Med. 2020;46(12):2436–49.
3. Nici L, Mammen MJ, Charbek E, Alexander PE, Au DH, Boyd CM, et al. Pharmacologic Management of Chronic Obstructive Pulmonary Disease. An official American Thoracic Society clinical practice guideline. Am J Respir Crit Care Med. 2020;201(9):e56–69.

Chapter 76
Approach to Acute Exacerbation of Asthma in the ICU

76.1 Introduction

Acute exacerbations of asthma are life-threatening emergencies that necessitate prompt recognition and aggressive management in the intensive care unit (ICU). Patients often present with severe respiratory distress and are at significant risk of respiratory failure.

Acute severe asthma exacerbation can present with status asthmaticus (SA) and near-fatal asthma (NFA). SA is defined as exacerbation of asthma that doesn't respond readily to initial intensive bronchodilator therapy (15–30 minutes). NFA presents with acute respiratory failure (hypoxemia and/or hypercarbia, metabolic or respiratory acidosis), apnea, paradoxical breathing, and impaired level of consciousness. The primary objectives in managing these patients are to reverse airway obstruction, correct hypoxemia, address underlying inflammation, and prevent complications such as barotrauma and prolonged mechanical ventilation [1, 2] [Ref: Algorithm 76.1].

76.2 Initial Assessment

76.2.1 Evaluate for Signs of Respiratory Distress

- Clinical Signs:
- Inability to Speak: Difficulty speaking complete sentences due to breathlessness.
- Use of Accessory Muscles such as sternocleidomastoid, scalene, abdominal muscles

S. B. Mishra et al., *Mastering ICU Care*,
https://doi.org/10.1007/978-981-95-0179-3_76

- Paradoxical Breathing: Abnormal chest and abdominal movements during respiration.
- Severe Wheezing or Silent Chest: Diminished or absent breath sounds indicating minimal airflow.
- Altered Mental Status: Confusion or drowsiness suggesting hypoxia or hypercapnia.

76.2.2 Vital Signs and Monitoring

- Continuous Monitoring:
- Oxygen saturation (SpO_2).
- Heart rate and rhythm.
- Respiratory rate and pattern.
- Blood pressure.
- Peak Expiratory Flow Rate (PEFR):
- Obtain baseline PEFR to quantify airway obstruction severity.
- Useful for assessing response to therapy.

76.3 Diagnostic Workup

76.3.1 Laboratory Tests

- Complete Blood Count (CBC):
- Evaluate for infection (elevated WBC) or anemia.
- Arterial Blood Gas (ABG) or Venous Blood Gas (VBG):
- Assess acid-base status, oxygenation (PaO_2), and ventilation ($PaCO_2$).
- Serum Electrolytes:
- Potassium and Magnesium Levels:
- Monitor for hypokalemia and hypomagnesemia due to β_2-agonist therapy.
- Sputum Culture:
- If a bacterial infection is suspected.
- Electrocardiogram (ECG):
- Detect arrhythmias, ischemia, or effects of hypoxia and electrolyte imbalances.

76.3.2 Imaging Studies

- Chest Radiograph (X-ray):
- Rule out pneumothorax, pneumonia, atelectasis, or other complications.
- Especially important if chest pain, unilateral breath sounds, or fever is present.

76.3.3 *Pulmonary Function Testing*

- Peak Expiratory Flow Rate (PEFR):
- Provides rapid, objective measurement of airway obstruction.
- Essential for initial assessment and ongoing monitoring.

76.3.4 *Additional Investigations*

- D-dimer, echocardiography, and CT scan as appropriate.

76.4 Differential Diagnosis

- Consider Alternative Diagnoses:
- Pneumothorax: Sudden chest pain, absent breath sounds on one side.
- Pulmonary Embolism: Sudden dyspnea, chest pain, hypoxia.
- Heart Failure: Edema, jugular venous distention, crackles on auscultation.
- Anaphylaxis: Hives, hypotension, airway swelling.
- Upper Airway Obstruction: Stridor, hoarseness.

76.5 Management of Acute Asthma Exacerbation

76.5.1 *Oxygen Therapy*

- Goal SpO_2:
- Maintain ≥ (94–98% BTS 2017)(≥ 95% in pregnant women and cardiovascular patients).
- Delivery Methods:
- Nasal cannula, face mask, or high-flow oxygen devices.
- Avoid Hyperoxia:
- Prevent worsening ventilation-perfusion mismatch.

76.5.2 *Pharmacological Management*

76.5.2.1 Short-Acting β_2-Agonists (SABA)

- Continuous Nebulization:

- Salbutamol (Albuterol):
- Concentration: 5 mg/mL solution.
- Dose: 10–15 mg/hour via continuous nebulization.
- Terbutaline:
- Dose: 2.5 mg/hour via continuous nebulization.
- Intermittent Nebulization:
- Salbutamol: 2.5–5 mg every 20 minutes for three doses, then 2.5–10 mg every 1–4 hours as needed.
- Monitoring:
- Watch for tachycardia, tremors, hypokalemia, and arrhythmias.

76.5.2.2 Anticholinergics

- Ipratropium Bromide:
- Dose: 0.5 mg every 6 hours via nebulization.
- Benefits:
- Enhances bronchodilation when combined with β_2-agonists.
- May improve outcomes in severe exacerbations.

76.5.2.3 Systemic Corticosteroids

- Administration:
- Methylprednisolone:
- Dose: 1–2 mg/kg/day IV, divided every 6–8 hours.
- Transition to Oral Therapy:
- Prednisone:
- Dose: 40–60 mg/day for prolonged therapy.
- Rationale:
- Reduces airway inflammation and mucus production.
- Potentiates β_2-agonist effects.
- Early initiation is crucial.

76.5.2.4 Magnesium Sulfate

- Indication:
- Severe exacerbations resistant to initial bronchodilator therapy.
- Administration:
- Dose: 2 g IV infusion over 20–30 minutes.
- Mechanism:
- Relaxes airway smooth muscle.

76.5.2.5 Subcutaneous β_2-Agonists

- Terbutaline:
- Dose: 0.25 mg subcutaneously every 20 minutes for up to three doses.
- Indication:
- Rescue therapy when inhaled medications are ineffective or impractical.

76.5.3 Ventilatory Support

76.5.3.1 Non-Invasive Ventilation (NIV)

- Indications:
- Moderate to severe exacerbations not responding to medical therapy.
- Signs of increasing work of breathing or hypercapnia.
- BiPAP Settings:
- Inspiratory Positive Airway Pressure (IPAP): 10–15 cm H_2O.
- Expiratory Positive Airway Pressure (EPAP): 4–5 cm H_2O.
- Monitoring:
- Respiratory rate, SpO_2, ABGs, and mental status.
- Contraindications:
- Altered mental status, inability to protect the airway, hemodynamic instability.

76.5.3.2 MechanicalVentilation

- Indications:
- Severe respiratory acidosis (pH < 7.25).
- Altered consciousness.
- Respiratory arrest or exhaustion.
- Failure or contraindication of NIV.
- Airway Management:
- Endotracheal Tube Size: ≥ 8.0 mm for reduced resistance and easier suctioning.
- Ventilator Settings:
- Low Tidal Volumes: 6–8 mL/kg predicted body weight.
- Permissive Hypercapnia:
- Allow elevated $PaCO_2$ to maintain pH > 7.2.
- Reduces risk of barotrauma.
- Prolonged Expiratory Time:
- I:E ratio of 1:3 to 1:4 to minimize air trapping.
- Plateau Pressures:
- Keep <30 cm H_2O to prevent lung injury.
- Sedation and Paralysis:

- May be necessary to synchronize the patient with the ventilator.
- Use cautiously and monitor for side effects.
- Monitoring:
- Frequent ABGs, ventilator parameters, and lung mechanics [3].

76.5.4 Adjunct Therapies

76.5.4.1 Ketamine

- Indications:
- Refractory cases not responding to standard treatments
- Administration:
- Bolus: 1–2 mg/kg IV
- Infusion: 0.5–1 mg/kg/hour
- Benefits:
- Bronchodilation, sedation, analgesia
- Minimal respiratory depression

76.5.4.2 Volatile Anesthetics

- Agents:
- Isoflurane, sevoflurane.
- Indications:
- Life-threatening bronchoconstriction unresponsive to conventional therapy.
- Considerations:
- Requires specialized equipment.
- Monitor for hypotension and arrhythmias.

76.5.4.3 Heliox Therapy

- Composition:
- Helium-oxygen mixtures (70:30 or 80:20).
- Mechanism:
- Lower density reduces airway resistance and breathing work.
- Indications:
- Severe airflow obstruction.
- Limitations:
- Limited oxygen content; not for significant hypoxemia.

76.5.5 Evaluate Blood Gas (pH) and Monitor Progress

76.5.5.1 Non-Severe Acidosis (pH ≥ 7.25)

- Management:
- Continue aggressive medical therapy.
- Consider or continue NIV.
- Monitoring:
- Close observation for signs of deterioration.

76.5.5.2 Severe Acidosis (pH 7.25)

- Management:
- Proceed to mechanical ventilation.
- Rationale:
- Indicates respiratory failure requiring advanced support.

76.5.6 Prevention and Post-Discharge Planning

76.5.6.1 Personalised Asthma Action Plans

- Components:
- Daily management instructions.
- Symptom monitoring guidelines.
- Step-by-step actions for exacerbations.
- Emergency contact information.

76.5.6.2 Patient and Family Education

- Topics:
- Proper inhaler and spacer technique.
- Medication adherence is important.
- Trigger identification and avoidance.
- Recognition of early exacerbation signs.

76.5.6.3 Maintenance Therapy

- Inhaled corticosteroids.
- Long-acting β_2-agonists.

- Leukotriene modifiers.
- Adherence:
- Emphasize consistent use to prevent exacerbations.

76.5.6.4 Follow-Up Care

- Appointments:
- Schedule regular visits with healthcare providers.
- Assessment:
- Monitor asthma control.
- Adjust treatment plans as needed.
- Referrals:
- Consider pulmonology or allergy specialists for uncontrolled asthma [4].

76.6 Conclusion

Managing acute asthma exacerbations in the ICU demands a comprehensive and systematic approach. Early recognition and prompt initiation of aggressive bronchodilator therapy, oxygen supplementation, and anti-inflammatory treatment are vital. Careful monitoring and appropriate ventilatory support are essential to prevent respiratory failure and minimize complications like barotrauma. Adjunct therapies such as ketamine, volatile anesthetics, and heliox may be beneficial in refractory cases. Post-discharge planning, including personalized asthma action plans and patient education, is crucial to reduce future exacerbations and hospital readmissions. A multidisciplinary team approach enhances patient outcomes and promotes long-term asthma control.

Algorithm 76.1: Approach to acute exacerbation of asthma in the ICU

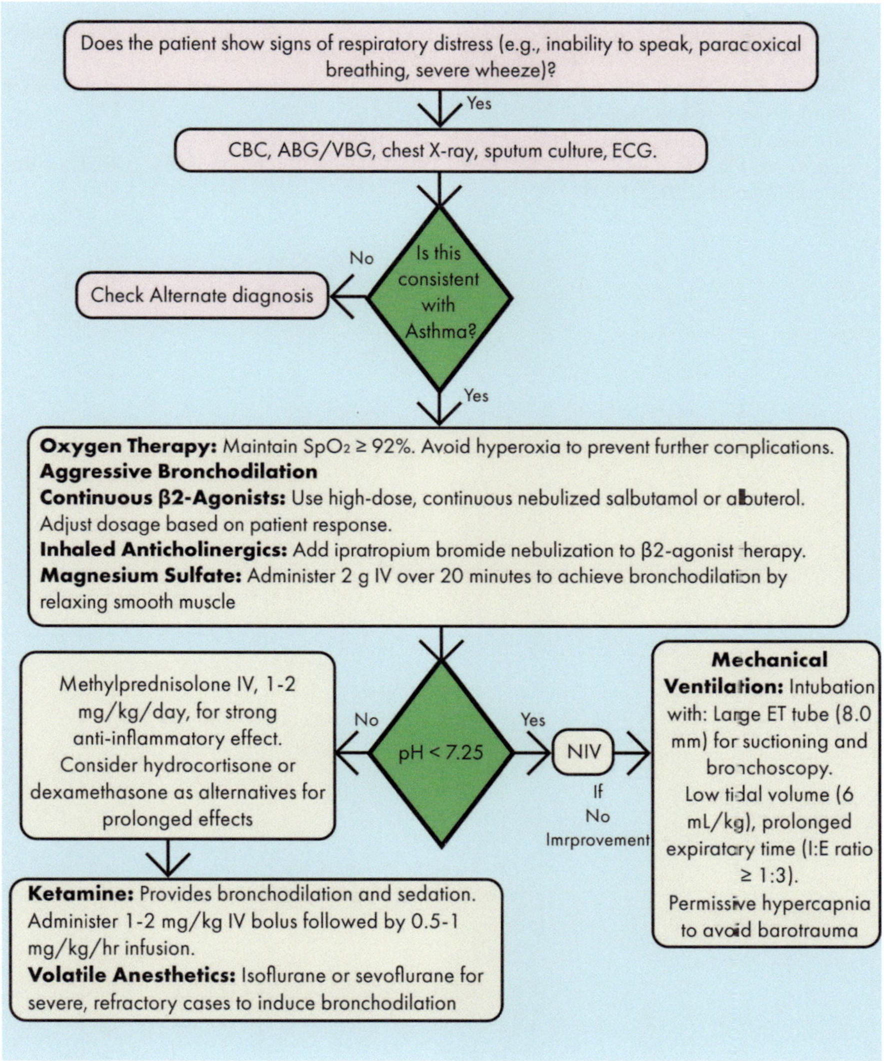

Bibliography

1. Louie S, Morrissey BM, Kenyon NJ, Albertson TE, Avdalovic M. The critically ill asthmatic--from ICU to discharge. Clin Rev Allergy Immunol. 2012;43(1–2):30–44.
2. Talbot T, Roe T, Dushianthan A. Management of acute life-threatening asthma exacerbations in the intensive care unit. Appl Sci. 2024;14(2)
3. Mosnaim G. Asthma in adults. N Engl J Med. 2023;389(11):1023–31.
4. Schivo M, Phan C, Louie S, Harper RW. Critical asthma syndrome in the ICU. Clin Rev Allergy Immunol. 2013;48:31.

Chapter 77
Approach to Acute Respiratory Distress Syndrome (ARDS) in the ICU

77.1 Introduction

Acute respiratory distress syndrome (ARDS) is a severe, life-threatening condition characterized by acute onset of hypoxemia and bilateral pulmonary infiltrates, not fully explained by cardiac failure or fluid overload. It often complicates critical illnesses such as abdominal trauma and requires prompt recognition and management to reduce morbidity and mortality. This algorithm provides a systematic approach to ARDS management in the intensive care unit (ICU), emphasizing personalized strategies based on ARDS phenotypes, evidence-based interventions, and emerging therapies [1, 2] [Ref: Algorithm 77.1].

77.2 Diagnosis

77.2.1 Diagnosis Based on Berlin Definition of ARDS

ARDS diagnosis is based on the following criteria:

- Acute Onset: Symptoms develop within 7 days of a known clinical insult.
- Bilateral Opacities: Detected on chest imaging (X-ray or CT scan), not fully explained by effusions, lobar/lung collapse, or nodules.
- Respiratory Failure Not Fully Explained by Cardiac Failure or Fluid Overload: Requires objective assessment (e.g., echocardiography) to exclude hydrostatic edema.
- Hypoxemia Severity (based on PaO_2/FiO_2 ratio with PEEP ≥5 cm H_2O):
- Mild: PaO_2/FiO_2 200–300 mmHg.

S. B. Mishra et al., *Mastering ICU Care*,
https://doi.org/10.1007/978-981-95-0179-3_77

- Moderate: PaO_2/FiO_2 100–200 mmHg.
- Severe: PaO_2/FiO_2 < 100 mmHg [3, 4]. Updated global definition: In non-intubated patients, ARDS can also be diagnosed when supported by HFNO at ≥30 L/min or NIV/CPAP with ≥5 cm H_2O of end-expiratory pressure. Modified definition for resource-limited settings: ARDS may be diagnosed if SpO_2/FiO_2 ≤ 315 (when SpO_2 ≤ 97%), without requiring a minimum PEEP or oxygen flow rate.

Additionally, phenotyping ARDS into hyperinflammatory and hypoinflammatory types can guide therapeutic approaches, as different phenotypes may respond variably to treatments like corticosteroids or PEEP adjustments.

77.2.2 Lung Ultrasound (LUS) Diagnosis of ARDS: (LUS ARDS Score)

Combining LUS aeration score and LUS findings specific for ARDS (pleural abnormalities/subpleural consolidation).

LUS aeration score varies from 0 to 3.

Score 0: Presence of A-lines
Score 1: Presence of B-lines less than 50% of the pleura
Score 2: Presence of B-lines more than 50% of the pleura
Score 3: Presence of consolidation

LUS ARDS score is useful for assessing the severity of ARDS at admission for monitoring the response by lung aeration on a daily basis.

77.3 Management

77.3.1 Initial Stabilization with Noninvasive Ventilation (NIV)

Consider NIV or High-Flow Nasal Cannula (HFNC) in patients with mild to moderate ARDS:

- Goal: Improve oxygenation while avoiding intubation.
- Monitoring: Closely observe for signs of NIV failure, such as worsening hypoxemia or increased work of breathing.
- Risks: Delayed intubation can worsen outcomes; therefore, NIV should be used cautiously, especially in early and severe ARDS.

77.3.2 Tidal Volume Adjustment in Mechanical Ventilation

Initiate Lung-Protective Ventilation:

- Low Tidal Volume (LTV): Set at 6 mL/kg of predicted body weight.
- Adjustments for High Chest Wall Elastance or Obesity: May require modification of tidal volumes to ensure adequate ventilation without overdistension.
- Plateau Pressure: Keep ≤30 cm H_2O to minimize barotrauma.
- Driving Pressure Optimization: Aim to reduce driving pressure (plateau pressure minus PEEP) to lower the risk of ventilator-induced lung injury (VILI) [5].

77.3.3 Positive End-Expiratory Pressure (PEEP) Strategy

Individualize PEEP Settings:

- Use of Esophageal Manometry: To estimate transpulmonary pressure and tailor PEEP accordingly.
- Avoid Routine Lung Recruitment Maneuvers: Unless guided by expert opinion or in cases of refractory hypoxemia.
- Balance: Adequate PEEP improves alveolar recruitment, but excessive PEEP can cause hemodynamic instability and overdistension [6].

77.3.4 Neuromuscular Blockade

Consider Early Neuromuscular Blockade in severe ARDS:

- Timing: Early administration (within 48 h) can improve patient-ventilator synchrony.
- Benefits: Reduces VILI by preventing asynchrony and high transpulmonary pressures.
- Duration: Use the minimal effective duration to reduce risks associated with prolonged paralysis [7].

77.3.5 Corticosteroid Therapy

Assess the Use of Corticosteroids:

- Role: Can reduce inflammation and ventilator days in certain ARDS phenotypes.
- Risks: Monitor for secondary infections, hyperglycemia, and other side effects.
- Evidence: Recent studies suggest benefits in early administration but require careful patient selection.

77.3.6 Prone Positioning

Implement Early Prone Positioning in severe ARDS ($PaO_2/FiO_2 < 150$ mmHg):

- Duration: At least 16 h per day.
- Mechanisms:
- Improves ventilation-perfusion matching.
- Promotes more homogeneous distribution of stress and strain.
- Enhances alveolar recruitment.
- Monitoring: Watch for potential complications like pressure sores, dislodgement of tubes, or hemodynamic changes [8].

77.3.7 Refractory Hypoxemia and Consideration of ECMO

Evaluate for Extracorporeal Membrane Oxygenation (ECMO):

- Criteria:
- Severe hypoxemia ($PaO_2/FiO_2 < 80$ mmHg) despite optimal mechanical ventilation and adjunctive therapies.
- Hypercapnia with acidosis (pH <7.20) refractory to conventional management.
- Contraindications: Uncontrolled bleeding, irreversible organ failure, or contraindications to anticoagulation.
- Resource Considerations: ECMO requires specialized equipment and trained personnel; consider transfer to a specialized center if necessary.

77.3.8 Conservative Fluid Management

Implement Strategies to Reduce Pulmonary Edema:

- Maintain a Negative Fluid Balance:
- Use diuretics if hemodynamically stable.
- Restrict fluid intake while ensuring adequate tissue perfusion.
- Monitor Parameters:
- Urine output.
- Hemodynamic status (e.g., via central venous pressure or echocardiography).
- Lactate levels as a marker of perfusion

77.3.9 Adjunctive Measures and Emerging Therapies

Investigate Emerging Therapies:

- Mesenchymal Stem Cells: Potential anti-inflammatory effects; currently under clinical trials.

- Extracorporeal CO_2 Removal: May allow ultra-protective ventilation strategies.
- Immunomodulators: Therapies targeting specific inflammatory pathways.
- Note: These therapies are experimental and not recommended for routine use outside of clinical trials.

77.3.10 Lessons from COVID-19 and ARDS Management

Apply Insights from COVID-19 ARDS:

- Lung-Protective Ventilation: Remains cornerstone therapy.
- High-Flow Nasal Cannula (HFNC): Effective in certain patients to improve oxygenation and reduce the need for intubation.
- Awake Prone Positioning: Can enhance oxygenation in spontaneously breathing patients.
- Adaptation: Tailor interventions based on individual patient response and emerging evidence.

77.3.11 Long-Term Outcomes and Post-ARDS Care

Recognize Post-ARDS Syndrome:

- Pulmonary Fibrosis: Can result in long-term respiratory dysfunction.
- Cognitive Dysfunction: Monitor for delirium and long-term cognitive deficits.
- Quality of Life Issues: Address physical weakness, psychological impact, and social reintegration.
- Follow-Up Care: Implement multidisciplinary rehabilitation programs to support recovery.

77.4 Conclusion

Management of ARDS in the ICU requires a comprehensive and individualized approach. By incorporating ARDS phenotyping, optimizing ventilatory strategies, and utilizing adjunctive therapies judiciously, clinicians can improve patient outcomes. Emerging therapies offer hope but require further research. Lessons learned from the COVID-19 pandemic have enriched our understanding and management of ARDS. Attention to long-term outcomes is crucial for supporting patients beyond the ICU.

Algorithm 77.1: Approach to acute respiratory distress syndrome (ARDS) in the ICU

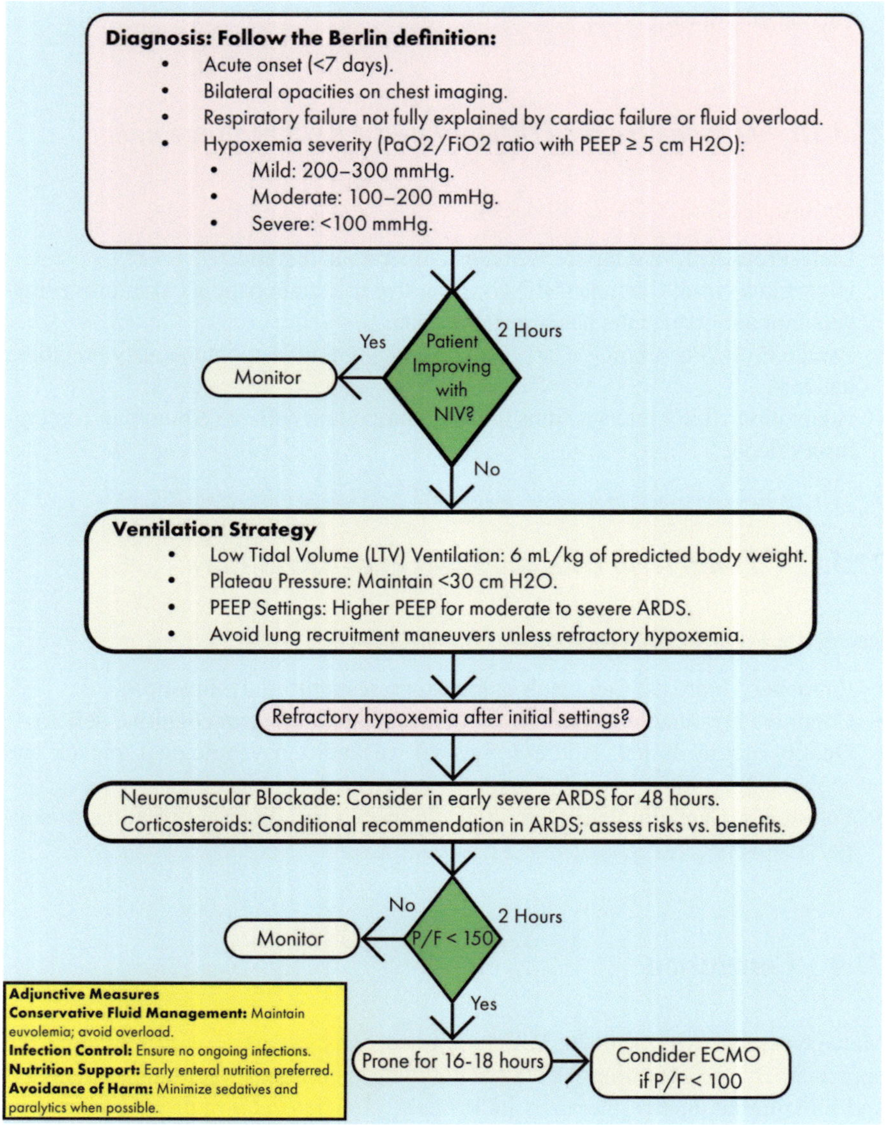

Bibliography

1. Grasselli G, Calfee CS, Camporota L, Poole D, Amato MBP, Antonelli M, et al. ESICM guidelines on acute respiratory distress syndrome: definition, phenotyping and respiratory support strategies. Intensive Care Med. 2023;49(7):727–59.
2. Qadir N, Sahetya S, Munshi L, Summers C, Abrams D, Beitler J, et al. An update on management of adult patients with acute respiratory distress syndrome: an official American Thoracic Society clinical practice guideline. Am J Respir Crit Care Med. 2024;209(1):24–36.
3. Cho YJ, Moon JY, Shin ES, Kim JH, Jung H, Park SY, et al. Clinical practice guideline of acute respiratory distress syndrome. Tuberc Respir Dis (Seoul). 2016;79(4):214–33.
4. Fan E, Del Sorbo L, Goligher EC, Hodgson CL, Munshi L, Walkey AJ, et al. An official American Thoracic Society/European Society of Intensive Care Medicine/Society of Critical Care Medicine clinical practice guideline: mechanical ventilation in adult patients with acute respiratory distress syndrome. Am J Respir Crit Care Med. 2017;195(9):1253–63.
5. Fujishima S. Guideline-based management of acute respiratory failure and acute respiratory distress syndrome. J Intensive Care. 2023;11(1):10.
6. Tasaka S, Ohshimo S, Takeuchi M, Yasuda H, Ichikado K, Tsushima K, et al. ARDS clinical practice guideline 2021. J Intensive Care. 2022;10(1):32.
7. Quigley N, Gagnon S, Fortin M. Aetiology, diagnosis and treatment of moderate-to-severe haemoptysis in a North American academic centre. ERJ Open Res. 2020;6(4):00204-2020.
8. Griffiths MJD, McAuley DF, Perkins GD, Barrett N, Blackwood B, Boyle A, et al. Guidelines on the management of acute respiratory distress syndrome. BMJ Open Respir Res. 2019;6(1):e000420.

Chapter 78
Approach to Setting Tidal Volume in ARDS Patients in the ICU

78.1 Introduction

Acute respiratory distress syndrome (ARDS) is a life-threatening condition marked by severe hypoxemia and decreased lung compliance due to diffuse alveolar damage. Mechanical ventilation is a cornerstone in the management of ARDS; however, inappropriate ventilator settings can exacerbate lung injury, leading to ventilator-induced lung injury (VILI). Over the past decades, ventilation strategies in ARDS have evolved significantly, shifting from high tidal volume (VT) approaches to protective ventilation strategies aimed at minimizing VILI. Landmark studies, such as the ARDSNet trial, have established the use of low VT (6 mL/kg predicted body weight [PBW]) as standard care, significantly reducing mortality and improving patient outcomes [1, 2] [Ref: Algorithm 78.1].

78.2 Understanding Elastic Components and their Influence

The mechanics of the respiratory system are determined by the combined elastance of the lungs and the chest wall. Chest wall elastance (ECW) plays a crucial role in influencing respiratory system compliance (CRS) and, consequently, the interplay between VT and driving pressure (ΔP). In patients with altered ECW—such as those with obesity, abdominal distension, or pleural effusions—the chest wall's reduced compliance can lead to increased ΔP for a given VT. This underscores the importance of assessing ECW, as it affects the distribution of pressures between the lungs and the chest wall, especially under varying positive end-expiratory pressure (PEEP) settings. Recognizing the impact of ECW allows clinicians to adjust ventilator settings more precisely to reduce the risk of overdistension and VILI.

S. B. Mishra et al., *Mastering ICU Care*,
https://doi.org/10.1007/978-981-95-0179-3_78

78.3 Dynamic and Static Driving Pressure Assessment

Driving pressure is a surrogate marker of the stress applied to the lungs during mechanical ventilation. It can be assessed using static measurements, such as plateau pressure minus PEEP, or dynamic measurements, using peak inspiratory pressure minus PEEP. Static ΔP reflects the pressure applied to the alveoli during a pause in airflow and is considered more accurate in assessing alveolar stress. Dynamic ΔP, on the other hand, includes resistive pressures and may overestimate alveolar stress. Both measurements have been correlated with patient outcomes, with higher ΔP associated with increased mortality. Understanding the differences between static and dynamic ΔP is essential for optimizing ventilator settings and tailoring them to individual patient needs.

78.4 Individualized Approaches Beyond Fixed Tidal Volumes

Recent evidence suggests that the universal application of a fixed VT of 6 mL/kg PBW may not be optimal for all ARDS patients. The proportion of aerated lung tissue varies among patients, and VT settings could be individualized based on CRS to reflect the functional size of the lung. Patients with higher compliance may tolerate slightly higher VT without increasing ΔP beyond safe limits, whereas those with low compliance may require further reductions in VT to prevent excessive lung stress. Individualizing VT settings based on the estimated proportion of aerated lung can enhance lung protection and improve outcomes, moving beyond a one-size-fits-all approach.

78.5 Utilizing Imaging and Advanced Monitoring

Advanced imaging techniques and monitoring tools play a pivotal role in tailoring ventilation strategies. Electrical impedance tomography (EIT) and computed tomography (CT) scans provide real-time and detailed assessments of lung ventilation distribution and mechanics. By integrating these tools, clinicians can identify areas of the lung that are overdistended or under-ventilated, allowing for adjustments in VT and PEEP to promote more homogeneous ventilation. Additionally, stress index analysis can help detect tidal recruitment and overdistension during ventilation, further guiding the optimization of ventilator settings.

78.6 Consideration of Ultra-Protective Ventilation

The concept of ultra-protective ventilation, involving VT less than 6 mL/kg PBW, has emerged as a potential strategy to reduce VILI further. This approach is mainly considered in severe ARDS cases where even low VT may result in high ΔP. Ultra-protective ventilation often necessitates adjuncts like extracorporeal carbon dioxide removal ($ECCO_2R$) to manage hypercapnia resulting from reduced minute ventilation. While promising, the feasibility and long-term benefits of ultra-protective ventilation remain subjects of ongoing research and debate, and its application should be individualized based on patient condition and available resources.

78.7 Influence of Injury Patterns and Positional Therapy

The severity and pattern of lung injury significantly influence the VT-ΔP relationship and patient outcomes. Inhomogeneous lung involvement leads to regional differences in compliance and ventilation distribution, as seen in ARDS. Interventions like prone positioning can enhance alveolar recruitment in dorsal lung regions, improving oxygenation and reducing VILI. Prone positioning has been shown to affect the VT-ΔP relationship by promoting more uniform ventilation and decreasing ΔP. Understanding these dynamics is essential for optimizing ventilator settings with positional therapies, ultimately improving gas exchange and patient survival.

78.8 Regional Stress Variability and Limitations of Global Measurements

Global measurements of ΔP and CRS may not accurately reflect regional lung mechanics due to the heterogeneous nature of ARDS. Regions of the lung may experience different levels of stress and strain, leading to localized overdistension or collapse despite acceptable global parameters. This regional variability necessitates more refined metrics and monitoring techniques to detect and mitigate regional lung stress. Advanced imaging and monitoring can help identify these discrepancies, allowing for adjustments that target specific lung regions and further reduce the risk of VILI.

78.9 Historical Evolution and Evidence-Based Practices

The approach to ventilating ARDS patients has evolved considerably over the years. Initially, high VT ventilation was common practice aimed at correcting hypoxemia and hypercapnia. However, this strategy was associated with high mortality rates due to the exacerbation of lung injury. The landmark ARDSNet study in 2000 demonstrated that lower VT ventilation (6 mL/kg PBW) significantly reduced mortality and set a new standard of care. Subsequent research has focused on refining ventilation strategies, emphasizing the importance of ΔP, individualized VT settings, and adjunctive therapies. This evolution reflects a growing understanding of ARDS's complex interplay between mechanical ventilation and lung pathology.

78.10 Conclusion

Optimizing tidal volume in ARDS patients requires a nuanced, physiologically informed approach that considers individual patient characteristics, lung mechanics, and the potential for regional variations in lung stress. Starting with a baseline VT of 6 mL/kg PBW remains a foundational strategy; however, adjustments based on ΔP, ECW, CRS, and advanced monitoring can enhance lung protection. By integrating imaging techniques, considering ultra-protective ventilation when appropriate, and acknowledging the influence of injury patterns and positional therapy, clinicians can tailor ventilation strategies to minimize VILI and improve patient outcomes. The ongoing evolution of evidence-based practices underscores the importance of continuous research and adaptation in the management of ARDS.

Algorithm 78.1: Approach to setting tidal volume (VT) in ARDS patients in the ICU

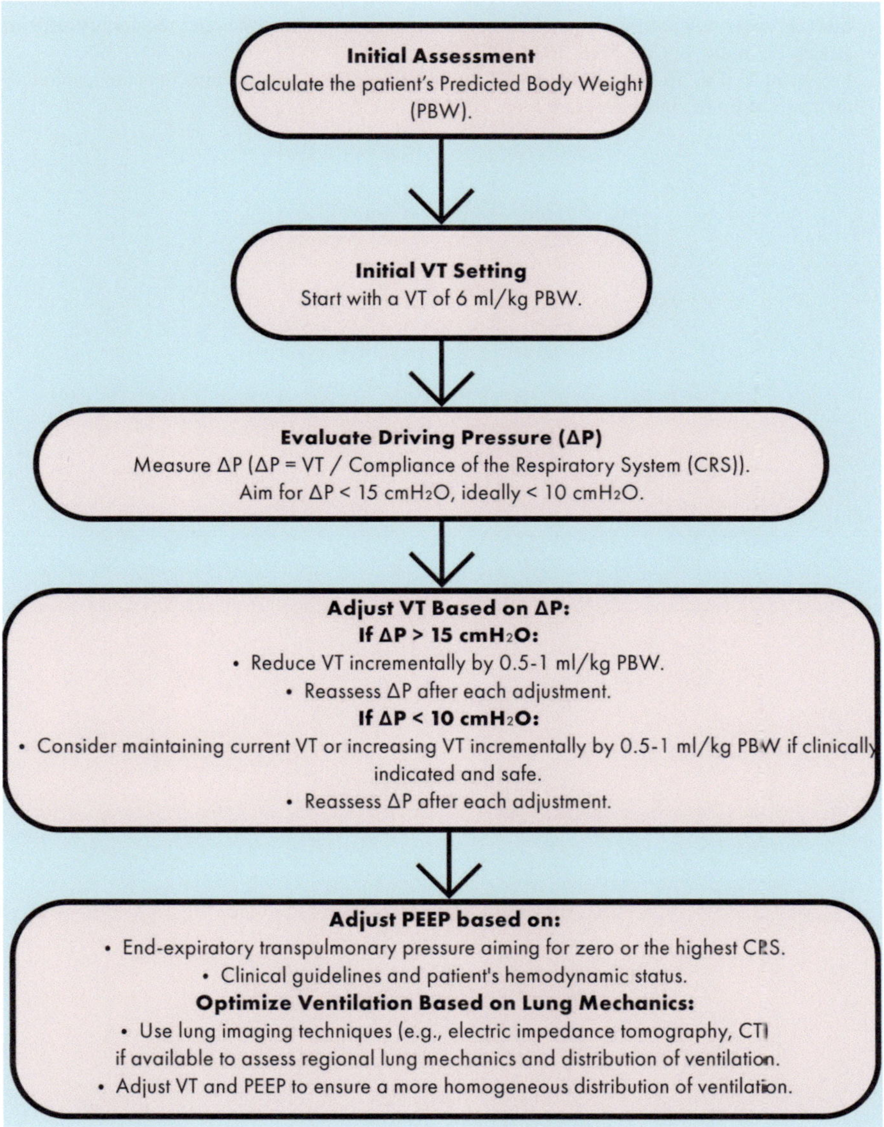

Bibliography

1. Grasselli G, Calfee CS, Camporota L, Poole D, Amato MBP, Antonelli M, et al. ESICM guidelines on acute respiratory distress syndrome: definition, phenotyping and respiratory support strategies. Intensive Care Med. 2023;49(7):727–59.
2. Pellegrini M, Del Sorbo L, Ranieri VM. Finding the optimal tidal volume in acute respiratory distress syndrome. Intensive Care Med. 2024;50(7):1154–6.

Chapter 79
Approach to Setting PEEP in ARDS Patients in the ICU

79.1 Introduction

Acute respiratory distress syndrome (ARDS) is a severe condition characterized by diffuse alveolar damage, reduced lung compliance, and hypoxemia. Positive end-expiratory pressure (PEEP) is a crucial component of mechanical ventilation in ARDS, aiming to maintain alveolar recruitment, improve oxygenation, and prevent ventilator-induced lung injury. However, setting the appropriate PEEP level requires balancing the benefits of alveolar recruitment against the risks of overdistension and hemodynamic compromise [1, 2] [Ref: Algorithm 79.1].

79.2 Setting PEEP

79.2.1 Ensure the Patient Is Fully Sedated or Paralyzed If Required

- Adequate sedation and/or paralysis reduce patient-ventilator dyssynchrony, allowing controlled delivery of mechanical ventilation. This is especially important when titrating PEEP to prevent erratic pressure changes due to spontaneous breathing efforts.
- Use neuromuscular blocking agents (NMBAs) only if necessary, as excessive paralysis carries risks of critical illness myopathy. Monitor sedation depth using validated scales [3].

S. B. Mishra et al., *Mastering ICU Care*,
https://doi.org/10.1007/978-981-95-0179-3_79

79.2.2 Evaluate Lung Recruitability and Obtain Baseline Values

- Utilize imaging techniques (e.g., CT scans, electrical impedance tomography [EIT]) or bedside evaluations of compliance changes during incremental PEEP trials [4]. This determines the potential for alveolar recruitment. Record the baseline PaO_2/FiO_2, compliance, cardiac output, and mean arterial pressure (MAP).

79.2.3 Assess Patient Stability

- Stable Hemodynamics: Adequate MAP without significant dependence on vasoactive agents.
- Minimal oxygenation requirement adjustments: Stable PaO_2/FiO_2.
- If Unstable: Use lower PEEP to avoid worsening hemodynamics and to minimize barotrauma risks. Reassess after stabilization [5].

79.2.4 Evaluate P/F Ratio (<100 or ≥100)

- $P/F < 100$:
- Severe ARDS likely benefits from higher PEEP to achieve alveolar recruitment and improve oxygenation.
- Initiate with a PEEP of 24 cm H_2O, then gradually reduce in 2 cm H_2O increments, observing for clinical and physiological improvements (e.g., oxygenation or compliance).
- $P/F \geq 100$:
- For moderate ARDS, set low PEEP (6 cm of H_2O) [6].

79.2.5 Monitoring During PEEP Titration

79.2.5.1 Key Parameters

- Oxygenation: Improvements in PaO_2 or PaO_2/FiO_2 suggest effective alveolar recruitment.
- Compliance: Better static compliance indicates optimal lung mechanics with current PEEP.
- Hemodynamics: Monitor for cardiac output reduction or hypotension due to high intrathoracic pressures compressing venous return.
- Overdistension: Watch for plateau pressures >30 cm H_2O, as this indicates risk of barotrauma.

79.2.5.2 Action for Complications

- Reduce PEEP if signs of hemodynamic compromise or overdistension emerge.
- Optimize fluid status and vasoactive support as needed [7, 8].

79.2.6 Reassessment

- Rationale: Changes in patient position, lung pathology, or ventilator settings can alter lung recruitability.
- Frequency: Reassess PEEP settings with any clinical or ventilatory changes to ensure optimal management.
- Tools: Repeat imaging or compliance evaluations to determine the need for adjustment.

79.2.7 Establish Optimal PEEP

- The goal is to identify the PEEP level that provides:
- The best lung compliance.
- Adequate oxygenation with the least FiO_2 requirement.
- Minimal adverse effects, such as overdistension or hemodynamic instability.
- Once identified, maintain this PEEP and continue monitoring patient progress.

Reassess the PEEP setting after every change in ventilator setting or any change in patient positioning in bed.

79.2.8 Other Methods

1. ARDS.net PEEP FiO_2 table: There are specific PEEP as per the FiO_2 requirement [9]
   Lower PEEP/higher FiO_2 table

FiO_2	0.3	0.4	0.4	0.5	0.5	0.6	0.7	0.7	0.7	0.8	0.9	0.9	0.9	1
PEEP	5	5	8	8	10	10	10	12	14	14	14	16	18	18–24

   Higher PEEP/lower FiO_2

FiO_2	0.3	0.3	0.3	0.3	0.3	0.4	0.4	0.5	0.5	0.5–0.8	0.8	0.9	1	1
PEEP	5	8	10	12	14	14	16	16	18	20	22	22	22	24

2. Empirical peep: Based on clinical experience and then titrated according to oxygenation and lung mechanics.
3. Recruitment to inflation ratio: PEEP is abruptly reduced by 10 cm of H_2O from 15 to 5. It is calculated as compliance of recruited lung divided by compliance at low PEEP. Recruited volume is the difference of volume during the abrupt fall and the anticipated volume based on compliance at low PEEP.

4. Esophageal manometry: PEEP is adjusted by measuring the esophageal pressure (surrogate of transpulmonary pressure (TPP))—prevents lung collapse and minimizes lung stress. TPP = Plateau pressure—Esophageal pressure ($P_{(plat)} - P_{es}$). Adjust PEEP so that TPP at end-expiration is 0–10. The disadvantages are that it relies on the esophageal balloon position. These readings will not be accurate due to heterogeneity in ARDS patients. P_{es} overestimates pleural pressure in the well-aerated regions of the lung and underestimates it in the dependent regions of the lung.
5. CT scan: PEEP is set depending on the gasless tissue under high and low pressure. Sequential CT scans are done to see the PEEP at which the greatest volume of the lung is recruited.
6. Lung ultrasound: PEEP is set according to reaeration tissue.
7. Electrical impedance tomography (EIT): It offers real-time, bedside imaging of regional lung ventilation, enabling clinicians to assess the distribution of air within the lungs. This tool is particularly useful for titrating PEEP, as it helps identify the optimal level that minimizes both alveolar collapse and overdistension, thereby promoting more uniform and protective ventilation.
8. PEEP should be titrated to the level that results in the smallest difference between arterial and end-tidal CO_2 levels, indicating the point at which physiological dead space is minimized.
9. PEEP slightly above the lower inflection point of the pressure volume curve—not practical to use the hysteresis loop for calculating PEEP.
10. Driving pressure (Dp): It is calculated by subtracting the positive end-expiratory pressure (PEEP) from the plateau pressure (Pplat) (Pplat—PEEP). Target driving pressure below 15 cm of H_2O for improved outcome and mortality.
11. Mechanical power (MP) is a comprehensive measure of the energy transferred from the ventilator to the patient's respiratory system over time. It accounts for the work required to overcome airway resistance during gas movement, the effort needed to inflate the lungs and chest wall, and the energy necessary to counteract the recoil forces associated with end-expiratory pressure, such as PEEP. MP = 0.098 × tidal volume × respiratory rate (Δ Pinsp + PEEP). Higher MP denotes higher work by the ventilator and thus higher chances of ventilator-induced lung injury. The mechanical power is directly proportional to the mortality and outcomes.

79.3 Conclusion

The systematic titration of PEEP in ARDS requires individualized assessment of lung recruitability, oxygenation, and hemodynamics. The algorithm emphasizes starting with stabilization, reassessing lung recruitability, and titrating PEEP based on severity (PaO_2/FiO_2). Continuous monitoring and reassessment are crucial for achieving the optimal balance between oxygenation improvement and adverse effects. This structured approach aligns with evidence-based practices to improve patient outcomes while minimizing ventilator-induced complications.

Algorithm 79.1: Approach to setting PEEP in ARDS patients in the ICU

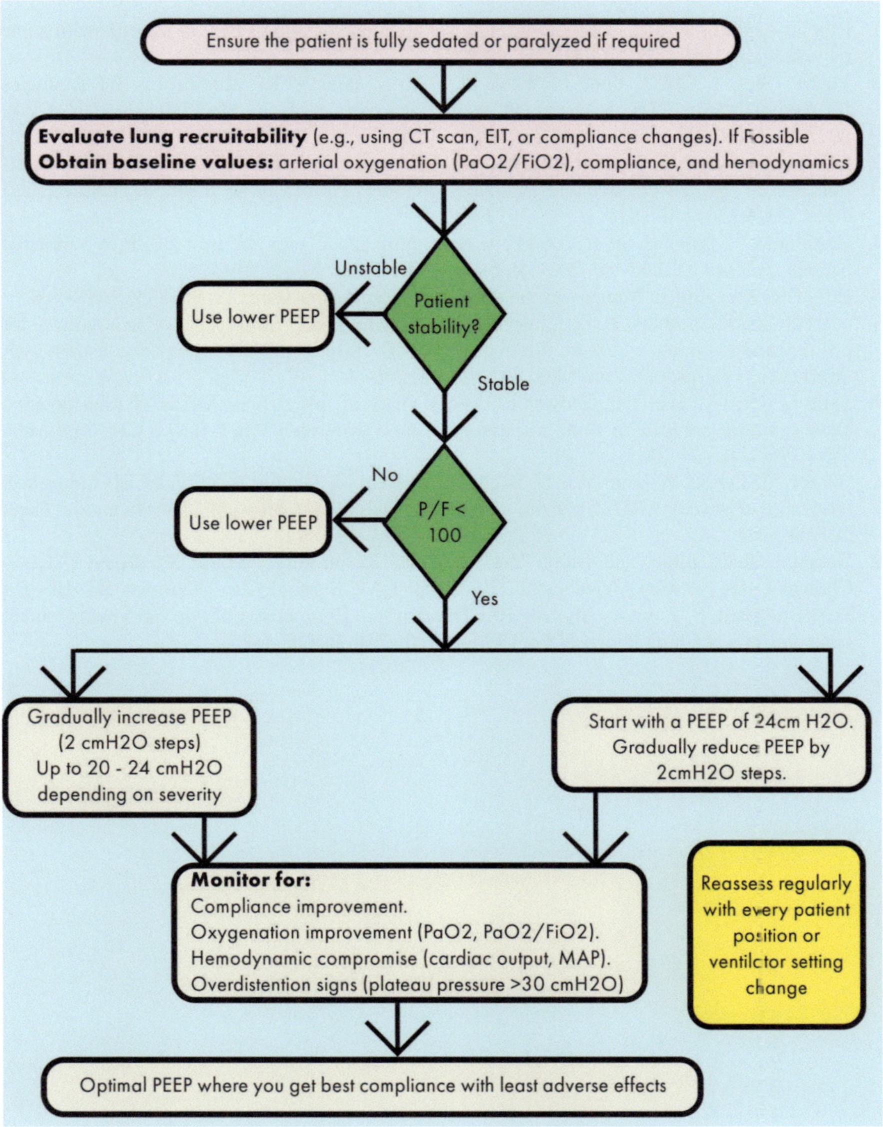

Bibliography

1. Heunks L, Piquilloud L, Demoule A. How we approach titrating PEEP in patients with acute hypoxemic failure. Crit Care. 2023;27(1):415.
2. Yu M, Deng Y, Cha J, Jiang L, Wang M, Qiao S, et al. PEEP titration by EIT strategies for patients with ARDS: a systematic review and meta-analysis. Med Intensiva (Engl Ed). 2023;47(7):383–90.
3. Edginton S, Kruger N, Stelfox HT, Brochard L, Zuege DJ, Gaudet J, et al. Methods for determination of optimal positive end-expiratory pressure: a protocol for a scoping review. BMJ Open. 2023;13(8):e071871.
4. Gattinoni L, Marini JJ. In search of the holy grail: identifying the best PEEP in ventilated patients. Intensive Care Med. 2022;48(6):728–31.
5. Hess DR. Recruitment Maneuvers and PEEP titration. Respir Care. 2015;60(11):1688–704.
6. van der Zee P, Somhorst P, Endeman H, Gommers D. Electrical impedance tomography for positive end-expiratory pressure titration in COVID-19-related acute respiratory distress syndrome. Am J Respir Crit Care Med. 2020;202(2):280–4.
7. Sahetya SK, Goligher EC, Brower RG. Fifty years of research in ARDS. Setting positive end-expiratory pressure in acute respiratory distress syndrome. Am J Respir Crit Care Med. 2017;195(11):1429–38.
8. Bergez M, Fritsch N, Tran-Van D, Saghi T, Bounkim T, Gentile A, et al. PEEP titration in moderate to severe ARDS: plateau versus transpulmonary pressure. Ann Intensive Care. 2019;9(1):81.
9. National Heart, Lung, and Blood Institute Acute Respiratory Distress Syndrome (ARDS) Clinical Trials Network, Wiedemann HP, Wheeler AP, Bernard GR, Thompson BT, Hayden D, deBoisblanc B, Connors AF, Hite RD, Harabin AL. Comparison of two fluid-management strategies in acute lung injury. N Engl J Med. 2006;354(24):2564–75.

Chapter 80
Approach to Patient-Ventilator Asynchrony in the ICU

80.1 Introduction

Ventilator asynchrony is a prevalent challenge in critical care medicine, with an incidence ranging from 10% to 85%. This mismatch between a patient's respiratory efforts and the ventilator's delivered breaths is associated with poor clinical outcomes, including prolonged ICU stays, increased mortality rates, and respiratory muscle dysfunction. Both patient-related factors—such as respiratory drive variations due to sepsis or acute respiratory distress syndrome (ARDS)—and ventilator-related factors like trigger sensitivity and flow settings contribute to asynchrony. Early recognition and management are crucial to optimize patient comfort, improve ventilator efficiency, and enhance clinical outcomes [1, 2] [Ref: Algorithm 80.1].

80.2 Identify Symptoms of Asynchrony

- Overview: Recognize signs of ventilator asynchrony, such as increased respiratory distress, tachypnea, hemodynamic instability, or visible discordance between patient effort and ventilator cycling.
- Rationale: Early detection prevents escalation of respiratory insufficiency and associated complications.
- Action: Confirm clinical suspicion by initiating waveform analysis for real-time detection and classification of asynchrony types [3].

S. B. Mishra et al., *Mastering ICU Care*,
https://doi.org/10.1007/978-981-95-0179-3_80

80.3 Proceed to Waveform Analysis and Monitoring

- Waveform Evaluation: Continuously monitor flow-time, pressure-time, and volume-time waveforms to identify patterns indicative of asynchrony.
- Importance: Waveform analysis is the cornerstone for diagnosing specific types of asynchrony. Advanced tools like esophageal pressure monitoring and diaphragmatic electromyography can be employed to confirm asynchrony when waveform analysis is inconclusive [4].
- Clinical Note: Incorporate esophageal manometry or diaphragm electrical activity monitoring to enhance detection accuracy.

80.4 Types of Asynchrony and Specific Interventions

80.4.1 Check Triggering Asynchronies

Ineffective Efforts

- Definition: Occurs when the ventilator fails to deliver a breath despite the patient's inspiratory effort, making it the most common type of asynchrony, especially in patients with auto-PEEP.
- Cause: Auto-PEEP, inadequate trigger sensitivity, or high respiratory drive.
- Intervention:
- Adjust trigger sensitivity to ensure the ventilator detects patient efforts.
- Reduce auto-PEEP by optimizing expiratory time or titrating ventilatory settings.
- Consider adjusting positive end-expiratory pressure (PEEP) levels to counterbalance auto-PEEP [5].

Auto-Triggering

- Definition: The ventilator delivers breaths without any patient effort.
- Cause: Circuit leaks, excessive trigger sensitivity, or inappropriate flow settings.
- Intervention:
- Evaluate and correct circuit leaks.
- Adjust trigger sensitivity to prevent false triggering.
- Modify flow trigger settings to align with patient needs [6].

80.4.2 Flow Asynchrony

- Definition: A mismatch between the ventilator's inspiratory flow rate and the patient's demand.
- Diagnosis: Inspect flow-time waveforms for abnormalities such as rapid deceleration or prolonged inspiratory phases.
- Management:
- Increase Flow: Adjust the inspiratory flow rate or switch to pressure-support ventilation to better match the patient's effort.
- Reduce Flow: Decrease tidal volumes or inspiratory pressures in patients demonstrating excessive flow demands.

80.4.3 Cycling Asynchrony

Premature Cycling

- Definition: The ventilator terminates inspiration before the patient completes their inspiratory effort.
- Management: Decrease the cycling-off percentage to extend the inspiratory time, allowing for complete breath delivery.

Delayed Cycling

- Definition: The ventilator continues delivering inspiration after the patient has finished their inspiratory effort.
- Management: Increase the cycling-off percentage to shorten the inspiratory time, preventing overdistension [7].

80.4.4 Double Triggering and Reverse Triggering

- Definition: Double triggering occurs when two consecutive breaths are triggered by a single patient effort; reverse triggering is when patient effort follows ventilator-delivered breaths. Both can contribute to lung injury due to excessive tidal volumes.
- Management:
- Adjust Tidal Volume: In ARDS patients, synchronize tidal volume adjustments to mitigate lung injury risks.
- Modify Inspiratory Time:
- For double triggering, increase inspiratory time to align with patient effort.
- For reverse triggering, reduce inspiratory time to prevent patient-ventilator mismatch.

80.5 Advanced Ventilatory Strategies

80.5.1 Optimize Ventilation Mode

- Switch to Proportional Modes: Utilize advanced modes like neurally adjusted ventilatory assist (NAVA) and proportional assist ventilation (PAV). These modes synchronize ventilator support with the patient's neural respiratory drive, reducing asynchrony.
- Advantages: Improved patient comfort, reduced work of breathing, and enhanced synchrony.
- Limitations: Limited widespread adoption due to complexity, equipment requirements, and the need for specialized training.

80.6 Address Patient Factors

- Underlying Issues: Identify and manage conditions contributing to respiratory drive mismatch, such as pain, anxiety, fever, or sepsis.
- Sedation Management: Avoid over-sedation to prevent respiratory muscle dysfunction. Use minimal sedation unless severe asynchrony necessitates controlled ventilation.

80.7 Outcome Correlation and Quality Metrics

- Asynchrony Index (AI): Calculate the AI, defined as the number of asynchronous events divided by the total number of breaths (patient-triggered and ventilator-triggered), multiplied by 100%.
- Clinical Significance: An AI greater than 10% is linked with higher mortality and longer durations of mechanical ventilation.
- Quality Improvement: Routine calculation of AI can be part of quality improvement initiatives to enhance patient outcomes.
- Training: Implement structured training programs for healthcare providers to improve detection accuracy of asynchrony, as automation in this area remains underdeveloped.

80.8 Research and Emerging Trends

- Machine Learning Algorithms: Ongoing developments in machine learning offer promise for automated detection of asynchrony and predictive analytics for intervention planning.
- Personalized Ventilatory Settings: Encourage the inclusion of personalized ventilatory settings as part of future precision medicine approaches to optimize patient outcomes.
- Future Directions: Research into user-friendly interfaces and integration of advanced monitoring tools could facilitate wider adoption of advanced ventilatory modes.

80.9 Conclusion

Ventilator asynchrony is a multifactorial issue that significantly impacts patient outcomes in critical care settings. A systematic approach involving careful waveform analysis, precise adjustments to ventilator settings, and addressing underlying patient factors is essential for achieving optimal synchronization. Advanced ventilatory strategies, such as NAVA and PAV, offer promising solutions but require further integration into clinical practice. Monitoring tools like the Asynchrony Index and developments in machine learning hold potential for improving detection and management. Clinicians must remain vigilant and adaptive, as patient conditions and ventilator dynamics continuously evolve during ICU management. Implementing structured training and embracing emerging technologies will be pivotal in enhancing patient care and outcomes.

Algorithm 80.1: Approach to patient-ventilator asynchrony in the ICU

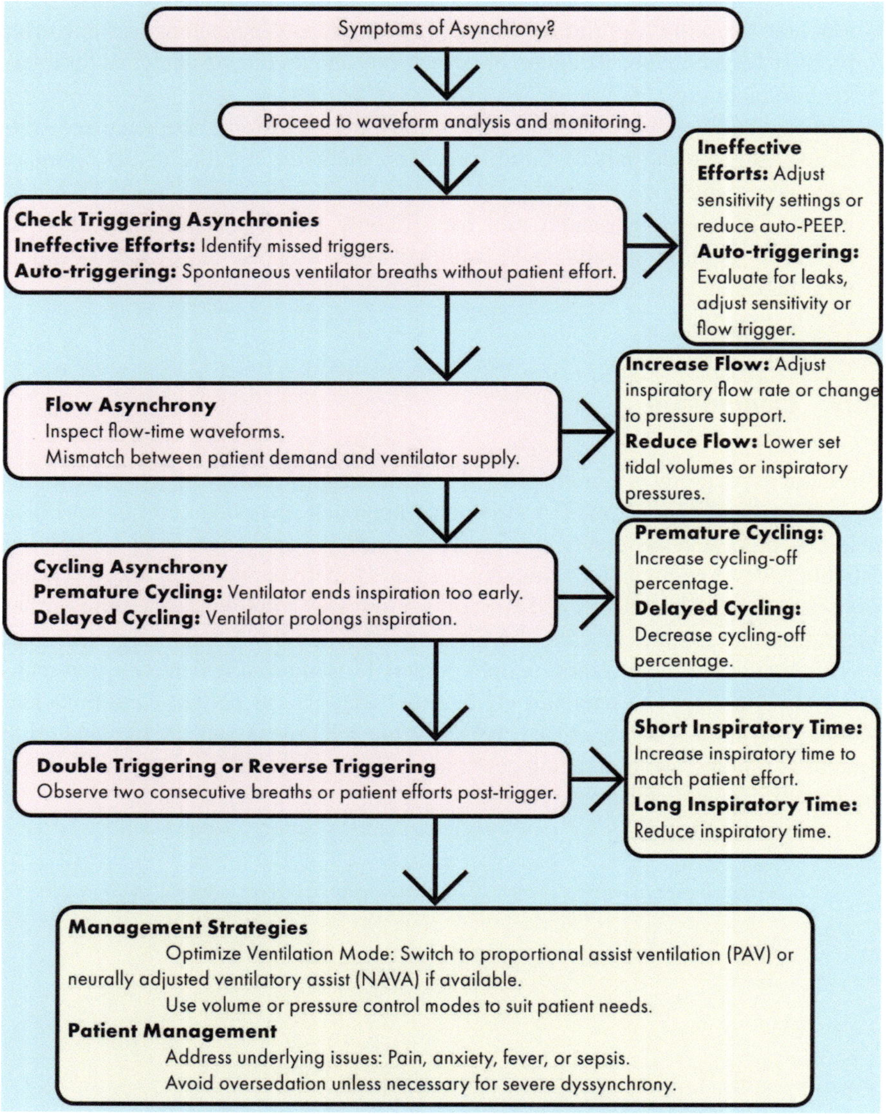

Bibliography

1. Holanda MA, Vasconcelos RDS, Ferreira JC, Pinheiro BV. Patient-ventilator asynchrony. J Bras Pneumol. 2018;44(4):321–33.
2. Saavedra SN, Barisich PVS, Maldonado JBP, Lumini RB, Gomez-Gonzalez A, Gallardo A. Asynchronies during invasive mechanical ventilation: narrative review and update. Acute Crit Care. 2022;37(4):491–501.
3. Mirabella L, Cinnella G, Costa R, Cortegiani A, Tullo L, Rauseo M, et al. Patient-ventilator asynchronies: clinical implications and practical solutions. Respir Care. 2020;65(11):1751–66.
4. Oto B, Annesi J, Foley RJ. Patient-ventilator dyssynchrony in the intensive care unit: a practical approach to diagnosis and management. Anaesth Intensive Care. 2021;49(2):86–97.
5. Bailey JM. Management of patient-ventilator asynchrony. Anesthesiology. 2021;134(4):629–36.
6. Subira C, de Haro C, Magrans R, Fernandez R, Blanch L. Minimizing asynchronies in mechanical ventilation: current and future trends. Respir Care. 2018;63(4):464–78.
7. Zhou Y, Holets SR, Li M, Cortes-Puentes GA, Meyer TJ, Hanson AC, et al. Etiology, incidence, and outcomes of patient-ventilator asynchrony in critically-ill patients undergoing invasive mechanical ventilation. Sci Rep. 2021;11(1):12390.

Chapter 81
Approach to Weaning from Mechanical Ventilation

81.1 Introduction

Weaning from mechanical ventilation is a pivotal process in the care of critically ill patients, transitioning them from ventilatory support to spontaneous breathing. This involves detailed assessment and management to minimize the risks of respiratory failure, airway obstruction, or cardiovascular instability. A structured, evidence-based approach ensures optimal outcomes while addressing potential challenges [1, 2] [Ref: Algorithm 81.1].

81.2 Detailed Categorization of Weaning

Patients can be categorized into three distinct groups, as defined by the International Consensus Conference:

- Simple Weaning: Patients who successfully transition after the first spontaneous breathing trial (SBT).
- Difficult Weaning: Patients requiring up to three SBTs or within 7 days of the first trial.
- Prolonged Weaning: Patients needing more than three SBTs or more than 7 days to achieve successful weaning [3].

S. B. Mishra et al., *Mastering ICU Care*,
https://doi.org/10.1007/978-981-95-0179-3_81

81.3 Key Considerations in the Weaning Process

1. Has the underlying cause of intubation improved?

   - Rationale: Ensure resolution or significant improvement of the condition requiring ventilatory support (e.g., ARDS, sepsis, or cardiac failure).
   - Clinical Considerations:
   - Improvement in infections, oxygenation, or hemodynamic stability.
   - Minimal vasopressor or sedative requirements.
   - Management: Continue ventilation if the condition persists, focusing on daily reassessment.

2. Are physiological parameters adequate?

   - Criteria for Stability:
   - Hemodynamic Stability: No significant inotropic or vasopressor support.
   - Oxygenation: $PaO_2/FiO_2 > 150$, PEEP ≤ 5 cm H_2O.
   - Mental Status: Alertness for spontaneous breathing and airway protection.
   - Muscle Strength: Adequate respiratory power.
   - Electrolyte Balance: Correct hypokalemia, hypophosphatemia, or hypomagnesemia.
   - Management: Optimize physiological parameters and reassess daily [4].

3. Is the patient tolerating a spontaneous breathing trial (SBT)?

   - Procedure: Conduct SBT using a T-piece, low-pressure support, or automatic tube compensation for 30–120 min.
   - Criteria for Success:
   - Respiratory rate < 35/min, $SpO_2 \geq 90\%$, heart rate < 140 bpm.
   - No signs of distress (e.g., agitation, accessory muscle use).
   - Management of Failure:
   - Address specific causes (e.g., airway resistance, fluid overload, anxiety).
   - Use adjuncts like bronchodilators or diuretics and initiate rehabilitation for ICU-acquired weakness.

4. Pathophysiological Insights into Weaning Challenges.

   - Diaphragmatic Dysfunction: Address ventilator-induced respiratory muscle fatigue through diaphragmatic training and gradual ventilatory support reduction.
   - Cardiovascular Effects: Loss of intrathoracic pressure during weaning can lead to increased preload and afterload, causing cardiovascular instability [5, 6].

5. Enhanced Weaning Parameters.

   - Utilize advanced predictive tools, including:
   - Heart Rate Variability (HRV): Indicates autonomic readiness for weaning.

- Diaphragmatic Thickening Fraction (DTF) via Ultrasound: Reflects diaphragmatic function and fatigue levels.

6. Proceed to Extubation Readiness Evaluation.
   Key Assessments:
   - Presence of a strong cough to ensure effective secretion clearance.
   - Airway patency via cuff-leak test to rule out airway edema.
   - Minimal secretions and intact airway protection.
   - Management: Return to ventilation if criteria are unmet and address barriers like airway edema with corticosteroids or secretion management strategies.
7. Proceed with Extubation.
   - Steps: Extubate and monitor closely for post-extubation respiratory failure.
   - Post-Extubation Care:
   - Use prophylactic noninvasive ventilation (NIV) or high-flow nasal oxygen in high-risk patients.

81.4 Addressing Primary Causes of Weaning Failure

1. Respiratory Causes.
   - Diaphragmatic Dysfunction: Implement respiratory muscle training.
   - Increased Airway Resistance: Optimize bronchodilators and secretion management.
2. Cardiovascular Causes.
   - Heart Failure/Volume Overload: Manage with diuretics and preload/afterload optimization.
3. Neurological and Psychological Causes.
   - Anxiety/Sedation: Titrate sedatives and employ anxiety-relief measures.
4. Nutritional and Muscular Causes.
   - Malnutrition/Myopathy: Provide nutritional support and physical therapy.

81.5 Role of Multidisciplinary Collaboration

- A dedicated team involving respiratory therapists, nurses, and physiotherapists ensures optimal outcomes by addressing all aspects of the weaning process.

81.6 Rehabilitation Protocols and Prevention of Extubation Failure

- Early Mobilization: Strengthens respiratory muscles and reduces ICU-acquired weakness.
- Post-Extubation Strategies: Include prophylactic NIV and cuff-leak tests to prevent respiratory failure.

81.7 Conclusion

Weaning from mechanical ventilation is a structured, multidisciplinary process requiring meticulous evaluation and management at each stage. Incorporating advanced predictive measures, rehabilitation protocols, and evidence-based practices ensures success in this critical transition while preventing complications and optimizing outcomes.

Algorithm 81.1: Approach to weaning from mechanical ventilation

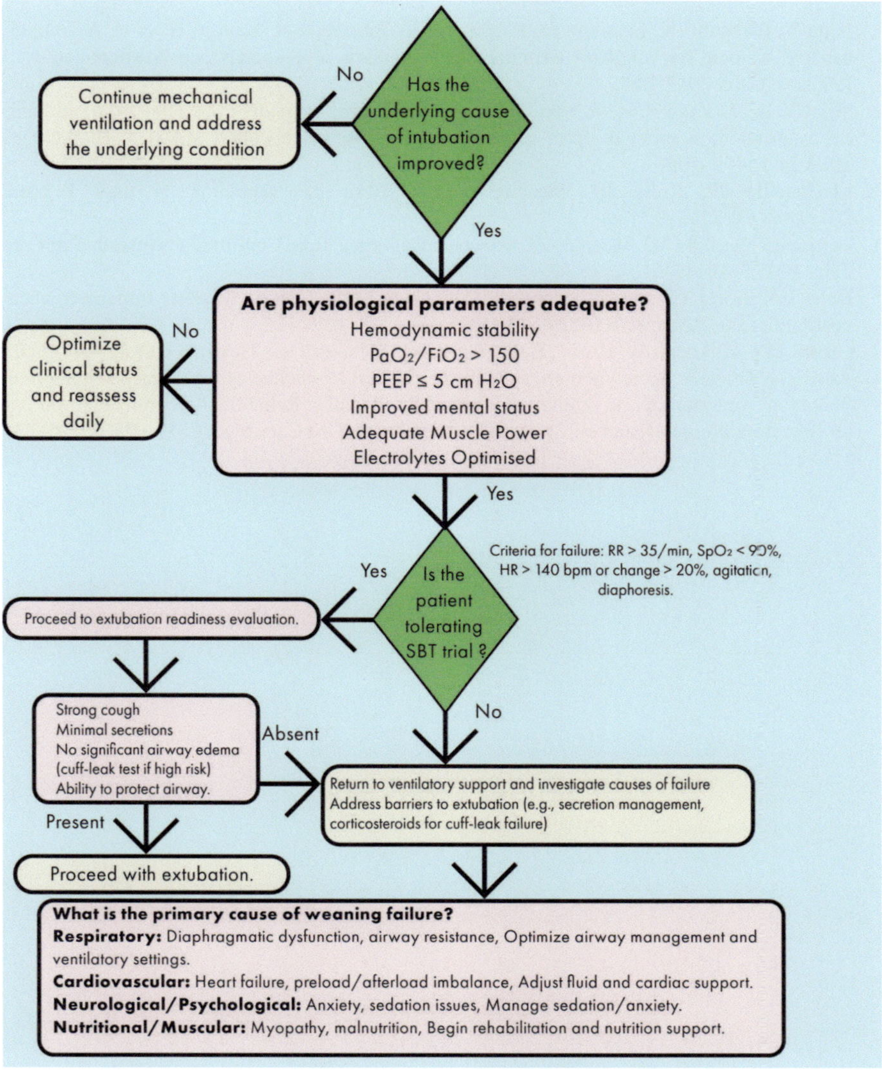

Bibliography

1. Nitta K, Okamoto K, Imamura H, Mochizuki K, Takayama H, Kamijo H, et al. A comprehensive protocol for ventilator weaning and extubation: a prospective observational study. J Intensive Care. 2019;7:50.
2. Wang Y, Lei L, Yang H, He S, Hao J, Liu T, et al. Weaning critically ill patients from mechanical ventilation: a protocol from a multicenter retrospective cohort study. J Thorac Dis. 2022;14(1):199–206.
3. McConville JF, Kress JP. Weaning patients from the ventilator. N Engl J Med. 2012;367(23):2233–9.
4. Lermitte J, Garfield MJ. Weaning from mechanical ventilation. Contin Educ Anaesth Crit Care Pain. 2005;5(4):113–7.
5. Boles JM, Bion J, Connors A, Herridge M, Marsh B, Melot C, et al. Weaning from mechanical ventilation. Eur Respir J. 2007;29(5):1033–56.
6. Girard TD, Alhazzani W, Kress JP, Ouellette DR, Schmidt GA, Truwit JD, et al. An official American Thoracic Society/American College of Chest Physicians clinical practice guideline: liberation from mechanical ventilation in critically ill adults. Rehabilitation protocols, ventilator liberation protocols, and cuff leak tests. Am J Respir Crit Care Med. 2017;195(1):120–33.

Chapter 82
Approach to Tracheostomy Care in the ICU

82.1 Introduction

Tracheostomy care is critical in managing patients with prolonged respiratory needs or airway compromise. Proper management ensures patient safety, prevents complications such as infection, tube obstruction, or dislodgment, and supports recovery, including potential decannulation. A multidisciplinary team approach enhances the quality of care, reduces complications, and improves patient satisfaction by ensuring comprehensive management of all aspects of tracheostomy care [1] [Ref: Algorithm 82.1].

82.2 Multidisciplinary Tracheostomy Care Team

Effective tracheostomy management involves a multidisciplinary team comprising:

- Physicians: Oversee medical management and coordinate care.
- Nurses: Provide daily care, monitor for complications, and educate patients.
- Respiratory Therapists: Manage ventilator settings, humidification and secretion clearance.
- Speech and Language Therapists: Assist with communication and swallowing rehabilitation.
- Physiotherapists: Promote mobilization and respiratory exercises.

This team collaborates to address the complex needs of tracheostomized patients, facilitating comprehensive care planning, early detection of issues, and tailored interventions to enhance patient outcomes.

S. B. Mishra et al., *Mastering ICU Care*,
https://doi.org/10.1007/978-981-95-0179-3_82

82.3 Routine Assessment

Objective: Ensure the tracheostomy tube functions properly and the patient's respiratory status is stable.

Actions:

- Inspect the Tube Position and Patency:
- Confirm the tube is secured and unobstructed.
- Check for proper alignment to prevent airway obstruction or accidental decannulation.
- Evaluate the Stoma:
- Assess for signs of infection, granulation tissue, or skin breakdown.
- Redness, swelling, or purulent discharge requires immediate attention.
- Confirm Cuff Pressure (if applicable):
- Cuff Management:
- Monitor cuff pressure every 8 h or as per protocol.
- Maintain pressure between 20 and 30 cm H_2O to prevent aspiration and minimize tracheal mucosal damage.
- Risks:
- Overinflation can cause tracheal ischemia and necrosis.
- Underinflation increases the risk of aspiration.
- Implement strategies for cuff deflation during weaning to assess readiness for decannulation.
- Assess Respiratory Status:
- Monitor oxygen saturation, respiratory rate, and work of breathing.
- Detect early signs of respiratory distress or inadequate ventilation.
- Check for Overall Stability:
- Address systemic issues like sepsis or hemodynamic instability that may impact tracheostomy care [2].

82.4 Tube Selection

Selecting the appropriate tracheostomy tube is vital and should be based on the patient's anatomy and clinical needs:

- Standard Tubes: Suitable for general use.
- Adjustable-Length Tubes: For patients with unusual neck anatomy or tracheal depth.
- Fenestrated Tubes: Facilitate speech by allowing air to pass through the vocal cords.
- Subglottic Suction Tubes: Allow continuous or intermittent suctioning above the cuff, reducing the risk of ventilator-associated pneumonia.

Proper tube selection enhances patient comfort, facilitates communication, and reduces complications.

82.5 Humidification and Secretion Management

Rationale: Adequate humidification ensures airway secretions remain thin and manageable. Dry air can lead to thick mucus, increasing the risk of obstruction.

Actions:

- Verify Humidification Systems:
- Ensure devices like heated humidifiers or heat and moisture exchangers (HMEs) are functioning properly.
- Crucial for patients on ventilators or oxygen support.
- Assess Secretions:
- Monitor volume and consistency.
- Thick or excessive secretions may indicate dehydration, infection, or inadequate humidification.
- Evidence-Based Practices:
- Utilize subglottic suction tubes when appropriate.
- Implement protocols for secretion management, including chest physiotherapy and nebulization.

82.6 Patient Communication and Rehabilitation

Facilitating communication and addressing psychosocial aspects are essential components of tracheostomy care:

- Speaking Valves:
- Use one-way speaking valves (e.g., Passy-Muir valve) to enable phonation.
- Assess the patient's ability to tolerate the valve, ensuring airway patency and adequate ventilation.
- Role of Speech and Language Therapists:
- Provide interventions to optimize vocalization and swallowing.
- Address issues related to dysphagia and risk of aspiration.
- Psychosocial Support:
- Recognize the emotional impact of tracheostomy on patients.
- Offer counseling and support to address anxiety, depression, or body image concerns [3].

82.7 Emergency Preparedness

Being prepared for emergencies is critical in tracheostomy care:

- Guidelines for Emergency Management:
- Develop and follow standardized protocols.

- Include flowcharts for managing airway obstruction, accidental decannulation, bleeding, or infection.
- Tracheostomy Emergency Kit:
- Ensure a kit is available at the bedside at all times.
- Should include spare tracheostomy tubes (same size and one size smaller), obturator, suction catheters, syringes, and lubricants.
- Staff Training:
- Regularly train all caregivers on emergency procedures.
- Simulate scenarios to enhance readiness.

82.8 Airway Obstruction Management

Decision Point: Determine if the airway is compromised due to secretions, mucus plugs, or tube kinking.

If Yes:

- Perform Suctioning:
- Clear secretions to restore airway patency.
- Inspect the Tube:
- Check for kinks or external occlusions.
- Replace the tube if issues cannot be corrected.
- Emergency Protocols:
- If obstruction persists, escalate care immediately (may need bronchoscopy to assess the cause of obstruction).
- Follow emergency flowcharts and call for additional support.

If No:

- Proceed to Evaluate Tube Position and Potential Dislodgment.

82.9 Accidental Decannulation Management

Significance: Accidental decannulation is a medical emergency, especially in new or immature tracheostomies.

If Yes:

- Attempt Reinsertion:
- Reinsert the tracheostomy tube promptly.
- Use a smaller size tube if reinsertion is difficult.
- Utilize Stay Sutures:
- If available, use stay sutures to aid reinsertion.
- Emergency Airway Support:
- If reinsertion fails, initiate emergency airway management (may go for orotracheal intubation and place endotracheal tube beyond the tracheal stoma).

- Ensure oxygenation and call for anesthesiology or airway specialists.

  If No:

- Continue Monitoring and Address Other Potential Issues.

82.10 Weaning and Decannulation

Assess Readiness for Decannulation.
Criteria:

- Stable Respiratory Function:
- Maintain adequate oxygenation and ventilation without ventilator support.
- Effective Secretion Clearance:
- Demonstrate the ability to manage secretions independently.
- Airway Protection:
- Intact cough and swallow reflexes to prevent aspiration.
- No Upper Airway Obstruction:
- Confirmed via endoscopic evaluation.

  Actions:

- Implement Weaning Protocols:
- Use evidence-based practices such as gradual cuff deflation, downsizing tubes, and capping trials.
- Utilize T-pieces or high-flow oxygen systems as appropriate.
- Trial of Cuff Deflation:
- Gradually deflate the cuff to assess tolerance.
- Downsizing the Tracheostomy Tube:
- Replace with a smaller, uncuffed tube when feasible.
- Decannulation Readiness Testing:
- Perform capping trials (cap the tracheostomy tube and see if patient is able to breathe on his own by the side of the downsized tracheostomy tube and through nose and mouth without distress—normal breaths), monitoring closely for any signs of distress.

  Benefits of Protocolized Care:

- Improved Outcomes:
- Standardized weaning protocols reduce decannulation time and complications.

82.11 Decannulation Protocol for Tracheostomy Care

82.11.1 Initial Assessment

- Confirm that the patient meets the following criteria:
- Stable respiratory function without ventilatory support.

- Ability to effectively clear secretions.
- No ongoing upper airway obstruction.
- Sufficient cognitive ability to protect the airway.
- Conduct an endoscopic/bronchoscopic evaluation of the airway to confirm patency and absence of granulation tissue.

82.11.2 Trial of Cuff Deflation

- Gradually deflate the cuff to assess airway patency and tolerance.
- Monitor for:
- Respiratory distress (e.g., increased work of breathing, hypoxia).
- Effective handling of secretions.
- Adequate phonation and swallowing.
- If unsuccessful, reinflate the cuff and reassess the patient's readiness after further support or interventions.

82.11.3 Downsizing the Tracheostomy Tube

- Replace the current tracheostomy tube with a smaller, uncuffed tube to test the airway.
- Monitor for tolerance to the smaller tube:
- Ensure no evidence of respiratory compromise.
- Evaluate the ability to manage secretions without aspiration.

82.11.4 Decannulation Readiness Testing

- Perform a capping trial:
- Place a decannulation cap over the tracheostomy tube to simulate normal breathing.
- Monitor respiratory rate, oxygen saturation, and patient comfort during the trial.
- Duration of capping may vary from a few hours to overnight, depending on patient tolerance.

82.11.5 Decannulation

- If the capping trial is successful, proceed to remove the tracheostomy tube.
- Cover the stoma with an occlusive dressing.

- Advise the patient to apply gentle pressure over the stoma during coughing or speaking.

82.11.6 Post-Decannulation Monitoring

- Observe the patient for:
- Respiratory distress or stridor.
- Signs of upper airway obstruction.
- Provide humidified oxygen if required.
- Encourage mobilization and airway clearance exercises.

82.11.7 Stoma Care

- Keep the stoma site clean and dry.
- Allow the stoma to close naturally or refer for surgical closure if necessary.

82.11.8 Documentation and Education

- Record the decannulation process, including the patient's tolerance and any complications.
- Educate the patient and caregivers on:
- Recognizing signs of respiratory distress.
- Proper wound care for the healing stoma.

82.12 Conclusion

This systematic approach to tracheostomy care emphasizes regular assessment, early identification, and resolution of complications, and a structured pathway to decannulation. Key practices include maintaining humidification, monitoring airway patency, and adhering to decannulation criteria. Timely interventions and careful monitoring can prevent adverse outcomes and promote safe patient recovery.

Algorithm 82.1: Approach to tracheostomy care in the ICU

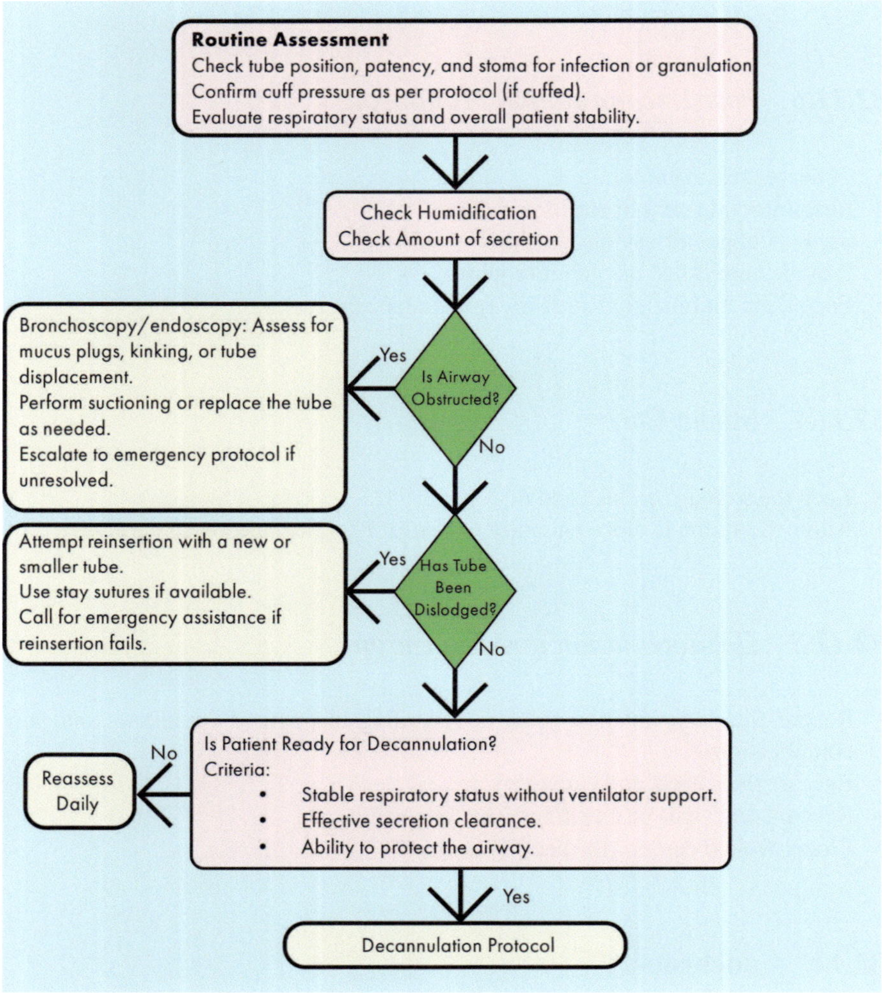

Bibliography

1. El-Anwar MW, Nofal AA, Shawadfy MA, Maaty A, Khazbak AO. Tracheostomy in the intensive care unit: a university hospital in a developing country study. Int Arch Otorhinolaryngol. 2017;21(1):33–7.
2. Lewith H, Athanassoglou V. Update on management of tracheostomy. BJA Educ. 2019;19(11):370–6.
3. Whitmore KA, Townsend SC, Laupland KB. Management of tracheostomies in the intensive care unit: a scoping review. BMJ Open Respir Res. 2020;7(1):e000651.

Chapter 83
Approach to Swallowing Dysfunction in the ICU

83.1 Introduction

Swallowing dysfunction, or dysphagia, is a critical concern in intensive care unit (ICU) patients. It is particularly prevalent among those with prolonged intubation, ICU-acquired weakness, or neurological impairments. Post-extubation dysphagia (PED) affects up to 62% of ICU patients and is associated with increased morbidity and mortality. Complications include aspiration pneumonia, malnutrition, dehydration, and prolonged hospital stays. Early recognition and comprehensive management are essential to mitigate these risks and optimize patient outcomes [1, 2] [Ref: Algorithm 83.1].

83.2 Epidemiological Insights

- Prevalence and Impact:
- PED: Affects up to 62% of ICU patients post-extubation.
- General Dysphagia: Occurs in up to 84% of patients with neurological impairments.
- Consequences: Increased risk of aspiration pneumonia, longer ICU stays, higher healthcare costs, and elevated mortality rates.

83.3 Detailed Risk Factors

- Key Question: Does the patient exhibit risk factors for dysphagia?
- Common Risk Factors:

S. B. Mishra et al., *Mastering ICU Care*,
https://doi.org/10.1007/978-981-95-0179-3_83

- Prolonged Intubation: Can cause laryngeal trauma and altered sensation, impairing swallowing reflexes.
- ICU-Acquired Weakness: Muscle weakness affects swallowing muscles.
- Reduced Sensorium: Cognitive or neurological deficits delay protective reflexes.
- Additional Risk Factors:
- Polypharmacy: Sedatives, anticholinergics, and other medications can impair swallowing.
- Altered Laryngeal Sensation: Due to intubation, leading to silent aspiration.
- Comorbidities:
- Chronic obstructive pulmonary disease (COPD).
- Diabetes mellitus.
- Hypertension.
- Others: Preexisting dysphagia, local malignancy/postsurgical medical conditions affecting anatomic structures of the swallowing tract, and/or considerable quantitative/qualitative reduction of consciousness.

  Action: If risk factors are present, proceed to bedside dysphagia screening.

83.4 Advanced Screening Techniques

Bedside tests for assessing swallowing dysfunction in ICU patients:

1. Yale Swallow Protocol:
   - Purpose: Screen for aspiration risk and swallowing safety.
   - Procedure:
   - Perform a brief cognitive screen to assess alertness.
   - Conduct an oral mechanism exam to evaluate the patient's ability to control and swallow saliva.
   - Administer a 90-mL water swallow challenge. The patient drinks water continuously without stopping.
   - Interpretation:
   - Pass: No coughing, choking, or voice changes after drinking.
   - Fail: Coughing, wet voice, or inability to complete the task indicates a risk of dysphagia.
2. Gugging Swallowing Screen (GUSS):
   - Purpose: Assess risk of aspiration and grade dysphagia severity.
   - Procedure:
   - Part 1: Indirect swallowing test (saliva swallowing). Assess for voluntary saliva swallow, drooling, or wet voice.
   - Part 2: Direct swallowing test with increasing textures (semisolids, liquids). Start with a small bolus size and progress as tolerated.
   - Interpretation:

- Assign scores based on performance (0–20 points). A higher score indicates better swallowing function and lower aspiration risk.
- Scores guide recommendations for oral or enteral feeding.

3. Three-Ounce Water Swallow Test:

- Purpose: Identify overt aspiration.
- Procedure:
- Provide 3 ounces (90 mL) of water.
- Instruct the patient to drink it without interruption.
- Interpretation:
- Pass: No coughing, choking, or wet voice during or after drinking.
- Fail: Any signs of coughing, choking, or altered voice indicate potential dysphagia.

4. Other tests: Post-Extubation Dysphagia Screening Tool, Bernese-ICU Dysphagia Algorithm, modified Volume Viscosity Swallow Test, Clinical Swallowing Examination (CSE).

Next Decision Point: Determine if the patient passes the screening.

83.5 Screening Outcome: Does the Patient Pass?

- Yes:
- Action: Initiate gradual reintroduction of oral intake.
- Start with safe textures and monitor for tolerance to prevent aspiration.
- Early oral intake improves patient morale and nutritional status and prevents translocation of gut bacteria.
- No:
- Action: Refer for instrumental evaluation to determine the nature and extent of dysphagia.

83.6 Instrumental Evaluations

- Refer for Instrumental Evaluation: Flexible endoscopic evaluation of swallowing (FEES), videofluoroscopic swallowing study (VFSS), ultrasonography, tissue Doppler imaging, high-resolution manometry, and oropharyngo-esophageal scintigraphy (OPES).
- Videofluoroscopic Swallowing Study (VFSS): Is done in the radiology room and a barium dye is given to assess all four stages of swallowing. Risk: Radiation exposure and difficulty to perform in ICU patients who cannot be mobilized.
- Benefits: Dynamic imaging to evaluate swallowing mechanisms and detect silent aspiration.

- Role: Identifies detailed pathophysiology of dysphagia.
- Fiber-optic Endoscopic Evaluation of Swallowing (FEES): Penetration and aspiration scale ranging from 1 to 8 is used, where 1 indicates no penetration and 8 indicates aspiration without coughing.
- Benefits: Direct visualization of pharyngeal and laryngeal structures during swallowing.
- Role: Detects structural abnormalities and aspiration events.

Next Decision Point: Determine if there are signs of aspiration or impaired swallowing mechanisms.

83.7 Management Algorithms

Are There Signs of Aspiration or Impaired Swallowing Mechanisms?

A. Yes:

- Implement Aspiration Precautions:
- Modified Diet: Thickened liquids, pureed foods.
- Nil per Oral (NPO) Status: If severe aspiration, risk is present.
- Alternative Nutrition: Nasogastric (NG) feeding, percutaneous endoscopic gastrostomy (PEG) [3, 4].
- Propose Evidence-Based Management Algorithms:
- Systematic Approach: Regular assessments, individualized care plans.
- **Handling Tracheostomized Patients**:
- Close observation of the patient's medical/health status, alertness, and cognition, including the impact of sedation, delirium, and agitation levels on their ability to actively participate.
- Cuff Management: Deflation trials—air flow through and air pressures through upper airway help in increasing sensation and thus reduce aspiration risk.
- Speaking Valves: Facilitate swallowing and vocalization.
- Minimize Risk and Further Complications: Elevating the head of the bed, dental brushing with antiseptic rinse and suctioning; patient mobilization.
- Reduce oral secretions.
- Swallowing maneuvers (e.g., supraglottic maneuver).
- Regular instrumental assessments to assess readiness for oral diet.
- Dislodging of tracheostomy *cannula* during active treatment needs to be mitigated.
- PES (Pharyngeal Electric Stimulation): For treatment of neurogenic dysphagia in stroke, traumatic brain injury, and desensitization following prolonged mechanical ventilation.
- Post-Extubation Dysphagia (PED):
- Specialized Protocols: Early screening post-extubation.

- Emerging Therapies:
- Pharyngeal Electrical Stimulation:
- Mechanism: Enhances neural pathways involved in swallowing.
- Evidence: Shows promise in improving swallowing function.
- Respiratory Muscle Strength Training:
- Mechanism: Strengthens muscles coordinating breathing and swallowing.
- Evidence: May reduce aspiration risk.
- Interdisciplinary Role:
- Speech-Language Pathologists (SLPs): Specialized assessment and therapy.
- Dietitians: Nutritional management tailored to swallowing ability.
- Occupational Therapists: Adaptive techniques for safe feeding.

B. No:

- Action: Initiate oral intake based on tolerance, with regular monitoring. Safe progression of diet to full oral intake.

83.8 Conclusion

Managing swallowing dysfunction in ICU patients is a comprehensive process requiring early recognition, advanced screening techniques, and a multidisciplinary approach. Incorporating detailed risk assessments, utilizing instrumental evaluations like FEES and VFSS, and adopting evidence-based management algorithms are crucial steps. Emerging therapies such as pharyngeal electrical stimulation and respiratory muscle strength training offer promising advancement in treatment. Overcoming barriers through education, protocol adherence, and collaboration enhances patient care. Emphasizing quality-of-life considerations ensures that long-term impacts are addressed, promoting overall well-being and recovery.

Algorithm 83.1: Approach to swallowing dysfunction in the ICU

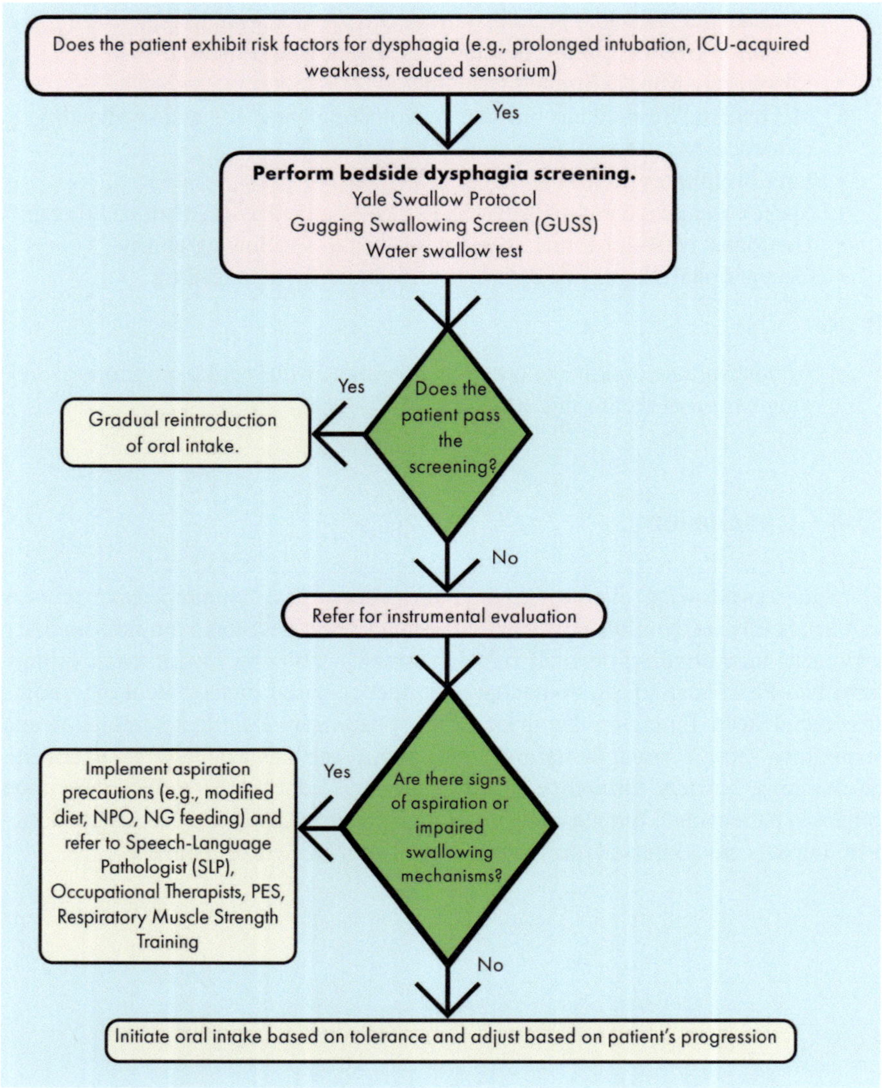

Bibliography

1. Demetriou M, Georgiou AM. Perspective on dysphagia screening, assessment methods, and protocols in intensive care units: an opinion article. Front Hum Neurosci. 2024;18:1375408.
2. Nielsen AH, Winding R, Busk BH, Noe L, Husted B, Kristensen GJ, et al. Nurse-led dysphagia screening in the intensive care unit – an implementation study. Aust Crit Care. 2024;38(1):101100.
3. Trapl M, Enderle P, Nowotny M, Teuschl Y, Matz K, Dachenhausen A, et al. Dysphagia bedside screening for acute-stroke patients: the Gugging Swallowing Screen. Stroke. 2007;38(11):2948–52.
4. Freeman-Sanderson A, Hemsley B, Thompson K, Rogers KD, Knowles S, Hammond NE, et al. Dysphagia in adult intensive care patients: results of a prospective, multicentre binational point prevalence study. Aust Crit Care. 2023;36(6):961–6.

Chapter 84
Approach to Airway Management in the ICU

84.1 Introduction

Airway management is a critical component of intensive care medicine (ICU), where prompt and effective intervention can significantly reduce morbidity and mortality. Patients in the ICU often require airway support due to inadequate oxygenation and ventilation or to protect against aspiration. Managing the airway in critically ill patients presents unique challenges, frequently due to physiological derangements and anatomical complexities. A structured approach—incorporating thorough assessment, preparation, and execution—is essential to optimize outcomes. Multidisciplinary teamwork, with clear communication and designated roles, enhances the efficiency and safety of airway interventions [1, 2] [Ref: Algorithm 84.1].

84.2 Assess Need for Airway Intervention

The initial step is to determine the necessity for airway management. Key considerations include:

- Oxygenation and Ventilation: Assess oxygen saturation (SpO_2), respiratory rate, and effort. Hypoxia ($SpO_2 < 90\%$) or hypercapnia (elevated $PaCO_2$) may necessitate airway intervention.
- Signs of Airway Obstruction: Look for stridor, severe respiratory distress, use of accessory muscles, or altered mental status due to hypoventilation or hypoxia.
- Neurological Status: A Glasgow Coma Scale (GCS) score of less than 8 or absent airway protective reflexes indicates the need for intubation to secure the airway [3].

S. B. Mishra et al., *Mastering ICU Care*,
https://doi.org/10.1007/978-981-95-0179-3_84

84.3 Preoxygenation Techniques

Optimizing preoxygenation is crucial to increase safe apnea time during intubation:

- High-Flow Nasal Oxygen (HFNO): Delivers heated and humidified oxygen at high flow rates (up to 60 L/min), providing apneic oxygenation and improving oxygenation in hypoxic patients.
- Noninvasive Ventilation (NIV): Using continuous positive airway pressure (CPAP) or bilevel positive airway pressure (BiPAP) can enhance preoxygenation, especially in patients with shunt physiology.
- Positive End-Expiratory Pressure (PEEP): Applying PEEP via a tight-fitting mask or circuit maintains alveolar recruitment, improving oxygenation in patients with atelectasis or pulmonary edema [4, 5].

84.4 Assess Risk Using Updated Algorithms

Risk stratification guides the airway management plan:

- MACOCHA Score: Incorporates factors like Mallampati score, obstructive sleep apnea, reduced cervical mobility, limited mouth opening, coma, hypoxemia, and anesthetist's experience to predict difficult intubation in ICU patients.
- American Society of Anesthesiologists (ASA) 2022 Guidelines: Provide updated recommendations on difficult airway management, emphasizing the importance of planning for both anticipated and unanticipated difficulties [6].

84.5 Physiologically Difficult Airway Management

Managing the physiologically difficult airway requires consideration of the patient's hemodynamic status and oxygenation:

- Hemodynamic Stability: Hypotension increases the risk of peri-intubation cardiac arrest. Pre-intubation optimization with fluid resuscitation and vasopressors may be necessary.
- Oxygenation: Severe hypoxemia increases the risk of desaturation during intubation. Enhanced preoxygenation techniques and apneic oxygenation strategies are essential.
- Medication Selection: Choose induction agents that minimize cardiovascular depression (e.g., ketamine) [7, 8].

84.6 Multidisciplinary Teamwork

Effective airway management in the ICU relies on a coordinated team approach:

- Designated Roles: Assign specific tasks to team members (e.g., primary operator, assistant, medication administration, monitoring).
- Shared Mental Model: Ensure all team members understand the plan, potential complications, and backup strategies.
- Communication: Use closed-loop communication to confirm tasks and relay critical information.

84.7 Management Based on Risk Assessment

Low-Risk Airway (Score 0–1)

- Technique: Perform rapid sequence intubation (RSI) with a videolaryngoscope and stylet.

Moderate-Risk Airway (Score 2–3)

- Pre-procedure Optimization: Address hypotension or hypoxemia before intubation using fluids, vasopressors, NIV, HFNO, and PEEP.
- Technique: Use RSI with a videolaryngoscope and stylet, with adjunct devices readily available.
- Key Considerations: Monitor closely for difficulty during intubation; have backup devices and plans prepared.

High-Risk Airway (Score 4–5)

- Delayed Sequence Intubation (DSI): Use sedation (e.g., ketamine) to facilitate preoxygenation in agitated or hypoxic patients.
- Team Coordination: Involve the most experienced personnel; prepare all necessary equipment, including tools for front-of-neck access (FONA).
- Rescue Plan: Ensure availability of advanced airway devices and have a clear plan for failed intubation.

84.8 Rescue Oxygenation

In cases of failed intubation or difficulty maintaining oxygenation:

- Second-Generation Supraglottic Airway Devices: Utilize devices like the i-gel or laryngeal mask airway (LMA) Supreme, which provide better seal pressures and allow for gastric access compared to traditional supraglottic airways.

- Advantages: Improved ventilation, reduced risk of aspiration, and the possibility of intubation through the device.
- Reassessment: If ventilation remains inadequate, reassess technique and consider alternative approaches or equipment.

84.9 Recognize and manage a CICO Situation

A "Cannot Intubate, Cannot Oxygenate" scenario requires immediate action:

- Identification: Failed intubation after multiple attempts, inability to oxygenate with face mask or supraglottic device, and persistent hypoxia ($SpO_2 < 80\%$).
- Preparation: Early recognition and readiness to proceed to emergency front-of-neck access.

84.10 Perform Front-of-Neck Airway (FONA)

Scalpel-Bougie-Tube Technique

1. Identify the Cricothyroid Membrane:
    - Palpate between the thyroid cartilage and cricoid cartilage.
2. Stabilize the Larynx:
    - Use the nondominant hand to hold the larynx firmly.
3. Make a Horizontal Incision:
    - Use a scalpel to make a transverse incision through the skin and cricothyroid membrane.
4. Insert the Bougie:
    - Direct the bougie through the incision into the trachea.
5. Railroad the Endotracheal Tube:
    - Advance a size 6.0–7.0 mm ETT over the bougie into the trachea.
6. Confirm Placement:
    - Verify tube placement with capnography and auscultation.

- Rationale: This technique provides a rapid and reliable method to establish a definitive airway when conventional methods fail.

84.11 Post-Intubation Care

Proper management after intubation is essential to prevent complications:

- Confirm Tube Placement:
- Use waveform capnography as the gold standard.
- Auscultate bilateral breath sounds and observe chest rise.
- Secure the ETT:
- Ensure the tube is properly secured to prevent displacement.
- Ventilation Settings:
- Adjust ventilator settings based on arterial blood gases and the patient's condition.
- Recruitment Maneuvers:
- Perform as needed to improve oxygenation, especially in patients with atelectasis.
- Monitoring:
- Continuous monitoring of vital signs, oxygenation, and ventilation parameters.

84.12 Complication Management

Preventing and managing complications is crucial during airway management:

- Aspiration:
- Preoxygenate and consider rapid sequence induction to minimize risk.
- Use cricoid pressure if indicated (controversial and based on provider preference).
- Hypoxia:
- Employ effective preoxygenation strategies.
- Minimize apnea time during intubation attempts.
- Cardiovascular Collapse:
- Anticipate hemodynamic changes; prepare vasopressors.
- Use induction agents with minimal cardiovascular effects.

84.13 Regional Challenges and Solutions

In resource-limited settings, adapt strategies to available resources:

- Equipment Limitations:
- Use available alternative devices, such as improvising with standard oxygen masks for preoxygenation.

84.14 Conclusion

A structured and systematic approach to airway management in the ICU is essential for patient safety and optimal outcomes. Incorporating thorough assessment, advanced preoxygenation techniques, and risk stratification allows for tailored strategies to address both anatomical and physiological challenges. Effective multidisciplinary teamwork and communication enhance the success of airway interventions. Staying updated with current guidelines and algorithms, along with regular training and preparedness, ensures that clinicians are equipped to handle both anticipated and unanticipated difficulties. In all settings, including resource-limited environments, adapting strategies to available resources and focusing on fundamental principles remain paramount.

Algorithm 84.1: Approach to airway management in the ICU

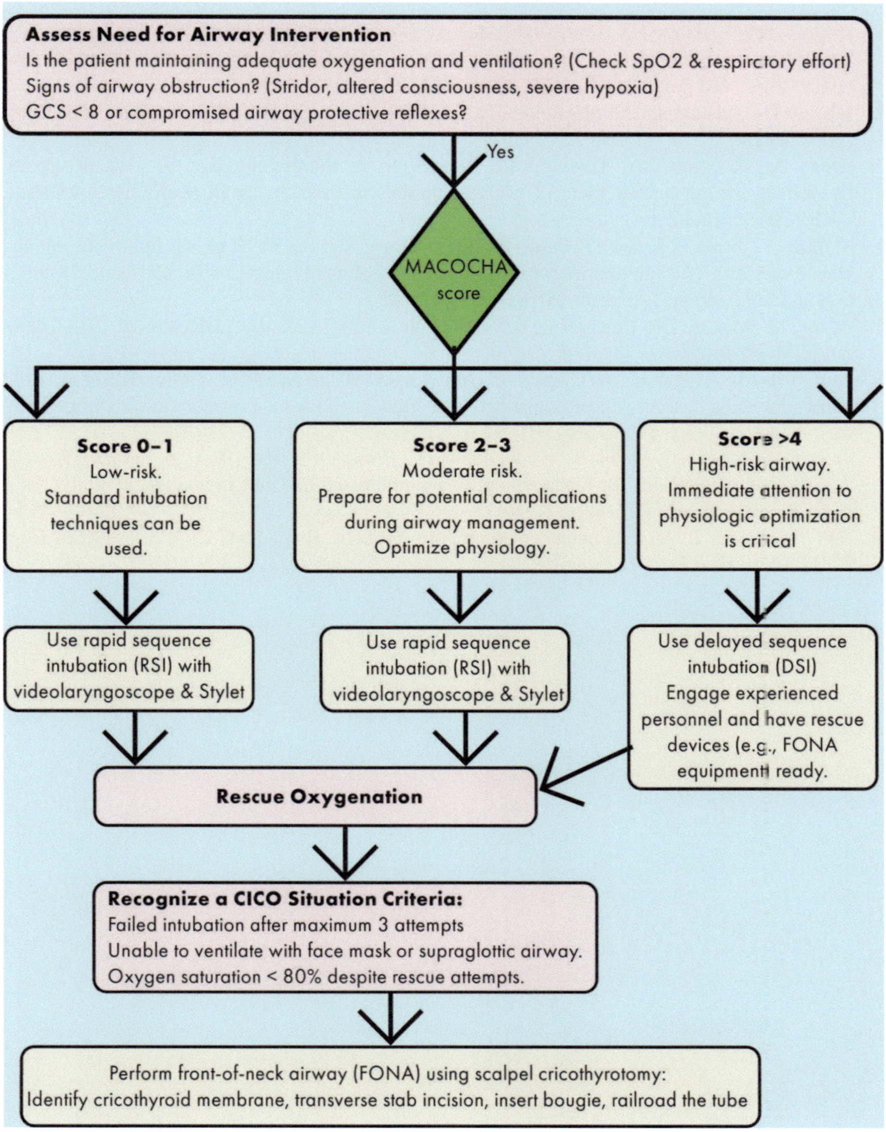

Bibliography

1. Admass BA, Endalew NS, Tawye HY, Melesse DY, Workie MM, Filatie TD. Evidence-based airway management protocol for a critical ill patient in medical intensive care unit: systematic review. Ann Med Surg (Lond). 2022;80:104284.
2. Jabaley CS. Managing the physiologically difficult airway in critically ill adults. Crit Care. 2023;27(1):91.
3. Higgs A, McGrath BA, Goddard C, Rangasami J, Suntharalingam G, Gale R, et al. Guidelines for the management of tracheal intubation in critically ill adults. Br J Anaesth. 2018;120(2):323–52.
4. Myatra SN, Shah A, Kundra P, Patwa A, Ramkumar V, Divatia JV, et al. All India difficult airway association 2016 guidelines for the management of unanticipated difficult tracheal intubation in adults. Indian J Anaesth. 2016;60(12):885–98.
5. Price TM, McCoy EP. Emergency front of neck access in airway management. BJA Educ. 2019;19(8):246–53.
6. Apfelbaum JL, Hagberg CA, Connis RT, Abdelmalak BB, Agarkar M, Dutton RP, et al. 2022 American Society of Anesthesiologists practice guidelines for management of the difficult airway. Anesthesiology. 2022;136(1):31–81.
7. Frerk C, Mitchell VS, McNarry AF, Mendonca C, Bhagrath R, Patel A, et al. Difficult Airway Society 2015 guidelines for management of unanticipated difficult intubation in adults. Br J Anaesth. 2015;115(6):827–48.
8. Natt B, Mosier J. Airway management in the critically ill patient. Curr Anesthesiol Rep. 2021;11(2):116–27.

Chapter 85
Approach to Pneumonia in the ICU

85.1 Introduction

Pneumonia remains a leading cause of morbidity and mortality among critically ill patients in the ICU. Early detection and appropriate therapeutic interventions are essential to optimize patient outcomes. Employing structured diagnostic criteria—such as those recommended by the Centers for Disease Control and Prevention (CDC) for ventilator-associated pneumonia (VAP) and other ICU-related pulmonary infections—helps clinicians differentiate VAP from other respiratory conditions and ensures consistency in clinical assessment and management strategies [1–3] [Ref: Algorithm 85.1].

The approach to pneumonia in the ICU involves:

- Differentiating infectious from noninfectious causes of respiratory symptoms.
- Categorizing the pneumonia type (community-acquired vs. nosocomial).
- Tailoring management based on clinical context and multidrug-resistant (MDR) pathogens risk.
- Implementing prevention strategies to reduce incidence.

85.2 Initial Assessment: Suspicion of Pneumonia

Patients presenting with fever, cough, dyspnea, purulent respiratory secretions, or a new infiltrate on chest imaging should prompt suspicion of pneumonia. However, these symptoms are nonspecific and may overlap with noninfectious conditions. Utilizing standardized surveillance criteria aids in accurate diagnosis. Early identification of the cause is crucial to avoid unnecessary antibiotics and promptly initiate appropriate therapy [4–6].

S. B. Mishra et al., *Mastering ICU Care*,
https://doi.org/10.1007/978-981-95-0179-3_85

85.3 Rule Out Non-Infectious Causes

- Noninfectious conditions like atelectasis, acute respiratory distress syndrome (ARDS), pulmonary embolism, or pulmonary edema can mimic pneumonia. Identifying these is critical as their treatment differs significantly.
- Approach: Use clinical judgment alongside diagnostic tools such as chest imaging, D-dimer tests, echocardiography, and biomarkers like procalcitonin to differentiate infectious and noninfectious causes. Advanced imaging techniques like lung ultrasound provide rapid bedside evaluation. A negative infectious workup should lead to reconsidering these diagnoses.

85.4 Timing of Symptoms

Community-Acquired pneumonia (CAP) vs. Nosocomial/Healthcare-Associated Pneumonia (HCAP)

- <48 h After Admission: Pneumonia developing within 48 h is classified as community-acquired pneumonia (CAP), typically caused by pathogens acquired outside the healthcare setting [7, 8].
- >48 h After Admission: Pneumonia occurring after 48 h is considered nosocomial. This includes hospital-acquired pneumonia (HAP) and ventilator-associated pneumonia (VAP), which are more likely to involve MDR pathogens.

85.5 Diagnostic Workup

For all suspected pneumonia cases in the ICU, a thorough diagnostic evaluation is necessary:

Gram stain and culture of respiratory secretions, along with blood cultures, should be obtained before starting antibiotics in select high-risk cases. These include patients with severe CAP, those receiving empirical therapy for *Pseudomonas aeruginosa* or Methicillin-Resistant Staphylococcus Aureus (MRSA) individuals with prior infections due to these organisms, and patients who have received parenteral antibiotics within the past 90 days [9].

Severe community-acquired pneumonia is identified by clinical indicators reflecting significant physiological compromise. A diagnosis is made when one high-risk feature or three or more moderate-risk features are observed.

High-Risk Features (Major Criteria):

- Presence of septic shock that mandates vasopressor administration.
- Acute respiratory failure requiring initiation of mechanical ventilation.

Moderate-Risk Features (Minor Criteria):

- Rapid breathing with respiratory rate > 30/min.
- Oxygenation impairment with a PaO_2/FiO_2 ratio below 250.
- Imaging showing infiltrates across multiple lobes.
- Changes in mental status, such as confusion or disorientation.
- Elevated urea levels (BUN >20 mg/dL), indicating renal involvement.
- Low white cell count (<4000 cells/mm^3), suggesting immune suppression.
- Reduced platelet count (<100,000/mm^3), reflecting hematologic dysfunction.
- Core body temperature below 36.8 °C, indicating hypothermia.
- Low blood pressure necessitating fluid resuscitation.

This scoring framework assists in identifying patients who may require intensive care admission and aggressive intervention.

- Blood Cultures: Essential to identify bacteremia or sepsis. Obtain two sets.
- Sputum Culture: For non-intubated patients to identify the causative organism.
- Endotracheal Aspirates: For intubated patients, noninvasive methods like endotracheal aspirates (colony forming unit 10^5 is considered significant) are recommended over invasive procedures like bronchoalveolar lavage (BAL—10^4 colony-forming unit is significant) unless clinically justified. This aligns with recent recommendations favoring less invasive diagnostics for suspected HAP/VAP. Protected specimen brush is another method for obtaining culture (10^3 colony-forming unit is significant).
- Chest Imaging: Chest X-rays are first-line; CT scans may assess complications like empyema, abscesses, or ARDS.
- Advanced Imaging: Lung ultrasound is valuable for rapid bedside differentiation between infectious and noninfectious causes.
- Biomarkers: Procalcitonin aids in distinguishing bacterial infections from other inflammatory causes.
- Urinary Antigen Tests: Useful for detecting *Legionella* and *Pneumococcus* in severe CAP.
- Viral PCR: Consider if a viral etiology (e.g., influenza, SARS-CoV-2) is suspected based on clinical or epidemiological factors.

A sterile culture of respiratory secretions in the absence of a new antibiotic in the past 72 h generally rules out bacterial pneumonia, but viral or *Legionella* infection can be possible.

HCAP: is suspected if the patient has a radiographic infiltrate that is new or progressive, along with new onset of fever, purulent sputum, leukocytosis, and decline in oxygenation. The findings without chest infiltrates on radiography should be considered as tracheobronchitis.

85.6 Risk Assessment for Multidrug-Resistant (MDR) Pathogens

- Risk Factors: Prior antibiotic use (usually in the last 90 days), prolonged hospitalization (5 days or more), recent healthcare exposure (hospitalization for 2 days or more in the preceding 90 days), immunosuppression, severe comorbidities, or local epidemiology indicating a high prevalence of MDR organisms, chronic dialysis within 30 days.

85.7 Management

Community-Acquired Pneumonia

Severe CAP Without MRSA or *Pseudomonas* Risk.

For patients with severe CAP who do not have risk factors for MRSA or *Pseudomonas aeruginosa*, empiric therapy should consist of a β-lactam in combination with a macrolide. Suitable β-lactams include:

- Ampicillin-sulbactam (1.5–3 g IV every 6 h).
- Cefotaxime (1–2 g IV every 8 h).
- Ceftriaxone (1–2 g IV once daily).

Macrolide options include:

- Azithromycin (500 mg once daily).
- Clarithromycin (500 mg twice daily).

If macrolides are contraindicated, levofloxacin (750 mg daily) or moxifloxacin (400 mg daily) may be considered as alternatives. However, to preserve fluoroquinolones for use in drug-resistant tuberculosis, they are typically avoided in our setting. In such cases, doxycycline (100 mg twice daily) is a suitable option.

Empirical MRSA Coverage.

When MRSA is suspected, initiate one of the following:

- Vancomycin: 15 mg/kg IV every 12 h, with dosing adjusted by therapeutic drug monitoring.
- Linezolid: 600 mg IV or oral every 12 h.

Empirical *Pseudomonas* Coverage.

In patients at risk for *Pseudomonas aeruginosa*, select one of these agents:

- Piperacillin-tazobactam: 4.5 g every 6 h.
- Cefepime: 2 g every 8 h.
- Ceftazidime: 2 g every 8 h.
- Aztreonam: 2 g every 8 h.
- Meropenem: 1 g every 8 h.
- Imipenem: 500 mg every 6 h.

De-escalation to pathogen-directed therapy is recommended as soon as microbiological results become available to reduce unnecessary broad-spectrum exposure.

Additional Considerations

- Corticosteroids are reserved for patients with ongoing septic shock and are not part of routine management.
- Oseltamivir may be added if influenza is suspected based on clinical signs or seasonal trends.
- Antibiotic therapy duration should be guided by clinical recovery and should not be less than 5 days.

Healthcare-Associated Pneumonia

In HCAP, the likelihood of multidrug-resistant pathogens is higher, particularly in those with healthcare exposure or other risk factors. Initial treatment should offer broad-spectrum coverage tailored to the local antibiogram and commonly includes agents effective against:

- *Pseudomonas aeruginosa.*
- *Klebsiella pneumoniae.*
- *Acinetobacter* species.
- Methicillin-resistant *Staphylococcus aureus* (MRSA).

Appropriate empirical agents may involve:

- Carbapenems.
- Polymyxins.
- Ceftazidime-avibactam.
- Vancomycin.
- Additional agents as guided by culture results and institutional resistance data.

85.7.1 Day 3 Reassessment of Antibiotics

- Evaluate Clinical Improvement: Reduction in leukocyte count, temperature normalization, and improved oxygenation indicate a positive response.
- De-escalation: Tailor antibiotics based on culture results.
- If No Improvement:
- Escalate Antibiotics: Consider broader-spectrum agents if the patient deteriorates.
- Reassess Diagnosis: Investigate complications like empyema, abscess, or alternative diagnoses.
- Additional Diagnostics: Repeat cultures, imaging, or consider bronchoscopy to identify resistant or atypical pathogens.

Duration 5–7 days

85.7.2 Continuation of Therapy

If the patient shows improvement with a reduction in leukocyte count by $\geq 2 \times 10^9$/L and clinical stabilization, continue the current antibiotic regimen for the recommended duration.

85.7.3 Escalation of Care

Patients failing to improve despite appropriate antibiotics require thorough reassessment:

- Repeat Cultures and Imaging: Identify persistent or new pathogens.
- Evaluate Alternative Diagnoses: Consider fungal or viral infections, or noninfectious causes like malignancy.

85.7.4 Special Populations

- Immunocompromised Patients: May present atypically and are at higher risk for opportunistic infections. Empirical therapy should cover a broader range of pathogens, including fungi and viruses.
- Patients with Severe Comorbidities: Conditions like chronic lung disease or renal failure may require adjusted dosing or alternative therapies.

85.7.5 Outcomes and Metrics

Track outcomes to evaluate the effectiveness of implemented strategies:

- Mortality Rates: Monitor pneumonia-associated mortality in the ICU.
- Duration of Ventilation: Assess the length of mechanical ventilation required.
- ICU Length of Stay: Evaluate pneumonia's impact on ICU resources.
- Incidence of VAP/HAP: Regular surveillance aids in quality improvement.
- Antibiotic Usage Patterns: Monitoring supports antibiotic stewardship efforts.

85.8 Conclusion

A systematic and standardized approach to pneumonia in the ICU enhances patient care by ensuring accurate diagnosis, appropriate management, and effective prevention strategies. Key components include:

- Differentiating infectious from noninfectious causes early using clinical assessment, biomarkers, and imaging.
- Classifying pneumonia into CAP or nosocomial based on symptom timing and applying CDC-defined surveillance criteria.
- Assessing MDR pathogen risk using structured frameworks and tailoring empirical therapy accordingly, guided by local antibiograms.
- Implementing antibiotic stewardship principles, including de-escalation based on microbiological data and clinical response.
- Employing prevention strategies and strict infection control protocols to reduce pneumonia incidence.
- Evaluating treatment response using standardized criteria and adjusting management as needed.
- Considering special populations who may require different management approaches.
- Tracking outcomes and metrics to continuously improve care quality and patient outcomes.

By integrating these practices, healthcare providers can reduce morbidity, mortality, and the risk of antibiotic resistance associated with pneumonia in critically ill patients.

Algorithm 85.1: Approach to pneumonia in the ICU

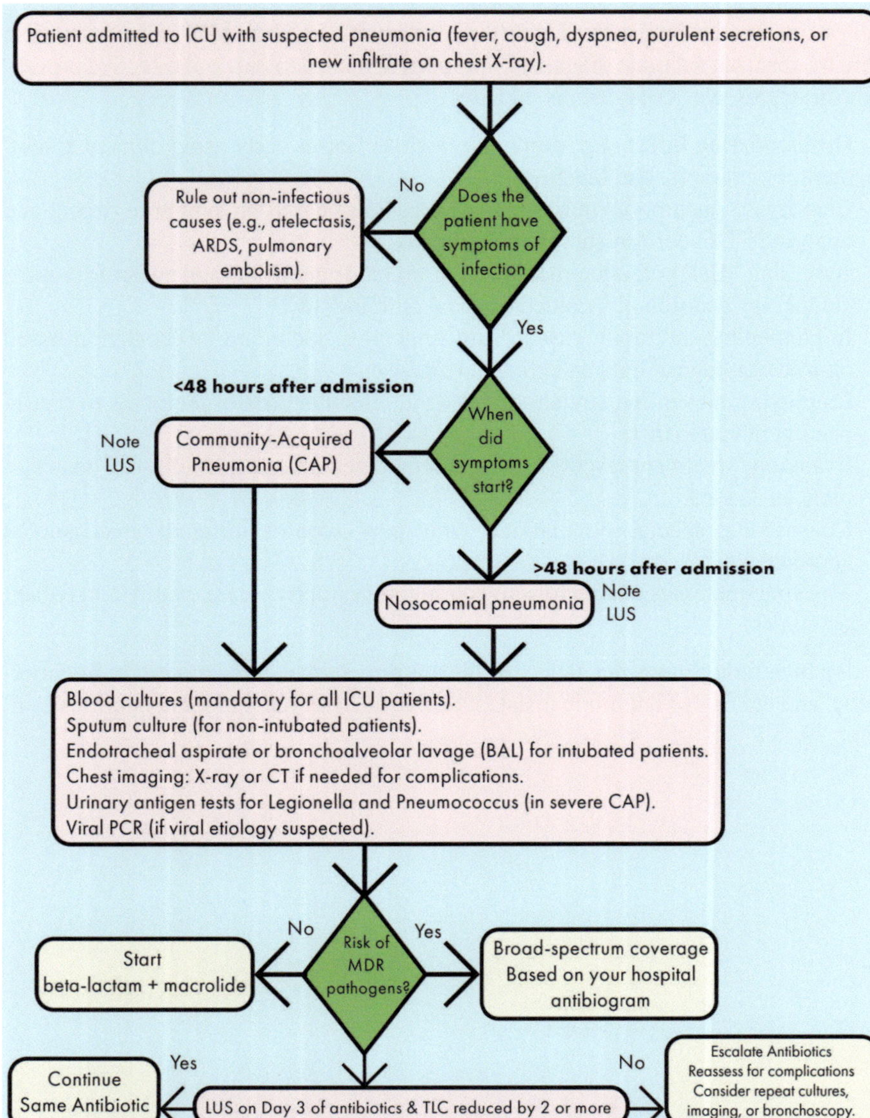

Bibliography

1. American Thoracic Society, Inefectious Diseases Society of America. Guidelines for the management of adults with hospital-acquired, ventilator-associated, and healthcare-associated pneumonia. Am J Respir Crit Care Med. 2005;171(4):388–416.
2. Gupta D, Agarwal R, Aggarwal AN, Singh N, Mishra N, Khilnani GC, et al. Guidelines for diagnosis and management of community- and hospital-acquired pneumonia in adults: joint ICS/NCCP(I) recommendations. Lung India. 2012;29(Suppl 2):S27–62.
3. Thimmaiah G, Pandey N, Prinja S, Jain K, Biswal M, Agarwal R, et al. Ventilator-associated pneumonia – what price does the public health system pay? Lung India. 2024;41(4):278–83.
4. Kalil AC, Metersky ML, Klompas M, Muscedere J, Sweeney DA, Palmer LB, et al. Management of adults with hospital-acquired and Ventilator-associated pneumonia: 2016 clinical practice guidelines by the Infectious Diseases Society of America and the American Thoracic Society. Clin Infect Dis. 2016;63(5):e61–e111.
5. Torres A, Niederman MS, Chastre J, Ewig S, Fernandez-Vandellos P, Hanberger H, et al. International ERS/ESICM/ESCMID/ALAT guidelines for the management of hospital-acquired pneumonia and ventilator-associated pneumonia: guidelines for the management of hospital-acquired pneumonia (HAP)/ventilator-associated pneumonia (VAP) of the European Respiratory Society (ERS), European Society of Intensive Care Medicine (ESICM), European Society of Clinical Microbiology and Infectious Diseases (ESCMID) and Asociacion Latinoamericana del Torax (ALAT). Eur Respir J. 2017;50(3):1700582.
6. Torres A, Niederman MS, Chastre J, Ewig S, Fernandez-Vandellos P, Hanberger H, et al. Summary of the international clinical guidelines for the management of hospital-acquired and ventilator-acquired pneumonia. ERJ Open Res. 2018;4(2):00028-2018.
7. Sharma BB, Singh V. Indian pneumonia guidelines. Lung India. 2012;29(4):307–8.
8. Martin-Loeches I, Torres A, Nagavci B, Aliberti S, Antonelli M, Bassetti M, et al. ERS/ESICM/ESCMID/ALAT guidelines for the management of severe community-acquired pneumonia. Eur Respir J. 2023;61(4):615–32.
9. Mandell LA. Severe community-acquired pneumonia (CAP) and the Infectious Diseases Society of America/American Thoracic Society CAP guidelines prediction rule: validated or not. Clin Infect Dis. 2009;48(4):386–8. https://doi.org/10.1086/596308.

Chapter 86
Approach to Pleural Effusion in the ICU

86.1 Introduction

Pleural effusion, an abnormal accumulation of fluid in the pleural space, is a common and potentially serious condition in ICU settings. Studies indicate a prevalence of up to 60% among critically ill patients, with significant associations with mortality. It arises from diverse causes such as infection, malignancy, or systemic illnesses, often presenting with dyspnea, hypoxia, and reduced breath sounds. Management involves prompt identification, accurate diagnosis, and tailored interventions to mitigate adverse outcomes [1, 2] [Ref: Algorithm 86.1].

86.2 Initial Assessment

- Clinical Presentation: Symptoms include dyspnea and hypoxia. Signs include diminished breath sounds, or dullness to percussion, signaling pleural effusion.
- Early recognition is essential to prevent complications such as respiratory failure, empyema, or tension hydrothorax [3].

86.3 Confirmation of Pleural Effusion

- Imaging:
- Thoracic Ultrasound (TUS): Preferred modality in the ICU due to its bedside applicability and superior sensitivity over chest X-rays. Detection rates exceed those of chest radiography and rival CT scans, making it indispensable. Real-time

S. B. Mishra et al., *Mastering ICU Care*,
https://doi.org/10.1007/978-981-95-0179-3_86

visualization facilitates rapid diagnosis and guided interventions, especially in mechanically ventilated patients [4].
- Significant Effusion: Defined by a pleural fluid depth ≥2 cm on TUS with adverse respiratory effects.

86.4 Evaluation of Effusion Type

- Classification: Use Light's Criteria to differentiate transudative and exudative effusions:
- Pleural protein/serum protein ratio >0.5.
- Pleural LDH/serum LDH ratio >0.6.
- Pleural LDH > 2/3 the upper limit of normal serum LDH.
- Advanced Diagnostics:
- Pleural fluid elastance and Starling's equation help in understanding pleural fluid dynamics.
- Mechanical ventilation complicates effusion diagnosis; strategies include dynamic TUS and pleural pressure monitoring.

86.5 Management Based on Effusion Type

- Transudative Effusions: Commonly linked to systemic conditions like heart failure or cirrhosis.
- Management: Address the underlying condition rather than direct drainage.
- Exudative Effusions: Associated with infections, malignancy, or inflammation.
- Actions: Diagnostic thoracentesis for further analysis; therapeutic drainage if indicated [5].

86.6 Therapeutic Interventions

- Indications: Symptomatic relief or unclear etiology.
- Guidelines:
- pH < 7.2 or Glucose <60 mg/dL: Suggests infection, requiring immediate drainage.
- Empyema: Purulent fluid mandates chest tube placement.
- Advanced Techniques:
- Intrapleural Fibrinolytics: Effective for complex parapneumonic effusions and empyemas, reducing surgical referrals.
- Early Drainage: Improves oxygenation and PaO_2/FiO_2 ratios [6].

86.7 Special Situations and Complications

- Hemothorax:
- Large-bore drainage for significant blood loss (>1500 mL initially or >200 mL/h).
- Prevents complications like fibrothorax and hemodynamic instability.
- Chylothorax:
- Milky fluid appearance with elevated triglycerides confirms the diagnosis.
- Managed with drainage and nutritional modifications, including low-fat diets or parenteral nutrition.
- Malignant Effusions:
- Recurrent effusions may require pleurodesis, indwelling catheters, or repeated thoracentesis.
- Focus on palliative measures to enhance quality of life.
- Complications of Drainage:
- Includes infection or visceral injury. Strategies to mitigate risks involve ultrasound-guided procedures and aseptic techniques [7].

86.8 Pathophysiology Insights

- Fluid Turnover:
- Governed by hydrostatic and oncotic pressures across the pleural membrane.
- Imbalances lead to effusion formation, with critical contributions from systemic and localized factors.

86.9 Multidisciplinary Collaboration

- Complex cases (e.g., empyema or malignancy) may require input from thoracic surgeons, interventional radiologists, or pulmonologists to ensure optimal outcomes.

86.10 Prognostic Implications

- Pleural effusion complicates ICU prognostication by increasing mortality risk and impeding mechanical ventilation weaning. Its presence underscores the need for vigilant monitoring and timely management.

86.11 Conclusion

Effective management of pleural effusion in the ICU demands a structured approach encompassing early recognition, precise diagnosis, and evidence-based interventions. Incorporating advanced imaging modalities, multidisciplinary collaboration, and updated management strategies ensures optimal patient outcomes while minimizing complications.

Algorithm 86.1: Approach to pleural effusion in the ICU

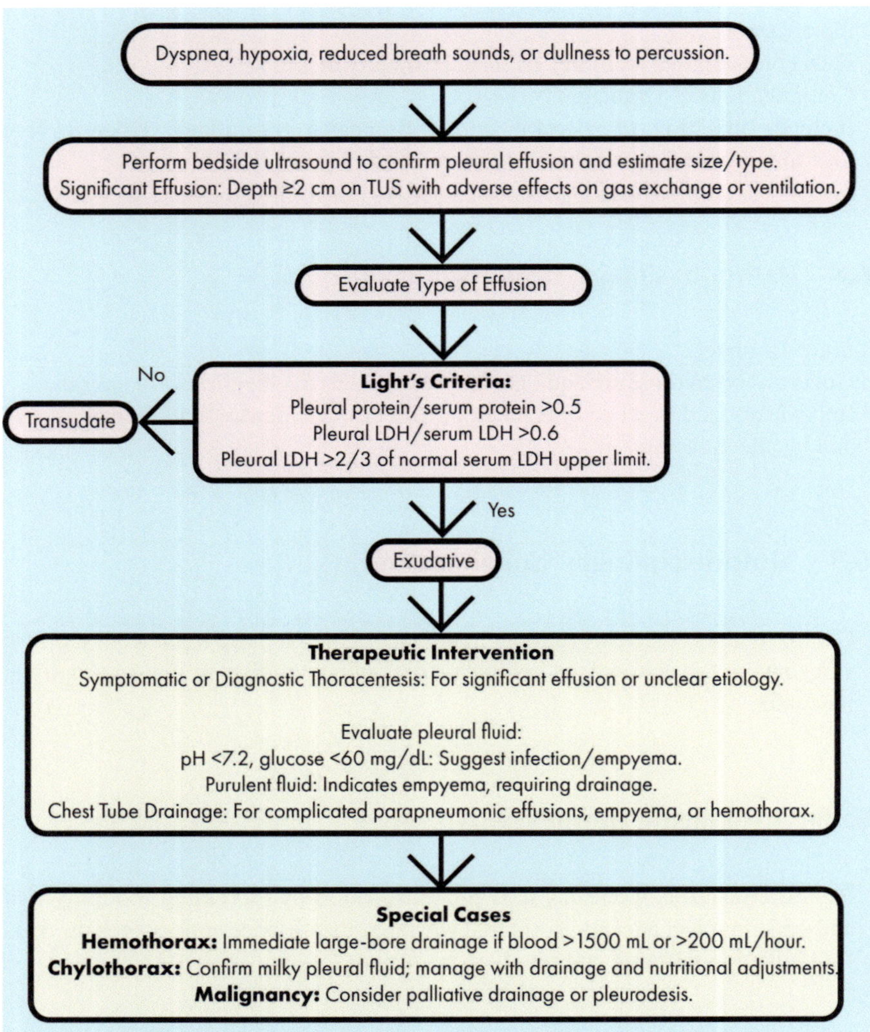

Bibliography

1. Fysh ETH, Smallbone P, Mattock N, McCloskey C, Litton E, Wibrow B, et al. Clinically significant pleural effusion in intensive care: a prospective multicenter cohort study. Crit Care Explor. 2020;2(1):e0070.
2. Bediwy AS, Al-Biltagi M, Saeed NK, Bediwy HA, Elbeltagi R. Pleural effusion in critically ill patients and intensive care setting. World J Clin Cases. 2023;11(5):989–99.
3. Hu K, Chopra A, Kurman J, Huggins JT. Management of complex pleural disease in the critically ill patient. J Thorac Dis. 2021;13(8):5205–22.
4. Maslove DM, Chen BT, Wang H, Kuschner WG. The diagnosis and management of pleural effusions in the ICU. J Intensive Care Med. 2013;28(1):24–36.
5. Paramasivam E, Bodenham A. Pleural fluid collections in critically ill patients. Contin Educ Anaesth Crit Care Pain. 2007;7(1):10–4.
6. Bates D, Yang N, Bailey M, Bellomo R. Prevalence, characteristics, drainage and outcome of radiologically diagnosed pleural effusions in critically ill patients. Crit Care Resusc. 2020;22(1):45–52.
7. Brogi E, Gargani L, Bignami E, Barbariol F, Marra A, Forfori F, et al. Thoracic ultrasound for pleural effusion in the intensive care unit: a narrative review from diagnosis to treatment. Crit Care. 2017;21(1):325.

Chapter 87
Approach to Empyema in the ICU

87.1 Introduction

Empyema, defined as the accumulation of pus within the pleural cavity, is a severe complication of infections such as pneumonia or sepsis. It is associated with significant morbidity and requires prompt identification and management to prevent progression and complications like fibrothorax or respiratory failure. The management of empyema in the intensive care unit (ICU) necessitates a multidisciplinary approach involving early recognition, accurate staging, and appropriate therapeutic interventions tailored to patient-specific factors [1, 2] [Ref: Algorithm 87.1].

87.2 Etiology and Risk Factors

Understanding the etiology and risk factors is crucial for early detection and prevention of empyema.

- Poor Oral Hygiene and Aspiration Disorders: Aspiration of oropharyngeal secretions containing anaerobic bacteria can lead to empyema, especially in patients with poor oral hygiene or swallowing disorders.
- Chronic Diseases: Conditions such as diabetes mellitus and cardiovascular disease compromise immune function, increasing susceptibility to infections that can progress to empyema.
- Immunosuppression: Patients with HIV, malignancies, or those on immunosuppressive therapy are at higher risk due to decreased immune defenses. In immunocompromised patients, fungi like *Candida* and *Aspergillus* species can cause empyema.

S. B. Mishra et al., *Mastering ICU Care*,
https://doi.org/10.1007/978-981-95-0179-3_87

- Hospital-Acquired Causes: Post-thoracic surgery complications and infections with methicillin-resistant *Staphylococcus aureus* (MRSA) significantly contribute to empyema in hospitalized patients.

87.3 Bacteriology

A thorough understanding of the microbiological agents involved is essential for effective treatment.

- Anaerobic Organisms: These are frequently implicated in empyema, particularly in cases associated with aspiration and poor dental hygiene. Anaerobes have a higher incidence in empyema compared to other pleural infections.
- Fungal Empyema: In immunocompromised patients, fungi like *Candida* and *Aspergillus* species can cause empyema, requiring antifungal therapy.
- Advanced Diagnostic Techniques: DNA amplification methods, such as polymerase chain reaction (PCR), enhance pathogen identification, especially for fastidious organisms not easily detected by conventional cultures [3].

87.4 Staging/Classification

Empyema due to pneumonia can be classified into three stages based on the progression of the disease:

- Exudative stage/Stage 1: Free-flowing exudate and does not contain bacteria per se. White cell count is usually low, and lactate dehydrogenase (LDH) level is less than half of the serum levels. pH and the glucose levels are mostly normal.
- Fibrinopurulent Stage/Stage 2: Bacterial invasion into the pleural space leading to triggering of the immune cascade resulting in fibrin deposition and loculation. In this stage there is usually a drop in pH to <7.2 and glucose levels below 40 mg/dL. The LDH levels are unusually high (>1000 IU/L). Presence of pus in this stage is called empyema.
- Chronic Organizing Stage/Stage 3: Fibrosis sets in leading to pleural fibrotic cortex formation leading to impaired lung function and prevention of re-expansion.

87.5 Laboratory

Send for complete blood count, liver function tests, renal function tests, coagulation studies, pleural fluid analysis (cytology, pH, protein levels, LDH, adenosine deaminase levels, Gram's stain, cultures). Blood cultures (depending if patient is in sepsis). Tracheal/sputum cultures should also be sent.

87.6 Imaging and Diagnostics

Accurate imaging is critical for diagnosis, staging, and guiding interventions.

- Thoracic Ultrasound (TUS): TUS is instrumental in assessing pleural effusions, detecting loculations, and guiding pleural procedures with real-time imaging.
- Computed Tomography (CT) Scan: Provides detailed images of the pleural space, identifying loculations, pleural thickening, and underlying lung pathology.
- Positron Emission Tomography (PET) and Magnetic Resonance Imaging (MRI): Recommended for complex cases, PET scans help differentiate empyema from malignancy, while MRI offers superior soft tissue contrast without radiation exposure.

87.7 Treatment Strategies

Advancements in medical and surgical therapies have improved empyema management.

- Antimicrobial Therapy: Initiate broad-spectrum antibiotics covering aerobic and anaerobic bacteria, adjusting based on culture results. Consider MRSA coverage in hospital-acquired cases.
- Intrapleural Fibrinolytic Therapy: The combination of tissue plasminogen activator (tPA) and deoxyribonuclease (DNase) has shown efficacy in breaking down fibrinous septations, enhancing chest tube drainage in complex cases [4].
- Tube Thoracostomy: Pleural fluid LDH >1000 IU/L, glucose <40 mg/dL, or a loculated pleural effusion suggests that the pleural effusion is unlikely to resolve with antibiotics alone and thus one should aim for tube thoracostomy.
- Minimally Invasive Techniques:
- Video-Assisted Thoracoscopic Surgery (VATS): Allows for direct visualization, drainage, and debridement with less morbidity compared to open thoracotomy, especially beneficial in chronic empyema.
- Vacuum-Assisted Closure (VAC): Used in managing chronic empyema cavities, promoting granulation tissue formation and reducing infection risk.

87.8 Special Situations and Considerations

- Post-Pneumonectomy Empyema: Management includes individualized open surgical techniques such as open window thoracostomy or muscle flap transposition to obliterate the empyema cavity.
- Stage-Specific Management.

Empyema progresses through three stages, each requiring tailored interventions.

87.8.1 Exudative Stage

- Treatment:
- Initiate broad-spectrum antibiotics with anaerobic coverage. Antibiotic should be based on patient's history and clinical condition and local antimicrobial resistance pattern.

For community acquired, second- or third-generation cephalosporin (e.g., Ceftriaxone) plus Metronidazole or Aminopenicillin plus beta-lactamase inhibitor (Ampicillin sulbactam).

For hospital acquired/post-procedural—methicillin-resistant *Staphylococcus aureus* (MRSA) and *Pseudomonas* cover should be given (e.g., Cefepime plus vancomycin and metronidazole or vancomycin plus piperacillin tazobactam).

The antibiotic should be de-escalated according to culture sensitivity data as soon as it is available.

- Close monitoring: Invasive drainage may not be required if the effusion is small and the patient is stable.

87.8.2 Fibrinopurulent Stage

- Treatment:
- Continue targeted antimicrobial therapy.
- Drainage Options:
- Image-Guided Chest Tube Placement: First-line intervention for draining loculated fluid.
- Intrapleural Fibrinolytics: Administer tPA and DNase to enhance drainage in complex loculations.
- VATS: Considered if chest tube drainage fails or the patient deteriorates.
- Rationale: Effective drainage prevents progression to the chronic stage and facilitates lung re-expansion [5].

87.8.3 Chronic Organizational Stage

- Treatment:
- Decortication: Surgical removal of the thick pleural peel via VATS or open thoracotomy to restore lung expansion and prevent long-term respiratory dysfunction.
- Ensuring Lung Re-expansion: Throughout all stages, it is crucial to ensure the lung re-expands properly to prevent persistent spaces that can harbor infection.

87.9 Outcomes and Prognosis

Understanding prognostic factors guides treatment intensity and anticipates outcomes.

- Prognostic Factors:
- Severity of Illness: Higher morbidity in patients with significant comorbidities or immunosuppression.
- Promptness of Intervention: Early diagnosis and treatment improve prognosis.
- Pathogen Virulence: Infections with resistant or virulent organisms may worsen outcomes.
- Scoring Systems and Biomarkers:
- Utilize tools like the RAPID score to predict mortality risk and guide treatment decisions.
- Monitor biomarkers such as C-reactive protein (CRP) and procalcitonin to assess response to therapy.

A clinical risk score—RAPID score (Table 87.1)—has been designed taking age, albumin levels, urea levels, infection acquired (community/acquired), and

Table 87.1 RAPID score

Variable	Value	Score
Age (years)	<50	0
	50–70	1
	≥70	2
Albumin (g/dL)	≥2.7	0
	≤2.7	1
Urea (mg/dL)	<30	0
	30–48	1
	≥48	2
Infection	Community acquired	0
	Hospital acquired	1
Purulence	Non-purulent	0
	Purulence	1

purulence of pleural fluid as variables. All variables have a minimum score of 0, whereas age and urea have a maximum score of 2, and the rest have 1. As per the score, high risk (score 5–7) has a 3-month mortality rate of 43.8%, medium risk (score 3–4) has 10.8%, and low risk (score 0–2) has 1.4%.

87.10 Conclusion

Managing empyema in the ICU requires a systematic, stage-based approach tailored to individual patient needs. Early recognition, accurate staging, and timely interventions—including antimicrobial therapy, drainage procedures, and surgical options—are essential. Imaging advancements like TUS, CT, PET, and MRI enhance diagnosis and guide management. Intrapleural fibrinolytics and minimally invasive techniques like VATS and VAC therapy have improved outcomes, particularly in complex or chronic cases. Special considerations for post-pneumonectomy emphasize the need for individualized care strategies. Ensuring lung re-expansion and preventing long-term complications are critical for improving patient outcomes.

Algorithm 87.1: Approach to empyema in the ICU

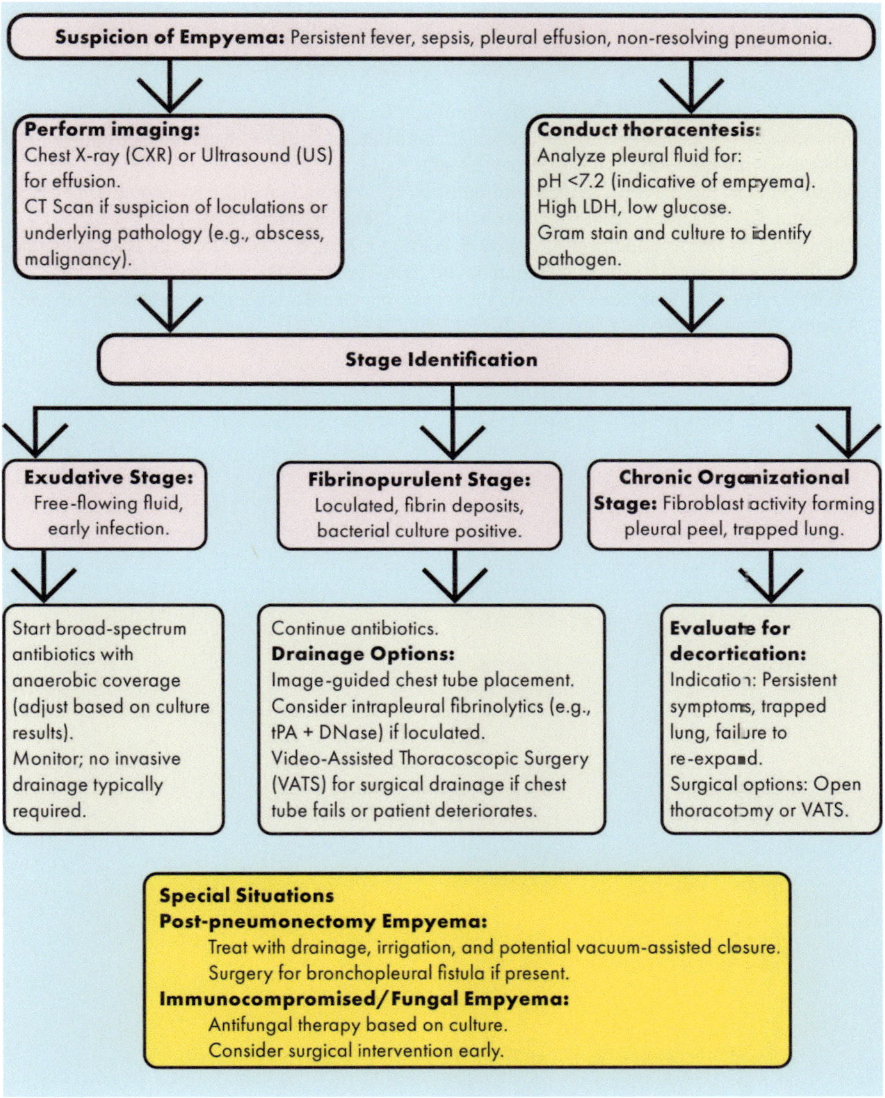

Bibliography

1. Scarci M, Abah U, Solli P, Page A, Waller D, van Schil P, et al. EACTS expert consensus statement for surgical management of pleural empyema. Eur J Cardiothorac Surg. 2015;48(5):642–53.
2. Shen KR, Bribriesco A, Crabtree T, Denlinger C, Eby J, Eiken P, et al. The American Association for Thoracic Surgery consensus guidelines for the management of empyema. J Thorac Cardiovasc Surg. 2017;153(6):e129–46.
3. Wang X. 26th international symposium on intensive care and emergency medicine. Brussels, Belgium. 21–24 March 2006. Abstracts. Crit Care. 2006;10(Suppl 1):P1–472.
4. Balfour-Lynn IM, Abrahamson E, Cohen G, Hartley J, King S, Parikh D, et al. BTS guidelines for the management of pleural infection in children. Thorax. 2005;60(Suppl 1):i1–21.
5. Walters J, Foley N, Molyneux M. Pus in the thorax: management of empyema and lung abscess. Contin Educ Anaesth Crit Care Pain. 2011;11(6):229–33.

Chapter 88
Approach to Management of Pneumothorax in the ICU

88.1 Introduction

Pneumothorax is a critical condition characterized by the presence of air in the pleural cavity, leading to partial or complete lung collapse. In the intensive care unit (ICU), timely recognition and effective management are vital, especially in patients with respiratory distress or hemodynamic instability. This chapter provides a comprehensive approach to managing pneumothorax in the ICU, incorporating detailed indications and contraindications, procedural techniques, post-procedural care, and considerations for training and nursing perspectives [1, 2] [Ref: Algorithm 88.1].

88.2 Initial Assessment of Clinical Signs

- Key Considerations: Conduct a thorough clinical assessment to determine the patient's stability.
- Unstable Features:
- Respiratory Distress: Severe dyspnea, increased respiratory rate, hypoxia.
- Hemodynamic Instability: Tachycardia, hypotension, signs of shock.
- Rationale: This step establishes the urgency of intervention and guides immediate management decisions.

88.3 Indications and Contraindications

- Indications for Chest Drain Insertion:
- Ventilated Patients with Pneumothorax: Positive pressure ventilation can exacerbate pneumothorax, necessitating prompt chest drain placement.

S. B. Mishra et al., *Mastering ICU Care*,
https://doi.org/10.1007/978-981-95-0179-3_88

- Large Secondary Spontaneous Pneumothorax (SSP): Patients with underlying lung disease and significant air accumulation require immediate intervention.
- Contraindications:
- Dense Pleural Adhesions: Can make drain insertion difficult and increase the risk of complications.
- Uncorrected Coagulopathy: Increases the risk of bleeding; coagulopathy should be corrected prior to the procedure if possible.

88.4 Use of Ultrasound Guidance

- Role of Real-Time Ultrasound:
- Site Selection and Needle Placement: Ultrasound aids in identifying the optimal insertion site, especially in patients with complex effusions or uncertain anatomy.
- Benefits:
- Reduces the risk of organ injury.
- Improves the success rate of drain placement.
- Application: Particularly useful in patients with adhesions, obesity, or distorted chest wall anatomy [3].

88.5 Pre-Procedural Considerations

- Consent and Patient Preparation:
- Informed Consent: Discuss the procedure, benefits, and potential complications such as infection, bleeding, and organ injury with the patient or their surrogate decision-maker.
- Aseptic Technique: Strict adherence to aseptic protocols minimizes the risk of infection.
- Premedication:
- Analgesia: Administer appropriate pain control measures.
- Anxiolytics: Consider sedation to reduce patient anxiety and movement during the procedure.

88.6 Drain Insertion Techniques

- Techniques Overview:
- Seldinger Technique (Guidewire Method):
- Indication: Preferred for small-bore ($\leq$14 Fr) chest drains.
- Procedure: Involves needle insertion, guidewire placement, dilation, and drain insertion.

- Advantages: Less traumatic, smaller incision, suitable for pneumothorax and simple effusions.
- Blunt Dissection Technique:
- Indication: Used for large-bore drains (>14 Fr), often necessary for draining thick pleural fluids or empyemas.
- Procedure: A small incision and blunt dissection through the intercostal muscles into the pleural space.
- Advantages: Allows placement of larger drains, better for viscous fluids.
- Safe Triangle for Drain Placement:
- Boundaries:
- Anterior Border: Lateral edge of pectoralis major muscle.
- Posterior Border: Anterior edge of latissimus dorsi muscle.
- Inferior Border: Line horizontal to the nipple (fifth intercostal space).
- Importance: Minimizes the risk of injury to underlying structures such as nerves, vessels, and organs.

88.7 Management of Unstable Patients

- Immediate Intervention:
- Lung Ultrasound:
- Findings: The "barcodesign" (absence of pleural sliding) and "lung point" confirm pneumothorax (M mode).
- Chest Drain Insertion:
- Action: Do not delay insertion for further imaging in life-threatening cases.
- Guidance: Use ultrasound guidance if time permits.

88.8 Management of Stable Patients

- Diagnostic Imaging:
- Chest X-Ray (CXR):
- Purpose: Confirm diagnosis, assess pneumothorax size, detect mediastinal shift or other complications.
- Computed Tomography (CT) Scan:
- Indication: Consider if CXR is inconclusive or for detailed assessment in complex cases.
- Immediate Action for Tension Pneumothorax:
- Signs: Mediastinal shift, severe respiratory compromise, cardiovascular collapse.
- Intervention: Perform needle decompression (mainly in primary spontaneous pneumothorax) followed by chest tube insertion.

88.9 Size-Based Evaluation

- Classification:
- Small Pneumothorax:
- Definition: Rim <2 cm between lung margin and chest wall or <20% lung collapse.
- Management: May consider conservative treatment or needle aspiration in primary spontaneous cases.
- Large Pneumothorax:
- Definition: Rim ≥2 cm or ≥20% lung collapse.
- Management: Chest drain insertion is typically required [4].

88.10 Primary Spontaneous Pneumothorax (PSP)

- Characteristics:
- Occurs in patients without underlying lung disease, often young and otherwise healthy.
- Management:
- Small PSP:
- Needle Aspiration: First-line treatment to evacuate air.
- Observation: If asymptomatic and small, some cases may be managed conservatively.
- Failed Aspiration or Symptomatic Patients:
- Chest Drain Insertion: If aspiration is unsuccessful or symptoms persist.
- Prognosis: Generally favorable with appropriate management.

88.11 Secondary Spontaneous Pneumothorax (SSP)

- Characteristics:
- Occurs in patients with underlying lung conditions such as COPD, cystic fibrosis, or pulmonary fibrosis.
- Higher risk due to limited pulmonary reserve.
- Management:
- Chest Drain Insertion:
- Recommended regardless of pneumothorax size due to the risk of deterioration.
- Needle aspiration is often insufficient as the leak persists due to fragile lung tissue and is usually not recommended.

88.12 Post-Procedural Care

- Monitoring Protocols:
- Assess for Complications:
- Air Leaks: Check for continuous bubbling in the water seal chamber.
- Infection: Monitor insertion site for signs of infection.
- Blocked Drains: Ensure adequate drainage and patency of the tube.
- Suction Application:
- Indication: May be applied to facilitate lung re-expansion, especially in cases of persistent air leaks (Maximum—20 cms of H_2O).
- Drainage Monitoring:
- Fluid Characteristics: Note volume, color, and consistency.
- Removal Criteria:
- Resolved Pneumothorax: No air leak and full lung expansion on imaging.
- Minimal Drainage: Less than 200 mL in 24 h for pleural effusions.

88.13 Management of Complications

- Persistent Air Leak or Failure of Lung Expansion:
- Low-Pressure Suction: Apply to aid lung re-expansion.
- Advanced Interventions:
- Video-Assisted Thoracic Surgery (VATS): For repair of air leaks, resection of blebs or bullae.
- Chemical Pleurodesis: Instillation of agents (e.g., talc) to adhere the lung to the chest wall.
- Chest Drain Dislodgement:
- Immediate Action: Cover the site with an occlusive dressing and prepare for reinsertion if necessary.
- Drainage Cessation:
- Assessment: Check for kinks or obstructions.
- Intervention: Flush the drain or replace if needed.

88.14 Nursing Perspectives

- Routine Assessments:
- Vital Signs: Monitor respiratory rate, oxygen saturation, heart rate, and blood pressure.
- Drain Site Care: Inspect for signs of infection or dislodgement.
- Securing Drains:

- Fixation: Ensure the drain is securely taped and anchored to prevent accidental removal.
- Dressing Changes: Maintain sterile technique during dressing changes.
- Patient Positioning:
- Optimal Positioning: Encourage semi-Fowler's position to promote drainage and prevent tube kinking.
- Mobility: Assist with ambulation as appropriate, ensuring the drain remains secure.

88.15 Conclusion

Effective management of pneumothorax in the ICU requires a systematic approach that prioritizes rapid assessment, precise diagnosis, and tailored intervention. Detailed understanding of indications and contraindications, proficiency in various drain insertion techniques, and adherence to pre- and post-procedural protocols are essential. Incorporating ultrasound guidance enhances safety and success rates. Addressing complications promptly and involving multidisciplinary teams, including nursing staff, optimizes patient outcomes. Continuous training and adherence to best practices ensure high standards of care and minimize the risk of adverse events.

Algorithm 88.1: Approach to management of pneumothorax in the ICU

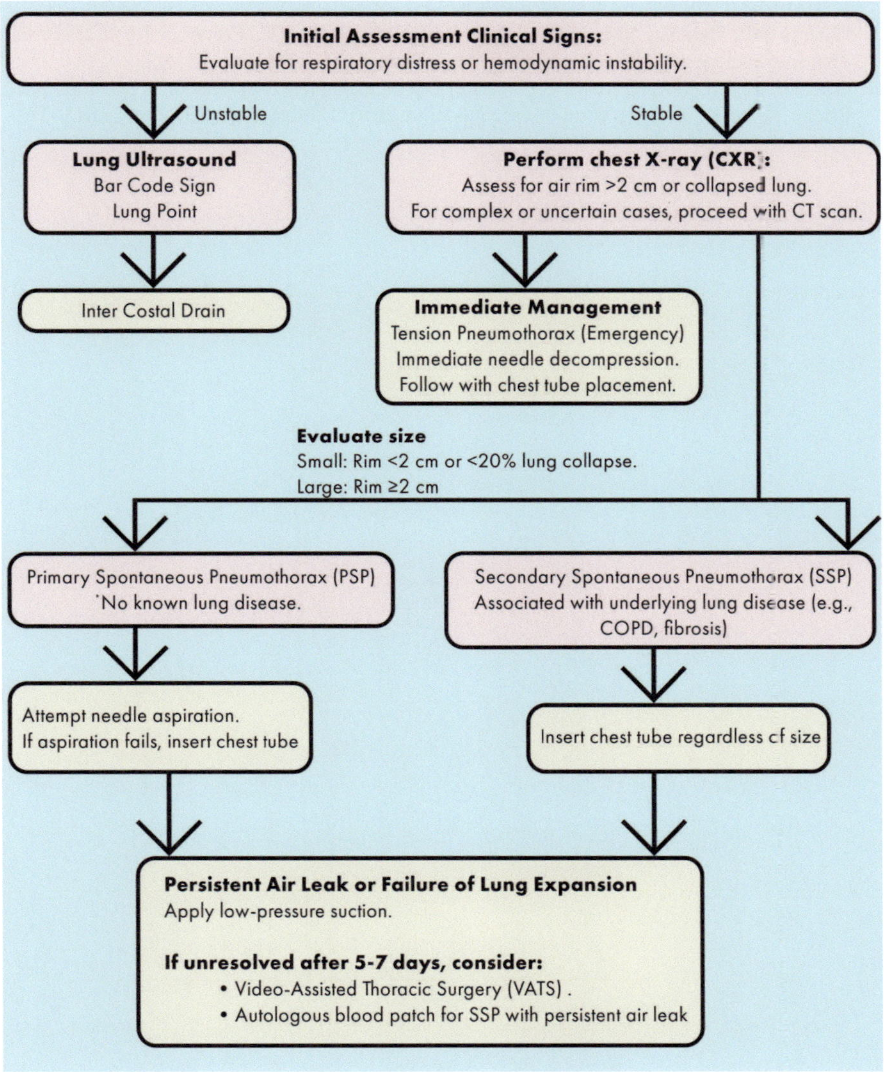

Bibliography

1. Jouneau S, Ricard JD, Seguin-Givelet A, Bige N, Contou D, Desmettre T, et al. SPLF/SMFU/SRLF/SFAR/SFCTCV guidelines for the management of patients with primary spontaneous pneumothorax. Ann Intensive Care. 2023;13(1):88.

2. Walker S, Hallifax R, Ricciardi S, Fitzgerald D, Keijzers M, Lauk O, et al. Joint ERS/EACTS/ESTS clinical practice guidelines on adults with spontaneous pneumothorax. Eur Respir J. 2024;63(5):2300797.
3. Roberts ME, Rahman NM, Maskell NA, Bibby AC, Blyth KG, Corcoran JP, et al. British Thoracic Society guideline for pleural disease. Thorax. 2023;78(11):1143–56.
4. MacDuff A, Arnold A, Harvey J, Group BTSPDG. Management of spontaneous pneumothorax: British Thoracic Society pleural disease guideline 2010. Thorax. 2010;65(Suppl 2):ii18–31.

Chapter 89
Approach to Interstitial Lung Disease in the ICU

89.1 Introduction

Interstitial lung disease (ILD) comprises a diverse group of disorders characterized by varying degrees of fibrosis and inflammation within the lung parenchyma. Patients with ILD are at increased risk for acute respiratory decompensation, particularly in the intensive care unit (ICU) setting. Managing these patients is challenging due to the complexities of their chronic condition and the potential for life-threatening complications such as pneumothorax. Clinicians must balance the need for prompt diagnosis and treatment with the risks associated with invasive procedures [1, 2] [Ref: Algorithm 89.1].

89.2 Initial Assessment: Is the Patient a Known Case of ILD?

- Yes: For patients with a known ILD diagnosis, management begins by assessing potential causes of acute decompensation while considering the underlying disease trajectory, subtype of ILD, and previous functional status.
- No: In undiagnosed patients, a thorough clinical history and targeted diagnostics are essential to identify or rule out ILD, considering the limitations and risks of invasive procedures in critically ill patients.

S. B. Mishra et al., *Mastering ICU Care*,
https://doi.org/10.1007/978-981-95-0179-3_89

89.3 Clinical History and Workup for Undiagnosed Patients

89.3.1 Key History Points

- Exposure History: Investigate occupational exposures (e.g., asbestos, silica), environmental factors (e.g., bird proteins, mold), and drug-related triggers (e.g., amiodarone, methotrexate).
- Autoimmune Screening: Assess for symptoms suggestive of connective tissue diseases. Laboratory tests may include antinuclear antibodies (ANA), extractable nuclear antigens (ENA) panel, and rheumatoid factor [3].

89.3.2 Laboratory Investigations

- Complete blood count.
- A comprehensive metabolic panel, including liver and kidney function tests and serum electrolytes.
- Electrocardiogram.
- Arterial blood gases.
- Transthoracic echocardiogram, cardiac enzymes—to rule out cardiac causes of hypoxia and breathlessness.
- CT pulmonary angiography: If acute worsening of conditions and development of shock. Patients with idiopathic pulmonary fibrosis (IPF) are more prone to deep vein thrombosis and pulmonary embolism(PE).

89.3.3 Imaging and Diagnostics

- High-Resolution Computed Tomography (HRCT):
- Fibrotic ILDs: Idiopathic pulmonary fibrosis(IPF)/usual interstitial pneumonia.
- Usual Interstitial Pneumonia (UIP): Characterized by subpleural, basal-predominant reticulation with honeycombing and traction bronchiectasis.
- Inflammatory ILDs: Nonspecific interstitial pneumonia, hypersensitivity pneumonitis.
- Nonspecific Interstitial Pneumonia (NSIP): Presents with ground-glass opacities and a more uniform distribution, minimal honeycombing (typically bilateral and symmetrically distributed in the lower zones).
  - Hypersensitivity Pneumonitis:

    Subacute: Diffuse ground-glass opacification, ill-defined centrilobular nodules, and lobular areas of decreased attenuation on images performed at end-expiration.

    Chronic: Reticular abnormalities and traction bronchiectasis, with a predominance in the upper and middle lung fields, and frequently shows a peribronchovascular accentuation with subpleural sparing. Honeycombing is observed in up to 69% of the cases. Centrilobular nodules, air trapping, and/or a mosaic pattern in a patient with a fibrosing lung disease are good clues to the diagnosis of CHP.

89.3.4 Challenges in Diagnosing ILD in Critically Ill Patients:

- Risks of Invasive Diagnostics: Procedures like bronchoalveolar lavage (BAL) and lung biopsy carry increased risks, including bleeding, pneumothorax, and worsening respiratory failure.
- Alternative Strategies: Utilize noninvasive imaging and postpone invasive diagnostics until the patient stabilizes, if possible [4].

89.4 Identifying Acute Decompensation Causes in Known ILD Patients

Common Causes

1. Pneumothorax: May require urgent intervention based on severity.
2. Pulmonary embolism.
3. Infection: Bacterial, viral, or opportunistic pathogens.
4. Cardiac Dysfunction: Pulmonary edema or heart failure.
5. Acute exacerbation of ILD (AE-ILD).
6. Aspiration.
7. Drug toxicity [5].

89.5 Ruling Out Reversible Causes of Decompensation

89.5.1 Diagnostic Workup

- CT Chest: High-resolution imaging to assess for new infiltrates, pneumothorax size, PE, or other abnormalities.
- Laboratory Tests:
- Cardiac Markers: B-type natriuretic peptide (BNP), troponin levels.
- Infection Markers: C-reactive protein (CRP), procalcitonin, complete blood count.
- Blood Cultures: If sepsis is suspected.
- Echocardiography: Evaluate for left ventricular dysfunction, valvular abnormalities, or pulmonary hypertension.

89.5.2 Management of Reversible Causes

- Pulmonary Edema:
- Management: Administer diuretics, optimize fluid balance, and address underlying cardiac issues.
- Infection:
- Management: Initiate empiric broad-spectrum antibiotics tailored to likely pathogens and local resistance patterns.
- Aspiration:
- Management: Supportive care; consider antibiotics if secondary infection is suspected, and implement measures to prevent further aspiration.
- Drug Toxicity:
- Management: Discontinue offending agents and provide supportive care.
- Pulmonary Embolism:
- Management: Initiate anticoagulation therapy promptly [4].

89.6 Management of AE-ILD

89.6.1 Definition

An acute, clinically significant respiratory deterioration characterized by new, widespread alveolar abnormality on imaging, not fully explained by cardiac failure or fluid overload.

89.6.2 Treatment Approach

- High-Dose Corticosteroids:
- Regimen: Methylprednisolone 500–1000 mg daily for 3 days, followed by a gradual taper.
- Immunosuppressants:
- Cyclophosphamide: Consider in non-IPF ILDs with severe inflammation.
  Dose: 500–1000 mg every 4 weeks or 1–2 mg/kg/day orally.
- Antifibrotic Agents:
- Nintedanib and Pirfenidone:

  – Dose: Nintedanib—150 mg twice a day.

    Pirfenidone—1800–2400 mg/day in divided doses, 200 mg three tablets thrice a day
- Role: Shown to slow disease progression in fibrotic ILDs like IPF.
- Potential Benefits During Acute Exacerbations: May reduce the rate of decline in lung function, though evidence during acute exacerbations is limited [6].

89.6.3 Supportive Care

- Oxygen Therapy: Aim to maintain adequate oxygenation using the least invasive methods.
- Advanced Respiratory Support:
- High-Flow Nasal Cannula (HFNC): Preferred for its ability to deliver humidified oxygen at high flow rates with precise FiO_2 control. Benefits: Better tolerated, reduces dead space, and provides consistent oxygen delivery.
- Indications: Hypoxemic respiratory failure without significant hypercapnia.
- Noninvasive Ventilation (NIV): Benefits: Provides positive pressure ventilation, which may be beneficial in select patients.
- Limitations: Poor tolerance due to discomfort, risk of air leaks, and may delay necessary intubation.
- Invasive Mechanical Ventilation (IMV):
- Limited Utility: High risk of mortality; reserved for cases where it serves as a bridge to lung transplantation or when acute reversible factors are identified.
- Ventilation Strategies: Employ low tidal volumes (4–6 mL/kg of predicted body weight) and limit plateau pressures to reduce ventilator-induced lung injury.

89.7 Risk Stratification and Prognosis

Prognostic Factors

- HRCT Features:
- Honeycombing: Suggests advanced fibrosis and is associated with higher mortality.
- Extent of Fibrosis: Greater extent correlates with increased risk of acute exacerbations and death.

  Mortality Rates and Outcomes

- IPF Patients:
- Higher Mortality: Acute exacerbations have in-hospital mortality rates exceeding 50%.
- Non-IPF ILDs:
- Variable Outcomes: Some subtypes respond better to immunosuppressive therapy, improving survival rates [7].

89.8 Reversible Triggers

- Pulmonary Edema: Optimize cardiac function, use diuretics.
- Infection: Early identification and targeted antimicrobial therapy.
- Aspiration: Preventive strategies and supportive care.

- Drug Toxicity: Identify and discontinue the offending agent.

  Flowchart for Diagnosing and Managing Acute Exacerbations

- Consider Including: A visual aid to guide clinicians through the assessment and management process, emphasizing the identification of reversible causes and appropriate interventions.

89.9 Special Considerations

- Decision-Making: Shared decision-making with patients and families regarding treatment options and goals of care.
  Palliative Care Integration

- Symptom Management: Address dyspnea, anxiety, and other distressing symptoms.
- Advance Care Planning: Discuss prognosis and end-of-life preferences early in the care continuum.

89.10 Emerging Therapies and Research

Experimental Therapies and Biomarkers

- KL-6: A serum biomarker elevated in ILD; under investigation for early disease activity detection and monitoring.
- Telomere Biology: Short telomeres are associated with familial ILD and worse outcomes; research is ongoing into targeted therapies.

  Genetics in ILD

- Familial Cases: Genetic mutations (e.g., in surfactant proteins, telomerase) contribute to disease pathogenesis.
- Syndromic ILD: Understanding genetic factors may lead to personalized treatment strategies [3].

89.11 Conclusion

Managing acute decompensation in ILD patients within the ICU is complex and requires a comprehensive, patient-centered approach. Differentiating between fibrotic and inflammatory ILDs is crucial for guiding therapy, and HRCT imaging plays a vital role in this distinction. Managing acute exacerbations involves ruling out reversible causes, employing immunosuppressive or antifibrotic therapies as appropriate, and carefully selecting respiratory support strategies to minimize further lung injury. A multidisciplinary team is essential for addressing the multifaceted needs of these patients, including consideration for lung transplantation and integration of palliative care. Ongoing research into emerging therapies and genetic underpinnings holds promise for improving outcomes in this challenging patient population.

Algorithm 89.1: Approach to interstitial lung disease in the ICU

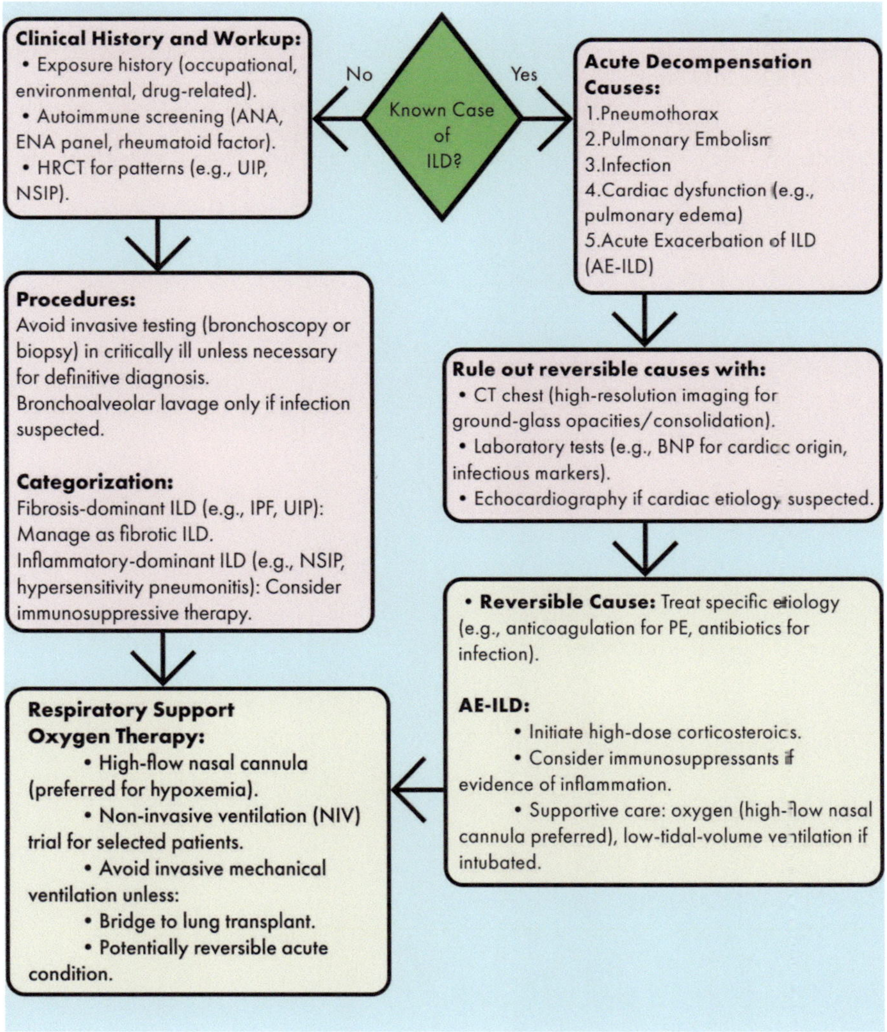

Bibliography

1. Hayat Syed MK, Bruck O, Kumar A, Surani S. Acute exacerbation of interstitial lung disease in the intensive care unit: principles of diagnostic evaluation and management. World J Crit Care Med. 2023;12(3):153–64.
2. Dhanani Z, Gupta R. The management of interstitial lung disease in the ICU: a comprehensive review. J Clin Med. 2024;13(22):6657.
3. Charokopos A, Moua T, Ryu JH, Smischney NJ. Acute exacerbation of interstitial lung disease in the intensive care unit. World J Crit Care Med. 2022;11(1):22–32.
4. Faverio P, De Giacomi F, Sardella L, Fiorentino G, Carone M, Salerno F, et al. Management of acute respiratory failure in interstitial lung diseases: overview and clinical insights. BMC Pulm Med. 2018;18(1):70.
5. Montesi SB, Fisher JH, Martinez FJ, Selman M, Pardo A, Johannson KA. Update in interstitial lung disease 2019. Am J Respir Crit Care Med. 2020;202(4):500–7.
6. Krishnan A, Janz DR, Lammi MR. ICU management of the patient with fibrotic interstitial lung disease. CHEST Crit Care. 2023;1(3):100020.
7. Hadley R, Hyzy R. Critically ill patients with interstitial lung disease. Clin Chest Med. 2015;36(3):497–510.

Chapter 90
Approach to Hemoptysis in the ICU

90.1 Introduction

Hemoptysis, the expectoration of blood originating from the respiratory tract, is a potentially life-threatening condition requiring rapid assessment and intervention in the ICU setting. Its prevalence and causes vary globally, reflecting differences between developed and developing countries. In developing nations, infectious diseases like tuberculosis are the most common causes of hemoptysis due to higher incidence rates and limited healthcare resources. Conversely, in developed countries, malignancies, bronchiectasis, and chronic inflammatory conditions are more prevalent etiologies [1].

Defining massive hemoptysis poses a significant challenge because of variability in volume thresholds and clinical consequences. Traditionally, massive hemoptysis has been described as bleeding exceeding 100–600 mL over 24 h. However, even smaller volumes can be life-threatening if they lead to airway obstruction or severe hypoxemia. Therefore, any hemoptysis that compromises ventilation or oxygenation warrants immediate medical attention [2, 3] [Ref: Algorithm 90.1].

90.2 Pathophysiology

Understanding the vascular origins of hemoptysis is crucial for effective management. Hemoptysis primarily arises from two circulatory systems:

- Bronchial Circulation: Originating from the systemic circulation, the bronchial arteries supply nutrients to the airways and are under systemic blood pressure. Hemorrhage from these vessels can be profuse due to the higher pressure, leading to significant bleeding.

S. B. Mishra et al., *Mastering ICU Care*,
https://doi.org/10.1007/978-981-95-0179-3_90

- Pulmonary Circulation: This low-pressure system is responsible for gas exchange in the alveoli. Bleeding from the pulmonary arteries is less common but can occur in conditions like pulmonary embolism, arteriovenous malformations, or pulmonary hypertension.

Differentiating between these sources helps guide therapeutic interventions, as bronchial artery hemorrhages may respond well to bronchial artery embolization (BAE), while pulmonary artery bleeding may require alternative approaches [4, 5].

90.3 Etiology

Pulmonary: Bronchiectasis, infections (tuberculosis, fungal, necrotizing pneumonia, mycetoma, lung abscess), malignancy (bronchogenic carcinoma, bronchial adenoma), vascular (arteriovenous malformation, Dieulafoy lesions, aortic aneurysm erosion), iatrogenic (bronchoscopy, pulmonary artery catheter), trauma.
Immunological: Systemic lupus erythematosus, Wegener's granulomatosis, Goodpasture's syndrome, microscopic polyarteritis, amyloidosis, Bechets disease.
Cardiovascular: Mitral stenosis, endocarditis, pulmonary edema, bronchial artery aneurysm, pulmonary embolism.
Bleeding Disorders: Disseminated intravascular coagulation, thrombocytopenia.

90.4 Algorithmic Approach to Management

A systematic, algorithmic approach enhances the efficiency of diagnosing and treating hemoptysis. The workflow emphasizes airway management, hemodynamic stabilization, localization of bleeding, and definitive interventions.

Step 1: Assessing Airway Compromise

- Key Question: "Is the patient's airway compromised?"

This is the most critical step, as significant bleeding can obstruct the airway, leading to hypoxemia or aspiration.

- Indicators of Compromise: Stridor, respiratory distress, large volumes of blood in the oropharynx, inability to clear secretions, decreased oxygen saturation.
- Action Plan:
- Immediate Airway Management:
- Proceed with endotracheal intubation using a large-bore tube (≥8.0 mm) to facilitate suctioning of clots and secretions.

- In cases requiring lung isolation to prevent blood spillage into the unaffected lung, use a double-lumen endotracheal tube or bronchial blockers.
- Rigid Bronchoscopy:
- Employ rigid bronchoscopy in difficult cases for better airway control, suction capabilities, and removal of large clots.
- Ensure continuous monitoring of oxygenation and ventilation parameters.

Step 2: Evaluating Hemodynamic Stability

- Key Question: "Is the patient hemodynamically stable?"

Hemodynamic instability suggests significant blood loss, necessitating urgent resuscitation.

- Indicators of Instability: Hypotension, tachycardia, altered mental status, signs of shock, decreased urine output.
- Action Plan:
- Resuscitation Measures:
- Initiate intravenous fluid replacement to maintain perfusion.
- Transfuse blood products to correct anemia and restore oxygen-carrying capacity.
- Correct Coagulopathies:
- Administer fresh frozen plasma, platelets, vitamin K, or procoagulant agents as indicated.
- Consider vasopressor support if hypotension persists despite fluid resuscitation.
- Implement invasive hemodynamic monitoring for ongoing assessment.

Step 3: Prioritizing Urgent Interventions

- Key Question: "If the patient is unstable, what urgent measures should be taken?"

For unstable patients, the focus shifts to rapidly identifying and stopping the bleeding source.

- Action Plan:
- Bronchoscopy:
- Flexible Bronchoscopy:
- Provides direct visualization of the bleeding site.
- Allows for suctioning of clots.
- Facilitates therapeutic interventions, such as:
- Application of topical vasoconstrictors (e.g., epinephrine), Nd:YAG laser or argon plasma coagulation.
- Use of topical hemostatic agents like fibrin glue.
- Balloon tamponade to compress bleeding vessels.
- Rigid Bronchoscopy:
- Preferred in massive hemoptysis for better airway control and removal of large clots.

- Pharmacologic Interventions:
- Tranexamic Acid:
- Administer antifibrinolytic agents intravenously or via nebulization to promote clot stability.
- Topical Hemostatic Agents:
- Apply agents such as thrombin or fibrin sealants during bronchoscopy.
- Bronchial Artery Embolization (BAE):
- Coordinate with interventional radiology for urgent BAE to control bleeding from bronchial arteries.
- BAE is less invasive than surgery and has a high success rate in controlling hemorrhage.
- Surgical Intervention:
- If bronchoscopic and endovascular measures fail or are unavailable, consult thoracic surgery.
- Surgical options include lobectomy or pneumonectomy, depending on the bleeding source and patient stability [6, 7].

Step 4: Imaging and Localization of Bleeding Source

- Key Question: "Is the patient hemodynamically stable and the airway secure?"

Once stabilized, imaging studies are critical to guide further interventions.

- Imaging Modalities:
- CT Angiography (CTA):
- Importance:
- Preferred modality for accurately localizing the bleeding source.
- Identifies underlying pathologies (e.g., tumors, bronchiectasis, vascular anomalies).
- Detects both bronchial and non-bronchial systemic arteries involved in bleeding.
- Advantages over Bronchoscopy:
- Noninvasive.
- Visualizes areas beyond the reach of the bronchoscope.
- Provides a roadmap for interventional radiologists during BAE.
- Emerging Technologies:
- Multi-row detector CT scanners enhance image quality and diagnostic accuracy.
- Chest X-ray:
- Useful as an initial tool but less sensitive and specific.
- May reveal infiltrates, masses, or other structural abnormalities.
- Action Plan:
- Based on imaging findings, plan targeted interventions such as embolization or surgery.
- Investigations: Complete blood count, coagulation profile, renal function tests, liver function tests, sputum/endotracheal secretions for gram stain, culture, acid fast bacilli detection, CBNAAT (nucleic acid amplification—tuber-

culosis), fungal culture, cytology, blood grouping, and cross matching. Imaging and bronchoscopy (discussed below). One may also send disease-specific investigations if there is a suspicion (e.g., antinuclear antibody tests).

Step 5: Controlling the Bleeding

- Key Focus: Definitive control of the bleeding after localization.
- Interventional Radiology:
- Bronchial Artery Embolization (BAE):
- First-line therapy for bleeding from the bronchial circulation.
- Procedure:
- Catheterization of the bronchial arteries under fluoroscopic guidance.
- Embolization using materials like polyvinyl alcohol particles, coils, or gel foam.
- Advancements:
- Newer embolic agents and techniques have improved success rates and reduced complications.
- Bronchoscopy:
- Continue to utilize for therapeutic interventions if bleeding persists.
- Repeat procedures may be necessary for ongoing management.
- Pharmacologic Therapy:
- Maintain antifibrinolytic therapy with agents like tranexamic acid.
- Adjust medications based on coagulation profiles and bleeding status.
- Surgical Options:
- Indications:
- Failure of bronchoscopic and endovascular interventions.
- Anatomically localized disease amenable to resection.
- Life-threatening hemorrhage requiring immediate control.
- Procedures:
- Lobectomy, segmentectomy, or pneumonectomy, depending on the extent of disease.
- Risks:
- High morbidity and mortality, especially in unstable patients.
- Requires thorough evaluation of surgical risks versus benefits [8].

Step 6: Multidisciplinary Approach

Optimal management necessitates collaboration among various specialists to ensure comprehensive care.

- Team Members:
- Intensivists:
- Coordinate critical care management.
- Oversee hemodynamic support and ventilatory strategies.
- Pulmonologists:
- Perform bronchoscopies.
- Manage respiratory complications.
- Interventional Radiologists:

- Conduct imaging studies and perform BAE.
- Utilize advanced embolization techniques.
- Thoracic Surgeons:
- Evaluate patients for surgical interventions.
- Perform operative procedures when indicated.
- Benefits:
- Enhances decision-making through shared expertise.
- Improves patient outcomes by streamlining interventions [9].
- Facilitates communication and coordination of care.

Step 7: Monitoring for Resolution

- Key Question: "Has the bleeding resolved post-treatment?"

Continuous assessment is essential to ensure effective control of hemoptysis.

- Indicators of Resolution:
- Stabilized vital signs.
- No new episodes of bleeding.
- Improved respiratory function.
- Normalizing laboratory values (e.g., hemoglobin, hematocrit).
- Action Plan:
- Ongoing Monitoring:
- Frequent reassessment of airway patency and breathing.
- Serial blood tests to monitor hemoglobin and coagulation status.
- Repeat Imaging:
- Follow-up CT scans or chest X-rays to assess for recurrent bleeding or complications.
- Adjust Supportive Care:
- Modify ventilator settings as the patient improves.
- Gradually wean off vasopressors and other supportive medications.

Step 8: Management of Recurrent Hemoptysis and Transition to Maintenance Therapy

- Recurrent Hemoptysis:
- Action Plan:
- Repeat Bronchial Artery Embolization:
- Effective for recurrent bleeding due to revascularization or missed vessels.
- Evaluate for Underlying Conditions:
- Investigate for diseases like aspergillosis, vasculitis, or bronchiectasis.
- Surgical Intervention:
- Consider in cases where embolization is unsuccessful or not feasible.
- Requires thorough risk assessment and patient optimization.
- Transition to Maintenance Therapy:
- Address Underlying Etiology:
- Infections:
- Initiate or adjust antibiotics for conditions like tuberculosis or pneumonia.
- Malignancies:

- Collaborate with oncology for chemotherapy, radiation therapy, or targeted treatments.
- Autoimmune Disorders:
- Implement immunosuppressive therapy for vasculitis or other inflammatory conditions.

90.5 Emerging Techniques and Innovations

Advancements in technology have enhanced the diagnosis and management of hemoptysis:

- Multi-row Detector CT:
- Embolization Techniques:
- Development of new embolic materials improves the safety and efficacy of BAE.
- Use of calibrated microspheres and liquid embolic agents allows for targeted vessel occlusion.
- Innovations in catheter design enhance navigation and reduce procedure time.
- Minimally Invasive Surgical Approaches:
- Video-assisted thoracoscopic surgery (VATS) offers less invasive options for surgical intervention.
- Reduces postoperative pain and accelerates recovery compared to open surgery.
- Pharmacologic Advances:
- Research into novel antifibrinolytic agents and topical hemostatics may provide additional tools for controlling bleeding.

These innovations hold promise for improving patient outcomes and expanding the availability of effective treatments worldwide.

90.6 Conclusion

Managing hemoptysis in the ICU demands a systematic, multidisciplinary approach prioritizing airway protection, hemodynamic stabilization, precise localization of bleeding, and definitive interventions. Rapid assessment and timely decision-making are critical to prevent catastrophic outcomes. The use of bronchoscopy and CT angiography serves as the cornerstone for diagnosis and initial management, while advanced therapies like bronchial artery embolization and surgical interventions address more severe cases. Collaboration among intensivists, pulmonologists, interventional radiologists, and thoracic surgeons is essential for optimizing patient care. Addressing global disparities in healthcare access remains a pivotal challenge, emphasizing the need for continued innovation and resource allocation to reduce the burden of hemoptysis worldwide.

Algorithm 90.1: Approach to hemoptysis in the ICU

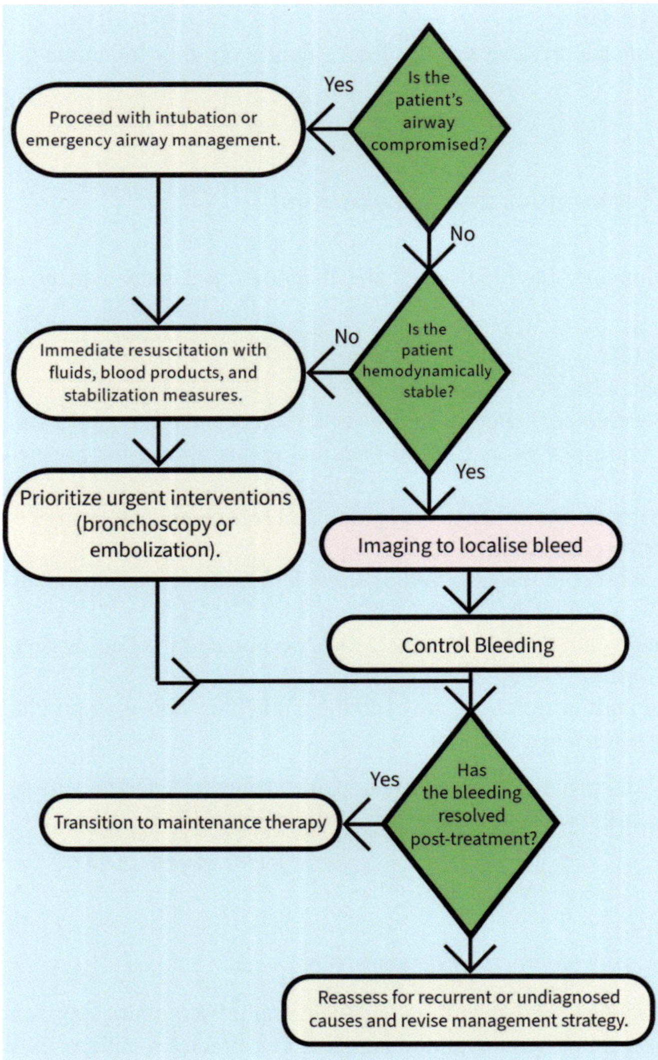

Bibliography

1. Chandler JK, Reid MM, Pitts L, Postigo Jasahui MR. Evaluation & management of clinically significant hemoptysis—a clinical practice review. AME Med J. 2024;9:1.
2. Park MS. Diffuse alveolar hemorrhage. Tuberc Respir Dis (Seoul). 2013;74(4):151–62.
3. Park JA. Treatment of diffuse alveolar hemorrhage: controlling inflammation and obtaining rapid and effective hemostasis. Int J Mol Sci. 2021;22(2):793.
4. Walz JM, McNamee CJ, Conlan AA. Hemoptysis in the intensive care unit: etiology and outcome in a series of 115 patients. Chest. 2004;126(4):869S.
5. Radchenko C, Alraiyes AH, Shojaee S. A systematic approach to the management of massive hemoptysis. J Thorac Dis. 2017;9(Suppl 10):S1069–86.
6. Fartoukh M, Khalil A, Louis L, Carette MF, Bazelly B, Cadranel J, et al. An integrated approach to diagnosis and management of severe haemoptysis in patients admitted to the intensive care unit: a case series from a referral centre. Respir Res. 2007;8(1):11.
7. Kathuria H, Hollingsworth HM, Vilvendhan R, Reardon C. Management of life-threatening hemoptysis. J Intensive Care. 2020;8:23.
8. de Prost N, Parrot A, Picard C, Ancel PY, Mayaud C, Fartoukh M, et al. Diffuse alveolar haemorrhage: factors associated with in-hospital and long-term mortality. Eur Respir J. 2010;35(6):1303–11.
9. Coviello E, Puma F, Pourmolkara D, Mandarano M, Napolitano AG. Massive, life-threatening hemoptysis due to localized granulomatosis with polyangiitis. J Cardiothorac Surg. 2023;18(1):239.

Part VIII
Miscellaneous

Chapter 91
Approach to Anemia in the ICU

91.1 Introduction

Anemia is a common and multifactorial condition encountered in critically ill patients, with potential consequences such as impaired oxygen delivery, increased cardiac workload, delayed wound healing, and worsened clinical outcomes. In the ICU, anemia often arises from acute blood loss, inflammation, impaired erythropoiesis, frequent phlebotomy, or nutritional deficiencies, making its evaluation and management a critical component of patient care. Understanding the complex interplay of these factors is essential for optimizing patient outcomes both during critical illness and after ICU discharge [1, 2] [Ref: Algorithm 91.1].

91.2 Hemoglobin Level Assessment

- Threshold: Begin with the measurement of hemoglobin (Hb). Current evidence supports a restrictive transfusion strategy, generally indicating red blood cell (RBC) transfusion when Hb levels are <7 g/dL, as it may improve oxygen delivery without increasing transfusion-related risks. For Hb ≥7 g/dL, further clinical evaluation is warranted before considering transfusion.
- Rationale: Transfusion thresholds should balance the risks of transfusion-associated complications—such as immunosuppression, transfusion-related acute lung injury (TRALI), and infections—with the benefits of improving oxygenation. Restrictive transfusion strategies have been associated with similar or better outcomes compared to liberal strategies in critically ill patients.

S. B. Mishra et al., *Mastering ICU Care*,
https://doi.org/10.1007/978-981-95-0179-3_91

91.3 Clinical Context and History Evaluation

- Key Considerations: Evaluate symptoms, underlying conditions, and clinical history to guide the diagnostic workup. Consider the following:
- Presence of active bleeding or hemodynamic instability.
- Past medical history of chronic diseases (e.g., chronic kidney disease, heart failure) or malnutrition.
- ICU-related factors such as frequent phlebotomy, inflammation, or renal dysfunction.
- Objective: Narrow down the likely etiology and initiate targeted diagnostic studies, while considering the patient's overall clinical status and comorbidities [3].

91.4 Pathophysiological Insights into Anemia in Critical Illness

Anemia in critically ill patients is multifactorial, resulting from a combination of decreased red blood cell (RBC) production, increased RBC loss, and shortened RBC lifespan. Key contributing factors include:

- Bleeding: Acute blood loss from overt sources such as gastrointestinal bleeding, surgical sites, or procedural punctures.
- Phlebotomy-Related Blood Loss: Frequent blood sampling can cumulatively result in significant blood loss, potentially amounting to a unit of blood per week.
- Inflammation and Anemia of Chronic Illness: Inflammatory cytokines like interleukin-1 (IL-1), interleukin-6 (IL-6), and tumor necrosis factor-alpha (TNF-alpha) impair erythropoiesis and iron metabolism. IL-6 stimulates the production of hepcidin, a hormone that reduces iron availability by inhibiting intestinal iron absorption and trapping iron within macrophages.
- Erythropoiesis Impairment: Suppression of erythropoietin production and resistance to erythropoietin action occur during critical illness and inflammation, further reducing RBC production. Renal dysfunction exacerbates this impairment due to decreased erythropoietin synthesis.
- Nutritional Deficiencies: Deficiencies of iron, vitamin B_{12}, and folate are common due to poor nutritional intake and increased metabolic demands.

91.5 Evaluation of Common Causes

The evaluation should be systematic, considering each potential cause:

Bleeding

- Action: Assess for overt bleeding sources such as gastrointestinal bleeding (via stool occult blood test or endoscopy), surgical wounds, and catheter sites.

- Diagnostic Imaging: Perform imaging studies if occult bleeding is suspected but not evident clinically.
- Rationale: Acute blood loss is a leading cause of anemia in the ICU and requires prompt identification and management.

Phlebotomy-Related Loss

- Action: Quantify the volume of blood drawn daily. Implement strategies to minimize blood loss, such as using pediatric-sized tubes, point-of-care testing, and consolidating laboratory tests.
- Rationale: Cumulative blood loss from frequent phlebotomy can significantly contribute to anemia, potentially equating to a unit of blood per week.

Inflammation and Anemia of Chronic Illness

- Action: Measure inflammatory markers (e.g., IL-6, CRP), iron studies (ferritin, transferrin saturation), and hepcidin levels if available.
- Rationale: Inflammation leads to anemia of chronic illness, characterized by impaired iron utilization and decreased erythropoiesis due to cytokine-mediated effects and elevated hepcidin levels.

Erythropoiesis Impairment

- Action: Assess erythropoietin levels and renal function tests. Evaluate for bone marrow suppression.
- Rationale: Suppressed erythropoietin production and resistance to its effects are common in critical illness, especially with renal dysfunction and inflammatory cytokines interfering with erythropoiesis.

Nutritional Deficiencies

- Action: Measure serum levels of iron, vitamin B_{12}, and folate. Interpret iron studies cautiously, as ferritin is an acute-phase reactant and may be elevated in inflammation despite iron deficiency.
- Rationale: Nutritional deficiencies contribute to anemia, with microcytic anemia suggesting iron deficiency and macrocytic anemia indicating vitamin B_{12} or folate deficiency.

91.6 Diagnostic Workup

After identifying potential causes, further diagnostics include:

Peripheral Blood Smear

- Action: Examine morphology for signs of hemolysis (e.g., schistocytes), megaloblastic changes, or other abnormalities.
- Rationale: Provides clues to underlying causes such as hemolysis or nutritional deficiencies.

Reticulocyte Count

- Action: Assess reticulocyte count to evaluate bone marrow response.
- Rationale: A low reticulocyte count indicates decreased RBC production, whereas a high count suggests active RBC production in response to anemia.

Coagulation Profile

- Action: Evaluate coagulation parameters to rule out disseminated intravascular coagulation (DIC) or other bleeding disorders.
- Rationale: Important in patients with active bleeding or unexplained anemia.

- Ultrasonography might be necessary in patients who have suffered trauma or have undergone recent surgery or in coagulopathic patients with no other obvious source of bleeding. A high LDH and reticulocyte count and/or positive Coombs test might suggest hemolysis.

91.7 Management Strategies

Management is tailored to the underlying cause, with a focus on minimizing risks and promoting recovery.

Transfusion Strategies

- Restrictive vs. Liberal Transfusion: Adopt a restrictive transfusion strategy, transfusing RBCs when Hb <7 g/dL, unless specific conditions warrant higher thresholds (e.g., acute coronary syndrome, severe hypoxia).
- Evidence: Studies have shown that restrictive strategies are associated with similar or improved outcomes compared to liberal strategies, reducing exposure to transfusion-related risks.

Acute Blood Loss

- Action: Control bleeding sources promptly. Stabilize hemodynamics with fluids and vasopressors as needed.
- Correction of Coagulopathies: Administer platelets, fresh frozen plasma (FFP), or specific factor concentrates as indicated.

Phlebotomy-Related Anemia

- Action: Implement blood conservation strategies, minimize unnecessary blood draws, and utilize point-of-care testing when feasible.

Inflammation and Anemia of Chronic Illness

- Action: Address the underlying inflammatory or infectious conditions aggressively.
- Erythropoiesis-Stimulating Agents (ESAs): Consider ESAs in select patients, acknowledging limitations and risks such as thromboembolic events and hypertension.

- Iron Supplementation: Evaluate the use of intravenous iron therapy, especially when oral absorption is impaired, while being cautious of risks like infections or anaphylaxis with certain formulations.

Erythropoiesis Impairment

- Action: Optimize renal function where possible. Consider ESAs in patients with chronic kidney disease.
- Monitoring: Regularly monitor Hb levels and adjust therapy accordingly [4].

Nutritional Deficiencies

- Iron Supplementation.
- Action: Administer intravenous iron in cases of confirmed deficiency, especially when oral iron is ineffective or contraindicated.
- Caution: Be aware of potential adverse effects and monitor for hypersensitivity reactions.
- Vitamin B_{12} and Folate Supplementation.
- Action: Provide appropriate supplementation for deficiencies.

Post-ICU Anemia Management

- Awareness: Recognize that anemia often persists after ICU discharge, potentially impacting physical function, quality of life, and rehabilitation.
- Follow-Up: Arrange for continued monitoring and management of anemia in the outpatient setting, integrating strategies to facilitate recovery.

91.8 Special Considerations for Subgroups

Patients with Heart Failure

- Impact: Anemia can exacerbate heart failure symptoms due to decreased oxygen delivery and increased cardiac workload.
- Management: Careful fluid management and consideration of ESAs under specialist guidance.

Chronic Kidney Disease (CKD) Patients

- Impact: CKD patients often have anemia due to decreased erythropoietin production and iron utilization.
- Management: ESAs and iron supplementation are mainstays, with close monitoring for complications.

Postsurgical Patients

- Impact: Blood loss during surgery contributes to anemia; optimizing Hb levels preoperatively and minimizing intraoperative blood loss are critical.
- Management: Employ blood conservation techniques and consider cell salvage when appropriate.

91.9 Addressing Persistent Post-ICU Anemia

- Prevalence: Anemia frequently persists after ICU discharge, with recovery often taking weeks to months.
- Impact: Persistent anemia can lead to decreased exercise capacity, fatigue, and reduced quality of life.
- Rehabilitation Planning: Recognize the importance of addressing anemia in post-ICU care to enhance recovery and rehabilitation outcomes.
- Long-Term Monitoring: Implement follow-up plans to monitor Hb levels and adjust treatment as needed.

91.10 Pathophysiological Summary

Anemia in critical illness is multifactorial, involving:

- Decreased RBC Production: Due to impaired erythropoiesis from inflammation, reduced erythropoietin production, and nutritional deficiencies.
- Increased RBC Loss: From overt bleeding and frequent phlebotomy.
- Shortened RBC Lifespan: Resulting from hemolysis or the effects of inflammatory cytokines.

91.11 Conclusion

Managing anemia in the ICU requires a comprehensive and systematic approach that addresses the underlying causes while minimizing risks associated with interventions. Adopting a restrictive transfusion strategy, minimizing iatrogenic blood loss, correcting nutritional deficiencies, and managing inflammation are key components. Understanding the multifactorial nature of anemia in critical illness allows for targeted therapies, improving patient outcomes both during critical illness and in the recovery phase. Special attention should be given to vulnerable subgroups, and plans should be made for ongoing management of anemia after ICU discharge to facilitate full rehabilitation.

Algorithm 91.1: Approach to anemia in the ICU

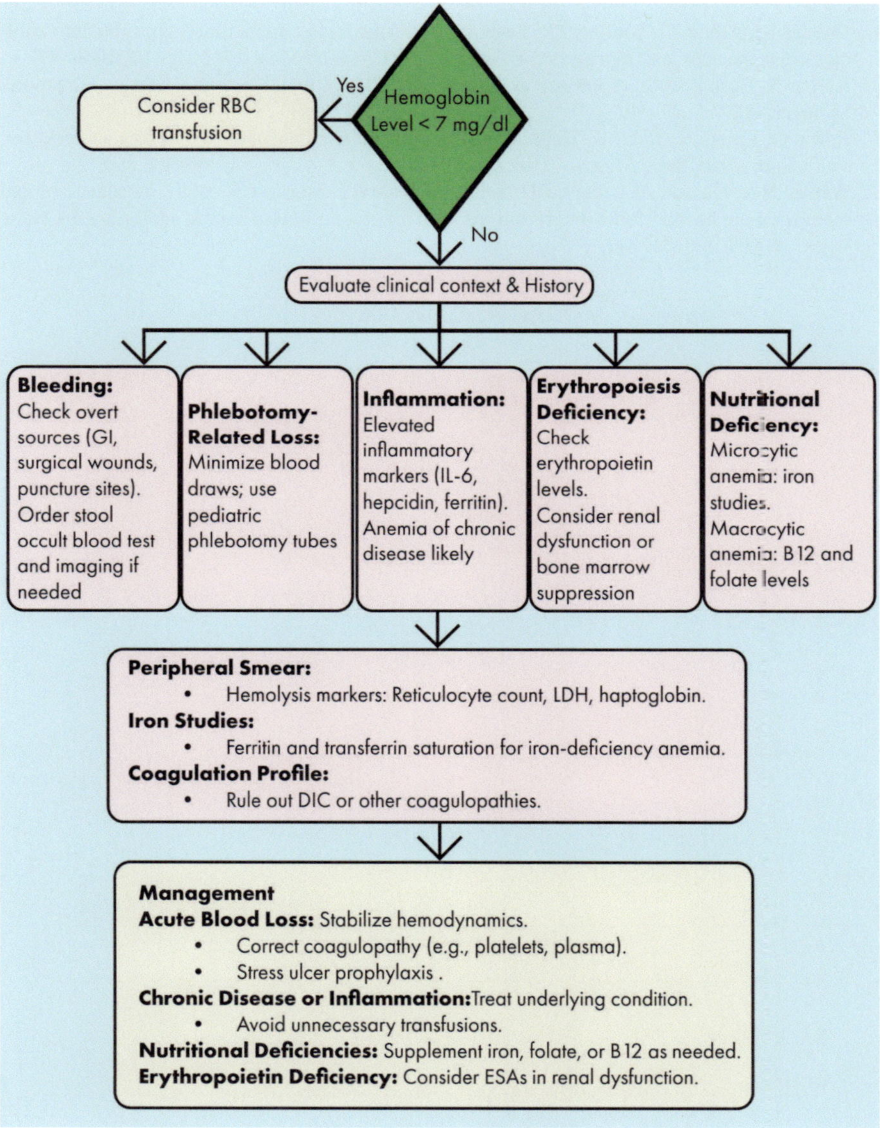

Bibliography

1. Hayden SJ, Albert TJ, Watkins TR, Swenson ER. Anemia in critical illness: insights into etiology, consequences, and management. Am J Respir Crit Care Med. 2012;185(10):1049–57.
2. Kumar N, Borkotoky A. Approach to anemia in ICU. In: Critical care hematology. Singapore: Springer; 2024. p. 47–59.
3. Rawal G, Kumar R, Yadav S, Singh A. Anemia in intensive care: a review of current concepts. J Crit Care Med (Targu Mures). 2016;2(3):109–14.
4. Warner MA, Hanson AC, Frank RD, Schulte PJ, Go RS, Storlie CB, et al. Prevalence of and recovery from anemia following hospitalization for critical illness among adults. JAMA Netw Open. 2020;3(9):e2017843.

Chapter 92
Approach to Thrombocytopenia in the ICU

92.1 Introduction

Thrombocytopenia, defined as a platelet count below 150×10^9/L, is a prevalent concern in the intensive care unit (ICU), affecting up to 41% of critically ill patients. The incidence varies significantly across different ICU settings—medical, surgical, cardiac—and among diverse patient demographics due to varying underlying conditions, interventions, and comorbidities. Thrombocytopenia is more than a laboratory anomaly; it is closely associated with adverse outcomes such as increased mortality, heightened bleeding risk, and a greater need for organ support therapies [1, 2] [Ref: Algorithm 92.1].

A systematic and nuanced approach is essential to promptly identify the etiology of thrombocytopenia, guide targeted management, and improve patient outcomes.

92.2 Confirm True Thrombocytopenia

- Rationale: Before initiating a workup, it is crucial to ensure that the thrombocytopenia is genuine and not an artifact (pseudothrombocytopenia).
- Key Considerations:
- Platelet Count Verification: Confirm that the platelet count is below 150×10^9/L.
- Exclude Pseudothrombocytopenia:
- Peripheral Smear Examination: Look for platelet clumping, giant platelets, or platelet satellitism, which may indicate laboratory artifacts.
- Repeat Testing: If clumping is observed, repeat the platelet count using a citrated or heparinized blood sample to eliminate EDTA-induced clumping.
- Management: If pseudothrombocytopenia is confirmed, no further investigation is needed.

S. B. Mishra et al., *Mastering ICU Care*,
https://doi.org/10.1007/978-981-95-0179-3_92

92.3 Evaluate Platelet Trajectory

- Rationale: Assessing the trend of platelet counts over time (platelet trajectory) provides valuable diagnostic and prognostic information.
- Key Considerations:
- Acute vs. Chronic Decline:
- Acute Drop (1–2 Days): Suggests conditions like disseminated intravascular coagulation (DIC), thrombotic microangiopathies (TMAs), or immune-mediated thrombocytopenias.
- Gradual Decline: May indicate bone marrow suppression, chronic liver disease, or sepsis.
- Predictive Value: Studies have shown that certain platelet trajectories correlate with increased mortality and morbidity. For instance, a persistent decline may predict worse outcomes.
- Action: Regular platelet count monitoring to detect significant changes and intervene promptly [3].

92.4 Explore Underlying Pathophysiological Mechanisms

- Rationale: Understanding the mechanisms leading to thrombocytopenia aids in narrowing down the differential diagnosis.
- Mechanisms Specific to ICU Patients:
- Decreased Production:
- Bone Marrow Suppression: Due to chemotherapy, radiation, severe infections, or infiltrative diseases like leukemia
- Nutritional Deficiencies: Vitamin B12 or folate deficiency impairs megakaryocyte function.
- Increased Consumption:
- DIC: Thrombin-mediated platelet activation leads to widespread microthrombi formation.
- Sepsis: Systemic inflammation accelerates platelet consumption.
- Extracellular Histones: Released during cell death, they can activate platelets and promote thrombosis.
- HELLP Syndrome (Hemolysis Elevated Liver Enzyme Low Platelet).
- Immune-Mediated Destruction:
- Heparin-Induced Thrombocytopenia (HIT): Antibodies against platelet factor 4-heparin complexes cause platelet activation and thrombosis.
- Immune Thrombocytopenic Purpura (ITP): Autoantibody-mediated platelet destruction.

- Drug-Induced Thrombocytopenia: Certain drugs can trigger immune-mediated platelet destruction.
  - Antimicrobials- Piperacillin, vancomycin, linezolid, trimethoprim/sulfamethoxazole, aztreonam.
  - Other- Phenytoin, Valproic acid, Aspirin, Ranitidine, Frusemide, Haloperidol.
- Thrombotic Microangiopathies (TMAs):
- Thrombotic Thrombocytopenic Purpura (TTP): Due to ADAMTS13 deficiency, leading to accumulation of ultra-large von Willebrand factor multimers and microthrombi.
- Hemolytic Uremic Syndrome (HUS): Often related to endothelial damage from shiga-toxin producing bacteria.
- Sequestration:
- Splenomegaly: Enlarged spleen traps platelets, reducing circulating counts.
- Portal Hypertension: Common in liver disease, leading to hypersplenism.
- Pseudothrombocytopenia:
- Laboratory Artifact: EDTA-induced platelet clumping falsely lowers automated platelet counts [4].

92.5 Detailed Etiological Framework

- Classification of Thrombocytopenia:
- Decreased Production:
- Bone Marrow Disorders: Aplastic anemia, myelodysplastic syndromes.
- Nutritional Deficiencies: B12, folate, iron.
- Increased Consumption:
- DIC, Sepsis, Massive Hemorrhage: Accelerated platelet use.
- Mechanical Devices: ECMO, intra-aortic balloon pumps causing platelet activation.
- Immune-Mediated Destruction:
- HIT, ITP, Drug-Induced Thrombocytopenia: Immune system targets platelets.
- Hemophagocytic Lymphohistiocytosis (HLH): Hyperinflammatory state causing phagocytosis of blood cells.
- Sequestration:
- Splenomegaly, Cirrhosis: Platelet pooling in an enlarged spleen.
- Pseudothrombocytopenia:
- Laboratory Artifacts: Platelet clumping in vitro.
- Rarer Causes:
- HLH: Consider in patients with persistent fever, cytopenias, organomegaly, and high ferritin levels.
- Drug-Induced Thrombocytopenia: Suspect in patients with new medications; common culprits include quinine, antibiotics, anticonvulsants.
- Other TMAs: Atypical HUS, often associated with complement pathway dysregulation.

92.6 Advanced Diagnostic Insights

- Peripheral Smear Evaluation:
- Microangiopathic Hemolysis: Presence of schistocytes indicates TMA or DIC.
- Giant Platelets: May suggest a myeloproliferative disorder or inherited platelet disorders.
- Laboratory Tests:
- Coagulation Profile: PT/INR, aPTT, fibrinogen, D-dimer for DIC assessment.
- ADAMTS13 Activity: Low levels (<10%) support TTP diagnosis.
- HIT Testing: ELISA for PF4-heparin antibodies and functional assays like serotonin release assay.
- Diagnostic Algorithms:
- DIC: Prolonged PT/INR, low fibrinogen, elevated D-dimer.
- TTP: Severe thrombocytopenia, microangiopathic hemolytic anemia, normal coagulation tests.
- HUS: Similar to TTP but often with renal failure; stool cultures may identify shiga-toxin.

92.7 Management Algorithm Enhancements

- Treat the Underlying Cause:
- Sepsis: Prompt antibiotic therapy, source control, supportive care.
- DIC: Address the trigger (e.g., infection, malignancy), replace coagulation factors cautiously.
- HIT: Discontinue heparin, initiate alternative anticoagulation (argatroban, bivalirudin).
- TTP: Urgent plasma exchange, steroids, and possibly rituximab.
- HUS: Supportive care; eculizumab for atypical HUS.
- HLH: Immunosuppressive therapy (steroids, etoposide), treat underlying infection or malignancy.
- Platelet Transfusion Guidelines:
- Prophylactic Transfusion:
- Counts $<10 \times 10^9$/L: Recommended to prevent spontaneous bleeding.
- Higher Thresholds: For patients with fever, sepsis, or coagulopathy, consider transfusion at $<20 \times 10^9$/L.
- Therapeutic Transfusion:
- Active Bleeding: Maintain platelet count $>50 \times 10^9$/L.
- Invasive Procedures:
- Major Surgery or Lumbar Puncture: Target $>50 \times 10^9$/L.
- Neurosurgery or Ophthalmic Surgery: Target $>100 \times 10^9$/L.
- Patients undergoing central line insertion: Target $>20 \times 10^9$ cells/L.
- Risks and Considerations:
- Transfusion Reactions: Allergic reactions, febrile nonhemolytic reactions.

- Alloimmunization: Reduced efficacy of future transfusions.
- Thrombosis Risk: In HIT or TTP; platelet transfusions may exacerbate thrombosis.
- Condition-Specific Management:
- Avoid Platelet Transfusion:
- HIT and TTP: Platelet transfusions are generally contraindicated unless life-threatening bleeding occurs.
- ECMO Patients:
- Anticoagulation Management: Balance between preventing circuit thrombosis and minimizing bleeding risk.
- Platelet Count Targets: Maintain platelet counts >50 × 10^9/L to reduce bleeding complications [5].

92.8 Emerging Insights

- Recent Studies:
- PLOT-ICU Study:
- Objective: Evaluated the efficacy and safety of prophylactic platelet transfusions in ICU patients.
- Findings: Restrictive transfusion strategy (transfusing at lower platelet counts) was non-inferior regarding bleeding events and reduced transfusion-related complications.
- Implications: Supports individualized transfusion strategies and reconsideration of transfusion thresholds.
- Ongoing Research:
- Novel Therapeutics: Agents targeting specific pathways like complement inhibitors in atypical HUS.
- Biomarkers: Identifying early detection and prognosis markers, such as elevated histone levels indicating endothelial damage.

92.9 Conclusion

Thrombocytopenia in the ICU represents a complex interplay of factors that can significantly impact patient outcomes. A comprehensive approach—starting from confirming true thrombocytopenia to exploring advanced diagnostic insights and understanding pathophysiological mechanisms—is essential for effective management. Incorporating recent evidence from studies like the PLOT-ICU trial and emerging therapies can refine treatment strategies.

Individualizing patient care by considering specific etiologies, severity, patient age, and comorbid conditions enhances the efficacy of interventions and minimizes risks. By staying abreast of emerging insights and maintaining a patient-centered focus, healthcare providers can improve survival rates and quality of care for critically ill patients with thrombocytopenia.

Algorithm 92.1: Approach to thrombocytopenia in the ICU

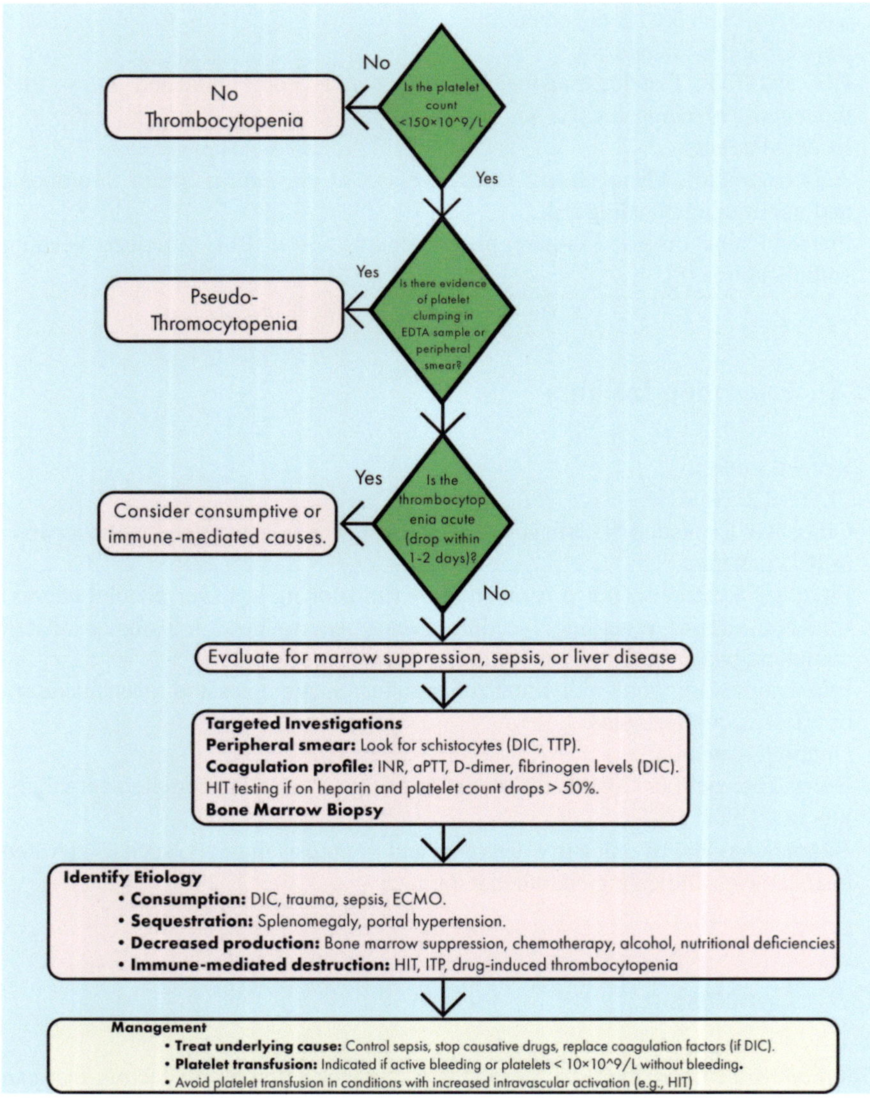

Bibliography

1. Anthon CT, Pene F, Perner A, Azoulay E, Puxty K, Van De Louw A, et al. Thrombocytopenia and platelet transfusions in ICU patients: an international inception cohort study (PLOT-ICU). Intensive Care Med. 2023;49(11):1327–38.
2. Patil KR, Patil RB. Approach to thrombocytopenia in ICU. In: Critical care hematology. Singapore: Springer; 2024. p. 75–85.
3. Vincent JL, Castro P, Hunt BJ, Jorres A, Praga M, Rojas-Suarez J, et al. Thrombocytopenia in the ICU: disseminated intravascular coagulation and thrombotic microangiopathies-what intensivists need to know. Crit Care. 2018;22(1):158.
4. Ostadi Z, Shadvar K, Sanaie S, Mahmoodpoor A, Saghaleini SH. Thrombocytopenia in the intensive care unit. Pak J Med Sci. 2019;35(1):282–7.
5. Greinacher A, Selleng S. How I evaluate and treat thrombocytopenia in the intensive care unit patient. Blood. 2016;128(26):3032–42.

Chapter 93
Approach to Pancytopenia in the ICU

93.1 Introduction

Pancytopenia, characterized by the simultaneous reduction of hemoglobin, neutrophils, and platelets below critical levels, is a significant clinical concern in the ICU. It reflects a broad spectrum of pathophysiological processes ranging from bone marrow suppression to peripheral destruction of blood elements. Effective management requires a systematic approach to diagnosis and treatment, as the causes can range from nutritional deficiencies to life-threatening conditions like disseminated intravascular coagulation (DIC) or hemophagocytic lymphohistiocytosis (HLH). This chapter provides a comprehensive approach to pancytopenia in critically ill patients, incorporating advanced diagnostic tools, management strategies, and considerations for special populations and emerging conditions [1, 2] [Ref: Algorithm 93.1].

93.2 Criteria

The following thresholds define Pancytopenia:

- Hemoglobin: <10 g/dL.
- Absolute neutrophil count (ANC): <1500/μL.
- Platelet count: <100,000/μL.

These thresholds should prompt immediate investigation to determine the underlying cause, especially in the ICU where patients are vulnerable to rapid deterioration.

S. B. Mishra et al., *Mastering ICU Care*,
https://doi.org/10.1007/978-981-95-0179-3_93

93.3 Etiological Classification

A thorough understanding of the potential causes is essential for effective management. The etiologies can be broadly classified into inherited syndromes, acquired conditions, nutritional deficiencies, autoimmune processes, infections, and other systemic diseases.

Inherited Syndromes
- Fanconi Anemia: A genetic disorder leading to bone marrow failure, congenital anomalies, and increased cancer risk.
- Dyskeratosis Congenita: A telomere maintenance disorder causing bone marrow failure, skin abnormalities, and pulmonary fibrosis.

Acquired Conditions
- Paroxysmal Nocturnal Hemoglobinuria (PNH): A stem cell disorder causing hemolysis, thrombosis, and bone marrow failure.
- Myelodysplastic Syndromes (MDS): Clonal hematopoietic stem cell disorders leading to ineffective hematopoiesis and risk of transformation to acute myeloid leukemia.
- Aplastic Anemia: Immune-mediated destruction of hematopoietic stem cells resulting in pancytopenia.

Nutritional Deficiencies
- Vitamin B12 and Folate Deficiency: Lead to megaloblastic anemia characterized by macrocytic red blood cells and ineffective erythropoiesis.
- Copper Deficiency: Causes neutropenia and anemia due to impaired hematopoiesis.
- Zinc Toxicity: Excess zinc interferes with copper absorption, leading to secondary copper deficiency and cytopenias.

Autoimmune Processes
- Systemic Lupus Erythematosus (SLE): Autoantibody-mediated destruction of blood cell lines.
- Felty's Syndrome: A triad of rheumatoid arthritis, neutropenia, and splenomegaly resulting in increased peripheral destruction.

Infections
- Sepsis and Cytokine Storms: Lead to bone marrow suppression and increased peripheral destruction.
- Viral Infections: Such as HIV, EBV, and emerging viruses like SARS-CoV-2 (COVID-19), can cause bone marrow suppression and cytokine-induced damage.

Hypersplenism
- Portal Hypertension: Causes splenomegaly and sequestration of blood cells.
- Infiltrative Diseases: Such as sarcoidosis or malignancies leading to splenic enlargement and cytopenias.

Hemophagocytic Lymphohistiocytosis (HLH)

- HLH: A life-threatening hyperinflammatory syndrome characterized by excessive activation of macrophages and cytotoxic T cells, leading to hemophagocytosis and pancytopenia.

HLH should be considered in patients with unremitting fevers and hyperferritinemia. The probability of HLH can be calculated via the H-score.

Iatrogenic

Chemotherapy, radiotherapy, antibiotics such as chloramphenicol, trimethoprim, and linezolid. Other medications like azathioprine, methotrexate, carbamazepine, and valproate.

Geographic and Epidemiological Variations

- Megaloblastic Anemia in South Asia: Higher prevalence due to dietary habits and malnutrition.
- Infectious Causes in Endemic Areas: Such as malaria, leishmaniasis, and certain viral infections contributing to pancytopenia.

93.4 Initial Workup

The patient's medical history should be thoroughly reviewed to identify potential causes of the disease. This includes evaluating symptoms such as fever, night sweats, weight loss, jaundice, fatigue, recurrent bleeding, and infections. A past history of drug or toxin exposure should be taken to investigate iatrogenic causes of pancytopenia. Travel history may indicate a tropical infection leading to hypersplenism. Physical examination should include assessment for lymphadenopathy, hepatomegaly, or splenomegaly.

The diagnostic workup aims to distinguish between central (bone marrow) and peripheral causes of pancytopenia. Early identification is crucial in the ICU to prevent rapid deterioration.

Complete Blood Count (CBC)

- Quantifies Cytopenias: Determines the severity and combination of low cell lines.
- Mean Corpuscular Volume (MCV): Assesses for macrocytosis or microcytosis, suggesting nutritional deficiencies or hemoglobinopathies.

Peripheral Blood Smear

- Cell Morphology: Identifies abnormal shapes, sizes, or inclusions in blood cells.
- Blasts and Dysplastic Cells: Suggestive of leukemias or MDS.
  Schistocytes: Indicate microangiopathic hemolytic anemia.

Reticulocyte Count

- Bone Marrow Activity: Low reticulocyte count suggests decreased production; high count indicates peripheral destruction or hemolysis.

Bone Marrow Examination

- Aspiration and Biopsy: Essential for diagnosing bone marrow disorders, infiltrative diseases, or malignancies.
- Cytogenetics and Flow Cytometry: Provide detailed information on cell lineage and genetic abnormalities.

Advanced Diagnostic Tools

- Next-Generation Sequencing (NGS): Detects genetic mutations associated with MDS, HLH, and inherited bone marrow failure syndromes.
- Molecular Diagnostics: Identify specific gene mutations (e.g., TP53, RUNX1) guiding prognosis and therapy.
- Immature Platelet Fraction (IPF) or Reticulated Platelet Count: Differentiate between decreased production and increased destruction of platelets.

93.5 Pathophysiological Insights

Autoimmune Processes

- Mechanism: Autoantibodies target blood cell antigens leading to their destruction.
- SLE: Autoantibodies against nuclear components cause complement-mediated lysis of cells.
- Treatment Implications: Immunosuppressive therapies reduce antibody production and inflammation.

Sepsis and Cytokine Storms

- Impact on Hematopoiesis: Pro-inflammatory cytokines suppress bone marrow function.
- Peripheral Destruction: Activation of the coagulation system and endothelial damage lead to consumption of blood cells.
- Critical Care Context: Management controls infection and modulates the immune response.

93.6 Management

Effective management involves supportive care and addressing the underlying cause.

Supportive Care

- Transfusion Thresholds:
- Hemoglobin: Maintain above 7 g/dL in stable patients; higher thresholds for those with cardiovascular disease.
- Platelets: Transfuse when <10,000/μL or < 20,000/μL if febrile or bleeding risk is high.
- Infection Management:

- Empirical Antibiotics: Early initiation in neutropenic fever.
- Antifungal and Antiviral Prophylaxis: Consider in prolonged neutropenia.
- Growth Factors:
- G-CSF: Stimulates neutrophil production in neutropenia.
- Thrombopoietin Receptor Agonists: Eltrombopag promotes platelet production, especially in aplastic anemia.

Targeted Therapies
- Aplastic Anemia:
- Immunosuppressive Therapy: Combination of antithymocyte globulin (ATG) and cyclosporine.
- Eltrombopag: Enhances hematopoiesis in refractory cases.
- Autoimmune Cytopenias:
- Corticosteroids: First-line therapy to reduce immune-mediated destruction.
- Rituximab: Monoclonal antibody against CD20 for steroid-refractory cases.
- Advanced Immunomodulatory Therapies: Such as azathioprine or mycophenolate mofetil.
- Myelodysplastic Syndromes (MDS):
- Hypomethylating Agents: Azacitidine or decitabine improve blood counts and delay progression.
- Lenalidomide: Effective in del(5q) MDS subtype.
- Hemophagocytic Lymphohistiocytosis (HLH):
- HLH-94 Protocol: Dexamethasone and etoposide-based regimen.
- Emerging Therapies: Targeted treatments like emapalumab (an interferon-gamma blocker).

Interventions for Refractory Cases
- Hematopoietic Stem Cell Transplantation (HSCT):
- Curative Potential: Especially in inherited bone marrow failure syndromes and severe aplastic anemia.
- Considerations: Patient's age, comorbidities, and availability of a suitable donor.
- Splenic Embolization or Splenectomy:
- Indications: Hypersplenism causing severe cytopenias unresponsive to medical therapy.
- Risks: Post-splenectomy infections; prophylactic vaccinations recommended.

Special Populations

Pediatric Patients
- Distinct Presentations: Higher likelihood of inherited syndromes like Fanconi anemia or dyskeratosis congenita.
- Management Considerations:
- Genetic Counseling: For family planning and risk assessment.
- Growth and Development Monitoring: Addressing endocrine and developmental issues.

- HSCT: Often considered earlier due to the progressive nature of inherited disorders.

Elderly Patients
- Myelodysplastic Syndromes Prevalence: Increases with age.
- Comorbidities: Affect treatment choices and tolerability.
- Management Strategies:
- Less Intensive Therapies: Adjusted doses of hypomethylating agents.
- Supportive Care Focus: Quality of life and symptom management.

Supportive Care Protocols in the ICU

Transfusion Strategies
- Individualized Thresholds: Based on patient's hemodynamic status, bleeding risk, and comorbidities.
- Leukoreduced and Irradiated Blood Products: Reduce the risk of transfusion reactions and graft-versus-host disease.

Infection Management
- Neutropenic Precautions: Protective isolation, strict hand hygiene.
- Empirical Antimicrobials: Broad-spectrum antibiotics initiated promptly.
- Antifungal and Antiviral Agents: For high-risk patients.

Organ Support
- Renal Replacement Therapy: If acute kidney injury develops due to sepsis or HLH.
- Mechanical Ventilation: For respiratory failure, often complicated by infections or pulmonary hemorrhage.

93.7 Emerging Conditions and Contexts

COVID-19 and Other Viral Pandemics
- Bone Marrow Suppression: Direct viral effects or immune-mediated damage leading to cytopenias.
- Cytokine Storms: Exacerbate pancytopenia and require immunomodulatory therapies.
- Management:
- Antiviral Treatments: As per evolving guidelines.
- Immunotherapies: Tocilizumab (IL-6 inhibitor) used in cytokine release syndrome.

Sepsis-Induced Pancytopenia

- Pathophysiology: Overwhelming infection leads to bone marrow suppression and increased consumption.
- Therapeutic Apheresis: Considered in severe cases of hyperinflammation.

93.8 Conclusion

The approach to pancytopenia in the ICU necessitates a comprehensive and systematic evaluation to identify the underlying cause promptly. Incorporating advanced diagnostic tools like NGS and molecular diagnostics enhances the accuracy of diagnoses such as MDS and HLH. Understanding the pathophysiological mechanisms, particularly in autoimmune processes and cytokine storms, guides targeted therapy.

Management strategies should be refined to include targeted therapies like eltrombopag for aplastic anemia and advanced immunomodulatory treatments for autoimmune cytopenias. Interventions for refractory cases, including hematopoietic stem cell transplantation and splenic embolization, should be considered.

Special attention is required for pediatric and elderly populations, acknowledging their distinct presentations and management needs. Additionally, emerging conditions like COVID-19 necessitate adaptability in management approaches due to their impact on bone marrow function.

Early intervention with appropriate supportive care protocols, tailored for ICU patients—including transfusion thresholds and infection management strategies—is critical. A structured algorithm ensures systematic assessment and guides appropriate interventions, ultimately improving patient outcomes in this critical setting.

Algorithm 93.1: Approach to pancytopenia in the ICU

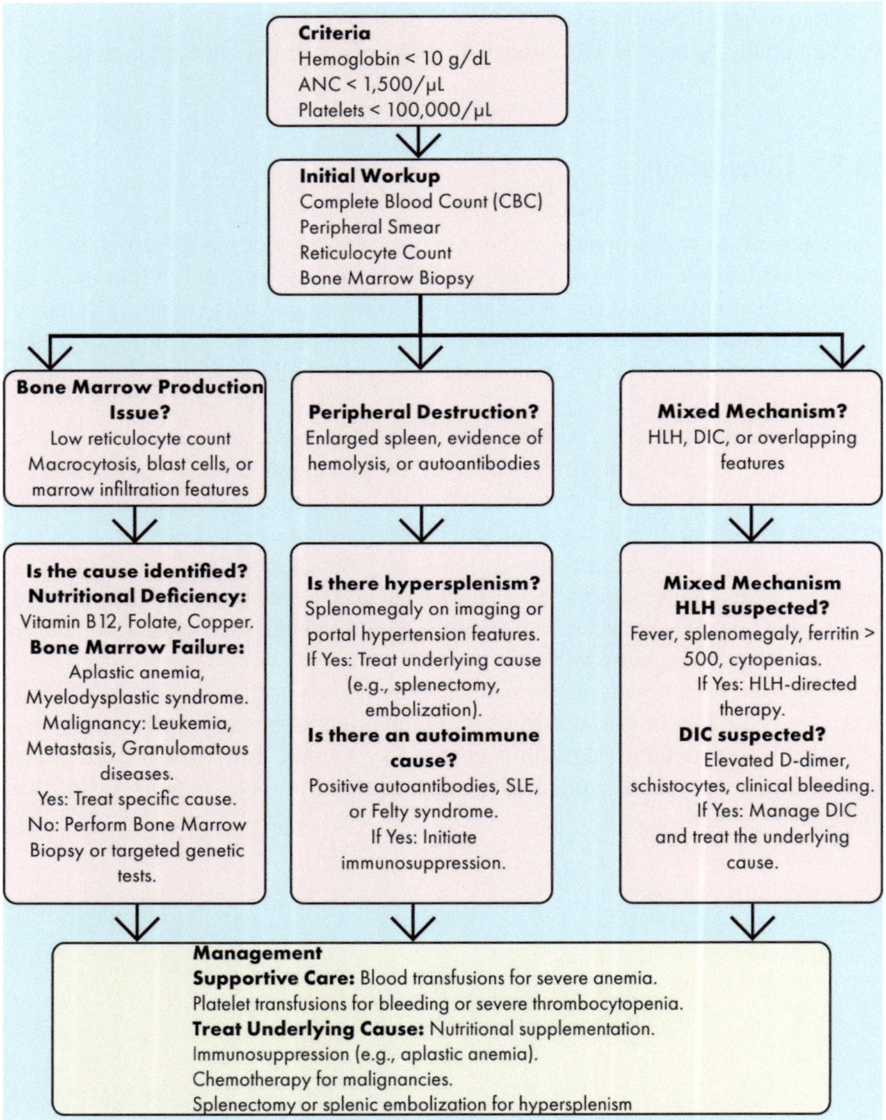

Bibliography

1. Gnanaraj J, Parnes A, Francis CW, Go RS, Takemoto CM, Hashmi SK. Approach to pancytopenia: diagnostic algorithm for clinical hematologists. Blood Rev. 2018;32(5):361–7.
2. Chew S, Kamangar M. Approach to pancytopenia: from blood tests to the bedside. Clin Med (Lond). 2024;24(5):100235.

Chapter 94
Approach to Massive Transfusion in the ICU

94.1 Introduction

Massive transfusion (MT) is a critical intervention in the management of severe hemorrhage, frequently encountered in trauma, perioperative, obstetric emergencies, and other critical care settings. It involves rapidly replacing blood products to restore circulating volume, oxygen-carrying capacity, and hemostasis. Early and structured intervention is crucial, as uncontrolled bleeding can lead to the "triad of death": hypothermia, acidosis, and coagulopathy [1, 2] [Ref: Algorithm 94.1].

94.2 Historical Perspective and Evolution

The development of massive transfusion protocols (MTPs) has its roots in military medicine during World Wars I and II. The high incidence of traumatic injuries and hemorrhage on the battlefield necessitated efficient blood replacement strategies. These military practices emphasized rapid, coordinated transfusion efforts to save lives under extreme conditions. Over time, the principles derived from these experiences transitioned into civilian medicine, establishing standardized MTPs in hospitals worldwide. The evolution reflects a growing understanding of the importance of timely and balanced transfusion therapy in managing massive hemorrhage [3].

94.3 Definitions of Massive Transfusion

Various definitions of massive transfusion exist, reflecting the dynamic and urgent nature of severe bleeding. Traditional definitions include:

S. B. Mishra et al., *Mastering ICU Care*,
https://doi.org/10.1007/978-981-95-0179-3_94

- Replace more than 10 units of packed red blood cells (PRBCs) within 24 h.
- Loss of one blood volume within 24 h.

Dynamic definitions, which better capture clinical urgency, include:

- Replacement of 50% of total blood volume within 3 h.
- Transfusion of more than 4 units of PRBCs in 1 h with ongoing bleeding.

Understanding these definitions aids in the early recognition and timely activation of MTPs.

94.4 Predictive Tools

Early identification of patients likely to require massive transfusion improves outcomes. Predictive tools include:

- Assessment of Blood Consumption (ABC) Score: Considers factors like penetrating injury, systolic blood pressure <90 mmHg, heart rate >120 bpm, and a positive Focused Assessment with Sonography for Trauma (FAST) exam.
- Shock Index: Calculated as heart rate divided by systolic blood pressure; values >0.9 indicate significant hypovolemia [4].

These tools assist clinicians in making prompt decisions regarding MTP activation.

94.5 Institutional Protocols

Institutional MTPs facilitate effective communication among multidisciplinary teams, ensure the rapid availability of blood products, and standardize care. Key components include:

- Clear activation criteria and procedures.
- Defined roles and responsibilities for team members.
- Guidelines for blood product ratios and adjunctive therapies.

Standardized protocols minimize delays and reduce variability in patient care during emergencies.

94.6 Clinical Contexts

Massive transfusion may be required in various clinical scenarios:

- Trauma: Severe injuries, especially penetrating trauma, can lead to life-threatening hemorrhage.
- Obstetric Hemorrhage: Conditions like placenta previa, uterine atony, or ruptured ectopic pregnancy necessitate rapid intervention.
- Gastrointestinal Bleeding: Massive bleeding from varices or ulcers requires prompt management.
- Perioperative Crises: Surgical complications may result in unexpected significant blood loss.

Each scenario demands specific considerations regarding patient management and transfusion strategies.

94.7 Immediate Assessment of Blood Product Availability

Upon recognizing significant hemorrhage:

- If blood products are available: Initiate transfusion using a balanced ratio (commonly 1:1:1) of PRBCs, plasma, and platelets to mimic whole blood and reduce coagulopathy risk.
- If not immediately available: Begin resuscitation with crystalloids while urgently arranging for blood products.

Timely transfusion is crucial to address hypovolemia and coagulopathy effectively.

94.8 Evaluation of Coagulation Parameters

Assess coagulation status using:

- Laboratory Tests: Prothrombin time (PT)/International Normalized Ratio (INR), activated partial thromboplastin time (aPTT), fibrinogen levels, platelet counts.
- Thromboelastography (TEG) or Rotational Thromboelastometry (ROTEM): Provide real-time insights into clot formation, strength, and stability.

Abnormal parameters indicate the need for targeted therapy with plasma, platelets, cryoprecipitate, or fibrinogen concentrate.

94.9 Laboratory and Real-Time Monitoring

Continuous monitoring guides ongoing management:

- Hemoglobin and Hematocrit: Evaluate oxygen-carrying capacity.
- Lactate Levels: Reflect tissue perfusion and oxygenation.
- Electrolytes: Monitor calcium and potassium levels to detect hypocalcemia or hyperkalemia.
- TEG/ROTEM: Adjust transfusion therapy based on dynamic coagulation profiles.

Regular assessment ensures appropriate and effective intervention [5].

94.10 Adjunctive Therapies

Adjunctive measures enhance hemostasis:

- Tranexamic Acid (TXA): Early administration reduces mortality in trauma by inhibiting fibrinolysis.
- Calcium Supplementation: Corrects hypocalcemia due to citrate binding from transfused blood products, essential for coagulation and cardiac function.

The Joint Trauma System Clinical Practice Guideline (CPG) for Damage Control Resuscitation suggests that 1 g of calcium chloride or 3 g of calcium gluconate be administered to patients in hemorrhagic shock during or immediately after the first unit of blood product transfusion and then with ongoing resuscitation after every 4 units of blood products, with monitoring of iCa and repletion if <1.2 mmol/L

- Fibrinogen Concentrate or Cryoprecipitate: Addresses low fibrinogen levels critical for clot formation.

Four-factor prothrombin complex concentrate (4F-PCC): It is a pathogen-reduced, freeze-dried product that provides therapeutic levels of vitamin K-dependent clotting factors: factors II, VII, IX, and X. It has been suggested as a possible adjunct treatment to counteract the effects of trauma-induced coagulopathy (TIC). While 4F-PCC is commonly used to reverse anticoagulation caused by vitamin K antagonists (VKAs) or direct oral anticoagulants (DOACs) in cases of severe bleeding, it has also been employed in patients with TIC who are not on anticoagulants. Its advantages include quick correction of coagulopathy, the need for smaller infusion volumes, and reduced risks associated with transfusions. Due to these benefits, European guidelines recommend 4F-PCC as part of the management strategy for bleeding and coagulopathy after major trauma.

Evidence supports the early use of these therapies to improve patient outcomes.

94.11 Prevention of the Triad of Death

Preventing hypothermia, acidosis, and coagulopathy is vital:

- Hypothermia: Use warming devices and warmed fluids to maintain body temperature above 36 °C.
- Acidosis: Optimize ventilation and perfusion; consider bicarbonate therapy if necessary.
- Coagulopathy: Administer appropriate blood products guided by coagulation monitoring.

Addressing these factors reduces bleeding and improves survival.

94.12 Control of Bleeding Source

Definitive bleeding control is essential:

- Surgical Intervention: Expedient surgery may be necessary to control internal bleeding.
- Interventional Radiology: Techniques like embolization can manage bleeding in less accessible areas.
- Endoscopic Procedures: Useful in gastrointestinal bleeding for direct hemostasis.

Persistent hemorrhage requires a coordinated, multidisciplinary approach.

94.13 Complications of Massive Transfusion

Potential complications include:

- Citrate Toxicity and Hypocalcemia: Result from large volumes of citrate-preserved blood; monitor calcium levels and administer calcium gluconate or chloride as needed.
- Hyperkalemia: Due to potassium leakage from stored red blood cells; monitor serum potassium and manage accordingly.
- Immunological Reactions: Such as transfusion-related acute lung injury (TRALI) and transfusion-associated circulatory overload (TACO); recognize early signs and provide supportive care.
- Dilutional Coagulopathy: Caused by transfusion of PRBCs without adequate plasma or platelets; prevented by balanced transfusion ratios.

Awareness and prompt management of these complications are crucial.

94.14 Special Populations

94.14.1 Pediatric Patients

- Considerations: Smaller blood volumes necessitate precise dosing; higher risk of volume overload and hypothermia.
- Transfusion Strategies: Use weight-based calculations; utilize warmed blood products.

94.14.2 Obstetric Patients

- Considerations: Unique physiological changes in pregnancy affect hemodynamics and coagulation.
- Transfusion Strategies: Rapid volume replacement; consider uterotonic agents and coordination with obstetric specialists.

Tailoring transfusion strategies to these populations improves safety and efficacy.

94.15 Quality Improvement and Metrics

Implementing quality measures enhances MTP effectiveness:

- Performance Metrics: Track activation times, adherence to protocols, patient outcomes.
- Regular Audits: Identify deviations and areas for improvement.
- Education and Training: Ongoing staff education ensures familiarity with MTPs.

Continuous evaluation promotes optimal patient care and resource utilization.

94.16 Future Directions

Emerging advancements include:

- Use of Whole Blood: Reintroducing whole blood transfusions in civilian settings may simplify logistics and improve outcomes.
- Artificial Blood Products: Development of synthetic oxygen carriers and hemoglobin-based substitutes offers potential alternatives.
- Enhanced Monitoring Technologies: Point-of-care devices for real-time assessment may refine transfusion strategies.

Staying informed about these developments is essential for evolving practice.

94.17 Conclusion

Management of massive transfusion in the ICU requires early recognition, rapid MTP activation, and a coordinated multidisciplinary approach. Utilizing predictive tools, adhering to institutional protocols, and customizing strategies for specific clinical contexts enhance patient outcomes. Continuous monitoring, adjunctive therapies, and prevention of complications are integral to effective care. Special considerations for pediatric and obstetric populations, along with commitment to quality improvement, further optimize management. As advancements continue, integrating new technologies and practices will improve survival rates for patients requiring massive transfusion.

Algorithm 94.1: Approach to massive transfusion in the ICU

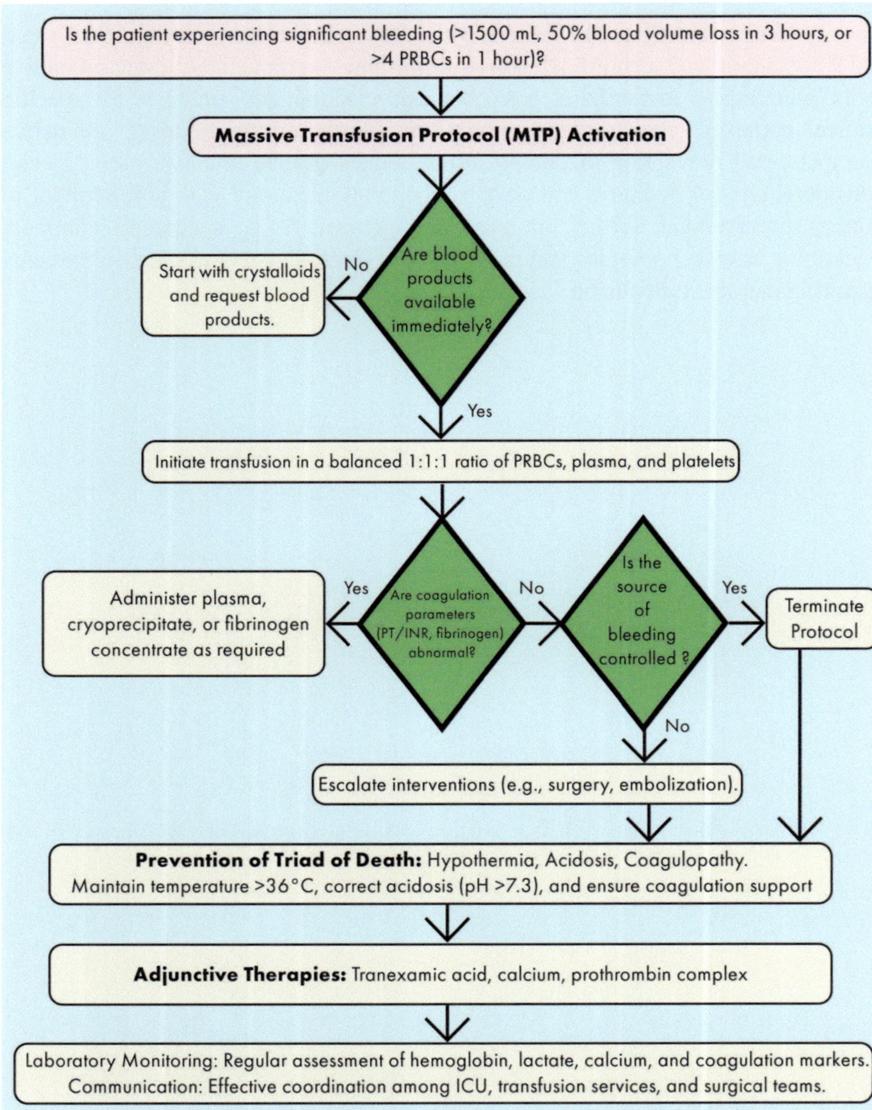

Bibliography

1. Moore SA, Raval JS. Massive transfusion: a review. Ann Blood. 2022;7:18.
2. Lin VS, Sun E, Yau S, Abeyakoon C, Seamer G, Bhopal S, et al. Definitions of massive transfusion in adults with critical bleeding: a systematic review. Crit Care. 2023;27(1):265.
3. Young PP, Cotton BA, Goodnough LT. Massive transfusion protocols for patients with substantial hemorrhage. Transfus Med Rev. 2011;25(4):293–303.
4. Patil V, Shetmahajan M. Massive transfusion and massive transfusion protocol. Indian J Anaesth. 2014;58(5):590–5.
5. Pham HP, Shaz BH. Update on massive transfusion. Br J Anaesth. 2013;111(Suppl 1):i71–82.

Chapter 95
Approach to General Poisoning in the ICU

95.1 Introduction

Poisoning remains a critical and potentially life-threatening presentation in the ICU, requiring prompt and systematic evaluation and intervention. Globally, poisoning accounts for a significant number of ICU admissions, with trends varying by region. Data from the American Association of Poison Control Centers (AAPCC) indicate thousands of poisoning incidents annually, highlighting both accidental and intentional exposures. Studies from India reveal a high prevalence of pesticide poisoning, often leading to severe outcomes due to the toxicity of agents involved and delays in treatment. Mortality rates are notably higher in intentional poisonings compared to accidental exposures, underscoring the urgency of effective management strategies [1–3].

General poisoning cases involve diverse toxins, each with specific clinical features and management protocols. This chapter outlines a structured approach to stabilize patients, assess risks, identify toxins, and initiate appropriate treatments, incorporating the latest recommendations and therapeutic innovations [Ref: Algorithm 95.1].

95.2 Initial Stabilization (ABCs)

- Airway: Assess and secure the airway to prevent aspiration and ensure adequate oxygenation. If compromised, consider endotracheal intubation. Common indications for intubation include altered mental status or airway obstruction. Advanced airway management strategies like Rapid Sequence Intubation (RSI) may be necessary for critically ill poisoned patients.

S. B. Mishra et al., *Mastering ICU Care*,
https://doi.org/10.1007/978-981-95-0179-3_95

- Breathing: Provide oxygen to address hypoxemia. Monitor for respiratory depression, which may suggest opioid or sedative-hypnotic toxicity. Mechanical ventilation may be required for severe cases.
- Circulation: Measure blood pressure, heart rate, and perfusion status. Administer IV fluids for hypotension. Vasopressors may be necessary if refractory shock occurs, especially in cardiotoxic overdoses (e.g., cyclic antidepressants). Continuous ECG monitoring is essential for early detection of arrhythmias.

95.3 Risk Assessment and Prioritization

Post-stabilization, a structured risk assessment is crucial to predict the toxicity course and tailor interventions:

- History and Exposure Details: Obtain information about the substance(s) involved, quantity, time of ingestion, and intent (accidental vs. intentional). Consider potential for mixed or unknown exposures.
- System-Based Diagnostic Approach:
- Cardiovascular: Assess for arrhythmias, conduction abnormalities, and signs of cardiotoxicity.
- Pulmonary: Evaluate for respiratory compromise or bronchospasm.
- Neurological: Monitor for altered mental status, seizures, or focal deficits.
- Gastrointestinal: Check for nausea, vomiting, abdominal pain, or bleeding.
- Renal and Hepatic: Assess for signs of organ dysfunction, such as decreased urine output or jaundice.
- Laboratory Tests: Order electrolytes, renal and liver function tests, blood glucose, arterial blood gases, and coagulation profiles. Obtain toxin-specific levels when indicated (e.g., acetaminophen, salicylates).
- Imaging and ECG: Perform ECG to detect cardiac abnormalities. Imaging studies may be required based on clinical suspicion (e.g., chest X-ray for aspiration).

95.4 Administer Coma Cocktail for Altered Mental Status

The "coma cocktail" targets reversible causes of unconsciousness in suspected poisoning:

- Dextrose: Administer if hypoglycemia is detected or suspected, as it can mimic severe poisoning.
- Thiamine: Give 100 mg IV to malnourished or alcoholic patients to prevent Wernicke's encephalopathy.
- Naloxone: Administer 0.04–2 mg IV for suspected opioid overdose to rapidly reverse respiratory depression. Titrate to improve respiratory function without precipitating withdrawal.

Note: The routine use of the coma cocktail is controversial and should be guided by clinical judgment.

95.5 Systematic Toxidrome Evaluation

A thorough assessment helps identify toxidromes, although overlapping presentations are common in mixed ingestions.

- Sedative-Hypnotics: CNS and respiratory depression, hypotension, bradycardia. Withdrawal may present with agitation and seizures.
- Opioids: Pinpoint pupils, respiratory depression, bradycardia, hypotension.
- Cholinergic: SLUDGE-M symptoms (Salivation, Lacrimation, Urination, Defecation, Gastrointestinal upset, Emesis, Miosis), bronchorrhea, bradycardia. Common in organophosphate poisoning.
- Anticholinergic: Hyperthermia, dry flushed skin, mydriasis, tachycardia, urinary retention, altered mental status ("hot as a hare, dry as a bone, red as a beet, mad as a hatter").
- Sympathomimetic: Agitation, tachycardia, hypertension, hyperthermia, mydriasis, diaphoresis. Seen with cocaine or amphetamine use.
- Serotonin Syndrome: Hyperreflexia, clonus, mydriasis, hyperthermia, autonomic instability.
- Withdrawal Syndromes: Alcohol or benzodiazepine withdrawal presents with tremors, hallucinations, tachycardia, hypertension, seizures.

Recognizing these patterns aids in narrowing down potential toxins and initiating appropriate treatments.

95.6 Supportive Measures

Adopt the Scandinavian method, emphasizing supportive care as the primary intervention:

- Symptom Management: Treat seizures with benzodiazepines, correct hypotension with fluids and vasopressors, manage arrhythmias per ACLS guidelines.
- Monitoring: Continuous observation of vital signs, neurological status, and organ function.
- Minimize Invasive Procedures: Avoid unnecessary interventions that may complicate the patient's condition.

95.7 Diagnostics

Understand the limitations and applications of toxicology screening:

- Limitations: Broad toxicology screens may not detect all substances and often do not impact acute management due to delayed results.
- Targeted Testing: Focus on specific toxins when identification will alter treatment (e.g., acetaminophen levels for N-acetylcysteine administration).
- ECG Monitoring: Essential for detecting cardiotoxic effects like QRS widening in tricyclic antidepressant overdose.

95.8 Decontamination and Operational Safety

- Activated Charcoal: Administer 1 g/kg (up to 50 g) for recent ingestions (within 1–2 h) if the airway is protected.
- Gastric Lavage: Rarely used; consider only for life-threatening ingestions within 1 h.
- Whole Bowel Irrigation: Use polyethylene glycol solutions for sustained-release preparations or substances not bound by charcoal (e.g., iron, lithium).

  Healthcare Worker Safety:

- Use personal protective equipment (PPE) during decontamination, especially with agents like organophosphates, to prevent secondary contamination.

95.9 Therapeutic Innovations

Lipid Emulsion Therapy:

- Indication: Overdose of lipophilic drugs (e.g., local anesthetics, certain antidepressants).
- Mechanism: Acts as a "lipid sink" to sequester fat-soluble toxins.
- Dose: Initial bolus of 1.5 mL/kg 20% lipid emulsion IV over 1 minute, followed by infusion.

  Extracorporeal Removal:

- Hemodialysis: Effective for methanol, ethylene glycol, lithium, salicylates.
- Hemoperfusion: Consider for high-molecular-weight or protein-bound toxins.
- Enhanced Elimination Techniques:
- Urinary Alkalinization: Useful for salicylate poisoning to enhance renal excretion.

95.10 Organ-Specific Management

Hepatic Failure:

- Acetaminophen Toxicity: Leads to coagulopathy and encephalopathy.
- Management: Early N-acetylcysteine administration, monitor liver function tests, consider liver transplantation in fulminant cases.

Cardiotoxicity:

- Tricyclic Antidepressants: Cause arrhythmias, hypotension.
- Management: Sodium bicarbonate therapy to narrow QRS complex, manage arrhythmias.

Renal Failure:

- Rhabdomyolysis: From prolonged immobilization or certain toxins.
- Management: Aggressive hydration, monitor electrolytes, consider dialysis.

95.11 Emerging Therapies and Guidelines

Stay updated with recent recommendations from key toxicology societies:

- American Academy of Clinical Toxicology (AACT).
- European Association of Poisons Centres and Clinical Toxicologists (EAPCCT).

These organizations provide evidence-based guidelines on managing specific toxins, dosing regimens, and new therapeutic interventions.

95.12 Tables and Quick-Reference Guides (Ref: Table 95.1).

Table 95.1 Common antidotes

Toxin	Antidote	Dose	Indications	Limitations
Acetaminophen	N-acetylcysteine	Oral: 140 mg/kg loading, then 70 mg/kg every 4 h (17 doses) IV: 150 mg/kg over 60 min, then 50 mg/kg over 4 h, then 100 mg/kg over 16 h	Elevated levels or ingestion >150 mg/kg	Best if started within 8 h of ingestion
Opioids	Naloxone	0.04–2 mg IV, repeat every 2–3 min as needed	Respiratory depression from opioids	May precipitate withdrawal
Benzodiazepines	Flumazenil	0.2 mg IV over 15 s, repeat up to 1 mg total	Known ingestion in non-tolerant patients	Risk of seizures in chronic users
Organophosphates	Atropine and Pralidoxime	Atropine: 1–2 mg IV every 5 min, Pralidoxine: 1–2 g IV over 30 min	Cholinergic symptoms	Monitor for atropine toxicity
Methanol/ethylene glycol	Fomepizole	15 mg/kg IV loading, then 10 mg/kg every 12 h	Toxic alcohol ingestion	Requires dialysis in severe cases
Digoxin	Digoxin-specific antibodies	Dose based on amount ingested or serum level	Life-threatening arrhythmias, hyperkalemia	Limited availability, costly
Beta-blockers/Ca channel blockers	Glucagon	3–10 mg IV bolus, followed by infusion	Refractory hypotension or bradycardia	May cause vomiting, hyperglycemia

95.13 Conclusion

A systematic approach to poisoning in the ICU enhances patient outcomes by ensuring prompt stabilization and targeted therapy. Prioritizing the airway, breathing, and circulation is crucial in the initial management of poisoned patients. A structured risk assessment helps predict the toxicity course and tailor interventions accordingly. Recognizing toxidromes enables clinicians to identify patterns and guide effective management strategies. Emphasizing supportive care through symptom management and continuous monitoring is fundamental. Judicious use of targeted diagnostics and laboratory tests assists in confirming suspected toxins and guiding treatment decisions. Incorporating therapeutic innovations, such as lipid emulsion therapy when appropriate, can improve patient outcomes. Promptly addressing organ-specific dysfunctions is essential to prevent further complications. Operational safety measures protect healthcare workers during decontamination procedures. Staying informed and adhering to current guidelines from toxicology societies ensures that management strategies are evidence-based and up-to-date. Early decontamination and elimination techniques, combined with supportive measures, are vital in preventing severe complications. Familiarity with this comprehensive approach is crucial for ICU providers managing toxicological emergencies.

Algorithm 95.1: Approach to general poisoning in the ICU

Initial Stabilization (ABCs)
Airway: Assess and secure if compromised.
Breathing: Provide oxygen; consider intubation if necessary.
Circulation: Monitor blood pressure and initiate IV fluids or vasopressors as required

↓

Administer coma cocktail for altered mental status
Dextrose (for hypoglycemia)
Thiamine (for malnourished or alcoholic patients)
Naloxone (for suspected opioid overdose)

↓

"SOCCER HALLS"
S - Sedative-hypnotic: CNS depression, respiratory depression, variable pupil size.
O - Opioid: Pinpoint pupils (miosis), respiratory depression, bradycardia.
C - Cholinergic: SLUDGE (Salivation, Lacrimation, Urination, Diarrhea, GI upset, Emesis), bradycardia, wheezing.
C - Cyclic antidepressant (anticholinergic): "Hot as a hare, dry as a bone, red as a beet, mad as a hatter" (hyperthermia, dry skin, flushed, delirium), tachycardia.
E - Ethanol or alcohol withdrawal: Agitation, tachycardia, tremors, seizures, confusion.
R - Sympathomimetic: Tachycardia, hypertension, dilated pupils (mydriasis), diaphoresis, ag tation.
H - Hallucinogenic: Hallucinations, mydriasis, tachycardia, hyperthermia, agitation.
A - Anticholinergic: Similar to cyclic antidepressant toxidrome.
L - Lithium or heavy metals: Tremor, confusion, GI distress, seizures (severe cases).
L - Local anesthetics (toxicity): CNS excitation followed by depression, seizures, arrhythmias
S - Serotonin Syndrome: Hyperreflexia, clonus, mydriasis, agitation, hyperthermia.

↓

Decontamination
Activated charcoal: For recent oral ingestions if no contraindications.
Gastric lavage: Rarely indicated; consider only for life-threatening cases.
Whole bowel irrigation: For extended-release drugs or heavy metal ingestion.

Focused Management
Antidotes: Administer specific antidotes based on identified toxin (e.g., N-acetylcysteine for acetaminophen, atropine for organophosphates) ⊠⊠⊠.
Enhanced elimination: Consider hemodialysis or hemoperfusion for toxins with high protein bound

Bibliography

1. Mokhlesi B, Leiken JB, Murray P, Corbridge TC. Adult toxicology in critical care: part I: general approach to the intoxicated patient. Chest. 2003;123(2):577–92.
2. Levine M, Brooks DE, Truitt CA, Wolk BJ, Boyer EW, Ruha AM. Toxicology in the ICU: part 1: general overview and approach to treatment. Chest. 2011;140(3):795–806.
3. Schwarz ES. Therapeutic approach to the critically poisoned patient. In: Critical care toxicology. Cham: Springer; 2017. p. 43–78.

Chapter 96
Approach to Organophosphate Poisoning in the ICU

96.1 Introduction

Organophosphate (OP) poisoning is a global health concern, particularly in rural areas of Asia and Africa, where pesticide use is prevalent. According to the World Health Organization (WHO), an estimated three million cases of pesticide poisoning occur annually, resulting in over 250,000 deaths. In developing countries, intentional self-poisoning is more common, whereas occupational exposure prevails in developed nations.

OP compounds inhibit acetylcholinesterase, leading to an accumulation of acetylcholine and overstimulation of nicotinic and muscarinic receptors. This biochemical mechanism results in a cholinergic crisis characterized by symptoms such as miosis, salivation, bronchorrhea, seizures, and neuromuscular dysfunction. Understanding the pathophysiology, timely diagnosis, and management strategies is critical for improving outcomes in the intensive care unit (ICU) [1–3]. [Ref: Algorithm 96.1].

Epidemiology

- Global Incidence: OP poisoning accounts for a significant proportion of pesticide-related morbidity and mortality worldwide. Rural agricultural communities in Asia and Africa experience the highest prevalence due to the accessibility of pesticides and limited regulations.
- Exposure Types:
- Occupational Exposure: Common in agricultural workers handling pesticides without adequate protective measures.
- Intentional Exposure: Suicide attempts through ingestion are a major issue in developing countries.
- Accidental Exposure: More frequent in children and nonagricultural settings in developed countries.

S. B. Mishra et al., *Mastering ICU Care*,
https://doi.org/10.1007/978-981-95-0179-3_96

Pathophysiology

OP compounds inhibit acetylcholinesterase by phosphorylating the serine hydroxyl group at the active site of the enzyme. This inhibition leads to:

- Accumulation of Acetylcholine: Excess acetylcholine overstimulates nicotinic and muscarinic receptors.
- Muscarinic Effects: Bronchorrhea, bronchospasm, bradycardia, miosis, salivation, lacrimation, urination, diarrhea.
- Nicotinic Effects: Muscle fasciculations, weakness, paralysis, tachycardia, hypertension.
- Enzyme Aging: Over time, the phosphorylated enzyme undergoes "aging," making reactivation by oximes like pralidoxime ineffective. This underscores the importance of timely oxime therapy, ideally within 6 h of exposure.

Diagnostic Tools

- Clinical Scoring Systems:
- Peradeniya Organophosphorus Poisoning (POP) Scale: Assesses severity based on pupil size, respiratory rate, heart rate, fasciculations, level of consciousness, and seizures.
- Laboratory Tests:
- Cholinesterase Assays: Measure plasma (butyrylcholinesterase) and red blood cell (acetylcholinesterase) activity.
- Limitations: Assays may not be readily available or standardized; levels do not always correlate with clinical severity.
- Differential Diagnosis: Rule out other causes of cholinergic symptoms, such as carbamate poisoning or nerve agent exposure.

96.2 Management Nuances

Step 1: Initial Assessment and Resuscitation

1. Suspect OP Poisoning:
    - Obtain history of exposure and identify clinical signs.
    - Early recognition is crucial for initiating life-saving interventions.
2. Airway Management:
    - Ensure airway patency; intubate if necessary due to excessive secretions or decreased consciousness.
    - Be prepared for difficult intubation due to bronchorrhea and laryngospasm.
3. Breathing:
    - Provide high-flow oxygen.
    - Use bronchodilators for bronchospasm.

4. Circulation:

  - Establish IV access.
  - Manage hypotension with isotonic fluids; vasopressors if unresponsive.

Step 2: Decontamination and Staff Safety

1. Personal Protective Equipment (PPE):

  - Healthcare providers should wear gloves, gowns, and masks to prevent secondary contamination.
  - Use decontamination facilities when available.

2. Remove Contaminated Clothing:

  - Cut off clothing to avoid further dermal absorption and reduce secondary exposure.

3. Skin Decontamination

  - Wash skin thoroughly with soap and water.
  - Avoid aggressive scrubbing to prevent skin damage.

4. Gastric Decontamination

  - Gastric Lavage: Consider within 1 hour of ingestion if airway is protected.
  - Activated Charcoal: Administer if the patient is alert or airway is secured.

Step 3: Advanced Therapies

1. Atropine:

  - Dosage: Start with 2–5 mg IV bolus; repeat every 5 min until muscarinic symptoms resolve (clear lung sounds, adequate oxygenation, dry mucous membranes).
  - Maintenance: Continuous infusion based on recurrence of symptoms.
  - Rationale: Competitive antagonist at muscarinic receptors, reversing muscarinic overstimulation.

2. Oxime Therapy (Pralidoxime):

  - Dosage:
  - Loading Dose: 1–2 g IV over 15–30 min.
  - Maintenance: 0.5–1 g/hour infusion.
  - Duration: Continue until clinical recovery, which may take several days.
  - Rationale: Reactivates acetylcholinesterase by removing the phosphate group before "aging" occurs.
  - Effective Agents: Pralidoxime is commonly used; obidoxime and asoxime are alternatives in certain regions.

3. Diazepam/Midazolam:

  - Indications: Seizure control, agitation, neuroprotection.
  - Dosage: Diazepam 5–10 mg IV; repeat as necessary.
  - Rationale: Benzodiazepines enhance GABAergic activity, providing anticonvulsant effects.

4. Magnesium Sulfate:

- Emerging Evidence: May provide neuroprotection by blocking NMDA receptors and reducing acetylcholine release.
- Dosage: 1–2 g IV over 15 min; monitor for hypotension and respiratory depression.

5. Butyrylcholinesterase Replacement Therapy:

- Experimental Therapy: Administering exogenous butyrylcholinesterase to scavenge OP compounds.
- Organophosphorus Hydrolases: Enzymes under investigation that degrade OP compounds.

Step 4: Monitoring and Management of Complications

1. Vital Signs and Respiratory Function:

- Continuous monitoring of heart rate, blood pressure, respiratory rate, and oxygen saturation.
- Frequent arterial blood gas analysis.

2. Neuromuscular Status:

- Assess for Signs of Intermediate Syndrome (IMS):
- Occurs 24–96 h post-exposure.
- Characterized by proximal muscle weakness, cranial nerve palsies, and respiratory failure.
- Management of IMS:
- Prolonged ventilatory support.
- Continued atropine and oxime therapy.
- Physical therapy to prevent muscle atrophy.

3. Delayed Neuropathy:

- Organophosphate-Induced Delayed Neuropathy (OPIDN):
- Occurs 1–3 weeks after exposure.
- Presents with distal motor-sensory polyneuropathy.
- Management:
- Supportive care.
- Rehabilitation services.

4. Cholinesterase Levels:

- Monitor plasma and RBC cholinesterase levels to assess treatment efficacy.
- Recognize that clinical improvement may lag behind laboratory normalization.

Step 5: Public Health and Interdisciplinary Collaboration

1. Regulatory Measures:
   - Pesticide Regulations: Advocacy for stricter controls and access restrictions can reduce incidence.
   - Public Awareness: Education on safe handling practices in agricultural settings.
2. Interdisciplinary Approach:
   - Collaboration among toxicologists, intensivists, emergency medicine specialists, and mental health professionals.
   - Implement protocols for mass casualty events involving nerve agents, as per national and WHO guidelines.

96.3 Conclusion

Managing organophosphate poisoning in the ICU requires a comprehensive approach that includes prompt recognition, decontamination, targeted pharmacologic therapy, and vigilant monitoring for complications. Advanced therapies like oxime administration and emerging treatments such as magnesium sulfate and butyrylcholinesterase replacement hold promise for improving outcomes. Public health initiatives and interdisciplinary collaboration are essential in reducing the incidence and improving the management of OP poisoning. By adhering to established guidelines and incorporating new evidence-based practices, healthcare providers can enhance patient care and outcomes in this critical area.

Algorithm 96.1: Approach to organophosphate poisoning in the ICU

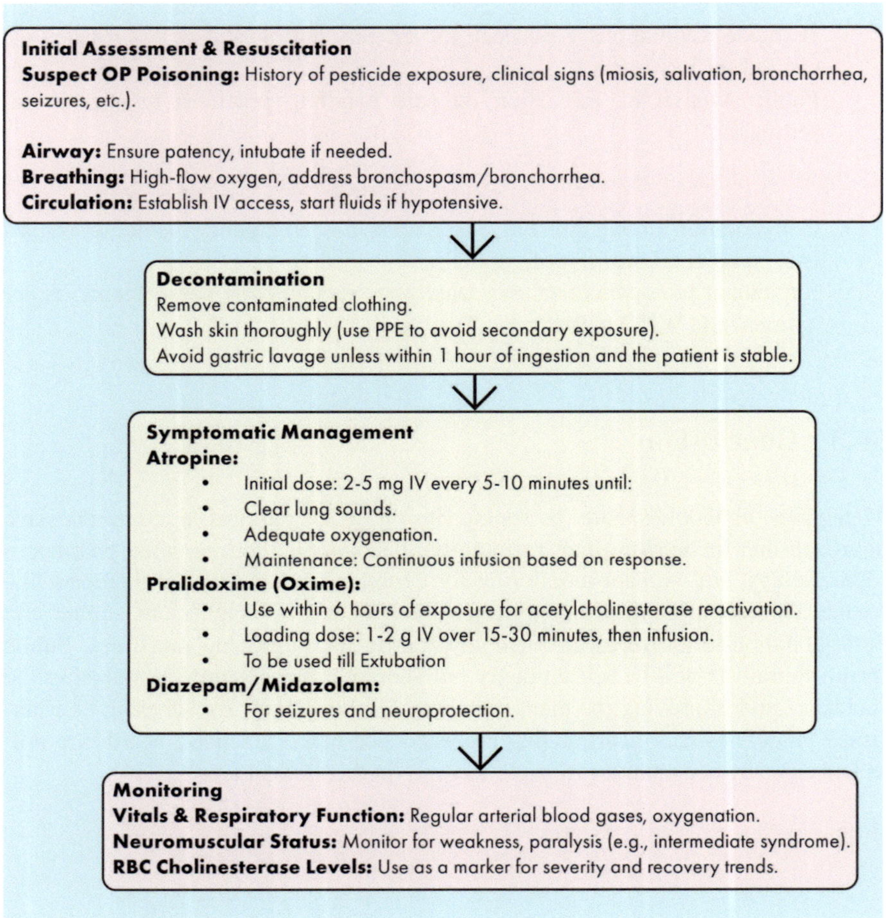

Bibliography

1. Eddleston M, Dawson A, Karalliedde L, Dissanayake W, Hittarage A, Azher S, et al. Early management after self-poisoning with an organophosphorus or carbamate pesticide – a treatment protocol for junior doctors. Crit Care. 2004;8(6):R391–7.
2. Eddleston M, Buckley NA, Eyer P, Dawson AH. Management of acute organophosphorus pesticide poisoning. Lancet. 2008;371(9612):597–607.
3. Hulse EJ, Haslam JD, Emmett SR, Woolley T. Organophosphorus nerve agent poisoning: managing the poisoned patient. Br J Anaesth. 2019;123(4):457–63.

Chapter 97
Approach to Paracetamol Poisoning in the ICU

97.1 Introduction

Paracetamol (acetaminophen) poisoning is a prevalent medical emergency worldwide and a leading cause of acute liver failure. Overdose can result from a single acute ingestion, repeated supratherapeutic doses, or chronic exposure. The risk of significant morbidity and mortality increases if not managed promptly and appropriately. Early recognition, risk stratification, and timely intervention are crucial. The cornerstone of management includes thorough patient assessment, application of the Rumack-Matthew nomogram (with revisions for high-risk populations), and administration of acetylcysteine. Recent advancements have led to updated guidelines and protocols, emphasizing considerations for special populations, modified-release formulations, and resource-limited settings [1, 2]. [Ref: Algorithm 97.1].

97.2 Risk Assessment

Effective management begins with a comprehensive risk assessment to determine the likelihood of hepatotoxicity and guide treatment decisions.

97.2.1 Patient History and Time of Ingestion

Key Actions
- Determine the Time and Circumstances of Ingestion:
- Establish the exact time of ingestion to apply the Rumack-Matthew nomogram accurately.

S. B. Mishra et al., *Mastering ICU Care*,
https://doi.org/10.1007/978-981-95-0179-3_97

- In cases of staggered or repeated ingestions, assess the duration and total amount consumed.
- Identify the Type of Formulation:
- Recognize if modified-release (MR) paracetamol was ingested, as it affects absorption and management.
- Assess Co-ingested Substances:
- Identify substances like anticholinergics or opioids that may delay gastric emptying and paracetamol absorption.
- Evaluate Symptoms and Clinical Status:
- Look for signs such as nausea, vomiting, abdominal pain, or altered mental status indicating toxicity or complications.

Paracetamol dosing may be associated with acute liver injury.

Acute single ingestion: ≥ 10 g or ≥ 200 mg/kg (whichever is less)

Repeated Supratherapeutic Ingestion:

≥ 10 g or ≥ 200 mg/kg (whichever is less) over a single 24-h period

≥ 12 g or ≥ 300 mg/kg (whichever is less) over a single 48-h period or ≥ a daily therapeutic dose (e.g., ≥4 g/day in adults) per day for more than 48 h in patients who also have abdominal pain or nausea or vomiting

Rationale

Understanding the type of ingestion (acute, staggered, or repeated supratherapeutic), the formulation involved, and any co-ingested substances is pivotal for determining hepatotoxicity risk and guiding timely intervention.

97.2.2 Populations with Altered Metabolism

Considerations for High-Risk Groups:

- Chronic alcoholics
- Patients with preexisting liver disease
- Malnourished individuals
- Patients taking enzyme-inducing medications

Rationale

These populations may have depleted glutathione stores or enhanced production of the toxic metabolite N-acetyl-p-benzoquinone imine (NAPQI), increasing their susceptibility to hepatotoxicity even at lower paracetamol doses.

97.3 Laboratory Tests

Recommended Tests

- Serum Paracetamol Concentration:
- Essential for applying the Rumack-Matthew nomogram in acute ingestions.
- Liver Function Tests (ALT/AST):
- Assess for hepatic injury; rising levels indicate hepatocellular damage.
- Coagulation Profile (PT/INR):
- Elevated INR may indicate progression to hepatic failure.
- Renal Function Tests (Serum Creatinine, BUN):
- Evaluate for potential acute kidney injury.
- Electrolytes and Glucose Levels:
- Identify metabolic derangements, such as hyponatremia.
- Arterial Blood Gas (ABG):
- Assess for acid-base disturbances.
- Additional Toxicology Screens:
- If co-ingestion is suspected.

Rationale

These investigations help stratify patients into low or high risk for hepatotoxicity, guide treatment decisions, and monitor for complications.

97.4 Management Pathways

Management should be tailored based on the type of ingestion, time since ingestion, patient-specific factors, and the presence of co-ingestants.

97.4.1 Acute Single Ingestion (<24 H)

Use of Rumack-Matthew Nomogram

- Standard Application:
- Plot serum paracetamol concentration against time since ingestion.
- If the level is above the treatment line (typically 150 μg/mL at 4 h), initiate acetylcysteine.
- Revised Nomogram for High-Risk Patients:
- For populations with altered metabolism, use a lower treatment threshold (e.g., 100 μg/mL at 4 h).

Rationale

The nomogram helps identify patients at risk of hepatotoxicity. Adjustments for high-risk populations ensure timely intervention.

97.4.2 Modified-Release Paracetamol Overdose

Challenges

- Extended Absorption Window:
- Peak serum levels may be delayed beyond 4 h.
- Potential for Double Peaks:
- Due to delayed and prolonged absorption.

Management Strategies

- Activated Charcoal:
- Administer up to 4 h post-ingestion, or later if delayed absorption is suspected.
- Serial Serum Paracetamol Levels:
- Measure at 4, 6, and 8 h post-ingestion.
- Initiate Acetylcysteine:
- Do not wait for levels if modified-release overdose is confirmed.
- Prolonged Acetylcysteine Administration:
- Extend treatment duration beyond standard protocols.

Rationale

Due to unpredictable absorption, early and prolonged treatment mitigates the risk of delayed hepatotoxicity.

Criteria for Liver Transplant (King's College Criteria)

I. Persistent acidosis (pH < 7.3) despite fluid resuscitation.

or

II. INR > 6 and creatinine >300 mmol/L with grade III or IV encephalopathy.

97.4.3 Massive Overdose

Criteria

- Ingestion of ≥ 30 g or ≥ 500 mg/kg (whichever is less).
- Serum paracetamol concentrations > double the nomogram line.

Management Strategies

- Higher-Dose Acetylcysteine Regimens:
- Increase the dose and duration.
- Consider Extracorporeal Elimination:
- Initiate hemodialysis in cases of mitochondrial dysfunction or persistent lactic acidosis.

Rationale

Massive overdoses may overwhelm detoxification mechanisms, necessitating aggressive interventions.

97.4.4 *Staggered and Repeated Supratherapeutic Ingestions (>24 H)*

Criteria

- Total dose >150 mg/kg over 24 h.
- Elevated ALT/AST levels.
- Serum paracetamol concentration > 20 μg/mL.

Management Strategies

- Initiate Acetylcysteine:
- Start treatment regardless of serum levels if clinical suspicion is high.
- Monitor Liver Function:
- Continue acetylcysteine until ALT/AST levels normalize.

Rationale

In repeated ingestions, toxicity may not correlate with serum levels, so clinical judgment is paramount.

97.4.5 *Management of High-Risk and Special Populations*

Pediatric Patients

- Adjusted Acetylcysteine Protocols:
- Use weight-based dosing to prevent adverse effects like hyponatremia.
- Monitoring:
- Close observation for fluid overload and electrolyte imbalances.

Pregnant Patients

- Safety of Acetylcysteine:
- Safe in all trimesters; treatment benefits outweigh risks.
- Fetal Monitoring:
- Consider obstetric consultation for fetal assessment.

Rationale

Tailoring treatment minimizes risks and maximizes benefits in vulnerable populations.

97.5 Treatment Protocol

97.5.1 *Activated Charcoal*

Indications

- Administer within 2–4 h of ingestion:

- Consider beyond 4 h for modified-release formulations or delayed gastric emptying.

Dosage
- Adults:
- 50 g orally
- Children:
- 1 g/kg orally (maximum 50 g).

Rationale
Activated charcoal reduces paracetamol absorption, decreasing the amount available for hepatotoxic metabolism.

97.5.2 Acetylcysteine Administration

Updated Two-Bag Protocol
- Bag 1:
- 200 mg/kg IV over 4 h.
- Bag 2:
- 100 mg/kg IV over the next 16 h.
- Total Dose:
- 300 mg/kg over 20 h.

Advantages over Traditional Three-Bag Protocol
- Simplifies Dosing:
- Reduces complexity and potential for errors.
- Reduces Adverse Reactions:
- Lower incidence of anaphylactoid reactions.

Higher Doses for Massive Ingestions
- Consider Increasing Dose:
- For ingestions >30 g or serum levels > double the nomogram line.
- Monitor Closely:
- Adjust based on clinical response and laboratory values.

Rationale
The two-bag regimen improves patient compliance and reduces side effects while ensuring effective detoxification.

97.5.3 Extracorporeal Techniques

Indications
- Massive Overdose:

- Extremely high serum paracetamol levels.
- Mitochondrial Dysfunction:
- Severe lactic acidosis unresponsive to standard therapy.

Methods
- Hemodialysis:
- Preferred method for extracorporeal elimination.

Rationale
Dialysis can remove paracetamol and its metabolites, particularly when hepatic metabolism is overwhelmed.

97.6 Monitoring and Criteria for Discontinuation

97.6.1 Ongoing Monitoring Protocols

Frequency of Measurements
- ALT/AST and INR:
- Every 12 h during acetylcysteine treatment.
- Serum Paracetamol Levels:
- As needed to assess ongoing absorption, especially in modified-release overdoses.
- Renal Function and Electrolytes:
- Regularly monitor for nephrotoxicity and electrolyte imbalances.

Rationale
Continuous monitoring detects worsening hepatic function and guides treatment adjustments.

97.6.2 Criteria for Discontinuation of Acetylcysteine

Stopping Criteria
- Decrease in ALT/AST:
- Levels falling by 25%–50% from peak values.
- Normalizing INR:
- Indicates improving liver function.
- Serum Paracetamol Concentration:
- Undetectable or < 10 μg/mL.
- Clinical Stability:
- No signs of hepatic failure or encephalopathy.

Rationale
Meeting these criteria indicates recovery, allowing safe cessation of acetylcysteine.

97.7 Special Considerations in Rural and Resource-Limited Settings

Simplified Management Protocols

- Empirical Treatment:
- Initiate acetylcysteine when paracetamol overdose is suspected.
- Use of Flowcharts:
- Provide visual aids for decision-making without extensive laboratory data.
- Community Education:
- Train healthcare workers on recognition and initial management.

Rationale

In the absence of laboratory testing, empirical treatment prevents delays that could worsen outcomes.

97.8 Algorithmic Approach

97.8.1 Decision-Making Flowchart for Paracetamol Poisoning

Step 1: Assess the Type of Ingestion

- Acute Single Ingestion.
- Modified-Release Formulation.
- Staggered or Repeated Supratherapeutic Ingestions.

Step 2: Determine Time since Ingestion

- <24 h: Use Nomogram for Acute Ingestions.
- >24 h: Consider Risk Factors and Clinical Presentation.

Step 3: Obtain Baseline Laboratory Tests

- Serum Paracetamol Concentration.
- ALT/AST Levels.
- INR and Renal Function.

Step 4: Apply Appropriate Guidelines

- Use Standard or Revised Nomogram for Acute Ingestions.
- Follow Modified-Release Protocols as Needed.
- Initiate Treatment in Repeated Ingestions if Criteria Met.

Step 5: Initiate Treatment

- Activated Charcoal if Within Timeframe.
- Acetylcysteine Using Updated Protocols.

Step 6: Monitor Patient

- Regular Laboratory Testing.
- Clinical Observations.

Step 7: Adjust Treatment

- Increase Acetylcysteine Dose for Massive Overdoses.
- Consider Extracorporeal Techniques if Indicated.

Step 8: Determine when to Discontinue Treatment

- Based on Clinical Improvement and Laboratory Criteria.

Rationale

An algorithmic approach ensures systematic assessment and management, improving patient outcomes by reducing the likelihood of oversight.

97.9 Conclusion

Management of paracetamol poisoning in the ICU requires a structured and comprehensive approach that accounts for the type of ingestion, patient-specific factors, and available resources. Early risk assessment using the standard or revised Rumack-Matthew nomogram guides timely initiation of acetylcysteine. Updated two-bag acetylcysteine protocols simplify dosing and reduce adverse reactions. Special considerations for high-risk populations, modified-release formulations, massive overdoses, and resource-limited settings enhance the effectiveness of interventions. Continuous monitoring and clear criteria for treatment discontinuation ensure patient safety. Utilizing algorithmic decision-making tools aids clinicians in providing optimal care across diverse clinical scenarios.

Algorithm 97.1: Approach to paracetamol poisoning in the ICU

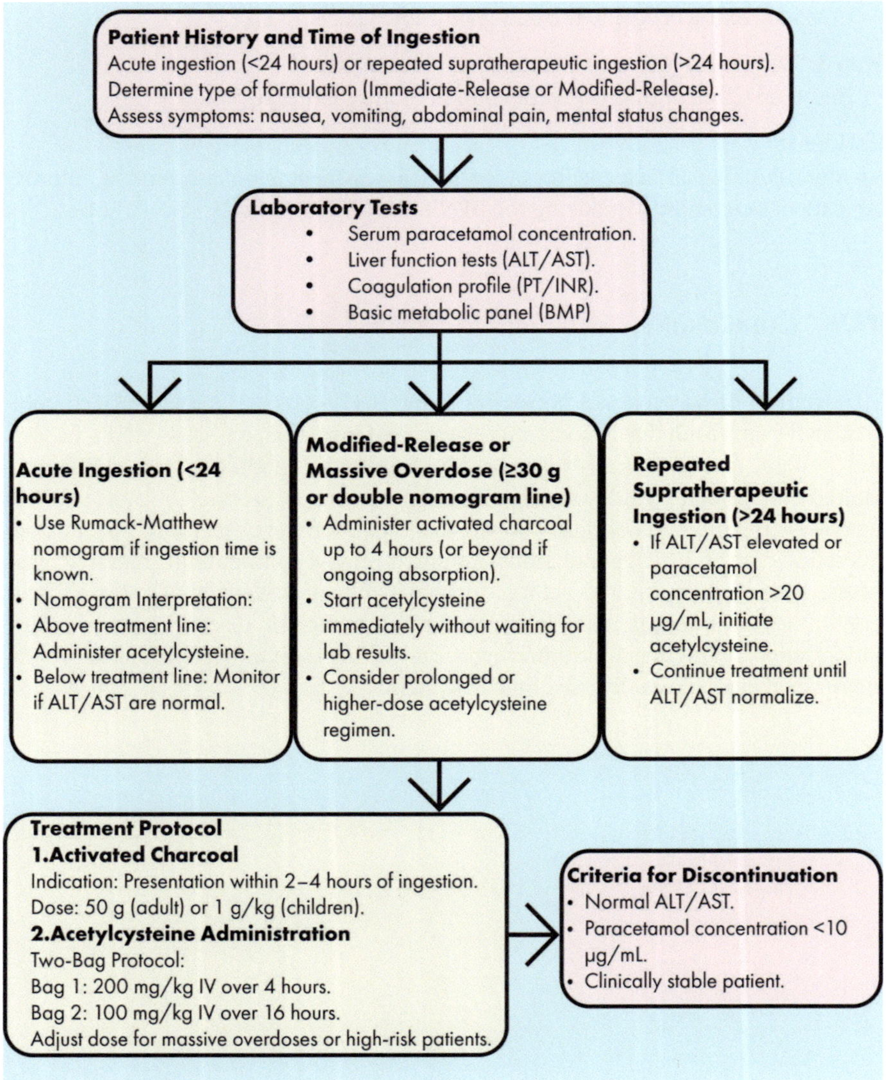

Bibliography

1. Chiew AL, Reith D, Pomerleau A, Wong A, Isoardi KZ, Soderstrom J, et al. Updated guidelines for the management of paracetamol poisoning in Australia and New Zealand. Med J Aust. 2020;212(4):175–83.
2. Dart RC, Mullins ME, Matoushek T, Ruha AM, Burns MM, Simone K, et al. Management of acetaminophen poisoning in the US and Canada: a consensus statement. JAMA Netw Open. 2023;6(8):e2327739.

Chapter 98
Approach to Snake Bite in the ICU

98.1 Introduction

Snake bites are a significant public health concern, particularly in tropical and subtropical regions, leading to substantial morbidity and mortality worldwide. The incidence of snake bites varies globally, with higher rates in rural and agricultural communities where humans and venomous snakes frequently interact. Certain regions have specific risk factors; for example, kraits often bite individuals during nocturnal settings, while viper and cobra bites are more common during agricultural activities. The demographics most affected are often those engaged in farming, herding, and other outdoor occupations, with children and young adults being particularly vulnerable [1].

Effective management of snake bites in the intensive care unit (ICU) requires a systematic approach that includes rapid assessment, stabilization, identification of envenomation syndromes, appropriate use of antivenom, and comprehensive supportive care. This chapter outlines the critical steps in managing snake bite patients in the ICU, emphasizing evidence-based practices and addressing challenges unique to different settings. [Ref: Algorithm 98.1].

98.2 First Aid Measures and Barriers to Treatment

First aid measures play a crucial role in the outcome of snake bite victims. Immediate and appropriate actions can significantly reduce morbidity and mortality.

Key Recommendations

- Avoid Harmful Traditional Practices:
- Do not perform incisions, suction, or apply tourniquets to the bite site.

S. B. Mishra et al., *Mastering ICU Care*,
https://doi.org/10.1007/978-981-95-0179-3_98

- These methods are ineffective in preventing venom spread and can cause additional harm, such as ischemia, necrosis, and increased risk of infection.
- Immobilization and Reassurance:
- Immobilize the affected limb with a splint and keep it at heart level to slow venom absorption.
- Reassure the patient to reduce anxiety and prevent increased circulation.
- Rapid Transport:
- Prioritize prompt transportation to the nearest healthcare facility equipped to manage snake bites.
- Delays in receiving antivenom can worsen outcomes.

Barriers to Treatment

- Transportation Challenges:
- Rural areas may lack adequate transportation, leading to delays in reaching medical care.
- Cost of Treatment:
- The expense of antivenom and ICU care can be prohibitive, discouraging timely medical intervention.
- Cultural Beliefs:
- Traditional healers and beliefs may lead patients to seek ineffective remedies instead of medical care.

Rationale
Educating communities about effective first aid measures and addressing barriers to treatment are essential components in improving snake bite outcomes. Avoiding harmful practices and ensuring rapid access to antivenom can significantly reduce mortality and morbidity.

98.3 Identification and Syndromic Approach

Accurate identification of the snake species is often challenging and sometimes impossible. Therefore, a syndromic approach focusing on clinical manifestations is crucial in managing snake bite envenomation.

Key Points

- Focus on Clinical Symptoms:
- Base management decisions on the patient's presenting signs and symptoms rather than relying solely on snake identification.
- Envenomation Syndromes:
- Neurotoxic Syndrome: Characterized by ptosis, diplopia, dysphagia, respiratory distress, and paralysis.
- Hemotoxic Syndrome: Presents with coagulopathy, spontaneous bleeding, hematuria, and hypotension.

- Cytotoxic Syndrome: Involves severe local tissue damage, swelling, blistering, and necrosis.

Rationale
A syndromic approach allows for timely and appropriate treatment, especially in regions where multiple venomous species coexist, and snake identification is unreliable.

98.4 History and Symptoms

Key Steps

- Confirm Occurrence and Timing:
- Determine the exact time of the bite to predict symptom evolution.
- Assess for Systemic Symptoms:
- Neurotoxic Signs: Ptosis, dysphagia, respiratory distress, and muscle weakness.
- Hemotoxic Signs: Bleeding tendencies, hematuria, hypotension, and bruising.
- Examine Bite Site:
- Look for local reactions such as swelling, erythema, blistering, and fang marks.

Rationale
Early identification of symptoms guides the urgency of interventions. Differentiating between systemic and local effects is critical for triaging and prioritizing treatment.

98.5 Laboratory Tests

Key Investigations

- Complete Blood Count (CBC):
- Check for anemia, leukocytosis, and platelet counts.
- Coagulation Profile:

20-Minute Whole Blood Clotting Test (20WBCT).

The 20-Minute Whole Blood Clotting Test (20WBCT) is a simple, rapid, and practical bedside test used to assess coagulopathy in patients suspected of hemotoxic snake envenomation, particularly in resource-limited settings. It is instrumental in detecting venom-induced consumption coagulopathy, which is common with bites from certain snake species like vipers.

Purpose

- Assess Coagulation Status:
- Detects the presence of coagulopathy caused by hemotoxic venoms that disrupt normal blood clotting mechanisms.

- Guide Antivenom Administration:
- A positive test indicates the need for antivenom therapy and helps in monitoring the effectiveness of treatment.

Procedure

1. Sample Collection:
    - Draw approximately 2 mL of fresh venous blood from the patient using standard phlebotomy techniques.
2. Use of Clean, Dry Glass Tube:
    - Place the blood into a new, clean, and dry glass test tube without any anticoagulant additives.
    - Important: Do not use plastic tubes, as they may interfere with clot formation due to their surface properties.
3. Undisturbed Clotting:
    - Leave the tube undisturbed at room temperature for 20 minutes.
    - Do not shake, stir, or move the tube during this period.
4. Assessment:
    - After 20 minutes, gently tilt the tube to check for clot formation.
    - Observe whether the blood has clotted or remains liquid.

Interpretation

- Normal Result (Negative Test):
- Clotted Blood: The blood has formed a solid clot that stays in place when the tube is tilted.
- Implication: Normal coagulation function; no significant hemotoxic envenomation affecting clotting.
- Abnormal Result (Positive Test):
- Unclotted Blood: The blood remains liquid and does not clot after 20 minutes.
- Implication: Presence of coagulopathy due to venom-induced defibrination; significant hemotoxic envenomation.

Clinical Significance

- Indicator for Antivenom Therapy:
- A positive 20WBCT is a strong indication for the administration of antivenom in patients bitten by snakes known to cause hemotoxic effects.
- Monitoring Treatment Efficacy:
- Repeating the test after antivenom administration can help assess the reversal of coagulopathy.
- Early Detection of Bleeding Risks:
- Identifies patients at risk of severe bleeding complications, allowing for timely supportive interventions.

Limitations and Considerations

- Standardization:
- Ensure strict adherence to the standardized procedure to avoid false results.
- Variations in blood volume, tube type, or timing can affect accuracy.
- Equipment:
- Use only clean, dry glass tubes; moisture or contaminants can interfere with clotting.
- Avoid using tubes previously exposed to anticoagulants.
- Temperature Factors:
- Perform the test at room temperature; extreme temperatures may alter clotting times.
- Not Comprehensive:
- The test detects gross coagulopathy but may not identify all coagulation abnormalities.
- Additional laboratory tests (e.g., PT, aPTT, fibrinogen levels) may be necessary for a comprehensive assessment.
- Patient Factors:
- Severe anemia, hypofibrinogenemia from other causes, or anticoagulant medications can influence results.

Advantages

- Simplicity and Accessibility:
- Requires minimal equipment and can be performed at the bedside.
- Ideal for use in rural or resource-poor settings where laboratory facilities are unavailable.
- Rapid Results:
- Provides timely information to guide immediate clinical decisions.

Rationale in Snake Bite Management

- Early Intervention:
- Facilitates prompt administration of antivenom and other supportive measures.
- Improved Outcomes:
- Reduces the risk of severe hemorrhagic complications and enhances patient recovery.
- Cost-Effective:
- Minimizes the need for more expensive and time-consuming laboratory tests in urgent situations.

Precautions

- Technique Accuracy:
- Ensure proper sample collection and handling to avoid contamination or activation of clotting pathways.
- Interpretation Caution:

- Be aware of potential false positives or negatives due to technical errors or patient-specific factors.
- Repeat Testing:
- If initial results are inconclusive, consider repeating the test to confirm findings.

Prothrombin Time (PT), Activated Partial Thromboplastin Time (aPTT)

- For detailed coagulation assessment.
- Renal Function Tests:
- Serum creatinine, blood urea nitrogen (BUN), electrolytes to detect acute kidney injury.
- Venom Antigen Detection Tests:
- Innovative diagnostic tools that help identify specific venom and guide antivenom selection.
- Electrolytes and Blood Gases:
- Identify metabolic disturbances.
- Imaging Studies:
- Ultrasound or MRI if compartment syndrome is suspected.

Rationale
Laboratory evaluation confirms the extent of systemic involvement, including coagulopathy and renal injury. Advanced diagnostics like venom antigen detection can enhance targeted treatment, while standardized bedside tests are crucial in resource-limited settings.

98.6 Local Wound Care and Compartment Syndrome Management

Local Wound Care

- Key Steps:
- Clean the Bite Area:
- Use antiseptics to reduce infection risk.
- Monitor for Signs of Infection:
- Redness, warmth, pus, or increased pain.
- Avoid Harmful Interventions:
- Do not apply ice, chemicals, or herbal remedies to the bite site.

Compartment Syndrome Management

- Identification:
- Signs and Symptoms:
- Severe pain out of proportion to injury, swelling, decreased distal pulses, paresthesia, and decreased motor function.
- Diagnosis:

- Use imaging modalities like ultrasound or MRI to assess muscle compartment pressures.
- Management:
- Immediate Medical Attention:
- Elevate the limb and remove any constrictive dressings or jewelry.
- Surgical Intervention:
- Fasciotomy may be required to relieve pressure and prevent tissue necrosis.

Rationale
Effective local wound care minimizes the risk of infection and tissue damage. Early identification and management of compartment syndrome are critical to prevent permanent disability.

98.7 Classification of Envenomation

Severity Levels

- No Envenomation:
- No local or systemic signs.
- Mild Envenomation:
- Local swelling confined to the bite site.
- Moderate Envenomation:
- Swelling extending beyond the bite site, mild systemic symptoms (e.g., nausea, mild hypotension).
- Severe Envenomation:
- Rapidly progressing swelling, severe systemic toxicity:
- Neurotoxicity: Respiratory paralysis, cranial nerve deficits.
- Hemotoxicity: Spontaneous bleeding, disseminated intravascular coagulation (DIC), shock.
- Cytotoxicity: Extensive local tissue necrosis.

Rationale
This classification directs antivenom administration and supportive measures. Severity grading ensures judicious use of resources and appropriate allocation of care.

98.8 Antivenom Use and Administration Guidelines

Indications

- Presence of Systemic Signs:
- Neurotoxic symptoms, coagulopathy, or significant hemodynamic instability.
- Progressive Local Symptoms:

- Rapidly spreading swelling, severe pain, or signs of compartment syndrome.

Dosage Considerations

- Standard Dosage:
- Mild Envenomation: Five vials.
- Moderate Envenomation: Five to ten vials.
- Severe Envenomation: Ten vials or more.
- Adjustments Based on Patient Factors:
- Body Weight:
- Dosage may be adjusted in pediatric patients.
- Pregnancy:
- Antivenom is safe and should not be withheld; dosage remains the same.
- Late Administration:
- Diminishing Efficacy Window:
- Antivenom is most effective when given within the first few hours after the bite.
- Efficacy decreases with time but should still be administered if signs of envenomation are present.

Administration

- Preparation:
- Dilute antivenom in 100–500 mL of normal saline.
- Infusion:
- Infuse over one hour.
- In severe cases, consider faster infusion under close monitoring.
- Monitoring for Adverse Reactions:
- Early Reactions:
- Anaphylaxis, urticaria, and bronchospasm.
- Management of Reactions:
- Stop the infusion temporarily.
- Administer antihistamines, corticosteroids, or epinephrine as needed.
- Restart the infusion at a slower rate once symptoms are controlled.

Rationale
Antivenom is the definitive treatment for neutralizing venom effects. Proper dosage and careful administration reduce the risk of adverse reactions while ensuring effective treatment.

98.9 Supportive Management

Multisystem Effects and Critical Complications

- Neurotoxic Envenomation:
- Interventions:
- Administer neostigmine and atropine to reverse neurotoxic effects.

Atropine 0.6 mg followed by neostigmine 1.5 mg to be given IV stat followed by neostigmine 0.5 mg with atropine every 30 minutes for five doses. Dose to be tapered at 1 hour, 2 hours, 6 hours, and 12 hours. The response is measured by recovery of ptosis. Positive response is defined as 50% or more recovery of ptosis in 1 hour. If there is no response after third dose, atropine neostigmine should be stopped.

- Provide ventilatory support in cases of respiratory paralysis.
- ICU Monitoring:
- Continuous respiratory and neurological monitoring.
- Hemotoxic Envenomation:
- Interventions:
- Transfuse blood products for bleeding or coagulopathy.
- Monitor for signs of DIC and treat accordingly.
- ICU Monitoring:
- Regular coagulation profile assessments.
- Acute Kidney Injury:
- Interventions:
- Maintain adequate hydration.
- Use diuretics cautiously.
- Initiate renal replacement therapy (dialysis) if indicated.
- ICU Monitoring:
- Monitor urine output, electrolytes, and renal function tests.
- Cardiovascular Support:
- Interventions:
- Manage hypotension with fluids and vasopressors as needed.
- ICU Monitoring:
- Continuous hemodynamic monitoring.

Rationale

Venom effects can lead to critical complications affecting multiple organ systems. Comprehensive supportive management addresses these complications, improving patient outcomes beyond what antivenom can achieve alone.

98.10 Rehabilitation and Long-Term Care

Key Components

- Physical Therapy:
- Restore function and mobility in affected limbs.
- Exercises to prevent contractures and muscle wasting.
- Psychological Support:
- Counseling to address trauma, anxiety, or depression resulting from the snake bite experience.
- Prosthetics and Assistive Devices:

- For patients with permanent disabilities or amputations.
- Follow-Up Care:
- Regular medical evaluations to monitor recovery and address ongoing complications.

Rationale
Rehabilitation services are essential for improving quality of life in snake bite victims who suffer long-term disabilities. Psychological support aids in coping with the emotional impact of the incident.

98.11 Preventive Strategies and Education

Public Health Initiatives

- Education Programs:
- Community education on snake bite prevention, first aid measures, and the importance of seeking medical care.
- Risk Reduction Strategies:
- Encourage the use of protective clothing and footwear during high-risk activities.
- Promote safe storage of food to prevent attracting snakes.
- Healthcare Infrastructure:
- Equip rural health centers with essential supplies, such as antivenom.
- Train healthcare workers in snake bite management.
- Collaboration with Traditional Healers:
- Engage local healers to encourage timely referral to medical facilities.

Rationale
Preventive strategies and education can significantly reduce the incidence of snake bites and improve early management, leading to better outcomes.

98.12 Monitoring and Reevaluation

Key Steps

- Regular Reassessment:
- Monitor vital signs, neurological status, and local wound progression.
- Laboratory Monitoring:
- Repeat 20WBCT every 6 hours until normalization.
- Monitor renal function, electrolytes, and coagulation profiles.
- Antivenom Doses:
- Administer additional antivenom if symptoms persist or worsen.
- Documentation:
- Maintain detailed records of clinical findings, interventions, and patient responses.

Rationale
Continuous monitoring ensures timely adjustments to the treatment plan. Regular reevaluation allows for early detection of complications and effectiveness of interventions.

98.13 Conclusion

Managing snake bites in the ICU demands a comprehensive, multidisciplinary approach that includes prompt first aid, accurate assessment, appropriate antivenom administration, and extensive supportive care. Addressing barriers to treatment and incorporating preventive strategies are essential for improving outcomes. By adhering to evidence-based protocols and emphasizing both acute management and long-term rehabilitation, healthcare providers can significantly reduce the morbidity and mortality associated with snake bites.

Algorithm 98.1: Approach to snake bite in the ICU

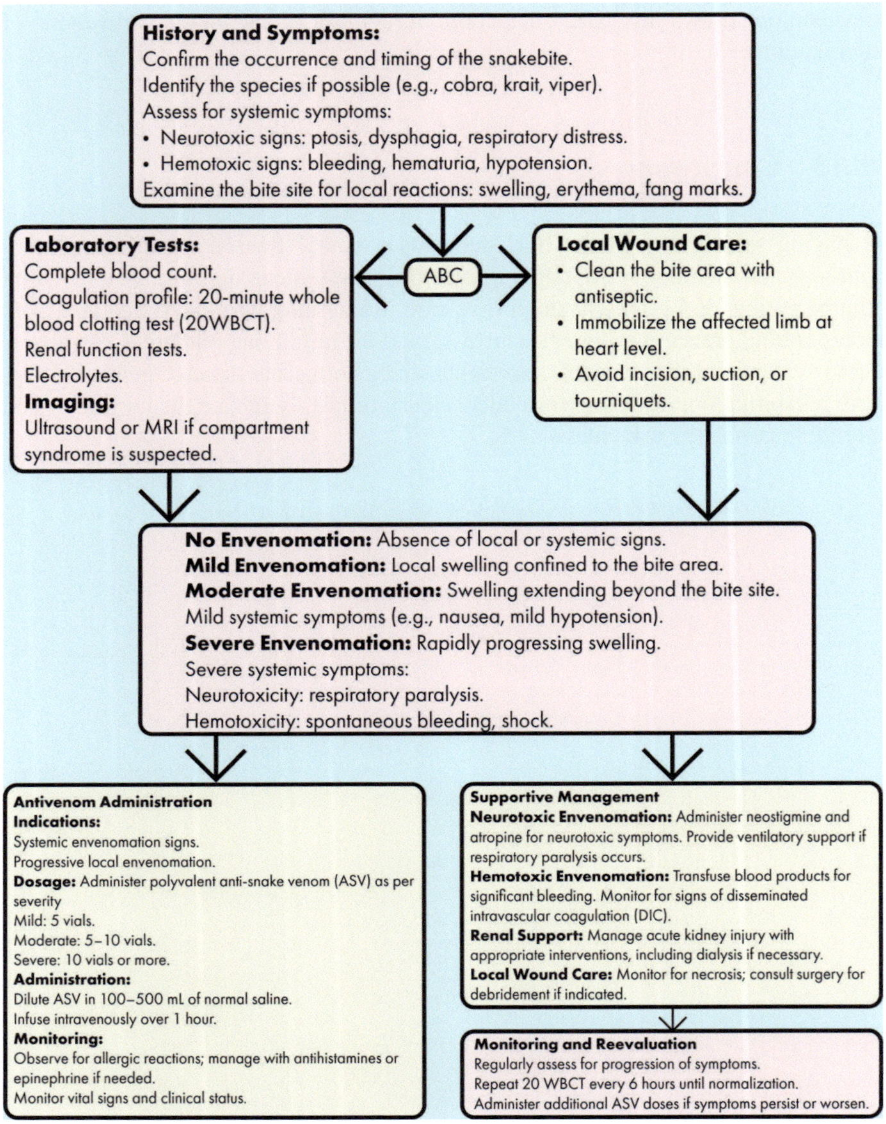

Bibliography

1. Ralph R, Faiz MA, Sharma SK, Ribeiro I, Chappuis F. Managing snakebite. BMJ. 2022;376:e057926.

Chapter 99
Approach to Fever in the ICU

99.1 Introduction

Fever in the intensive care unit (ICU) is a prevalent clinical challenge that necessitates prompt identification and management. It is crucial to distinguish between fever (an elevation in body temperature due to a regulated increase in the hypothalamic set point), pyrexia (often used interchangeably with fever but can imply sustained elevated temperature), and hyperthermia (an unregulated rise in body temperature due to excessive heat production or impaired heat dissipation). Each condition has specific clinical implications and requires different management strategies.

Fever can result from both infectious and noninfectious causes, with infections being a primary concern in critically ill patients. Mismanagement can lead to delayed diagnoses, unnecessary testing, and inappropriate treatments. Importantly, immunocompromised patients—such as those who are neutropenic or have undergone organ transplantation—may not mount robust febrile responses. Therefore, lower temperature thresholds are used to define fever in these populations [1–3] [Ref: Algorithm 99.1].

99.2 Initial Assessment and Temperature Confirmation

Accurate temperature measurement is critical to avoid over- or underestimating fever. The hierarchy of accuracy in temperature measurement methods is especially important in the ICU setting.

S. B. Mishra et al., *Mastering ICU Care*,
https://doi.org/10.1007/978-981-95-0179-3_99

Preferred Methods

- Central Thermistors: Pulmonary artery, bladder, or esophageal thermistors provide the most accurate core temperature measurements.
- Oral and Rectal Thermometers: Acceptable alternatives if central monitoring is unavailable.

Less Accurate Methods to Avoid

- Tympanic and Axillary Thermometers: These peripheral methods are less reliable, particularly in critically ill patients with altered hemodynamics.

Limitations in Certain ICU Scenarios

- Extracorporeal Therapies: Patients undergoing extracorporeal membrane oxygenation (ECMO) or continuous renal replacement therapy (CRRT) may have altered peripheral temperatures, affecting the accuracy of peripheral measurements.

Thresholds for Fever

- General ICU Population: A temperature of ≥38.3 °C (100.9 °F) sustained for at least 1 hour defines significant fever.
- Immunocompromised Patients: A lower threshold of ≥38.0 °C (100.4 °F) is often used due to their blunted febrile response.

If the threshold is not met, hourly monitoring for the next 6 hours is recommended [4].

99.3 Etiological Approach

A systematic clinical evaluation is essential to differentiate between infectious and noninfectious causes of fever. Creating a differential diagnostic framework can guide clinicians through potential etiologies specific to the ICU.

Clinical Evaluation

- History: Document recent surgeries, invasive procedures, catheter placements, medication changes, and known comorbidities.
- Physical Examination: Focus on signs of infection or inflammation, such as redness, swelling, discharge, or pain at catheter sites.

Infectious Causes

- Catheter-Related Infections
- Ventilator-Associated Pneumonia (VAP)
- Urinary Tract Infections (UTIs)
- Abdominal Abscesses

Noninfectious Causes (See Table 99.1 for Diagnostic Clues)

- Drug-Induced Fever
- Thromboembolic Events (acute myocardial infarction, fat embolism, venous thrombosis, lung infarction, stroke)
- Autoimmune Responses
- Transfusion Reactions
- Pancreatitis
- Adrenal Insufficiency
- Malignant Hyperthermia
- Neuroleptic Malignant Syndrome
- Nonconvulsive Status Epilepticus
- Serotonin Syndrome
- Thyroid Storm

99.4 Role of Biomarkers

Biomarkers can aid in differentiating between infectious and noninfectious causes of fever, guiding diagnosis and rationalizing antibiotic use.

- Procalcitonin (PCT): Elevated levels suggest bacterial infections and help distinguish bacterial sepsis from other causes of systemic inflammation.
- C-Reactive Protein (CRP): A nonspecific marker of inflammation; trends can help assess response to therapy.

Recommendations

- Use PCT levels to guide initiation and discontinuation of antibiotics in suspected bacterial infections.
- Monitor CRP trends in conjunction with clinical findings to evaluate treatment efficacy.

Table 99.1 Diagnostic clues for noninfectious causes

Noninfectious cause	Diagnostic clues
Drug-induced fever	Recent initiation of new medications; lack of infection signs
Thromboembolism	Unilateral leg swelling, dyspnea, hypoxia
Autoimmune responses	Joint pain, rash, elevated inflammatory markers
Transfusion reactions	Fever shortly after blood product administration

The use of PCT and CRP is done only when there is low to intermediate probability of bacterial infection in a critically ill patient with a new onset fever, but no clear focus of infection.

99.5 Microbiological Evaluation

Microbiological investigations are critical for identifying pathogens.

Blood Cultures

- Collect samples from two different sites sequentially. Ideal volume to be collected—60 mL in total. There should not be any time interval between the two collections.
- For patients with central venous catheters (CVC), collect paired samples from the catheter and peripheral vein to calculate the differential time to positivity. It is better to sample at least two lumens of CVC while sending cultures.
- Utilize rapid molecular diagnostics when available. This should be used only with blood cultures and not as isolated tests to confirm bacterial infections.

Specific Infections

- Urinary Tract Infections: Replace the urinary catheter before obtaining a culture sample to reduce contamination (i.e., culture to be obtained from new catheter).
- Ventilator-Associated Conditions: Consider bronchoalveolar lavage (BAL) for culture and nucleic acid amplification tests (NAATs). BAL is particularly valuable in ventilator-associated conditions.
- SARS-CoV-2 Testing: Include in workup during periods of high community transmission [5].

99.6 Imaging and Diagnostic Pathways

Imaging is pivotal when initial evaluations are inconclusive.

Chest Radiographs

- Routinely assess for pulmonary infections.

Ultrasonography

- Abdominal Ultrasound: Useful for detecting biliary sources of infection or abscesses.
- Doppler Ultrasound: Evaluate for deep vein thrombosis (DVT) in cases where thromboembolism is suspected.

Computed Tomography (CT)

- Abdominal CT: For suspected intra-abdominal infections or abscesses.
- CT Pulmonary Angiography: If pulmonary embolism is suspected.

Positron Emission Tomography/Computed Tomography (PET/CT)

- Considered when the fever source remains elusive after standard workup.

99.7 Therapeutic Recommendations

Antipyretic Use

- Nuanced Approach: Recognize that fever is a natural immune response. Over-suppression may impair host defenses.
- Indications for Antipyretics:
- Patient discomfort.
- Exacerbation of comorbid conditions (e.g., increased intracranial pressure, cardiac ischemia).
- Physical Cooling Methods: Can be used as complementary therapies, including cooling blankets or ice packs. This should be adopted only with antipyretics and not as the first line of management of raised temperature.

Aggressive Temperature Management

- Risks vs. Benefits: Recent studies suggest that aggressive temperature reduction may not improve outcomes and may be associated with adverse effects.
- Best Practices: Individualize temperature management based on patient condition and clinical context [6]

99.8 Economic and Practical Considerations

- Cost-Conscious Approach: Avoid reflexive ordering of tests without a guiding hypothesis.
- Patient-Centric Diagnostics: Prioritize tests that directly impact patient management.
- Stewardship Programs: Engage in antimicrobial stewardship to reduce unnecessary antibiotic use.

99.9 Special Populations

Immunocompromised Patients

- Neutropenic Patients: Use a lower fever threshold (≥38.0 °C or 100.4 °F).
- Organ Transplant Recipients: May have atypical presentations; maintain a high index of suspicion for opportunistic infections.

Diagnostic Protocols

- Early Broad-Spectrum Antibiotics: Consider in neutropenic fever after appropriate cultures are obtained.
- Customized Workup: May include fungal cultures, cytomegalovirus PCR, or other specialized tests.

99.10 Conclusion

Managing fever in the ICU requires a comprehensive and systematic approach. Accurate temperature measurement, utilizing the most reliable methods, is the first critical step. Differentiating between infectious and noninfectious causes through a structured framework ensures targeted diagnostics and treatments. The integration of biomarkers like procalcitonin and CRP can refine diagnostic accuracy and guide antibiotic stewardship. Advanced imaging modalities and procedures, such as PET/CT and bronchoalveolar lavage, play significant roles in identifying elusive sources of fever. Therapeutic interventions should balance the benefits of fever reduction with potential risks, avoiding unnecessary suppression of the immune response. Emphasizing a cost-conscious, patient-centric approach minimizes unnecessary testing and interventions. Special populations, including immunocompromised patients, require adjusted thresholds and tailored diagnostic protocols. By adhering to these comprehensive guidelines, clinicians can optimize care for febrile ICU patients, improving outcomes while efficiently utilizing resources.

Algorithm 99.1: Approach to fever in the ICU

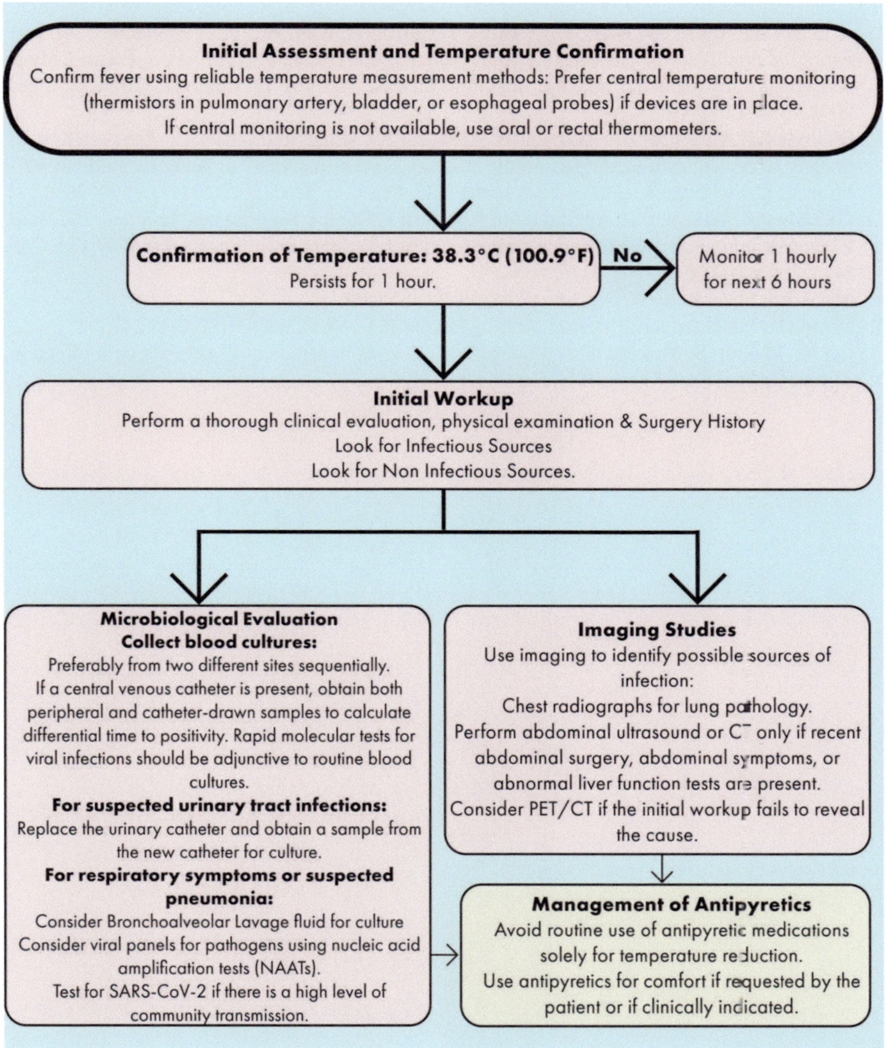

Bibliography

1. O'Grady NP, Barie PS, Bartlett JG, Bleck T, Carroll K, Kalil AC, et al. Guidelines for evaluation of new fever in critically ill adult patients: 2008 update from the American College of critical care medicine and the infectious diseases society of America. Crit Care Med. 2008;36(4):1330–49.
2. O'Grady NP, Alexander E, Alhazzani W, Alshamsi F, Cuellar-Rodriguez J, Jefferson BK, et al. Society of critical care medicine and the infectious diseases society of America guidelines for evaluating new fever in adult patients in the ICU. Crit Care Med. 2023;51(11):1570–86.
3. O'Grady NP, Alexander E, Alhazzani W, Alshamsi F, Cuellar-Rodriguez J, Jefferson BK, et al. Executive summary: guidelines for evaluating new fever in adult patients in the ICU. Crit Care Med. 2023;51(11):1566–9.
4. Marik PE. Fever in the ICU. Chest. 2000;117(3):855–69.
5. Niven DJ, Laupland KB. Pyrexia: aetiology in the ICU. Crit Care. 2016;20(1):247.
6. Egi M, Makino S, Mizobuchi S. Management of fever in critically ill patients with infection. J Emer Critical Care Med. 2018;2:10.

Chapter 100
Approach to Gram-Negative Multidrug-Resistant Organisms (MDROs) in the ICU

100.1 Introduction

Gram-negative multidrug-resistant organisms (MDROs) pose a significant challenge in intensive care units (ICUs) due to their capacity to resist multiple classes of antibiotics. Organisms such as extended-spectrum beta-lactamase-producing *Enterobacterales* (ESBL-E), carbapenem-resistant *Enterobacterales* (CRE), *Pseudomonas aeruginosa*, and *Acinetobacter baumannii* are associated with increased morbidity, mortality, and healthcare costs. The emergence of extensively drug-resistant (XDR) pathogens necessitates a comprehensive approach that includes updated susceptibility testing, optimized antimicrobial therapy, and preventive strategies. Prompt identification and individualized management are critical to improving patient outcomes [1, 2] [Ref: Algorithm 100.1].

Step 1: Confirm Diagnosis

1. Objective: Suspect MDRO infections based on clinical, epidemiological, and laboratory factors.

   - Clinical Clues: Previous healthcare exposure, recurrent infections, invasive devices, or inadequate response to conventional antibiotics.
   - Diagnostic Tools:
   - Cultures: Obtain specimens from blood, urine, respiratory secretions, or wound swabs based on the suspected source.
   - Rapid Diagnostic Testing: Utilize PCR-based assays or matrix-assisted laser desorption/ionization time-of-flight (MALDI-TOF) mass spectrometry for early identification.
   - Susceptibility Testing: Refer to the latest Infectious Diseases Society of America (IDSA) guidelines and joint Clinical and Laboratory Standards Institute (CLSI)/European Committee on Antimicrobial Susceptibility

S. B. Mishra et al., *Mastering ICU Care*,
https://doi.org/10.1007/978-981-95-0179-3_100

Testing (EUCAST) recommendations for specific testing methods and breakpoints, especially for agents like colistin and polymyxin B.
- Early and accurate pathogen identification directs targeted therapy, improves outcomes, and reduces unnecessary broad-spectrum antibiotic use.

Step 2: Determine Infection Type

1. Key Considerations:

- Site of Infection: Identify whether the infection involves the urinary tract, bloodstream, respiratory tract, central nervous system (CNS), or is of polymicrobial origin.
- Severity Assessment: Distinguish between complicated infections (e.g., complicated urinary tract infections [cUTIs] with obstruction, bacteremia, or ventilator-associated pneumonia) and uncomplicated cases.
- The type and location of infection influence the choice of empiric antibiotics, the need for adjunctive therapies like inhalation or intrathecal administration, and the urgency of interventions (e.g., source control).

Step 3: Initiate Empiric Therapy (Ref: Tables 100.1 and 100.2)

1. Factors Influencing Empiric Therapy:

- Severity of Illness: Critically ill patients require broader coverage until pathogen susceptibility is known.
- Local Resistance Patterns: Utilize local antibiograms and molecular epidemiology data to guide empiric therapy decisions, acknowledging regional variations in MDRO prevalence.
- Recent Antibiotic Exposure: Adjust empiric coverage based on prior treatments to minimize resistance selection.
- Patient-Specific Factors: Consider immune status, comorbidities, organ function, and pharmacokinetics/pharmacodynamics when selecting agents.

Step 4: Evaluate Pathogen and Susceptibility

1. Interpretation of Susceptibility Results:

- Updated Guidelines: Follow the latest IDSA and CLSI/EUCAST recommendations for susceptibility testing and breakpoint interpretations.
- If ESBL-E: Carbapenems (e.g., meropenem) are preferred. Alternatives may include ertapenem, trimethoprim-sulfamethoxazole (TMP-SMX), or fluoroquinolones if susceptible. (Refer Table 100.1).
- If CRE: Utilize novel beta-lactam/beta-lactamase inhibitor combinations like ceftazidime-avibactam or meropenem-vaborbactam. Cefiderocol may be considered based on susceptibility. (Refer Table 100.1).
- If difficult-to-treat *Pseudomonas aeruginosa*: Consider ceftolozane-tazobactam, cefiderocol, or imipenem-relebactam.
- If carbapenem-resistant *Acinetobacter baumannii* (CRAB): High-dose sulbactam-durlobactam is preferred. Polymyxins (colistin or polymyxin B) may be used as alternatives.
- If *Stenotrophomonas maltophilia*: TMP-SMX is the drug of choice; levofloxacin is an alternative.

Table 100.1 GNB organism and the preferred treatment

S. no.	Organism	Condition/scenario	Treatment
1a.	ESBL-E	Uncomplicated cystitis	**Preferred**—TMP-SMX **Alternative**—ciprofloxacin, levofloxacin, carbapenems, aminoglycoside (single dose), and oral fosfomycin (*E. coli* only)
b.		Pyelonephritis or complicated UTI	**Preferred**—TMP-SMX, ciprofloxacin, or levofloxacin **Alternative**—ertapenem, meropenem, and imipenem-cilastatin, and aminoglycosides
c.		Outside urinary tract	**Preferred**—meropenem, imipenem-cilastatin, or ertapenem **Transition**—oral TMP-SMX, ciprofloxacin, or levofloxacin if susceptible and good clinical response
2 a.	*Enterobacterales* with AmpC, e.g., *E. cloacae* complex, *K. aerogenes*, and *C. freundii*	Uncomplicated cystitis	**Preferred**—nitrofurantoin and TMP-SMX **Alternative**—ciprofloxacin, levofloxacin, or an aminoglycoside (as a single dose)
b.		Pyelonephritis or complicated UTI	**Preferred**—TMP-SMX, ciprofloxacin, or levofloxacin **Alternative**—aminoglycosides
c.		Outside urinary tract	**Preferred**—cefepime **Transition**—oral TMP-SMX, ciprofloxacin, or levofloxacin
3 a.	Carbapenem resistant *Enterobacterales* (CRE)	Uncomplicated cystitis	**Preferred**—nitrofurantoin, TMP-SMX, ciprofloxacin, or levofloxacin **Alternative**—aminoglycoside (as a single dose), oral fosfomycin (for *E. coli* only), colistin, ceftazidime-avibactam, meropenem-vaborbactam, imipenem-cilastatin-relebactam, cefiderocol, or colistin
b.		Pyelonephritis or complicated UTI	**Preferred—**TMP-SMX, ciprofloxacin, or levofloxacin if susceptible. Ceftazidime-avibactam, meropenem-vaborbactam, imipenem-cilastatin-relebactam, and cefiderocol **Alternative**—aminoglycosides

(continued)

Table 100.1 (continued)

S. no.	Organism	Condition/scenario	Treatment
c.		Outside urinary tract not producing carbapenemase (susceptible to meropenem and imipenem (i.e., MICs ≤1 μg/mL), but are not susceptible to ertapenem (i.e., MICs ≥1 μg/mL))	**Preferred**—extended-infusion meropenem (or imipenem-cilastatin)
d.		Outside urinary tract **not producing carbapenemase** with resistance to all carbapenems	**Preferred—**ceftazidime-avibactam, meropenem-vaborbactam, and imipenem-cilastatin-relebactam
e.		Outside urinary tract with **KPC** production	**Preferred**—meropenem-vaborbactam, ceftazidime-avibactam, and imipenem-cilastatin- relebactam **Alternative—**cefiderocol
f.		Outside urinary tract with **NDM** or other **MBL** production	**Preferred**—ceftazidime-avibactam in combination with aztreonam or cefiderocol
g.		Outside urinary tract with **OXA-48** like production	**Preferred**—Ceftazidime-avibactam **Alternative—**cefiderocol
4 a.	*Pseudomonas aeruginosa* difficult-to-treat resistance (DTR)	Susceptible to both traditional non-carbapenem β-lactam agents and carbapenems	**Preferred**—piperacillin-tazobactam, ceftazidime, cefepime, and aztreonam
		Not susceptible to any carbapenem agent but susceptible to traditional β-lactams	**Preferred**—piperacillin-tazobactam, ceftazidime, cefepime, and aztreonam—*high-dose extended-infusion therapy*
b.		Poor source control with *P. aeruginosa* isolates resistant to carbapenems but susceptible to traditional β-lactams	**Preferred—**ceftolozane-tazobactam, ceftazidime-avibactam, and imipenem-cilastatin-relebactam
c.		Uncomplicated cystitis	**Preferred—**ceftolozane-tazobactam, ceftazidime-avibactam, imipenem-cilastatin-relebactam, and cefiderocol **Alternative**—tobramycin or amikacin (as a single dose

(continued)

Table 100.1 (continued)

S. no.	Organism	Condition/scenario	Treatment
d.		Pyelonephritis or cUTI	**Preferred—**ceftolozane-tazobactam, ceftazidime-avibactam, imipenem-cilastatin-relebactam, and cefiderocol **Alternative**—tobramycin or amikacin once daily
e.		Outside of the urinary tract	**Preferred—**ceftolozane-tazobactam, ceftazidime-avibactam, and imipenem-cilastatin-relebactam **Alternative—**cefiderocol
f.		Produce **MBL** enzymes	**Preferred—**cefiderocol
5.	*Acinetobacter baumannii*	Carbapenem resistant	**Preferred—**sulbactam-durlobactam in combination with a carbapenem (i.e., imipenem-cilastatin or meropenem) **Alternative—**high-dose ampicillin-sulbactam (9 gm sulbactam) + 1 of polymyxin B, minocycline > tigecycline, or cefiderocol Polymyxin B + another agent High-dose Minocycline or Tigecycline + another agent Cefiderocol—refractory cases only
6.	*Stenotrophomonas maltophilia*		**Preferred** (a) Two of the following agents: cefiderocol, minocycline, TMP-SMX, or levofloxacin. oor (b) Ceftazidime-avibactam and aztreonam **Alternative—**cefiderocol as a component of combination therapy

Note:
TMP-SMX—trimethoprim-sulfamethoxazole
Tigecycline and eravacycline are alternative options when β-lactam agents are either not active or unable to be tolerated for the treatment of CRE urinary tract infections or bloodstream infections.
Ceftazidime-avibactam and aztreonam have to be given simultaneously using a three-way cannula
Refer Appendix 1 for dosing of each drug
MBL—metallo-beta-lactamase
NDM—New Delhi metallo-beta-lactamase
KPC—*Klebsiella pneumoniae* carbapenemase
OXA—oxacillinase
UTI—urinary tract infection

Table 100.2 Antibiotics and their dose

S. No.	Drug/antibiotic	Dose
1	TMP-SMX—trimethoprim-sulfamethoxazole	10–15 mg of trimethoprim/kg/day—in 2 or 3 divided doses (160 mg for uncomplicated cystitis on 2 divided dose)
2	Ciprofloxacin	IV—400 mg 3 times daily PO—750 mg twice daily In uncomplicated cystitis IV 400 mg twice daily or PO 500 mg twice daily
3	Levofloxacin	750 mg once daily
4	Amikacin (aminoglycoside)	15 mg/kg
5	Tobramycin (aminoglycoside)	7 mg/kg 5 mg/kg (uncomplicated cystitis)
6	Ertapenem	1 gm once daily over 30 min
7	Imipenem cilastatin	500 mg 4 times daily over 3 h infusion Over half an hour in uncomplicated cystitis
8	Meropenem	2 gm 3 times daily over 3 h infusion 1 gm 3 times daily over half hour in uncomplicated cystitis
9	Imipenem-cilastatin-relebactam	1.25 gm 4 times daily over 30 min
10	Meropenem vaborbactam	4 gm thrice daily over 3 h infusion
11	Ceftazidime avibactam	2.5 gm 3 times daily over 3 h infusion
12	Aztreonam	2 gm 3 times daily over 3 h infusion
13	Nitrofurantoin	100 mg twice daily
14	Cefepime	2 gm 3 times daily over 3 h infusion 1 gm in uncomplicated cystitis
15	Cefiderocol	2 gm 3 times daily over 3 h infusion
16	Fosfomycin	3 gm PO single dose for uncomplicated cystitis
17	Polymyxin B	See text
18	Colistin	See text
19	Ceftolozane tazobactam	3 gm 3 times daily over 3 h infusion 1.5 gm over 1 h in uncomplicated cystitis
20	Eravacycline	1 mg/kg per dose twice daily
21	Tigecycline	200 mg loading dose then 100 mg twice daily
22	Minocycline	200 mg twice daily
23	Ampicillin sulbactam	9 gm of sulbactam daily: 6 gm ampicillin +3 gm sulbactam 3 times daily over 4 h infusion or 27 gm ampicillin + sulbactam over 24 h infusion
24	Sulbactam durlobactam	1 gm each 4 times daily over 3 h infusion

2. Polymyxin Use and Dosing Guidelines:

   - Optimal Use: Reserve polymyxins for infections caused by XDR organisms when no safer, effective alternatives are available.
   - Dosing regimens:
   - Colistin (Polymyxin E):
   - Loading Dose: A loading dose is essential due to colistin's pharmacokinetics and to rapidly achieve therapeutic plasma concentrations. The recommended loading dose is nine million international units (MIU), which is approximately 300 mg of colistin base activity (CBA), administered intravenously over 30–60 min.
   - Maintenance Dose: The maintenance dosing depends on the patient's renal function. For patients with normal renal function (creatinine clearance [CrCl] $\geq$ 80 mL/min), the recommended maintenance dose is 4.5 MIU (150 mg CBA) every 12 h.
   - Renal Dosing Adjustments: Adjust maintenance doses for patients with impaired renal function:
   - CrCl 50–79 mL/min: 3 MIU (100 mg CBA) every 12 h.
   - CrCl 30–49 mL/min: 2.25 MIU (75 mg CBA) every 12 h.
   - CrCl 10–29 mL/min: 2.25 MIU (75 mg CBA) every 24 h.
   - CrCl<10 mL/min or on intermittent hemodialysis: 1.5 MIU (50 mg CBA) every 24 h, administered after dialysis, on dialysis days.
   - Continuous Renal Replacement Therapy (CRRT): May require dosing similar to patients with normal renal function; consult a specialist.
   - Critically Ill Patients: Due to altered pharmacokinetics in critically ill patients, they may require higher maintenance doses or more frequent dosing. Therapeutic drug monitoring (TDM) is recommended to adjust dosing based on plasma concentrations.
   - Polymyxin B:
   - Loading Dose: A loading dose is recommended to achieve effective plasma levels quickly. The suggested loading dose is 2.0–2.5 mg/kg (based on total body weight), administered intravenously over 1 h.
   - Maintenance Dose: The maintenance dose is 1.25–1.5 mg/kg every 12 h (based on total body weight).
   - Renal Dosing Adjustments: Polymyxin B is less affected by renal function because it is not significantly eliminated by the kidneys. Therefore, no dosage adjustment is generally necessary for patients with renal impairment, including those on dialysis.
   - Critically Ill Patients: Similar to colistin, critically ill patients may have altered drug clearance. TDM is advisable to ensure therapeutic levels without reaching toxicity.

Key Considerations

- Therapeutic Drug Monitoring (TDM):
- Purpose: TDM helps in optimizing dosing by measuring plasma drug concentrations, ensuring efficacy while minimizing toxicity.
- Recommendations: Regularly monitor colistin plasma levels, especially in critically ill patients or those with fluctuating renal function.
- Target Concentrations: Aim for a steady-state plasma concentration of colistin (as the active formed colistin base) between 2 and 4 mg/L for efficacy, while keeping below levels associated with increased toxicity.
- Toxicity Management:
- Nephrotoxicity:
- Risk Factors: High doses, prolonged therapy, concomitant use of other nephrotoxic agents (e.g., aminoglycosides, vancomycin), and preexisting renal impairment.
- Monitoring: Check serum creatinine and urine output at baseline and at least every 2–3 days during therapy.
- Management: If nephrotoxicity develops, consider dose adjustment, increased monitoring, or alternative therapies if possible.
- Neurotoxicity:
- Symptoms: Paresthesias, dizziness, ataxia, visual disturbances, and, rarely, neuromuscular blockade leading to respiratory failure.
- Monitoring: Assess for neurological symptoms regularly, especially in patients with risk factors such as high doses or concomitant neuromuscular blockers.
- Management: Discontinue or adjust dosing if significant neurotoxicity occurs.
- Administration tips:
- Infusion Rates: Administer colistin over 30–60 min and polymyxin B over 1 h to reduce the risk of infusion-related reactions.
- Compatibility: Ensure compatibility with other intravenous medications to prevent precipitation or inactivation.
- Preparation: Reconstitute according to manufacturer instructions, and use prepared solutions promptly to maintain stability.
- Pharmacokinetics and Pharmacodynamics:
- Colistin: It is administered as colistin methanesulfonate (CMS), an inactive prodrug converted to active colistin in the body. The conversion is slow and variable, necessitating a loading dose and careful maintenance dosing.
- Polymyxin B: Administered in its active form, leading to more predictable plasma concentrations and not requiring adjustment in renal impairment.
- Achieving adequate plasma concentrations is crucial for bactericidal activity against MDROs.
- Suboptimal dosing can promote the development of resistance.

Step 5: Consider Adjunctive Therapies

1. Combination Therapy Strategies:

   - Rationale for Combination Therapy: Combining polymyxins with other agents (e.g., rifampin, carbapenems, or tigecycline) may enhance efficacy against XDR pathogens like *Pseudomonas aeruginosa* and *Acinetobacter baumannii* and minimize resistance development.
   - Select combinations based on in vitro synergy studies and clinical evidence.

   Combination antibiotic therapy (i.e., the use of a β-lactam agent in combination with an aminoglycoside, fluoroquinolone, tetracycline, or polymyxin) is not suggested for the treatment of infections caused by CRE. Combination antibiotic therapy is not suggested for infections caused by DTR *P. aeruginosa* if susceptibility to ceftolozane-tazobactam, ceftazidime-avibactam, imipenem-cilastatin- relebactam, or cefiderocol has been confirmed.

2. Alternative Delivery Methods:

   - Inhalation Therapy: Consider aerosolized antibiotics (e.g., colistin) for respiratory infections to achieve high local concentrations while reducing systemic toxicity.
   - Intrathecal or Intraventricular Therapy: Utilize for CNS infections caused by MDROs when systemic therapy is inadequate.

3. Source Control:

   - Interventions: Drain abscesses, remove or replace infected devices, and debride infected tissues promptly.

4. Rationale: Adjunctive therapies address the infection comprehensively, enhancing antimicrobial effectiveness and improving patient outcomes.

Step 6: Transition to Oral Therapy

1. Criteria for Transition:

   - Clinical Stability: Improvement in hemodynamics and resolution of systemic signs of infection.
   - Effective Oral Options: Ensure availability of effective oral agents based on susceptibility, such as Fluoroquinolones or TMP-SMX.
   - Gastrointestinal Function: Confirm adequate absorption capability.
   - Patient Factors: Consider comorbidities and potential drug interactions.

2. Transitioning to oral therapy reduces the risks associated with prolonged intravenous access, lowers healthcare costs, and facilitates earlier discharge when appropriate.

Step 7: Duration of Therapy

1. Tailored duration based on infection type and patient response:

   - cUTI: Typically 5–7 days.
   - Bacteremia: Usually 7–14 days, depending on the source and patient factors.
   - Pneumonia: Generally 7–10 days.
   - MDRO Considerations: Evidence suggests that MDRO-associated infections may not always require extended durations compared to nonresistant infections.
   - TDM and Monitoring: Use TDM and clinical markers to guide therapy duration.

100.2 Conclusion

Managing Gram-negative MDROs in the ICU requires a multidisciplinary and patient-centered approach. Utilizing updated susceptibility testing methods and adhering to the latest guidelines ensures accurate pathogen identification and effective therapy selection. Empiric therapy should be guided by local resistance patterns, patient-specific factors, and a thorough understanding of pharmacokinetics and pharmacodynamics. Adjunctive strategies, including combination therapies and alternative delivery methods, play a crucial role in treating XDR pathogens. Therapeutic drug monitoring, especially for nephrotoxic agents like polymyxins, optimizes therapeutic outcomes while mitigating toxicity. Preventive strategies are equally important. Infection prevention measures such as antimicrobial stewardship programs, strict hand hygiene, and decolonization protocols help curb the transmission and emergence of MDROs. By emphasizing individualized therapy adjustments, source control, and judicious use of antibiotics, healthcare professionals can optimize patient outcomes while combating the growing threat of antimicrobial resistance in the ICU setting.

Algorithm 100.1: Approach to gram-negative multidrug-resistant organisms (MDROs) in the ICU

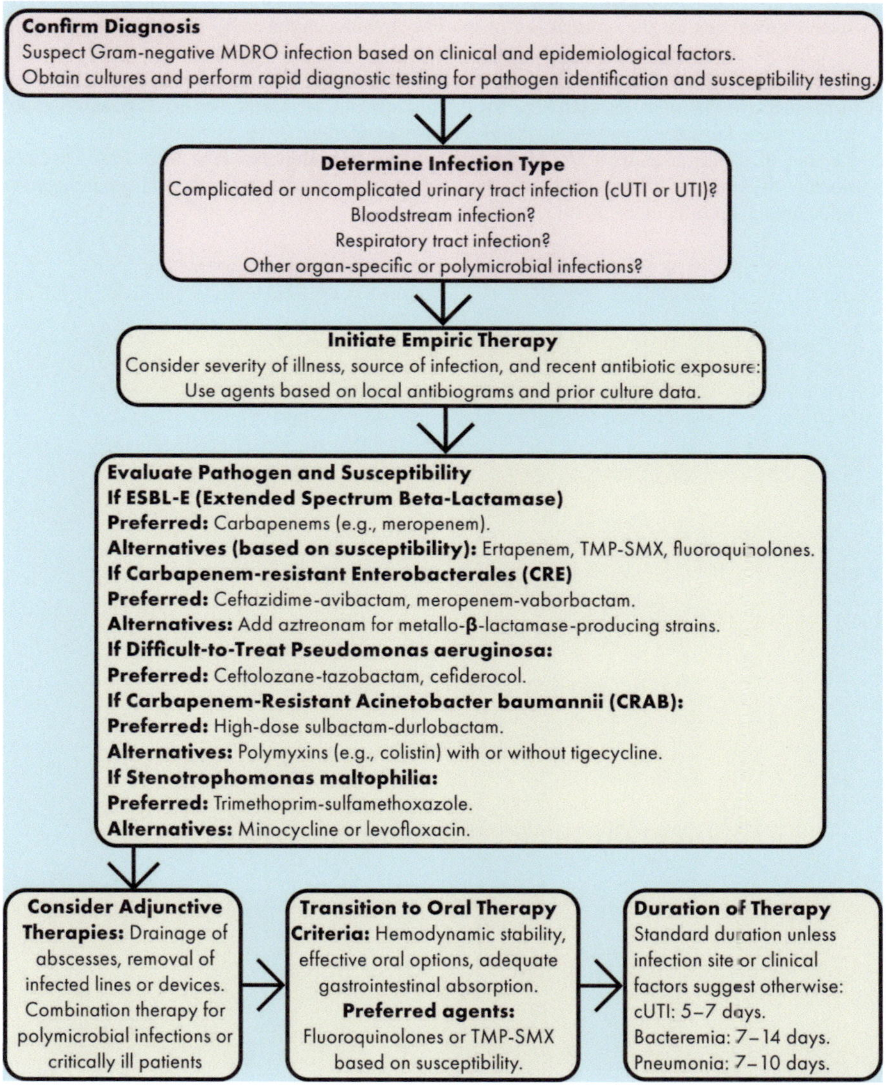

Bibliography

1. Tsuji BT, Pogue JM, Zavascki AP, Paul M, Daikos GL, Forrest A, et al. International consensus guidelines for the optimal use of the Polymyxins: endorsed by the American College of Clinical Pharmacy (ACCP), European Society of Clinical Microbiology and Infectious Diseases (ESCMID), Infectious Diseases Society of America (IDSA), International Society for Anti-infective Pharmacology (ISAP), Society of Critical Care Medicine (SCCM), and Society of Infectious Diseases Pharmacists (SIDP). Pharmacotherapy. 2019;39(1):10–39.
2. Tamma PD, Heil EL, Justo JA, Mathers AJ, Satlin MJ, Bonomo RA. Infectious Diseases Society of America 2024 guidance on the treatment of antimicrobial-resistant gram-negative infections. Clin Infect Dis. 2024;

Chapter 101
Approach to Candidemia in the ICU

101.1 Introduction

Candidemia is a significant bloodstream infection caused by *Candida* species, particularly affecting critically ill patients in the intensive care unit (ICU). The infection is associated with high morbidity and mortality, often due to delayed diagnosis and inappropriate treatment. Early identification and effective management are critical to improving outcomes.

Recent epidemiological trends have highlighted a rise in non-albicans species such as *Candida glabrata* and *Candida auris*, which often exhibit resistance to commonly used antifungals like fluconazole (azoles). Additionally, geographical variations in *Candida* species prevalence and resistance patterns necessitate region-specific management strategies. Understanding these patterns is essential for effective treatment and containment of the infection [1, 2] [Ref: Algorithm 101.1]

101.2 *Candida* Score and Colonization Index

1. *Candida* Score:

   The *Candida* Score is a clinical tool to identify ICU patients at high risk for invasive candidiasis (IC). It incorporates four parameters, with a total score of ≥3 suggesting a high risk for IC.

   Parameters

   1. Severe Sepsis: 2 points
   2. Total Parenteral Nutrition (TPN): 1 point
   3. Multifocal *Candida* Colonization: 1 point
   4. Surgery: 1 point

S. B. Mishra et al., *Mastering ICU Care*,
https://doi.org/10.1007/978-981-95-0179-3_101

Interpretation

- Score < 3: Low risk of invasive candidiasis
- Score ≥ 3: High risk of invasive candidiasis (sensitivity ~80%, specificity ~70%)

2. Colonization Index (CI):

The Colonization Index quantifies *Candida* colonization to predict the risk of IC. It is the ratio of the number of positive *Candida* culture sites to the total number of sites sampled.

Calculation

$$\text{Colonization Index}(\text{CI}) = \text{Number of positive}\,\textit{Candida}\,\text{colonization sites} \\ /\text{Total number of sites sampled}$$

- Threshold for Concern: CI ≥ 0.5 suggests significant colonization.
- Corrected Colonization Index (CCI): Adds weight to multifocal colonization.

$$\text{CCI} = \text{CI} \times 2(\text{if at least two sites are colonized})$$

Interpretation

- CI ≥ 0.5: Associated with increased risk of invasive candidiasis
- CCI ≥ 0.4–0.5: Stronger predictor of IC

Clinical Utility

- *Candida* Score and Colonization Index help in early identification of ICU patients who may benefit from empirical antifungal therapy.
- These tools complement clinical judgment and should be combined with other risk factors for optimal decision-making [3].

101.3 Monitor and Reassess Clinical Status Regularly

- Vigilance for candidemia is crucial for all ICU patients, especially those with risk factors such as recent surgery, central venous catheters (CVCs), hemodialysis, prolonged ICU stay, immunosuppression, or broad-spectrum antibiotic use. Immunocompromised patients, including neutropenic individuals, present unique challenges and may require tailored therapy.
- Candida Scoring Systems:
- Utilize validated tools like the *Candida* Score (≥3) or *Candida* Colonization Index (≥0.5) to evaluate the risk.
- These tools aid in the initiation of prophylactic or preemptive antifungal therapy.
- Implementing prophylactic or preemptive therapy in high-risk patients can reduce mortality but must be balanced against the potential for antifungal resistance due to unnecessary exposure.

- Advanced Diagnostic Modalities:
- Non-culture-Based Diagnostic Tools: Incorporate assays such as the beta-D-glucan test and PCR-based methods for early detection.
- Biomarkers in Preemptive Therapy: Monitor biomarkers to guide preemptive therapy strategies, aiming to initiate treatment before the onset of symptoms.
- Key Considerations:
- If the scoring criteria are not met and advanced diagnostics are negative, continue routine monitoring and reassess periodically.
- Prompt action is warranted when thresholds are crossed or if new risk factors emerge.

101.4 Initial Steps If Candidemia Is Suspected

- Removal of Central Venous Catheters (CVCs):
- If feasible, remove the CVC promptly, as it is often the source of candidemia.
- Early removal reduces fungal burden and prevents persistent infection.
- Blood Cultures:
- Obtain blood cultures from multiple sites to confirm the diagnosis and identify the *Candida* species and its susceptibility profile.
- Due to the rise of non-albicans species like *C. glabrata* and *C. auris*, which may be resistant to fluconazole, species identification is critical.
- Repeat cultures daily until clearance is documented.
- Additional Investigations:
- Transesophageal Echocardiography (TEE): Perform TEE to evaluate for *Candida*-associated endocarditis, a serious complication requiring prolonged therapy.
- Ophthalmologic Examination: Conduct regular ophthalmologic evaluations to rule out endophthalmitis.
- Infection Control Measures: Implement strict infection control practices to limit the spread of resistant species like *C. auris* within the ICU.
- These steps ensure the identification of infection sources and complications, guiding necessary adjustments in therapy and management strategies [4].

101.5 Management

101.5.1 Empirical Antifungal Therapy

- When to consider: Critically ill patients with risk factors and no other known cause of fever. Assess the various risk factors and send surrogate markers. Start empirical therapy if the patient is in septic shock with positive above said factors.

- Examples: ICU patients persistently febrile, but without microbiological evidence, ICU patients with positive (1,3)-β-D-glucan test
- Initiation of Therapy:
- First-Line Agents: Initiate empirical antifungal therapy promptly with echinocandins (e.g., caspofungin—loading dose of 70 mg, then 50 mg daily; micafungin—100 mg daily; anidulafungin—loading dose of 200 mg, then 100 mg daily) due to their broad spectrum of activity and efficacy against most *Candida* species, including resistant non-albicans strains.
- Alternative Agents:
- Fluconazole, 800 mg (12 mg/kg) loading dose, then 400 mg (6 mg/kg) daily—no recent azole exposure and are not colonized with azole-resistant *Candida* species.
- For patients intolerant to echinocandins or with resistant species, consider liposomal amphotericin B (3–5 mg/kg daily) or voriconazole.
- Therapeutic Drug Monitoring (TDM): Implement TDM for antifungals like voriconazole to optimize efficacy and minimize toxicity.
- Clinical Considerations:
- Tailoring Therapy: Adjust antifungal therapy based on susceptibility results as soon as they are available.
- Recommended duration: 2 weeks if improvement noticed. Discontinue empiric therapy if no improvement after 4–5 days and negative evidence of invasive candidiasis or negative results for non-culture-based assays.
- Timelines: Early initiation of appropriate antifungal therapy significantly improves survival rates. Delays in therapy are associated with increased mortality [5].
- Ongoing Assessment: Continue clinical and microbiological assessments to ensure the effectiveness of therapy and to detect any potential complications early [6].

101.5.2 Prophylactic and Preemptive Therapy

- Definition:
  - Prophylactic antifungal therapy: treatment of a patient without signs or symptoms of fungal disease. It is usually used when the benefit to the patient outweighs the development of resistance and adverse effects.

For example, recent abdominal surgery AND recurrent gastrointestinal perforations or anastomotic leakages; critically ill surgical patients with an expected length of ICU stay ≥3 day, ventilated for 48 h and expected to be ventilated for another ≥72 h, ventilated, hospitalized for >3 day, received antibiotics, CVC, and ≥ 1 of: parenteral nutrition, dialysis, major surgery, pancreatitis, systemic steroids, immunosuppression, hematological malignancies (acute myeloid leukemia and myelodysplastic syndrome with neutropenia>10 days), transplant (stem cell, lung, liver and heart transplant on immunosuppressants), and inherited immune disorders.

- Preemptive antifungal therapy: Used in patients who have a laboratory assay positive for invasive fungal infections (galactomannan assays, beta-D-glucan assays). It is a therapy triggered by microbiological evidence of candidiasis without proof of invasive fungal infection.

- Risk-Based Prophylaxis:
- In patients with persistent risk factors or those who are highly colonized, consider initiating prophylactic or preemptive antifungal therapy based on scoring systems like the *Candida* Colonization Index.
- Balancing Risks: Weigh the benefits of preventing invasive candidiasis against the potential for antifungal resistance due to unnecessary exposure.
- Clinical Considerations:
- Tailored Approach: Customize prophylactic strategies based on individual patient risks, local epidemiology, and resistance patterns.
- In the ICU with incidence of invasive candidiasis >5%: Inj Fluconazole 800 mg (12 mg/kg) loading dose, then 400 mg (6 mg/kg) daily or with echinocandins (dose mentioned above).
- Daily chlorhexidine bath may be considered.
- Avoiding Resistance: Use antifungal agents judiciously to minimize the development of resistant strains [7].

101.5.3 Definitive Therapy

Nonneutropenic Patients:

- Initial Therapy: Echinocandin (caspofungin: loading dose 70 mg, then 50 mg daily; micafungin: 100 mg daily; anidulafungin: loading dose 200 mg, then 100 mg daily).
- Not critically ill and unlikely to have fluconazole resistance: Fluconazole, intravenous or oral, 800 mg (12 mg/kg) loading dose, then 400 mg (6 mg/kg) daily.
- Alternative: Lipid formulation amphotericin B (AmB) (3–5 mg/kg daily).
- *C. glabrata*: Higher-dose fluconazole 800 mg (12 mg/kg) daily or voriconazole 200–300 (3–4 mg/kg) twice daily if susceptible.
- Reassess Therapy After 5–7 Days

De-escalation: If the patient is clinically stable and the isolate is confirmed to be fluconazole-susceptible and has negative repeat blood cultures following initiation of antifungal therapy, consider transitioning to fluconazole for step-down therapy.

- Continue antifungal therapy for at least 14 days after the first negative blood culture and resolution of symptoms.
- Extend treatment duration in cases involving endocarditis or endophthalmitis, following specialist recommendations.

- Neutropenic Patients:

  - Recommended Drug: Echinocandin (caspofungin: loading dose 70 mg, then 50 mg daily; micafungin: 100 mg daily; anidulafungin: loading dose 200 mg, then 100 mg daily).
  - Alternative: Lipid formulation amphotericin B (AmB) (3–5 mg/kg daily).
  - Not Critically Ill and Unlikely to Have Fluconazole Resistance: Fluconazole, intravenous or oral, 800 mg (12 mg/kg) loading dose, then 400 mg (6 mg/kg) daily.
  - Fluconazole Susceptible Isolates and Documented Bloodstream Clearance: Stepdown to fluconazole (400 mg (6 mg/kg) twice daily for 2 doses, then 200–300 mg (3–4 mg/kg) twice daily).
  - *C. krusei* Infection: Echinocandin, lipid formulation amphotericin B, or voriconazole.
  - Duration: 14 days after the first negative blood culture and resolution of symptoms.

- Abdominal Candidiasis:

  - Consider empiric therapy.
  - Source Control: Debridement with drain.
  - Drugs: Same as nonneutropenic patients.

- Cardiac:

  Native Valve Endocarditis:
  Lipid formulation AmB, 3–5 mg/kg daily, with or without flucytosine, 25 mg/kg four times daily, OR high-dose echinocandin (caspofungin 150 mg daily, micafungin 150 mg daily, or anidulafungin 200 mg daily).
  Similar step-down approach as mentioned in the above section.
  Voriconazole 200–300 mg (3–4 mg/kg) twice daily, or posaconazole tablets, 300 mg daily to be used if fluconazole resistant.
  Surgery: Valve replacement with 6 weeks of treatment after surgery.
  Prosthetic Valve Endocarditis.
  Same as native valve plus fluconazole 400–800 mg (6–12 mg/kg) daily for chronic suppression.

  Implantable Cardiac Device (ICD)

- Remove device.
- Drugs: Same as native valve endocarditis.
- Generator Pockets Infection: 4 weeks antifungal after device removal.
- ICD Wire: 6 weeks antifungal after wire removal.
- Candida Osteoarticular Infections
- Fluconazole, 400 mg (6 mg/kg) daily, for 6–12 months or an echinocandin (caspofungin 50–70 mg daily, micafungin 100 mg daily, or anidulafungin 100 mg daily) for at least 2 weeks followed by fluconazole, 400 mg (6 mg/kg) daily, for 6–12 months.
- Surgical debridement if necessary.
- Candida Septic Arthritis

- Same as osteoarticular infections.
- Mandatory surgical drainage and debridement.
- Candida Endophthalmitis
- All patients with candidemia should have a dilated retinal examination within the first week of therapy in nonneutropenic patients or after neutrophil count recovery in neutropenic patients.
- Consult ophthalmologist regarding treatment plan.
- Usual duration of antifungals (Fluconazole/Voriconazole/Liposomal Amphotericin B) is 4–6 weeks.
- Intravitreal injection of amphotericin B deoxycholate 5–10 μg/0.1 mL sterile water is used in macular involvement and in case of vitritis.
- Vitrectomy should be considered to decrease the organism burden and to allow the removal of fungal abscesses.
- CNS Candidiasis
- Liposomal AmB, 5 mg/kg daily, with or without oral flucytosine, 25 mg/kg four times daily.
- Stepdown: Fluconazole, 400–800 mg (6–12 mg/kg) daily after response to initial treatment.
- Duration: All signs and symptoms and CSF and radiological abnormalities have resolved.
- Urinary Tract Infection (UTI) with *Candida*
- Asymptomatic: Remove indwelling catheter; antifungals—oral fluconazole, 400 mg (6 mg/kg) daily, OR amphotericin B deoxycholate, 0.3–0.6 mg/kg daily if planning for urological procedures.
- Symptomatic:

  - Remove indwelling catheter.
  - Fluconazole-susceptible: Oral fluconazole 200 mg (3 mg/kg) daily for 2 weeks.
  - Fluconazole-resistant *C. glabrata*, *krusei*: Amphotericin B deoxycholate, 0.3–0.6 mg/kg daily for 1–7 days.

- Pyelonephritis:
- Fluconazole-susceptible: Oral fluconazole 200–400 mg (3–6 mg/kg) daily for 2 weeks.
- Fluconazole-resistant *C. glabrata*: AmB deoxycholate, 0.3–0.6 mg/kg daily for 1–7 days with or without oral flucytosine, 25 mg/kg four times daily.
- Fluconazole-resistant *C. krusei*: Amphotericin B deoxycholate, 0.3–0.6 mg/kg daily for 1–7 days.
- UTI with Fungal Balls: Surgical intervention plus antifungal therapy as in pyelonephritis. Amphotericin B deoxycholate irrigation (25–50 mg in 200–500 mL sterile water) if nephrostomy tube in situ.
- Moderate to Severe Oropharyngeal and Esophageal Candidiasis
- Oropharyngeal: Oral fluconazole, 100–200 mg daily, for 7–14 days (itraconazole—solution 200 mg daily/posaconazole suspension 400 mg twice daily for 3 days followed by 400 mg daily, for up to 28 days if refractory to fluconazole).

– Esophageal: Oral fluconazole, 200–400 mg (3–6 mg/kg) daily, for 14–21 days. IV fluconazole or 400 mg (6 mg/kg) daily, or an echinocandin (micafungin, 150 mg daily, caspofungin, 70 mg loading dose, then 50 mg daily, or anidulafungin, 200 mg daily) can also be given if oral therapy is not tolerated or cannot be given. Itraconazole solution, 200 mg daily, OR voriconazole, 200 mg (3 mg/kg) twice daily either intravenous or oral, for 14–21 days if disease is refractory to fluconazole.

101.6 Management of Complications

- Early Detection and Intervention:
- Regular Evaluations: Emphasize the importance of regular TEE and ophthalmologic examinations to detect complications such as endocarditis and endophthalmitis early.
- Specialist Involvement: Involve infectious disease specialists and other relevant consultants to manage complex cases effectively.
- Treatment Strategies:
- Extended Therapy: Implement prolonged antifungal therapy for patients with confirmed complications, following evidence-based guidelines.
- Surgical Intervention: Consider surgical management when indicated, such as valve replacement in endocarditis.

101.7 Multimodal Interventions

- Bundled Care Approaches:
- Infectious Disease Consultations: Engage infectious disease specialists early to optimize antifungal therapy and management plans.
- Central Venous Catheter Management: Implement protocols for the timely removal or replacement of CVCs and strict adherence to catheter care practices.
- Infection Control Practices:
- Preventing Spread: Apply rigorous infection control measures to prevent the transmission of resistant species like *C. auris* within the ICU.
- Education and Training: Provide ongoing staff education on hand hygiene, equipment disinfection, and isolation precautions.

101.8 Special Populations and Comorbidities

- Immunocompromised Patients:
- Tailored Therapy: Adjust antifungal regimens for immunocompromised patients, including those with neutropenia, to address their specific needs and risks.

- Close Monitoring: Intensify monitoring for signs of infection and response to therapy, given their higher risk for complications.
- Comorbid Conditions:
- Holistic Management: Consider the impact of comorbidities on treatment choices and patient outcomes, adjusting therapy as necessary.

101.9 Outcomes and Prognostic Indicators

- Mortality Rates:
- Species-Specific Outcomes: Recognize that ICU mortality rates associated with candidemia vary by *Candida* species, with higher mortality observed in infections caused by non-albicans species like *C. glabrata* and *C. auris*.
- Treatment Delays: Understand that delays in initiating appropriate antifungal therapy are linked to worse outcomes, reinforcing the need for rapid diagnosis and treatment.
- Recent Studies:
- Timeliness of Therapy: Incorporate findings from recent research highlighting that early antifungal therapy significantly reduces mortality rates.
- Prognostic Indicators: Utilize prognostic indicators to identify high-risk patients who may benefit from more aggressive interventions.

101.10 Conclusion

The management of candidemia in the ICU requires a comprehensive and systematic approach that incorporates early risk assessment, advanced diagnostic modalities, prompt initiation of appropriate antifungal therapy, and careful monitoring to guide treatment adjustments. Recognizing the rise of resistant non-albicans *Candida* species and geographical variations in prevalence and resistance patterns is essential for effective management. Removal of central venous catheters and thorough diagnostic evaluations are critical first steps. Echinocandins remain the preferred first-line agents in most cases, with transitions to alternative therapies based on susceptibility results and patient stability. Multimodal interventions, including bundled care approaches and infection control practices, play a vital role in improving outcomes. Special attention to immunocompromised patients and timely initiation of therapy are paramount. Adherence to these guidelines ensures optimal patient outcomes while minimizing complications and the development of antifungal resistance.

Algorithm 101.1: Approach to candidemia in the ICU

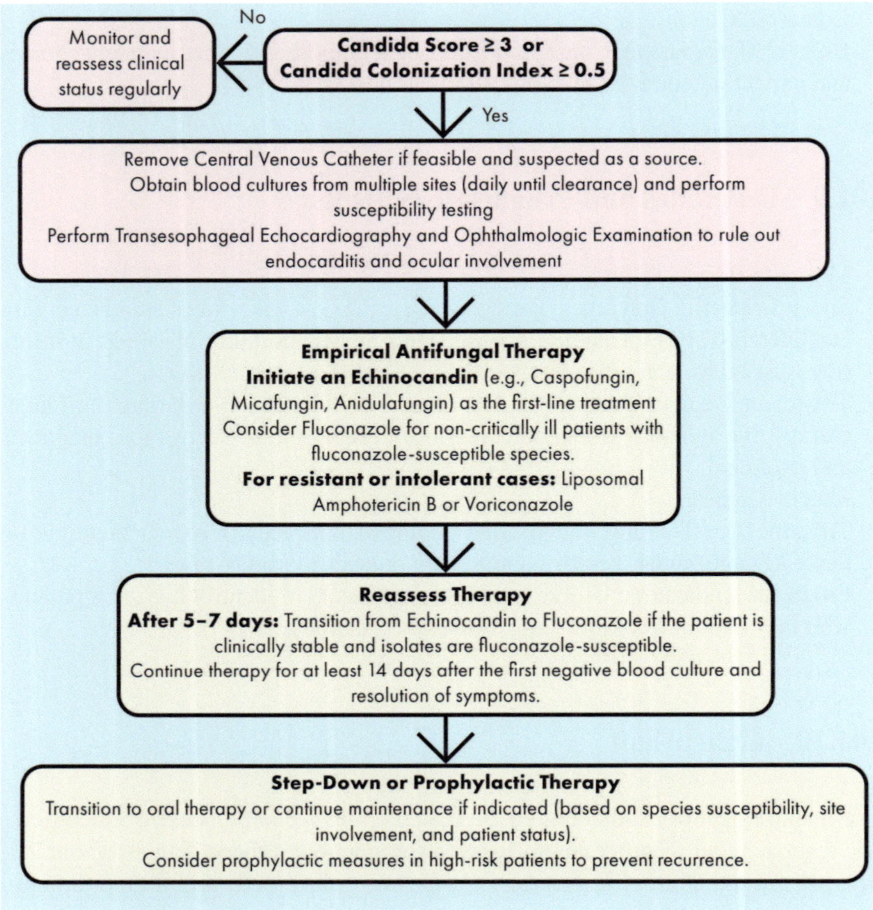

Bibliography

1. Pappas PG, Kauffman CA, Andes DR, Clancy CJ, Marr KA, Ostrosky-Zeichner L, et al. Clinical practice guideline for the Management of Candidiasis: 2016 update by the Infectious Diseases Society of America. Clin Infect Dis. 2016;62(4):e1–50.
2. Azim A, Ahmed A. Diagnosis and management of invasive fungal diseases in non-neutropenic ICU patients, with focus on candidiasis and aspergillosis: a comprehensive review. Front Cell Infect Microbiol. 2024;14:1256158.

3. Keighley C, Cooley L, Morris AJ, Ritchie D, Clark JE, Boan P, et al. Consensus guidelines for the diagnosis and management of invasive candidiasis in haematology, oncology and intensive care settings, 2021. Intern Med J. 2021;51(Suppl 7):89–117.
4. Hankovszky P, Tarsy D, Oveges N, Molnar Z. Invasive Candida infections in the ICU: diagnosis and therapy. J Crit Care Med (Targu Mures). 2015;1(4):129–39.
5. Cornely OA, Bassetti M, Calandra T, Garbino J, Kullberg BJ, Lortholary O, et al. ESCMID* guideline for the diagnosis and management of Candida diseases 2012: non-neutropenic adult patients. Clin Microbiol Infect. 2012;18(Suppl 7):19–37.
6. Martin-Loeches I, Antonelli M, Cuenca-Estrella M, Dimopoulos G, Einav S, De Waele JJ, et al. ESICM/ESCMID task force on practical management of invasive candidiasis in critically ill patients. Intensive Care Med. 2019;45(6):789–805.
7. Nascimento T, Inacio J, Guerreiro D, Patricio P, Proenca L, Toscano C, et al. Insights into Candida colonization in intensive care unit patients: a prospective multicenter study. J Fungi (Basel). 2024;10(6)

Chapter 102
Approach to Aspergillosis in the ICU

102.1 Introduction

Invasive aspergillosis (IA) is a severe fungal infection predominantly affecting immunocompromised individuals or those with critical illnesses. The condition is associated with high morbidity and mortality rates, especially in intensive care unit (ICU) settings, due to delayed diagnosis and limited treatment windows. Effective management of IA requires a structured approach that involves identifying at-risk patients, recognizing clinical and diagnostic clues, and initiating timely antifungal therapy [1, 2] [Ref: Algorithm 102.1].

102.2 Assessing Risk Factors

The first step is to determine if the patient has risk factors for IA. Key risk factors include:

Severe Respiratory Illness:

- Acute Respiratory Distress Syndrome (ARDS)
- Ventilator dependence
- Chronic Obstructive Pulmonary Disease (COPD)
- Viral pneumonias such as influenza and COVID-19

Immunosuppressive Therapy:

- Corticosteroids
- Chemotherapy (e.g., induction/reinduction regimens for acute leukemia)
- Immunomodulatory agents

S. B. Mishra et al., *Mastering ICU Care*,
https://doi.org/10.1007/978-981-95-0179-3_102

Underlying Conditions:

- Prolonged neutropenia
- Liver failure
- Subtle immune dysfunctions
- Hospitalized allogeneic HSCT recipients

ICU-Related Factors:

- Prolonged mechanical ventilation
- Use of broad-spectrum antibiotics

For patients without risk factors, monitor for new developments such as clinical deterioration or the emergence of new risk factors [3].

102.3 Assessing Clinical Signs

For at-risk patients, evaluate for clinical signs suggestive of IA:

- Fever unresponsive to broad-spectrum antibiotics
- Respiratory decline with worsening hypoxemia
- Hemoptysis or pleuritic chest pain

These signs, though nonspecific, raise suspicion for IA in critically ill patients, especially when unresponsive to standard therapies. If clinical signs are absent, reassess the patient only if new symptoms or risk factors develop.

102.4 Imaging Evaluation

CT scan: To be done when there is suspicion, regardless of chest radiograph findings. Obtain imaging studies, specifically a chest CT scan, to identify findings consistent with invasive pulmonary aspergillosis (IPA). Look for:

- Halo Sign: Ground-glass opacity surrounding a nodule.
- Wedge-Shaped Infarcts: Recently added as imaging criteria for probable IPA.
- Segmental or Lobar Consolidations: Inclusion enhances diagnostic sensitivity.
- Air Crescent Sign: May develop later in the disease

Bronchoscopy: Bronchoscopy and BAL should be done in patients with a suspicion of IPA (invasive pulmonary aspergillosis). BAL sample should be sent for routine culture and cytology as well as non-culture-based methods.

Imaging findings are often the first objective clues for IPA, as culture results may be delayed. The inclusion of wedge-shaped infarcts and segmental or lobar consolidations expands the radiological criteria, aiding in earlier diagnosis [4]. Consider alternative diagnoses but remain vigilant if clinical suspicion remains high.

102.5 Non-culture-Based Diagnostic Markers

Evaluate for fungal markers using advanced biomarker techniques:

- Galactomannan (GM) Assay:
- GM is not recommended for routine blood screening in patients receiving mold-active antifungal therapy or prophylaxis, but can be applied to bronchoscopy specimens.
- GM is an accurate marker for the diagnosis of IA in adults in certain patient subpopulations (hematologic malignancy, HSCT).
- β-D-Glucan Testing:
- Useful as a broad fungal biomarker (not specific for IA).
- *Aspergillus* PCR:
- Incorporated into the BM-AspICU algorithm for improved classification.
- Next-Generation Sequencing (NGS):
- Helpful in patients where biopsy is contraindicated.

Non-culture-based markers and molecular diagnostics like PCR and NGS enhance diagnostic sensitivity, especially in cases where imaging is inconclusive or invasive procedures are contraindicated. If markers are negative, move to step 5 (histopathological or sterile site identification).

102.6 Histopathology or Sterile Site Identification

If non-culture markers are inconclusive, attempt to identify *Aspergillus* in sterile body sites or tissue histopathology:

- Histopathological Examination:
- Look for hyphal structures or evidence of tissue invasion.
- Utilize rRNA sequencing when fungal invasion is observed.
- Sterile Site Sampling:
- Perform a biopsy or obtain fluid from a sterile site if clinically feasible.

Definitive diagnosis often requires direct visualization or isolation of the organism in sterile sites. Molecular diagnostics can provide additional confirmation. If no evidence is found, reconsider the diagnosis and evaluate for colonization or other conditions mimicking IA [1].

102.7 Initiating Antifungal Therapy

If IA is strongly suspected or confirmed, initiate antifungal treatment:

- First-Line Therapy:
- Voriconazole: Preferred due to its superior efficacy and tolerability.

- Dose: Loading dose of 6 mg/kg intravenous IV infusion or 400 mg BD orally for 24 hours, followed by a 4 mg/kg IV or 200 mg BID oral maintenance dose).
- Alternative Options:
- Isavuconazole: Effective against azole-resistant *Aspergillus fumigatus*.
- Loading dose: 372 mg PO/IV three times daily x six doses (48 hr).
- Maintenance: 372 mg PO/IV once daily.
- Liposomal Amphotericin B
- 3–5 mg/kg IV once daily
- Combination Therapy: Consider in refractory cases or when resistance is suspected.
- Susceptibility Testing:
- Essential for guiding therapy in the context of emerging azole resistance.
- Echinocandins:
- Echinocandins (micafungin or caspofungin) can be used in settings where azole and polyene antifungals are contraindicated.

Early initiation of appropriate antifungal therapy improves outcomes, reduces hospital costs, and shortens the length of stay. Awareness of azole resistance patterns is crucial for effective management. Reassess the diagnosis, consider susceptibility testing, and adjust therapy accordingly.

Adjunctive Measures:

- Reduce dose or avoid using immunosuppressive agents whenever possible.
- Colony-stimulating factors may be considered in neutropenic patients with diagnosed or suspected IA.
- Granulocyte Transfusion: in neutropenic patients with IA who are refractory or unlikely to respond to standard therapy, and for an anticipated duration of more than one week.
- Recombinant interferon-γ is recommended as prophylaxis in chronic granulomatous disease patients.
- Surgery for aspergillosis should be considered for localized disease that is easily accessible to debridement.

102.8 Monitoring Response to Therapy

Assess for clinical and radiological improvement following antifungal initiation:

- Clinical Improvement:
- Resolution of fever.
- Improved respiratory status.
- Radiological Improvement:
- Reduction in cavitary lesions or nodules.
- Serial monitoring of serum GM can be used; can also help to prognosticate.
- Therapeutic Drug Monitoring:

- Monitor antifungal drug levels to ensure therapeutic efficacy and minimize toxicity.

Continue antifungal therapy for 6–12 weeks, tailoring the duration to clinical response and patient-specific factors.

Reassess the diagnosis, consider combination antifungal therapy, explore emerging therapeutics, or evaluate for alternative conditions [2].

Refractory or Progressive Aspergillosis (Salvage Therapy)

- Individualized approach
- (i) Changing the class of antifungal, (ii) tapering or reversal of underlying immunosuppression when feasible, and (iii) surgical resection of necrotic lesions in selected cases.
- Antifungal from another class may be added to the ongoing regimen.
- Consider lipid formulations of AmB, micafungin, caspofungin, posaconazole, or itraconazole.

102.9 Host-Specific Tailoring

Customize diagnostic and therapeutic approaches based on the patient's immune status and comorbidities:

- Immune Status Assessment:
- Utilize the 2019 EORTC/MSGERC definitions for stratification.
- Comorbidity Considerations:
- Adjust treatment plans for patients with liver failure, renal impairment, or other significant comorbidities.

102.10 Extrapulmonary Aspergillosis

- CNS Aspergillosis: Primary Therapy: Voriconazole. Liposomal Amphotericin B in case of intolerance or refractory to Voriconazole.
- Endophthalmitis: Systemic oral or intravenous voriconazole plus intravitreal voriconazole or intravitreal AmB deoxycholate.
- Paranasal Sinus: Surgery and either systemic voriconazole or a Liposomal Amphotericin B.
- *Aspergillus* Endocarditis, Pericarditis, and Myocarditis: Early surgical intervention combined with Voriconazole or Liposomal Amphotericin B. Consider lifelong antifungal therapy post surgery/valve replacement surgery.
- *Aspergillus* Osteomyelitis and Septic Arthritis: Surgery along with Voriconazole.
- *Aspergillus* Peritonitis: Removal of peritoneal dialysis catheter plus Voriconazole.

- Esophageal, Gastrointestinal, and Hepatic Aspergillosis: Voriconazole and surgery to treat/prevent complications like perforation, obstruction, infarction, or hemorrhage.
- Renal Aspergillosis: Voriconazole plus surgery (decompression with local instillation of Amphotericin B deoxycholate in the presence of ureteric obstruction).

102.11 Management of Breakthrough Infections

- Aggressive and prompt attempt to establish a specific diagnosis with bronchoscopy and/or CT-guided biopsy.
- Therapeutic drug monitoring of Azole levels (if available).
- Change to an alternative class of antifungal with anti-*Aspergillus* activity.
- Reduction/Stop immunosuppression.

Empirical Treatment:

- High-risk patients with prolonged neutropenia with persisting febrile episodes not responding to broad-spectrum antibiotics.
- Avoid empirical therapy in neutropenia with <10 days duration.
- Use preemptive approach over empirical therapy: BAL fungal biomarkers such as GM or $(1 \rightarrow 3)$-β-D-glucan in.

102.12 Conclusion

Managing IA in the ICU requires a vigilant, stepwise approach focused on early identification, accurate diagnosis, and prompt treatment. Key principles include:

1. Recognizing High-Risk Patients Early:
   - Including emerging risk groups with subtle immune dysfunctions
2. Utilizing Advanced Diagnostic Tools:
   - Incorporating updated biomarkers, molecular diagnostics, and expanded imaging criteria
3. Initiating Appropriate Antifungal Therapy Promptly:
   - Considering azole resistance and tailoring therapy accordingly
4. Monitoring and Tailoring Treatment:
   - Based on patient-specific factors and treatment responses

Adherence to this comprehensive algorithm can improve outcomes by minimizing delays in diagnosis and treatment, reducing economic burdens, and enhancing patient prognoses through personalized care strategies.

Algorithm 102.1: Approach to aspergillosis in the ICU

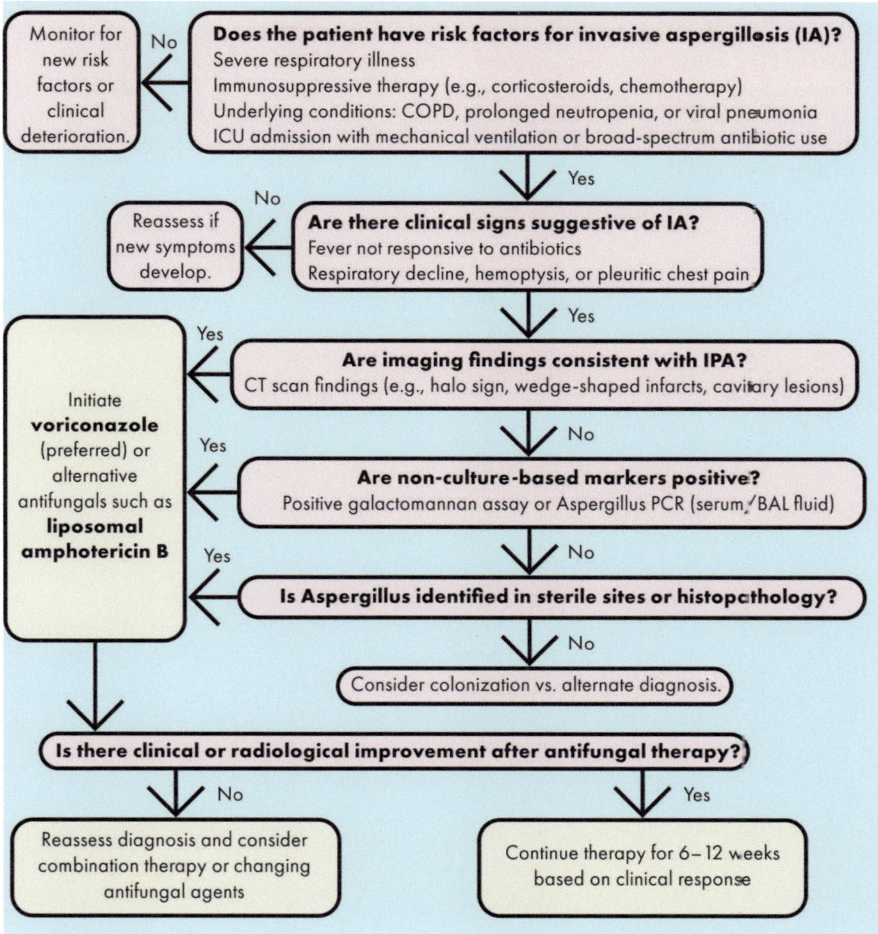

Bibliography

1. Bulpa P, Bihin B, Dimopoulos G, Taccone FS, Van den Abeele AM, Misset B, et al. Which algorithm diagnoses invasive pulmonary aspergillosis best in ICU patients with COPD? Eur Respir J. 2017;50(3):1700532.
2. Hamam J, Navellou JC, Bellanger AP, Bretagne S, Winiszewski H, Scherer E, et al. New clinical algorithm including fungal biomarkers to better diagnose probable invasive pulmonary aspergillosis in ICU. Ann Intensive Care. 2021;11(1):41.

3. Patterson TF, Thompson GR 3rd, Denning DW, Fishman JA, Hadley S, Herbrecht R, et al. Practice guidelines for the diagnosis and Management of Aspergillosis: 2016 update by the Infectious Diseases Society of America. Clin Infect Dis. 2016;63(4):e1–e60.
4. Jenks JD, Nam HH, Hoenigl M. Invasive aspergillosis in critically ill patients: review of definitions and diagnostic approaches. Mycoses. 2021;64(9):1002–14.
5. Vanderbeke L, Van Wijngaerden E, Maertens J, Wauters J, Lagrou K. Diagnosis of invasive Aspergillosis in intensive care unit patients. Curr Fungal Infect Rep. 2020;14(2):166–73.
6. Townsend L, Martin-Loeches I. Invasive Aspergillosis in the intensive care unit. Diagnostics (Basel). 2022;12(11)

Chapter 103
Approach to Tropical Infections in the ICU

103.1 Introduction

Tropical infections represent a significant challenge in the ICU due to their diverse etiologies and potential for severe outcomes. These infections are prevalent in specific geographic regions such as Southeast Asia, sub-Saharan Africa, and parts of South America, often exacerbated by environmental, occupational, or travel-related factors. Data from the GeoSentinel database highlight regions where infections like malaria, dengue, and rickettsial diseases are endemic. The monsoon season, characterized by heavy rainfall and flooding, is a peak time for certain infections such as leptospirosis and melioidosis, particularly in countries like India, Thailand, and northern Australia. Effective management in the ICU demands a structured approach to rapidly identify and treat the underlying pathogen while mitigating complications [1–4] [Ref: Algorithm 103.1].

103.2 Clinical Presentation

The initial assessment focuses on categorizing acute febrile illness based on associated clinical features:

- Fever, Rash, or Eschar:
- Suggestive of rickettsial infections (e.g., Scrub Typhus) or Dengue.
- Rash or eschar is an essential clinical clue; an eschar is particularly pathognomonic of rickettsial diseases.
- Fever with Respiratory Symptoms:
- Raises suspicion for Malaria, Leptospirosis, Melioidosis, or Tuberculosis.

S. B. Mishra et al., *Mastering ICU Care*,
https://doi.org/10.1007/978-981-95-0179-3_103

- Key differentials include malaria-associated pulmonary edema, leptospirosis-induced acute respiratory distress syndrome (ARDS), or severe pneumonia in melioidosis.
- Leptospirosis may progress to Weil's disease, characterized by jaundice, renal failure, hemorrhagic manifestations, severe acidosis, and atypical features like necrotizing pancreatitis.
- Fever with Shock or Bleeding Diathesis:
- Prioritize evaluating for Viral Hemorrhagic Fevers such as Dengue or severe Malaria.
- Shock may indicate capillary leak syndrome or sepsis, while bleeding points to thrombocytopenia or disseminated intravascular coagulation.
- Fever with Altered Mentation:
- Indicates possible Scrub Typhus, Dengue encephalitis, Tuberculosis meningitis, or Cerebral Malaria.
- Central nervous system involvement necessitates prompt imaging and lumbar puncture to rule out meningitis or encephalitis.
- Fever with Adrenal Insufficiency:
- Tuberculosis can cause adrenal insufficiency, leading to hypotension unresponsive to vasopressors.
- Consider adrenal insufficiency in patients with TB-related shock.
- Recent Travel to Endemic Areas:
- Helps narrow the diagnosis to regional infections like Japanese encephalitis or Malaria.
- Occupational or Environmental Exposure:
- Environmental cues, such as contact with soil or rodents, suggest Leptospirosis or Melioidosis.
- Melioidosis can present with severe pneumonia, septic shock, or abscess formation in various organs.

103.3 Laboratory Investigations

Laboratory workup is essential for identifying the pathogen and assessing organ dysfunction:

- General Tests:
- Include complete blood count (CBC), liver and renal function tests, and coagulation profile to assess systemic involvement.
- Findings such as thrombocytopenia (Dengue), elevated liver enzymes (Leptospirosis), or pancytopenia (severe Malaria) guide management.
- Specific Tests:
- Peripheral Smear/Rapid Diagnostic Test (RDT):
- Confirms Malaria; a peripheral smear also provides insight into parasite density.
- IgM ELISA or MAT (Microscopic Agglutination Test):

- Used to confirm Leptospirosis.
- For difficult-to-diagnose cases, advanced techniques like nested PCR can increase diagnostic yield.
- RT-PCR/NS1 Antigen, IgM ELISA:
- RT-PCR/NS1: Highly sensitive for early detection of Dengue.
- Early rapid diagnostic tests in endemic regions help reduce delays in management and improve outcomes.
- GeneXpert or (*Mycobacteria* Growth Indicator Tube) MGIT Culture:
- For diagnosing tuberculosis, especially in extrapulmonary cases.
- In suspected tuberculosis-related adrenal insufficiency, cortisol levels and Adrenocorticotrophic hormone (ACTH) stimulation tests may be necessary.
- Blood Culture:
- Identifies organisms in Melioidosis (*Burkholderia pseudomallei*) or Enteric fever.
- Whole-genome sequencing can be utilized for precise identification and antibiotic susceptibility profiling, especially in rickettsial infections.
- Scrub Typhus IgM ELISA:
- A specific test to confirm Scrub Typhus.

103.4 Imaging

Imaging complements laboratory investigations by identifying organ-specific involvement:

- Chest X-ray:
- Evaluate for ARDS or consolidation, which is common in Leptospirosis, Tuberculosis, Melioidosis, or secondary bacterial infections.
- Abdominal Ultrasound:
- Used to detect organomegaly, abscesses, or hepatosplenomegaly, which are hallmark features of Melioidosis, Enteric fever, or Malaria.
- Computed Tomography (CT scan)
- CT scan of thorax for Tuberculosis and CT scan of abdomen (with contrast) for Tuberculosis, Melioidosis.

103.5 Prognostic Indicators

Prognostic tools aid in risk stratification and guide management decisions:

- Leptospirosis:
- Tools like the SPiRO (Sequential Organ Failure Assessment for Leptospirosis) or THAI LEPTO score help predict severe disease and mortality risk.
- These scores consider factors such as age, organ dysfunction, and laboratory parameters.

- Dengue:
- The World Health Organization (WHO) classification stratifies patients into dengue without warning signs, with warning signs, and severe dengue, guiding monitoring and treatment intensity.
- Malaria:
- High parasite density, severe anemia, or cerebral involvement indicates a poor prognosis.

103.6 Initial Empiric Therapy

Early empiric therapy is vital while awaiting confirmatory diagnostics. Treatment selection is based on clinical suspicion:

- **Severe Malaria**: [5]
- Definition: Severe Malaria is defined as *Plasmodium parasitemia* plus one or more of the following:
  - Altered level of consciousness: Glasgow Coma Scale (GCS) score below 11 in adults
  - Prostration: Severe weakness rendering the patient unable to sit, stand, or walk without help
  - Recurrent seizures: More than two convulsive episodes within a 24-hour timeframe
  - Metabolic acidosis: Evidenced by a base deficit exceeding 8 mEq/L, plasma bicarbonate below 15 mmol/L, or venous lactate concentration of 5 mmol/L or higher
  - Hypoglycemia: Blood or plasma glucose <40 mg/dL
  - Severe malarial anemia: Hemoglobin concentration < 7 g/dL or a hematocrit of $\leq 20\%$ with a parasite count $>10{,}000/\mu L$ (count only for *P. falciparum*)
  - Renal impairment: Plasma or serum creatinine $>265\ \mu mol/L$ (3 mg/dL) or blood urea >20 mmol/L
  - Jaundice: Plasma or serum bilirubin >3 mg/dL with a parasite count $>100{,}000/\mu L$ (count only for *P. falciparum*).
  - Pulmonary edema: Radiologically confirmed or oxygen saturation $< 92\%$ on room air with a respiratory rate > 30/min
  - Significant bleeding refers to persistent or repeated bleeding episodes, such as from the nose, gums, or venipuncture sites, as well as gastrointestinal bleeding presenting as hematemesis or melena.
  - Shock is categorized as follows:
  - Compensated shock is indicated by a capillary refill time of 3 seconds or more, or a noticeable temperature gradient between the mid and proximal parts of the limb, without the presence of hypotension.
  - Decompensated shock is defined by a systolic blood pressure lower than 80 mmHg in adults.

  - Hyperparasitemia*:* *P. falciparum* parasitemia >10% (not to be considered in case of *vivax*). *P. knowlesi* > 100,000/μL or jaundice and parasite density > 20,000/μL.
  - Splenic rupture (a complication)

- IV Artesunate is the first-line therapy for *Plasmodium falciparum* malaria.
- Dose: 2.4 mg/kg body weight each dose, three doses in first 24 hours (0, 12, and 24 hours) and then once daily for three more days. At least 1 day of IV therapy is recommended. It may be switched to ACT [Artemisinin-based combination therapy, e.g., Artemether-lumefantrine (80 mg BD + 480 mg BD x 3 days), Artesunate-mefloquine (Artesunate 100 mg BD x 3 days + Mefloquine 750 mg on second day and 500 mg on third day), Artesunate-amodiaquine, Artesunate-sulfadoxine-pyrimethamine (Artesunate 100 mg BD x 3 days + Sulfadoxine 1500 mg and Pyrimethamine 75 mg single dose)] on day 2 if patient is able to take orally. This ACT should be given for 3 days.
- Adjunct therapies include managing complications like hypoglycemia, cerebral malaria, hyperpyrexia, convulsions, severe anemia, pulmonary edema, acute kidney injury, coagulopathy, metabolic acidosis or shock.
- **Leptospirosis**:
- IV Ceftriaxone (1 g IV every 24 hours) or Penicillin (1.5 MU IV every 6 hours) to address leptospiral sepsis. Doxycycline 100 mg BD or Azithromycin 500 mg once daily can also be given as second line of therapy.
- Consider doxycycline prophylaxis for high-risk exposures.
- **Dengue**:
- Supportive care with fluid resuscitation for plasma leakage syndrome.
- Platelet transfusion is indicated only for severe thrombocytopenia with active bleeding.
- Monitor for rare complications like encephalitis, which may require specific supportive measures.
- **Tuberculosis**:
- Initiate anti-TB therapy per resistance patterns or empiric regimens if drug sensitivity testing is pending.
- In cases of adrenal insufficiency, stress-dose steroids (hydrocortisone) may be necessary to manage hypotension and other symptoms.
- **Rickettsial Infections:**
- Doxycycline (100 mg IV twice daily) is effective against Scrub Typhus and other rickettsioses. Azithromycin is an alternative (500 mg IV once daily).
- In severe cases, a combination with Azithromycin may be beneficial.
- **Melioidosis:**
- IV Ceftazidime (2 g every 8 hour by a continuous infusion after a 2 g bolus) or Meropenem (1 g every 8 hour by a continuous infusion after a 1 g bolus) is critical for this potentially fatal infection. Most of the time, IV therapy extends to beyond 10 days. This is defined as the acute phase/intensive phase.

- Following initial intensive therapy, an eradication phase with oral antibiotics such as doxycycline and trimethoprim-sulfamethoxazole (160 mg/800 mg tablets; two tablets every 12 h) is essential to prevent relapses.
- Combination therapy (Co-trimoxazole+ Ceftazidime, Ceftazidime + Meropenem, Meropenem + Co-trimoxazole) may be given in case of poor clinical response to individual regimen. Combination therapy is important due to the organism's resistance patterns. The dose for IV Co-trimoxazole being 160 mg/800 mg–320 mg/1600 mg.
- Adjunctive therapies like granulocyte colony-stimulating factor (G-CSF) may be considered in septic shock to enhance neutrophil function. Adjunctive management also involves comprehensive supportive care for sepsis, which includes maintaining hemodynamic stability, ensuring proper blood glucose control, addressing respiratory and renal failure, and performing drainage of abscesses when feasible.

103.7 Conclusion

Managing tropical infections in the ICU requires a structured approach tailored to the clinical presentation, regional epidemiology, and individual patient factors. Recognizing symptom patterns and understanding the epidemiological context are crucial for early diagnosis. Comprehensive laboratory and imaging studies, including advanced diagnostic techniques, facilitate accurate identification of pathogens. Prognostic indicators and statistical tools aid in risk stratification and inform clinical decision-making. Initiating prompt empiric therapy and appropriate adjunctive treatments, while awaiting confirmatory diagnostics, improves patient outcomes. Early intervention and supportive care are pivotal in managing severe cases like Dengue, Malaria, or Melioidosis. Understanding the nuances of each condition and maintaining vigilance for complications—such as adrenal insufficiency or severe acidosis—are crucial for optimizing patient care.

Algorithm 103.1: Approach to tropical infections in the ICU

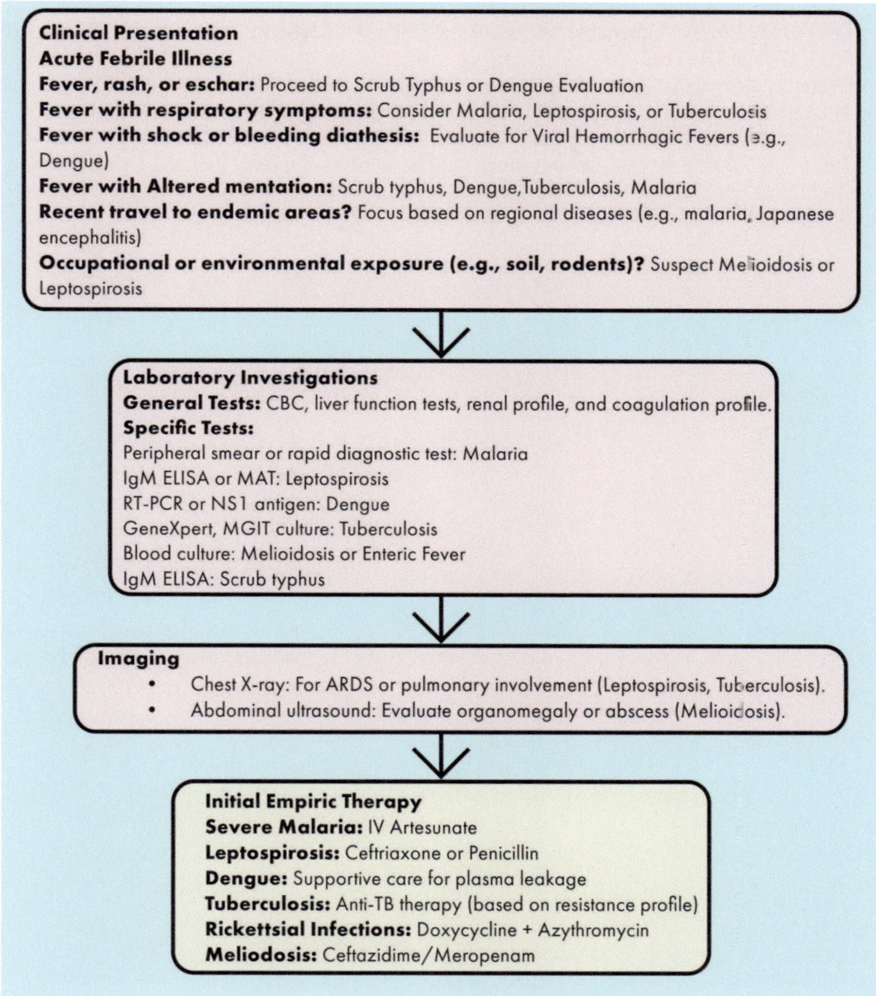

Bibliography

1. Basu S, Shetty A. Laboratory diagnosis of tropical infections. Indian J Crit Care Med. 2021;25(Suppl 2):S122–S6.
2. Chaudhry D, Tyagi D. Tuberculosis in intensive care unit. Indian J Crit Care Med. 2021;25(Suppl 2):S150–S4.
3. Hegde A. Malaria in the intensive care unit. Indian J Crit Care Med. 2021;25(Suppl 2):S127–S9.
4. Shastri PS, Taneja S. Dengue and other viral hemorrhagic fevers. Indian J Crit Care Med. 2021;25(Suppl 2):S130–S3.
5. WHO Guidelines for malaria. Geneva: World Health Organization; 2021.

Chapter 104
Approach to Liver Dysfunction in Pregnancy in the ICU

104.1 Introduction

Liver dysfunction during pregnancy is a challenging clinical scenario with a wide range of potential causes, varying in severity and urgency. It affects approximately 3% of pregnancies in developed countries, highlighting its clinical significance. Early recognition and appropriate management are critical to minimizing maternal and fetal morbidity and mortality. Management often requires a multidisciplinary approach involving hepatologists, obstetricians, and neonatologists to optimize outcomes for both mother and child [1, 2].

Pregnancy-specific liver disorders include hyperemesis gravidarum (HG), intrahepatic cholestasis of pregnancy (ICP), HELLP syndrome, and acute fatty liver of pregnancy (AFLP). In addition, non-pregnancy-specific causes such as viral hepatitis, autoimmune hepatitis, and biliary obstruction may mimic or exacerbate pregnancy-related liver dysfunction [Ref: Algorithm 104.1].

104.2 Normal Physiological Changes in Pregnancy

Understanding normal physiological changes in liver function tests during pregnancy is essential to differentiate between physiological alterations and pathological conditions.

- Serum Albumin: Decreased serum albumin levels occur due to hemodilution and increased plasma volume.
- Alkaline Phosphatase (ALP): ALP levels increase significantly because of placental production, which can elevate levels up to two to four times the normal upper limit.

S. B. Mishra et al., *Mastering ICU Care*,
https://doi.org/10.1007/978-981-95-0179-3_104

- Aminotransferases (AST/ALT) and Bilirubin: Generally, remain within normal limits during pregnancy. Any elevation should prompt further investigation as they may indicate underlying pathology [3].

104.3 Initial Assessment

Clinical Symptoms

Presenting symptoms often include nausea, vomiting, jaundice, pruritus, abdominal pain, and fatigue. These symptoms may overlap with normal pregnancy physiology or signal significant pathology.

Initial Laboratory Tests

- Liver Function Tests (LFTs): ALT, AST, bilirubin, ALP
- Coagulation Profile: To assess synthetic liver function
- Complete Blood Count (CBC): To identify associated hematologic abnormalities like anemia or thrombocytopenia [4]

104.4 Timing of Symptoms

Determining the gestational age and timing of symptoms can provide clues about the etiology:

- First Trimester Symptoms: Often linked to hyperemesis gravidarum
- Late Second/Third Trimester Symptoms: Consider ICP, HELLP syndrome, or AFLP
- Postpartum Symptoms: Evaluate for chronic liver disease, genetic predispositions, or autoimmune conditions [5]

104.5 Specific Disorders by Presentation

A. First Trimester: Hyperemesis Gravidarum (HG)

Key Features

- Persistent Nausea and Vomiting: With associated weight loss and dehydration
- LFTs: Elevated ALT > AST with mild jaundice
- Transient Hyperthyroidism: Occurs in up to 60% of cases due to high levels of hCG stimulating the thyroid

  Action
- Supportive Care:
- IV Fluids: Rehydration is essential.

- Antiemetics: Medications like ondansetron and metoclopramide can be used to control nausea and vomiting. However, European medicines agency does not allow use of ondansetron in the first trimester due to risk of newborns with defects such as cleft palate and cardiac septal defects (although <1%). Vitamin B6/Pyridoxine and Doxylamine (Antihistamine/H1 antagonist) combination can be used to reduce nausea during the first trimester of pregnancy.
- Nutritional Support: In severe cases, enteral or parenteral nutrition may be necessary.
- Rule Out Other Causes: If symptoms are atypical or severe, consider other diagnoses.

B. Pruritus and Hallmark Symptoms: Intrahepatic Cholestasis of Pregnancy (ICP)

Key Features

- Intense Pruritus: Especially on the palms and soles, without rash.
- Elevated Bile Acids: Levels are typically elevated (>10 μmol/L).
- Mild AST/ALT Elevation.
  Action
- Treatment:
- Ursodeoxycholic Acid (UDCA): To reduce bile acids and alleviate symptoms.
- Hydroxyzine (25 mg/d) or an aqueous cream with 1% menthol may be used to alleviate pruritus.
- Administration of *S*-adenosyl methionine in combination with ursodeoxycholic acid may increase its benefit.
- Monitoring:
- Regular Bile Acid Levels: Close monitoring is essential.
- Delivery Timing:
- Early Delivery Consideration: If bile acid levels exceed 40 μmol/L, consider early delivery after 37 weeks (no later than 38 weeks) to reduce the risk of stillbirth.
- Urgent Action: Bile acid levels ≥100 μmol/L may necessitate delivery as early as 34–36 weeks.
- Genetic Testing:
- ABCB11 and ABCB4 Mutations: In severe or recurrent cases, genetic testing may help identify mutations associated with bile salt transporters [6].

C. Hypertension or Severe Symptoms: HELLP Syndrome

Key Features

- Majority present in the third trimester (28–36 weeks)
- Hemolysis:
- Peripheral Smear: Schistocytes, indicating microangiopathic hemolytic anemia
- Low Haptoglobin: Due to hemolysis
- Elevated Liver Enzymes:
- AST/ALT: Elevated (>70 IU/L) is significant.
- Low Platelets:

- Thrombocytopenia: Platelet counts <100,000/mm^3.
  Action
- Immediate Stabilization:
- Magnesium Sulfate: For seizure prophylaxis if there is a risk of eclampsia.
- Blood Pressure Control: Using antihypertensive agents like labetalol or hydralazine.
- Corticosteroids:
- Role in Management: May improve maternal platelet counts and hepatic function, although their efficacy is still under investigation.
- Expedite Delivery:
- Definitive Treatment: Delivery of the fetus is the only cure and should be considered once the maternal condition is stabilized, regardless of gestational age.
  Complications
- Intra-parenchymal hemorrhage
- Liver infarction
- Subcapsular hematoma
- Hepatic rupture
- Hepatic failure

D. Acute Fatty Liver of Pregnancy (AFLP)

Key Features

- Symptoms:
- Nausea, vomiting, abdominal pain, and jaundice.
- Hypoglycemia: Due to impaired gluconeogenesis. It indicates a poor prognosis.
- Coagulopathy: Elevated PT/INR.
- Hyperbilirubinemia: Usually not >5 mg/dL
- Transaminitis: AST and ALT are elevated to around 300–500 times (lower than acute viral hepatitis levels)
- Imaging:
- Ultrasound or MRI: May reveal fatty infiltration of the liver.
  Swansea diagnostic criteria
  Six or more of the following without any alternative explanation:

1. Vomiting
2. Abdominal pain
3. Polydipsia/polyuria
4. Encephalopathy
5. High bilirubin (>14 mg/dl)
6. Hypoglycemia (< 70 mg/dl)
7. High uric acid (>340 μmol/L)
8. Leucocytosis (>11 × 10^6/L)
9. Ascites or bright liver on ultrasound
10. High AST/ALT (>42 IU/L)
11. High ammonia (>47 μmol/L)
12. High ammonia (>47 μmol/L)

13. Renal impairment (creatinine >150 μmol/L)
14. High ammonia (>47 μmol/L)
15. Coagulopathy (PT >14 s or aPTT>34 s)
16. Microvesicular steatosis on liver biopsy

Action

- Immediate Stabilization:
- IV Glucose: To correct hypoglycemia
- Correction of Coagulopathy: Using plasma products as needed
- Supportive Care: Intensive monitoring in a high-dependency unit
- Urgent Delivery:
- Definitive Treatment: Prompt delivery is necessary to prevent further maternal and fetal complications.
- Long-Term Follow-Up:
- Mitochondrial Dysfunction: AFLP is associated with defects in mitochondrial fatty acid oxidation, particularly LCHAD deficiency. Both mother and child may require genetic counseling and long-term monitoring.

4. Nonspecific Liver Abnormalities

If no clear etiology is identified, assess for conditions unrelated to pregnancy:

- Viral Hepatitis:
- Serologies: For HBV, HCV, HAV, HEV
- Autoimmune Hepatitis:
- Autoantibodies: ANA, SMA, anti-LKM1
- IgG Levels: May be elevated
- Biliary Obstruction:
- Ultrasound: To evaluate for gallstones or cholestasis
- Other Conditions:
- Budd-Chiari Syndrome: Hepatic vein thrombosis presenting with abdominal pain and hepatomegaly
- Autoimmune Liver Diseases: Such as primary biliary cholangitis
- Noninvasive Assessment:
- Elastography: Can assess liver fibrosis or steatosis safely during pregnancy Action
- Treat Underlying Condition:
- Antiviral Therapy: For viral hepatitis, considering pregnancy safety profiles
- Immunosuppressants: For autoimmune hepatitis, balancing maternal benefits and fetal risks
- Interventional Procedures: For biliary obstruction, such as ERCP if necessary

5. Postpartum and Chronic Liver Disease

Persistent symptoms beyond delivery may signal chronic liver disease or an underlying genetic predisposition:

- Conditions to Consider:
- Nonalcoholic Fatty Liver Disease (NAFLD)

- Autoimmune Hepatitis
- Chronic Viral Hepatitis
- Risk of Future Liver Disease:
- ICP: Women with a history of ICP have a higher risk of developing gallstones, hepatitis C, or NAFLD.
  Action
- Long-Term Follow-Up:
- Hepatology Referral: For ongoing management and monitoring
- Lifestyle Modifications: Diet and exercise recommendations
- Genetic Counseling: For conditions like AFLP or recurrent ICP

104.6 Conclusion

The management of liver dysfunction in pregnancy requires a systematic approach grounded in gestational age, symptomatology, and laboratory findings. Understanding normal physiological changes is crucial to differentiate between pathological and physiological alterations. Early identification of pregnancy-specific conditions such as hyperemesis gravidarum, ICP, HELLP syndrome, and AFLP is essential for optimal outcomes. A multidisciplinary team involving hepatologists, obstetricians, and neonatologists can provide comprehensive care. Postpartum follow-up is equally important to address persistent or chronic liver dysfunction and to mitigate future risks.

Algorithm 104.1: Approach to liver dysfunction in pregnancy in the ICU

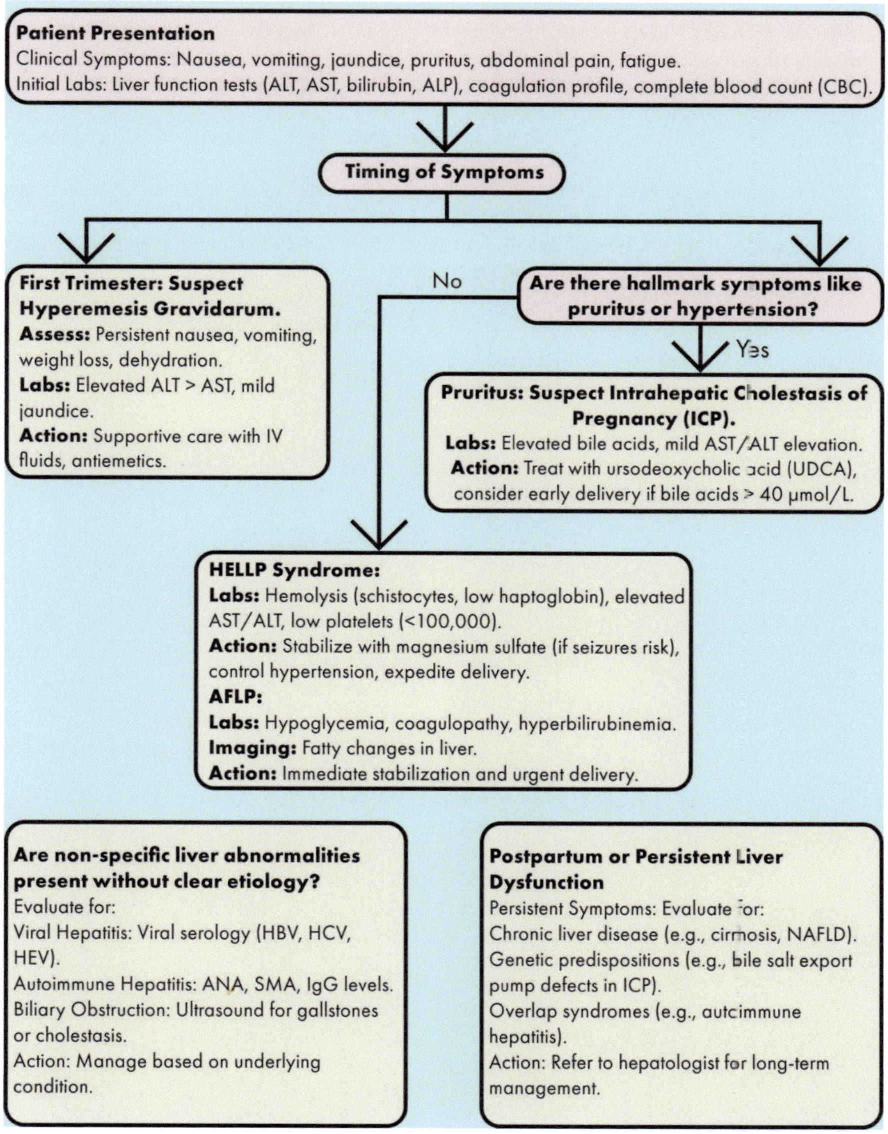

Bibliography

1. Shekhar S, Diddi G. Liver disease in pregnancy. Taiwan J Obstet Gynecol. 2015;54(5):475–82.
2. European Association for the Study of the liver. Electronic address eee, European Association for the Study of the L. EASL clinical practice guidelines on the management of liver diseases in pregnancy. J Hepatol. 2023;79(3):768–828.
3. Terrault NA, Williamson C. Pregnancy-associated liver diseases. Gastroenterology. 2022;163(1):97–117 e1.
4. Dajti E, Bruni A, Barbara G, Azzaroli F. Diagnostic approach to elevated liver function tests during pregnancy: a pragmatic narrative review. J Pers Med. 2023;13(9)
5. Morrison MA, Chung Y, Heneghan MA. Managing hepatic complications of pregnancy: practical strategies for clinicians. BMJ Open Gastroenterol. 2022;9(1):e000624.
6. Garcia-Romero CS, Guzman C, Cervantes A, Cerbon M. Liver disease in pregnancy: medical aspects and their implications for mother and child. Ann Hepatol. 2019;18(4):553–62.

Chapter 105
ICU Discharge Planning in the ICU

105.1 Introduction

Intensive care unit (ICU) discharge planning is a critical component of patient care that ensures a smooth and safe transition from the ICU to a general ward or home. Effective discharge planning minimizes complications, reduces readmission risks, and enhances long-term outcomes. This multifaceted process involves assessing both clinical and psychological readiness, enhancing communication strategies, and providing post-discharge support. A patient-centered approach, coupled with a multidisciplinary effort, is essential for optimizing recovery and ensuring continuity of care [1, 2] [Ref: Algorithm 105.1].

1. Assessment of Patient Readiness

   - Clinical Stability: Patients must demonstrate sustained stability in vital signs—heart rate, blood pressure, oxygen saturation, and respiratory rate—without requiring intensive monitoring or pharmacological support. Successful weaning from critical care interventions such as mechanical ventilation and vasopressors is essential.
   - Resolution of Acute Illness: The acute phase of the illness or injury should be under control, evidenced by resolved sepsis, improved organ function, or stabilized neurological status.
   - Functional Status: Assessing the patient's mobility, ability to perform basic tasks, and overall physical strength is crucial to ensure they can cope with the less intensive support available in general wards.
   - Psychological Readiness: The psychological state of the patient and their family plays a significant role in the transition. Addressing the "care shock" phenomenon—where patients experience anxiety and uncertainty about leaving the ICU—is vital. Strategies such as providing education on self-care,

S. B. Mishra et al., *Mastering ICU Care*,
https://doi.org/10.1007/978-981-95-0179-3_105

offering psychological support, and gradually disengaging from ICU-specific support systems can alleviate these concerns [3].

2. Communication with the Care Team

    - Multidisciplinary Discharge Planning Meeting: A comprehensive discussion involving ICU physicians, nurses, respiratory therapists, physical therapists, and other allied health professionals is essential to finalize the discharge decision. This collaborative approach ensures all aspects of the patient's care are considered.
    - Effective Communication Strategies: Emphasizing both verbal and written communication during the transition is crucial for continuity of care. Poor communication between ICU and ward teams is a major risk factor for adverse outcomes. Implementing standardized discharge summaries and checklists minimizes information loss and ensures accurate conveyance of the patient's status and care needs.
    - Patient and Family Engagement: Involving patients and their families in the discharge planning process enhances understanding and satisfaction. Clear explanations of the patient's condition, care requirements, and the rationale for transfer help in managing expectations and reducing anxiety [4].

3. Transfer Logistics

    - Structured Discharge Timing: Timing of discharge significantly impacts patient outcomes. Nighttime and weekend discharges are associated with higher readmission and mortality rates due to reduced staffing and resource availability. Policies should recommend daytime, well-resourced transitions to enhance safety and support.
    - Handoff Protocols: Utilizing structured handoff tools like SBAR (Situation-Background-Assessment-Recommendation) ensures accurate and complete communication of the patient's status and care needs. This reduces the risk of misunderstandings and errors during the transition.
    - Transport Safety: Ensuring safe transportation with appropriate equipment and staff support is essential, especially for patients with mobility challenges or residual clinical instability [4].

4. Post-ICU Care Plan

    - Monitoring Needs in the General Ward: Clearly outlining specific monitoring parameters—such as fluid balance, infection markers, or neurological status—is essential. The receiving team must be fully aware of these requirements to provide appropriate care.
    - Training for Ward Staff: Addressing disparities in care quality due to staffing and resource differences between the ICU and general wards is important. Training ward staff on managing high-acuity patients can mitigate these gaps and improve patient outcomes.

- Patient and Family Education: Providing education on disease management, medication administration, wound care, and self-monitoring techniques empowers patients and families to take an active role in recovery.

5. Early Identification of Risks for Readmission

- Use of Discharge Planning Tools: Developing and applying ICU discharge planning tools, such as prediction models for adverse events, triage frameworks, or peer support programs, enhances decision-making. Tools like APACHE II or LACE scores help assess readmission risk and guide post-ICU care strategies.
- Close Observation for High-Risk Patients: Patients identified as high-risk may require closer observation, including telemonitoring, early outpatient follow-ups, or temporary stays in step-down units for additional monitoring.

6. Follow-Up Planning

- Scheduled Outpatient Follow-Ups: Integrating follow-up protocols tailored to patient risk factors is essential. Early outpatient follow-up appointments can reduce readmissions by addressing complications promptly and adjusting care plans as needed.
- Long-Term Monitoring of Post-ICU Syndrome: Post-ICU syndrome, characterized by symptoms such as muscle weakness, cognitive dysfunction, delirium, or post-traumatic stress disorder (PTSD), requires long-term tracking. Identifying and managing these symptoms improves quality of life and functional recovery.
- ICU Outreach Services: ICU outreach teams play a vital role in post-discharge monitoring. They can track patients after discharge, provide interventions for emerging problems, and potentially avoid unnecessary readmissions [5].

7. Challenges in Transition

- Disparities in Care Quality: Differences in staffing levels and resources between the ICU and general wards can impact patient outcomes. Patients may experience reduced monitoring and support, leading to increased risks during the transition.
- Mitigating Gaps: Implementing strategies such as training ward staff on high-acuity patient care and ensuring adequate resources can help bridge these gaps. Promoting collaboration between ICU and ward teams enhances overall care quality.

8. Outcome Metrics and Continuous Improvement

- Measuring Discharge Outcomes: Implementing metrics such as patient satisfaction, readmission rates, and mortality provides valuable feedback on the effectiveness of discharge processes. Regular audits and feedback loops enable healthcare teams to identify areas for improvement.
- Quality Improvement Initiatives: Utilizing outcome data to inform quality improvement initiatives promotes evidence-based practices in discharge

planning. Continuous evaluation and adaptation of protocols enhance patient safety and care quality.

105.2 Conclusion

The ICU discharge process is a multifaceted approach that prioritizes patient safety, continuity of care, and long-term recovery. By systematically evaluating both clinical and psychological readiness, ensuring comprehensive communication, and addressing logistical and post-discharge considerations, healthcare teams can minimize the risk of adverse outcomes. Incorporating a multidisciplinary approach, utilizing discharge planning tools, and focusing on patient-centered strategies enhance the transition experience. Ongoing measurement of discharge outcomes and continuous improvement efforts are essential for optimizing care and reducing healthcare utilization.

Algorithm 105.1: ICU discharge planning

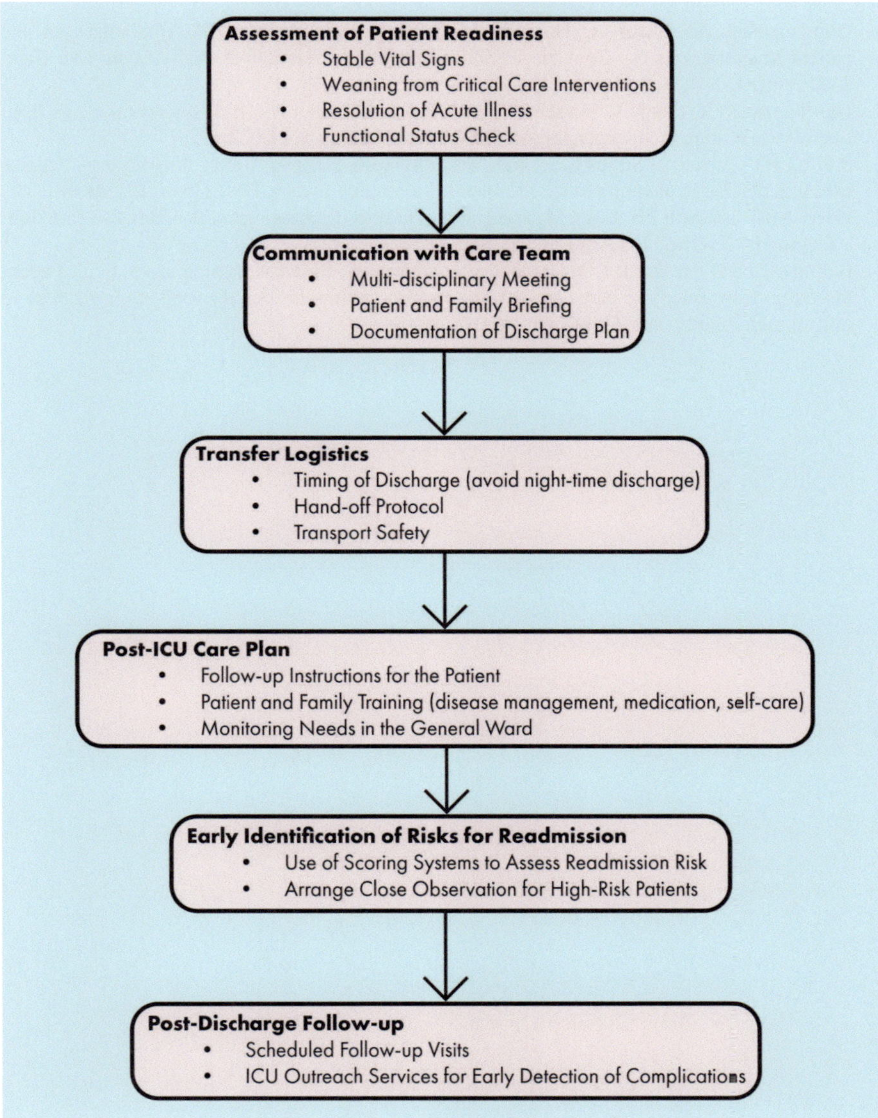

Bibliography

1. Ghorbanzadeh K, Ebadi A, Hosseini M, Madah SSB, Khankeh H. Challenges of the patient transition process from the intensive care unit: a qualitative study. Acute Crit Care. 2021;36(2):133–42.
2. Ghorbanzadeh K, Ebadi A, Hosseini MA, Madah S, Khankeh HR. Transition of patients from intensive care unit: a concept analysis. Int J Africa Nursing Sci. 2022:17.
3. Stelfox HT, Perrier L, Straus SE, Ghali WA, Zygun D, Boiteau P, et al. Identifying intensive care unit discharge planning tools: protocol for a scoping review. BMJ Open. 2013;3(4)
4. Herve MEW, Zucatti PB, Lima M. Transition of care at discharge from the intensive care unit: a scoping review. Rev Lat Am Enfermagem. 2020;28:e3325.
5. Plotnikoff KM, Krewulak KD, Hernandez L, Spence K, Foster N, Longmore S, et al. Patient discharge from intensive care: an updated scoping review to identify tools and practices to inform high-quality care. Crit Care. 2021;25(1):438.

Chapter 106
Family Communication in the ICU

106.1 Introduction

Effective communication with families in the Intensive Care Unit (ICU) is a cornerstone of compassionate and patient-centered care. Families often experience significant stress due to the critical condition of their loved ones, making clear, empathetic communication crucial. The ICU team must provide timely information, ensure transparency, and support families emotionally while involving them in shared decision-making. Recognizing the challenges and implementing structured communication frameworks, diverse modalities, and tailored approaches can enhance the quality of interactions and alleviate family distress [1, 2] [Ref: Algorithm 106.1].

1. Initial Contact and Introduction

   - Meet the Family: Initiate the relationship by introducing the ICU team, highlighting the collaborative nature involving physicians, nurses, social workers, and other specialists. Establishing trust from the outset sets the tone for open and constructive communication.
   - Explain Team Roles: Clarify who is responsible for various aspects of the patient's care. Understanding each team member's role reduces confusion and ensures families know who to approach for specific concerns.
   - Identify Key Family Members: Determine the primary decision-makers and spokespersons, especially when surrogate decision-making is required.
   - Understand Family Values and Obtain Consent: Assess family dynamics, cultural values, and preferences. Recognize and respect cultural differences during initial interactions, tailoring communication strategies accordingly to enhance family trust and involvement. Gain consent for care plans, ensuring alignment with the patient's and family's wishes.

2. Role of Nurses and Multidisciplinary Teams

S. B. Mishra et al., *Mastering ICU Care*,
https://doi.org/10.1007/978-981-95-0179-3_106

- Significant Role of Nurses: Acknowledge the crucial role nurses play in providing bedside updates and emotional support to families. Nurses often serve as the primary point of contact and can offer valuable insights into the patient's condition.
- Challenges Faced by Nurses: Address challenges such as staff constraints and communication barriers that may impact nurses' ability to provide thorough updates.
- Interdisciplinary Pre-briefings: Advocate for interdisciplinary pre-briefings before family meetings to align team goals and ensure consistent messaging. This collaborative approach enhances the effectiveness of communication and supports shared decision-making [3].

3. Routine Communication

- Provide Daily Updates: Deliver concise and jargon-free updates about the patient's condition, progress, and any changes in the treatment plan. Frequent informal bedside updates have been shown to improve family satisfaction, as noted in studies on contemporary ICU practices.
- Ensure Transparency in Care Plans: Clearly outline the goals of care, anticipated outcomes, and any potential challenges. Transparency builds trust and minimizes confusion or distrust later.
- Utilize Diverse Communication Modalities: Incorporate digital tools such as teleconferencing for family meetings, especially when family members cannot be physically present. This approach has demonstrated comparable satisfaction levels and ensures that all key individuals are informed and involved.

4. Empathy and Active Listening

- Listen to Family Concerns: Actively listen to family members' questions, worries, and feedback. This demonstrates respect for their role in the patient's care and validates their emotions.
- Acknowledge Emotions: Recognize and empathize with the family's feelings, such as fear, grief, or frustration. Statements like "I can see how difficult this must be for you" can help.
- Build Rapport: Consistent and empathetic communication fosters a sense of partnership between the medical team and the family, strengthening trust and cooperation.

5. Decision-Making Process

- Involve Family in Shared Decision-Making: Families should be integral to discussions about care plans, especially when decisions are complex or emotionally charged.
- Explain Risks, Benefits, and Outcomes: Use clear language to outline the implications of treatment options. Families should understand both the potential benefits and limitations of interventions.

- Review Advance Directives (if available): Respect predetermined wishes expressed in advance directives or living wills to guide care aligned with the patient's values.
- Integrate Family Preferences in Care Plan: When possible, incorporate family preferences into the patient's care, ensuring a collaborative approach. Tailoring communication strategies to respect cultural differences and family dynamics enhances trust and involvement in the decision-making process [4].

6. Special Communication

- End-of-Life Discussions
- Emphasize the VALUE Framework: Utilize the VALUE framework to foster empathy and reduce family distress during end-of-life discussions.
- V: Value Family Statements: Recognize and appreciate the family's insights and perspectives about the patient's life, values, and priorities.
- A: Acknowledge Emotions: Address emotional expressions compassionately, validating the family's feelings.
- L: Listen: Provide attentive listening without interruption, allowing families to express themselves fully.
- U: Understand the Patient as a Person: Engage in conversations that reflect an understanding of the patient's life beyond their illness.
- E: Elicit Questions: Encourage families to ask questions, ensuring they have the information needed to make informed decisions.
- Foster Empathy and Reduce Distress: By following the VALUE framework, healthcare providers can create a supportive environment that eases the emotional burden on families during challenging times.
- Breaking Bad News
- Follow the SPIKES Protocol: Implement the SPIKES protocol as a practical guide to deliver bad news effectively and compassionately:
- S: Set Up: Prepare the environment by choosing a private space, sitting down, and ensuring all key family members are present and emotionally ready.
- P: Perception: Assess the family's understanding of the situation before providing new information.
- I: Invitation: Invite the family to indicate how much detail they wish to receive.
- K: Knowledge: Deliver information clearly and succinctly, avoiding medical jargon.
- E: Emotions: Address emotional responses with empathy, allowing time for the family to process the information.
- S: Summary and Strategy: Recap the discussion and outline next steps, providing a clear plan moving forward.
- Practical Guide: Utilizing the SPIKES protocol ensures that the delivery of bad news is handled with sensitivity and professionalism, minimizing additional stress for the family [5].

7. Psychological Support and Education
    - Offer Emotional Support: Provide access to chaplains, counselors, or social workers who can assist families in coping with their emotions and stress.
    - Integrate Coping Strategies and Support Groups: Propose integrating coping strategies, support groups, and educational materials for families to mitigate stress and enhance understanding of the ICU environment.
    - Provide Educational Materials: Share resources such as brochures, websites, or videos that explain ICU procedures, equipment, and common medical terms to demystify the environment and reduce anxiety.
8. Cultural Competence and Tailored Approaches
    - Respect Cultural Differences: Stress the importance of respecting cultural differences and tailoring communication strategies accordingly.
    - Enhance Family Trust and Involvement: By acknowledging and integrating cultural values into communication, healthcare providers can enhance family trust and encourage active involvement in care decisions.
9. Documentation and Follow-Up
    - Document Family Interactions: Recommend detailed documentation of family interactions, including discussions about patient values, preferences, and decisions made. This guides continuity of care and supports shared decision-making among the healthcare team.
    - Schedule Follow-Up Communications: Set regular times to reconnect with families to provide updates or revisit decisions. This ensures ongoing support and avoids gaps in communication.
10. Addressing Challenges and Solutions
    - Identify Barriers: Acknowledge common barriers such as time constraints, language differences, and emotional stress in the ICU setting.
    - Practical Interventions:
    - Translation Services: Utilize professional translation services to overcome language barriers, ensuring accurate and clear communication.
    - Emotional Resilience Training for Staff: Implement training programs to equip staff with skills to manage their own emotional stress, enhancing their capacity to support families effectively.
    - Efficient Use of Time: Develop strategies to manage time constraints, such as delegating communication tasks appropriately within the multidisciplinary team.

106.2 Conclusion

Family communication in the ICU requires a structured and empathetic approach to address both informational and emotional needs. By fostering transparency, listening actively, and involving families in decision-making, the ICU team can build trust and improve overall care experiences. Implementing structured communication frameworks like VALUE and SPIKES, utilizing diverse communication modalities, respecting cultural differences, and addressing challenges proactively ensures that even the most challenging conversations are conducted with sensitivity and professionalism. Integrating support services, educational resources, and thorough documentation further enhances the family's ability to navigate the ICU environment, ultimately contributing to better outcomes for patients and their loved ones.

Algorithm 106.1: Family communication in the ICU

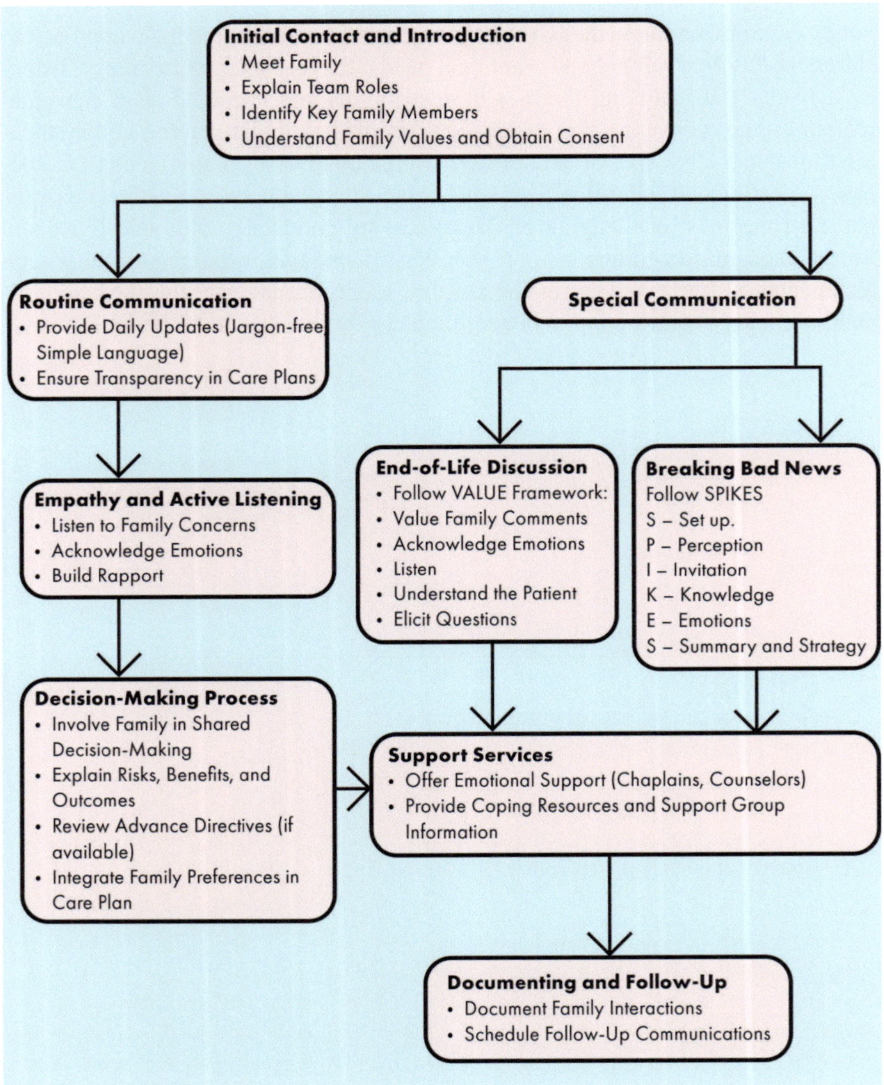

Bibliography

1. Scheunemann LP, Ernecoff NC, Buddadhumaruk P, Carson SS, Hough CL, Curtis JR, et al. Clinician-family communication about patients' values and preferences in intensive care units. JAMA Intern Med. 2019;179(5):676–84.

2. Reifarth E, Garcia Borrega J, Kochanek M. How to communicate with family members of the critically ill in the intensive care unit: a scoping review. Intensive Crit Care Nurs. 2023;74:103328.
3. Yoo HJ, Lim OB, Shim JL. Critical care nurses' communication experiences with patients and families in an intensive care unit: a qualitative study. PLoS One. 2020;15(7):e0235694.
4. Goneppanavar U. Communication in the intensive care unit. Indian J Resp Care. 2022;1(2):83–6.
5. Au SS, Roze des Ordons AL, Amir Ali A, Soo A, Stelfox HT. Communication with patients' families in the intensive care unit: a point prevalence study. J Crit Care. 2019;54:235–8.

Chapter 107
Approach to Burn Patients in the ICU

107.1 Introduction

Burn injuries are critical conditions requiring prompt and organized management due to their potential for systemic complications, including airway compromise, shock, infections, and long-term physical and psychological effects. Patients with significant burns, especially those involving inhalational injury or large total body surface area (TBSA) burns, require intensive care. Early interventions, both prehospital and within the ICU, are essential to improve outcomes [1, 2] [Ref: Algorithm 107.1].

107.2 Prehospital and Initial Management

Effective management of burn patients begins at the scene of injury.

First Aid

- Cooling the Burn Area: Immediate cooling of the burn area with tepid water (20–30 minutes) significantly reduces burn depth and progression. Avoid using ice-cold water or ice, as they can exacerbate tissue damage.
- Subatmospheric Pressure Dressings: The use of subatmospheric pressure dressings, such as vacuum-assisted closure (VAC) therapy, can minimize edema and improve outcomes in certain burn areas.

  Initial Evaluation

  The immediate priorities upon arrival align with the principles of Advanced Trauma Life Support (ATLS):
- Airway Assessment: Assess for signs of inhalational injury, such as soot in the airway, carbonaceous sputum, or stridor. Early intubation is critical if airway edema or inhalation injury is suspected.

S. B. Mishra et al., *Mastering ICU Care*,
https://doi.org/10.1007/978-981-95-0179-3_107

- Breathing: Exclude complications like pneumothorax or chest wall burns that could restrict respiration. Assess oxygenation and ventilation through clinical examination and arterial blood gases.
- Circulation: Establish vascular access with two large-bore IV cannulas or a central line if peripheral access is inadequate. This step ensures fluid resuscitation can begin promptly [3].

107.3 Resuscitation Strategies

Fluid resuscitation is paramount in managing burn shock.

Fluid Calculation

- Modified Brooke's formula: American Burn Association 2018 guidelines advocate 2 mL of Ringer's lactate (RL) per kg body weight times the % of TBSA for flame and scald injury, whereas 4 mL of RL per kg body weight times the % of TBSA for electric burn. The latest consensus recommends starting at lower fluid resuscitation rate (2 mL x weight x %TBSA) and then titrating and going higher as per response of individual patient (target urine output of 0.5 mL/kg/h minimum) [4].
- Colloid may be added in the first 24 hours to achieve target end points and thus reduce the need of high volume of crystalloid administration and leading to complications like "fluid creep" [4].
- Parkland Formula: Traditionally used for initial fluid estimation (4x %TBSA x body weight in kg).
- Half of this volume is given in the first 8 hours from the time of burn, and the remainder over the next 16 hours.

Limitations and Individualization

- Limitations of the Parkland Formula: Overreliance can lead to "fluid creep" and complications like abdominal compartment syndrome. Individualized fluid titration based on hemodynamic monitoring and laboratory markers is essential.
- Alternate Resuscitation Strategies:
- Permissive Hypovolemia: In select cases, accepting lower blood pressure to minimize fluid overload. The fluid resuscitation volume should rather target an output of 0.5 mL/kg body weight per hour 30–50 mL/h.
- Colloids: The use of colloids like human albumin after the first 24 hours can help maintain oncotic pressure and reduce total fluid volume [5].

Monitoring

- Urine Output: Aim for 0.5–1 mL/kg/h (30–50 mL/kg) as a marker of adequate perfusion and 75–100 mL/h until urine clears in case of pigment in urine.
- Hemodynamic Parameters: Monitor blood pressure, heart rate, central venous pressure, and lactate levels.

- Crystalloids: Use lactated Ringer's solution initially. Avoid over-resuscitation to prevent complications like pulmonary edema.

107.4 Secondary Evaluation

After stabilization, a detailed secondary evaluation is essential.

- Head-to-Toe Survey: Assess for associated injuries (e.g., fractures, trauma).
- Burn Estimation: Accurately determine the TBSA using tools like the Rule of Nines or Lund-Browder chart.
- Adjust the fluid administration based on targets rather than a definite pre-calculated volume. Use of Human Albumin early if targets are not achieved with adequate fluid resuscitation or there is a risk of fluid overload.
- Send laboratory tests, chest X-ray
- Pain and anxiety management
- Psychological support
- Wound care (Fig. 107.1)

- History (AMPLET):
- A: Allergies
- M: Medications
- P: Past medical history
- L: Last meal
- E: Events leading to the injury
- T: Tetanus history (if **Unknown or < 3 doses of tetanus toxoid:** Administer Tdap, Td, or DTaP and Tetanus Immune Globulin (TIG). **≥3 doses of tetanus toxoid:** Administer Tdap, Td, or DTaP if it has been more than 5 years since the last dose. TIG is not required.

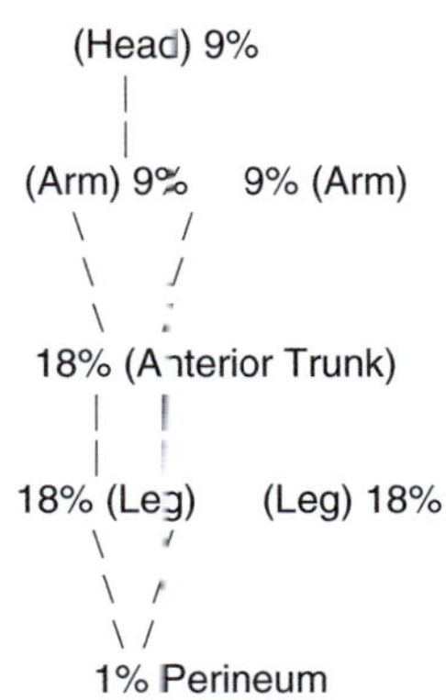

Fig. 107.1 Wallace's Rule of 9 for calculating % TBSA (Total body surface area)

107.5 Inhalation Injury Management

Inhalation injuries significantly increase morbidity and mortality.

- Oxygenation: Administer 100% oxygen to displace carbon monoxide.
- Diagnosis: Bronchoscopy is the gold standard.
- Nebulized Medications: Use nebulized heparin and N-acetylcysteine to reduce airway obstruction.
- Ventilation: Apply lung-protective strategies for patients with ARDS [6].

107.6 Pain and Sedation Management

Effective pain control is essential.

- Analgesia: Utilize multimodal approaches, including opioids and regional nerve blocks.
- Sedation: Adjust sedation levels to balance pain control with the need for patient interaction.

107.7 Nutritional Support

Burn patients experience a profound hypermetabolic response.

- Early Enteral Feeding: Initiate within 4–6 hours to mitigate hypermetabolism and support wound healing.
- Caloric Needs: Calculate based on predictive equations considering the burn size.
- Protein Requirement: 1.5–2 g of protein/kg/d
- Antioxidant vitamins (including vitamins E and C [ascorbic acid]) and trace minerals (including selenium, zinc, and copper) may improve patient outcome.
- Pharmacological Interventions:
- Beta-Blockers: Reduce hypermetabolic response (e.g., propranolol).

107.8 Infection Control

Burn wounds are highly susceptible to infection.

- Topical Antibiotics: Apply agents like silver sulfadiazine for full thickness burns and bacitracin for partial thickness burns.
- Systemic Antibiotics: Use only when there is evidence of infection to prevent resistance.
- Aseptic Techniques: Maintain strict asepsis during wound care [7].

107.9 Wound Care

Burn depth can be classified into partial (some, but not all layers of the skin are injured) or full thickness (all layers of the skin are injured).

Partial thickness can be first or second degree. A first-degree burn is a superficial injury limited to the epidermis and is characterized by redness, hypersensitivity, pain, and no skin sloughing. Whereas, second-degree burns involve the epidermis and part of the dermis. The skin may be red and blistered, wet, weepy, or whiter, yet edematous.

Full thickness burn is also called a third-degree burn in which there is destruction of the entire thickness of dermis and epidermis, including dermal appendages. This gives rise to the eschar formation.

Fourth-degree burns penetrate below the skin into the subdermal fat and are classified as fourth-degree burns. These burns also have an eschar on the surface.

Burn wounds have a zone of coagulation (central—maximum contact with source), zone of stasis, and zone of hyperemia (most peripheral).

- Clean the wound with soap or chlorhexidine and remove dirt and debris from wound.
- Limit exposed areas while dressing.
- Gently debride blisters >2 cms. Apply topical antimicrobial.

107.10 Advanced Surgical Interventions

Early surgical intervention can improve outcomes.

- Early Excision and Grafting: Perform within 48 hours to decrease the risk of sepsis and promote healing.
- Escharotomy/Fasciotomy: Indicated for circumferential burns causing compartment syndrome.

107.11 Monitoring and Prognostication

Effective monitoring aids in predicting outcomes.

- Scoring Systems:
- Revised Baux Score: Age + TBSA (%) + 17 (if inhalation injury present) to predict mortality.
- Abbreviated Burn Severity Index (ABSI): Considers age, gender, inhalation injury, depth, and TBSA. Ranges from 2 to 18 points, with a probability of survival ranging from $\geq$99% to $\leq$10%.
- Frailty Assessment:

- Rockwood Scale: Assesses frailty in older patients to refine prognostication.
- Belgian Outcome in Burn Injury (BOBI) Score: Uses absolute values of age and BSA(%).

107.12 Special Considerations

Chemical Burns

- Decontamination: Remove contaminated clothing and irrigate the area extensively.
- Neutralizing Agents: Use specific agents when appropriate (e.g., calcium gluconate for hydrofluoric acid burns).
  Electrical Burns
- Cardiac Monitoring: Monitor for arrhythmias due to potential myocardial injury.
- Internal Injuries: Assess for deep tissue damage not apparent on the skin.
  Radiation Burns
- Management: Similar to thermal burns but consider systemic radiation effects.
- Long-Term Monitoring: For potential radiation-induced complications [8].
  Coagulopathy
- Risk Assessment: Severe burns can lead to coagulopathy due to massive tissue destruction.
- Management: Monitor coagulation profiles; administer blood products as needed.

107.13 Psychological and Social Aspects

Long-term recovery extends beyond physical healing.

- Rehabilitation: Early physical therapy to prevent contractures and maintain function.
- Psychological Support: Address issues like PTSD, depression, and anxiety with counseling and support groups.
- Social Integration: Assist with vocational rehabilitation and community reintegration.

107.14 Technological Advances

Incorporate new technologies for improved care.

- Point-of-Care Ultrasound (POCUS): Use for dynamic resuscitation monitoring, assessing cardiac function, and detecting complications like pneumothorax.

107.15 Research and Emerging Therapies

- Hemofiltration: Potential for removing inflammatory mediators; current evidence is emerging.
- Stem Cell Therapy: Investigational use for enhancing wound healing.
- Artificial Skin Substitutes: Development of bioengineered tissues for grafting.

107.16 Conclusion

Managing burn patients in the ICU requires a structured, multidisciplinary approach, beginning with prehospital care and extending through resuscitation, surgical intervention, and long-term rehabilitation. Incorporating individualized resuscitation strategies, aggressive nutritional support, advanced surgical techniques, and psychological care can significantly improve patient outcomes. Utilizing scoring systems and technological advances aids in monitoring and prognostication, ensuring evidence-based, patient-centered care.

Algorithm 107.1: Approach to burn patients in the ICU

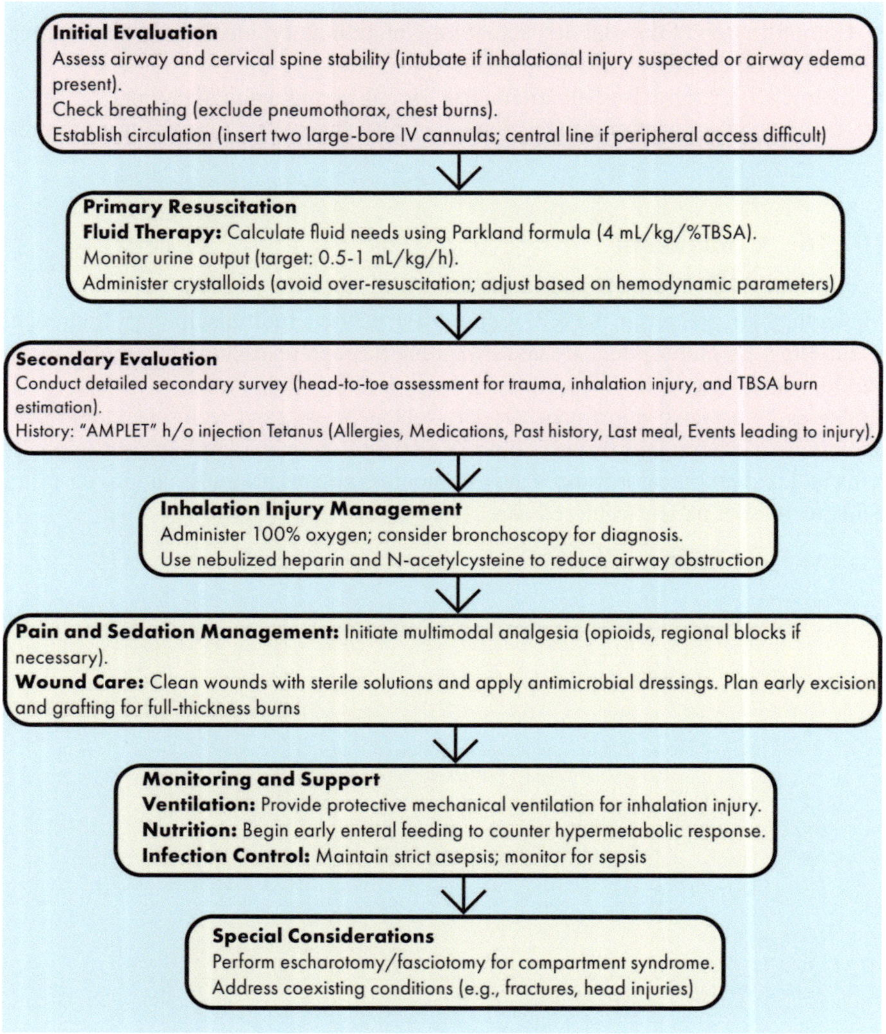

Bibliography

1. Vivo C, Galeiras R, del Caz MD. Initial evaluation and management of the critical burn patient. Med Intensiva. 2016;40(1):49–59.
2. McCann C, Watson A, Barnes D. Major burns: part 1. Epidemiology, pathophysiology and initial management. BJA Educ. 2022;22(3):94–103.

3. Datta PK, Roy Chowdhury S, Aravindan A, Saha S, Rapaka S. Medical and surgical Care of Critical Burn Patients: a comprehensive review of current evidence and practice. Cureus. 2022;14(11):e31550.
4. Cartotto R, Johnson LS, Savetamal A, et al. American burn association clinical practice guidelines on burn shock resuscitation. J Burn Care Res. 2024;45(3):565–89. https://doi.org/10.1093/jbcr/irad125.
5. Bishop S, Maguire S. Anaesthesia and intensive care for major burns. Cont Edu Anaesthesia Crit Care Pain. 2012;12(3):118–22.
6. Hilton PJ, Hepp M. The immediate care of the burned patient. BJA CEPD Reviews. 2001;1(4):113–6.
7. McGovern C, Puxty K, Paton L. Major burns: part 2. Anaesthesia, intensive care and pain management. BJA Educ. 2022;22(4):138–45.
8. Lorente JA, Amaya-Villar R. Update in the management of critically ill burned patients. Med Intensiva. 2016;40(1):46–8.

MIX
Papier aus verantwortungsvollen Quellen
Paper from responsible sources
FSC® C105338

If you have any concerns about our products,
you can contact us on
ProductSafety@springernature.com

In case Publisher is established outside the EU,
the EU authorized representative is:
Springer Nature Customer Service Center GmbH
Europaplatz 3, 69115 Heidelberg, Germany

Printed by Libri Plureos GmbH
in Hamburg, Germany